Encyclopedia of
FORENSIC AND LEGAL MEDICINE

Encyclopedia of
FORENSIC AND
LEGAL MEDICINE

EDITED BY

JASON PAYNE-JAMES
ROGER W BYARD
TRACEY S COREY
CAROL HENDERSON

ELSEVIER
ACADEMIC
PRESS

AMSTERDAM • BOSTON • HEIDELBERG • LONDON
NEW YORK • OXFORD • PARIS • SAN DIEGO
SAN FRANCISCO • SINGAPORE • SYDNEY • TOKYO

Elsevier Ltd., The Boulevard, Langford Lane, Kidlington, Oxford, OX5 1GB, UK

First edition 2005

Library of Congress Control Number: 2004113925

A catalogue record for this book is available from the British Library

ISBN 0-12-547970-0 (set)

This book is printed on acid-free paper
Printed and bound in Spain

EDITORS AND EDITORIAL ADVISORY BOARD

vi **EDITORS AND EDITORIAL ADVISORY BOARD**

Stephen Cordner
Victorian Institute of Forensic Medicine,
Southbank, VIC, Australia

Mary Fran Ernst
St Louis University School of Medicine
St Louis, MO, USA

David L Faigman
Hastings College of Law
University of California
San Francisco, CA, USA

Robert Forrest
University of Sheffield
Sheffield, UK

James L Frost
St Louis, MO, USA

Michael Graham
St Louis University HSC
St Louis, MO, USA

John A Henry
St Mary's Hospital
London, UK

A Wayne Jones
University Hospital
Linköping, Sweden

Alison Jones
Guy's and St Thomas' Hospital
London, UK

Tzipi Kahana
Division of Identification and
Forensic Sciences - DVI
Israel Police
Tel Aviv
Israel

Steven B Karch
Consultant Pathologist
Berkeley, CA, USA

Anthony Maden
Imperial College London
London, UK

Bernard Marc
Centre Hospitalier Compiegne
Compiegne, France

Kasinathan Nadesan
Hunter New England Pathology Services
Newcastle, NSW,
Australia

Torleiv Ole Rognum
University of Oslo
Oslo, Norway

Guy N Rutty
University of Leicester
Leicester, UK

Betty Spivack
University of Louisville
Louisville, KY, USA

Shigeyuki Tsunenari
Kumamoto University
Kumamoto,
Japan

Michael Welner
The Forensic Panel
New York, NY, USA

FOREWORD – A FORENSIC PERSPECTIVE

To comprehensively encompass the fields of both forensic medicine and legal medicine is an ambitious project indeed, as conventionally, the two disciplines are usually treated separately. Even "forensic medicine" itself is traditionally divided into autopsy pathology and the clinical aspects, so to produce anything more than an overview of the whole spectrum of the subject, is something that has probably never before been attempted in the English language.

The Editors have assembled an impressive array of contributors, each masters of their own topic and the result is an impressive work which deserves the highest praise, both to the authors and to those who have had to labor at editing to achieve a coherent whole – a feat which personal experience has taught me can be a daunting task. Having myself written about ten books on forensic medical topics, as well as contributions to many more, I can vouch for the fact that the most difficult job of all was editing a couple of multi-author volumes.

The content of this encyclopedia is diverse and comprehensive. The actual range can be seen from the very extensive chapter list and covers virtually every sub-discipline in forensic and legal medicine, from anthropology to botany, from malpractice to substance abuse. Some of the subjects dealt with, would be thought of as "forensic science" in the more compartmentalized attitude of Great Britain, but of course in very many countries, there is not the same demarcation of professional interests within their Institutes of Legal Medicine and thus this book avoids geographical restrictions, which in the past have always raised difficulties in writing for different parts of the world, which have markedly diverse medico-legal systems.

Some of the headings in the list of contents would seem unfamiliar to doctors of previous generations – examples might be "accreditation, digital evidence, crime-scene management, profiling, ritualistic crime, terrorism and torture" – but this underlines the evolutionary nature of all medical disciplines, in which legal medicine is no exception. In former years, many textbooks remained relatively static over numerous editions, following a conventional sequence of topics. Whereas forensic science developed almost explosively, the pace of progress in forensic pathology was slow and it seemed hardly worth buying new editions of established manuals. This has all changed and it is timely that such an ambitious work as this encyclopedia should seek to sweep all current knowledge into its grasp for the benefit of those doctors "at the sharp end" of forensic practice, who need to refer to any part of such a broad field of knowledge that now exists.

Professor Bernard Knight, CBE
Cardiff, UK
January 2005.

FOREWORD – A LEGAL PERSPECTIVE

Over my judicial career I have observed a tremendous number of changes in the law, scientific and medical practices, and society in general. DNA evidence is now commonplace in many criminal and family cases, domestic violence and child abuse are unfortunately still prevalent, and the notion of personal rights and freedoms for incapacitated children and adults is now becoming widely accepted. The courts are also becoming increasingly involved in difficult cases concerning individuals who, but for advances in life-prolonging technologies, might have reached a natural death much sooner. I am particularly pleased to see a single work that is relevant to all these topics, and with contributions by distinguished practitioners and authors from many disciplines. I am only disappointed that a work of this importance was not available long ago.

The Encyclopedia will be of use and interest to a wide-ranging audience. Judges, lawyers, medical practitioners, scientists and students will be among the many who will benefit from this single repository of knowledge. I especially welcome, as will many, the electronic version which will receive regular updates. This will ensure that the Encyclopedia remains at the forefront of legal, technological and medical developments and will be of continuing use over the years to come.

The number of cases requiring evidence or advice from medical and other forensic experts has increased over recent years. In some cases as many as nine experts have been involved, providing a variety of viewpoints. The Encyclopedia will be a valuable aid in explaining to judges, lawyers and many others engaged in the court process the technical language of forensic and legal medicine and will assist in elucidating the complex issues which arise for resolution in the courts.

Elizabeth Butler-Sloss

Dame Elizabeth Butler-Sloss, GBE
President of the Family Division
London, UK
January 2005.

PREFACE

The phrase "Forensic and Legal Medicine" may at first appear cumbersome. It does, however, enable all the areas that this Encyclopedia covers to be fully embraced. Global differences in terminology and cross-over with other healthcare and scientific disciplines mean that unlike many other medical specialties such as cardiology or gastroenterology – each with clear boundaries – there may be misunderstanding, both within and without the medical profession as to the vast scope of subject covered. "Forensic medicine" and "legal medicine" are terms that can be used interchangeably, and their specific use may vary from country to country. For many readers, the term "forensic medicine" is synonymous with that of forensic pathology (that specialty of medicine which investigates the cause of death). However, forensic pathology, although part of forensic medicine, is but a small part of the vast range of subjects with which forensic medicine practitioners may be involved. In the broadest terms forensic and legal medicine includes all areas where medicine interacts with the law (including criminal and civil law), judiciary, police bodies, investigative agencies, professional bodies and government or state bodies.

When developing this Enyclopedia the Editors and the Publishers had the objective of providing *the* major reference source of subjects related to forensic and legal medicine. This information is provided in separate chapters generally of about 3–5,000 words. Each chapter gives a source of specific Further Reading to which those requiring even more detailed information can be directed. The degree of interaction of those practising forensic and legal medicine with the law, the judiciary, police bodies, investigative agencies, professional, government and state bodies, will vary from country to country, and from jurisdiction to jurisdiction. Some forensic medicine specialists will be independent of state, government or judiciary, while others will not. Some will work full-time in their field, others part-time. Just a few examples of key areas where differences arise include the investigation of death, approaches to care of detainees in custody, structure of investigative of systems, and interpretation of human rights issues. Clearly it is not possible for a single work, even of this size to illustrate all the differences that exist in our complex world. As Editors, we have sought to identify the most relevant issues and give examples of how such systems, or topics work within a given country or region. There will of course be omissions – and these we apologise for any such in advance. We hope that readers will inform us directly of any information that they feel should have been included. The online version of the Encyclopedia will be updated at timely intervals. Any such suggestions from readers will be assessed and considered as we plan the new material to be included at each update, and will thus help the development and evolution of this work.

The main readership groups of the Encyclopedia are intended to be medical practitioners whose work comprises a forensic element (including forensic pathologists, medical examiners, forensic physicians, forensic odontologists, paediatricians, psychiatrists, psychologists, genitourinary medicine specialists, emergency medicine specialists and primary care physicians), others within the forensic setting (including scientists, toxicologists, anthropologists), legal practitioners (lawyers, advocates, attorneys, coroners, barristers and solicitors), the judiciary, police and related bodies, government and state bodies responsible for – or using the services of – forensic practitioners, research institutes and those undertaking (as educators or students) academic courses or training in medical law, forensic medicine, investigation of crime and related topics. The Editors also hope that those who require authoritative information about the wide range of topics included – such as journalists and campaigning bodies, will find the information contained within as a valuable and indispensable resource.

The Editors have to offer huge thanks to the international spectrum of respected authors of the chapters, for their patience in the production of this substantial work. Each author has been chosen because of their reputation and their expertise in their given topic. Some aspects of some chapters may be controversial – we hope and intend that this is so. Forensic and legal medicine is not a science of absolutes, and its purpose is best served when opinions and approaches to the often complex and sensitive topics of debate can be discussed freely, openly and reasonably without fear of intimidation, retribution or victimisation.

Our thanks must of course go to the publishers – Elsevier – and to the staff of the Major Reference Works Department. In particular, we must congratulate Mark Knowles for his patience and understanding throughout the project, as he as borne the brunt of the development and given the Editors unqualified and unhesitating support. As Editors we have been very grateful for his involvement from shortly after conception, through gestation, to delivery. Assisting Mark have been Tracey Mills, Eleanor Orchard, Sue Stokes, Davinia Hurn-Shanley and Mireille Yanow. Nick Fallon, Mark Listewnik and Carey Chapman were key in establishing and supporting the project through its development. In the production stages Sarah Parkin has been extremely active in identifying any concerns and providing solutions in the production of the work.

Jason Payne-James
Roger W Byard
Tracey S Corey
Carol Henderson
November, 2004

INTRODUCTION

The need for an understanding of the roles, responsibilities and relationships of practitioners of forensic and legal medicine – and those related specialties – in relation to issues outside the specific medical world has never been greater. There are many issues that are of huge relevance today, where the medical and related professions can have a multiplicity of roles. International terrorism is one example. The medical profession may be involved at a number of levels – the investigation of causes of death after an attack; the identification of human remains; the appropriate sampling of substances that may have evidential value; the care and assessment of terrorist suspects and their victims; the presentation of evidence to courts; and at a more local level, issues of consent for treatment of those unable to consent for themselves; and concern for the treatment of prisoners. Each of these issues requires independent, impartial and objective opinions which allow justice to be pursued appropriately and fairly. With this example the skills of forensic pathologists, forensic physicians, forensic anthropologists, forensic odontologists, forensic psychologists, forensic psychiatrists and forensic scientists may be required. Their findings and conclusions need to be given robustly, with emphasis given where facts or scientific research support an opinion, and clear guidance when such facts or research are either equivocal, or not available.

In some ways the forensic and legal medicine specialist may act as one of the gatekeepers within judicial systems. The recognition of the critical importance of such evidence has been highlighted worldwide where expert evidence has been challenged and impartiality has been questioned. Such challenges and questioning have put much focus on attempting to improve and clarify how, when and to what extent expert opinions in the forensic setting can be utilised, and different judicial systems apply a range of tests to such evidence to assess its integrity. This means that for all those working in forensic and legal medicine and its related specialties, and scientific or healthcare specialties, training, update training and audit and assessment has become a *sine qua non*. "Accreditation", "revalidation" and "standard setting" are terms that are used interchangeably worldwide. Training and education in medical law and forensic aspects of medicine are much more widely available and, increasingly, medical practitioners may be dually trained in medicine and law. However, there are few areas of medicine and healthcare now which are untouched by a need to understand certain aspects of forensic and legal medicine. All healthcare professionals need to be aware of, and put into practice, issues such as consent and confidentiality and apply these into their practice. Every medical or healthcare specialty has some aspect that may require specialist forensic and legal medical knowledge. In many areas this knowledge may be available from a forensic practitioner, but all practitioners need to be able to assist their patients in the absence of such a specialist. To give a number of examples: emergency medicine specialists need to be able to document accurately wounds that present for treatment, so that later interpretation in terms of modes of causation may be undertaken; those caring for the elderly need to recognise and document signs of elder abuse; similarly, paediatricians need to recognise and document signs of child abuse; genitourinary medicine specialists and gynaecologists need to be able to assess, document and provide management plans for victims of sexual assault; primary care physicians need to be able to assess and documents signs of domestic or interpersonal violence; psychiatrists and psychologists need to determine whether mentally vulnerable individuals are responsible for their actions; radiologists need to be able to recognise image appearances of non-accidental injury. All may have to present evidence in court to assist a court with their deliberations. The Encyclopedia provides sources of information to assist in all these functions, as well as giving examples of how court and legal systems compare in different jurisdictions worldwide.

The Encyclopedia endeavours to ensure that the cross-over of boundaries between different related but non-medical specialties, such as forensic toxicology, forensic psychology, forensic anthropology and forensic science are understood and defined. The interrelationship between these specialties is complex and the investigation of issues such as war crimes may require the skills of all these specialties and more.

The work undertaken by forensic practitioners must be based on a bedrock of an understanding of human rights and ethical principles. These principles are identified and referred to in the Encyclopedia; the Editors believe that these ethical principles should guide all those whose careers are primarily or even peripherally involved in the forensic and legal medicine setting.

Jason Payne-James
Roger W Byard
Tracey S Corey
Carol Henderson
November, 2004

GUIDE TO USE OF THE ENCYCLOPEDIA

Structure of the Encyclopedia

The material in the Encyclopedia is arranged as a series of entries in alphabetical order. Most entries consist of several articles that deal with various aspects of a topic and are arranged in a logical sequence within an entry. Some entries comprise a single article.

To help you realize the full potential of the material in the Encyclopedia we have provided three features to help you find the topic of your choice: a Contents List, Cross-References and an Index.

1. Contents List

Your first point of reference will probably be the contents list. The complete contents lists, which appears at the front of each volume will provide you with both the volume number and the page number of the entry. On the opening page of an entry a contents list is provided so that the full details of the articles within the entry are immediately available.

Alternatively you may choose to browse through a volume using the alphabetical order of the entries as your guide. To assist you in identifying your location within the Encyclopedia a running headline indicates the current entry and the current article within that entry.

You will find 'dummy entries' where obvious synonyms exist for entries or where we have grouped together related topics. Dummy entries appear in both the contents lists and the body of the text.

Example
If you were attempting to locate material on hair analysis for drugs via the contents list:

HAIR ANALYSIS *See* DNA: Hair Analysis; SUBSTANCE MISUSE: Hair Analysis

The dummy entry directs you to the Hair Analysis article, in the SUBSTANCE MISUSE entry. At the appropriate location in the contents list, the page numbers for articles under Substance Misuse are given.

If you were trying to locate the material by browsing through the text and you looked up Hair Analysis then the following information would be provided in the dummy entry:

Hair Analysis *See* **DNA:** Hair Analysis; **Substance Misuse:** Hair Analysis

Alternatively, if you were looking up Substance Misuse the following infrmation would be provided:

SUBSTANCE MISUSE

Contents
Medical Effects
Cocaine and Other Stimulants
Herbal Medicine
Heroin
Substitution Drugs
Sedatives
Miscellaneous Drugs
Urine Analysis
Hair Analysis
Alternative Body Fluids Analysis
Patterns and Statistics
Crime

2. Cross References

All of the articles in the Encyclopedia have been extensively cross-referenced.

The cross-references, which appear at the end of an article, serve three different functions. For example, at the end of the Anthropology: Archeology, Excavation and Retrieval of Remains article, cross-references are used:

  i. To indicate if a topic is discussed in greater detail elsewhere.

See Also

Anthropology: Bone Pathology and Ante-mortem Trauma; Cremated Bones; Overview; Role of DNA; Sex Determination; Taphonomy; **Autopsy:** Procedures and Standards; **Deaths:** Trauma, Musculo-skeletal System; **Death Investigation Systems:** United States of America; **Odontology:** Overview; **Post-mortem Changes:** Overview; **War Crimes:** Pathological Investigation; Site Investigation

 ii. To draw the reader's attention to parallel discussions in other articles.

See Also

Anthropology: Bone Pathology and Ante-mortem Trauma; Cremated Bones; Overview; Role of DNA; Sex Determination; Taphonomy; **Autopsy:** Procedures and Standards; **Deaths:** Trauma, Musculo-skeletal System; **Death Investigation Systems:** United States of America; **Odontology:** Overview; **Post-mortem Changes:** Overview; **War Crimes:** Pathological Investigation; Site Investigation

iii. To indicate material that broadens the discussion.

See Also

Anthropology: Bone Pathology and Ante-mortem Trauma; Cremated Bones; Overview; Role of DNA; Sex Determination; Taphonomy; **Autopsy:** Procedures and Standards; **Deaths:**

Trauma, Musculo-skeletal System; **Death Investigation Systems:** United States of America; **Odontology:** Overview; **Post-mortem Changes:** Overview; **War Crimes:** Pathological Investigation; Site Investigation

3. Index

The Index will provide you with the page number where the material is located, and the index entries differentiate between material that is a whole article, is part of an article or is data presented in a figure or table. Detailed notes are provided on the opening page of the index.

4. Contributors

A full list of contributors appears at the beginning of each volume.

CONTRIBUTORS

Aggrawal, A
Maulana Azad Medical College, New Delhi, India

Al-Alousi, L M
Leicester Royal Infirmary, Leicester, UK

Allden, K
Dartmouth Medical School, Hanover, NH, USA

Allison, S P
Queen's Medical Centre, Nottingham, UK

Anderson, R A
University of Glasgow, Glasgow, UK

Artecona, J
Tulane University School of Medicine, New Orleans, LA, USA

Asser, S M
Hasbro Children's Hospital, Providence, RI, USA

Baccino, E
Centre Hospitalier Universitaire de Montpellier, Montpellier, France

Baldwin, H B
Forensic Enterprises, Inc., Orland Park, IL, USA

Ballantyne, J
University of Central Florida, Orlando, FL, USA

Barley, V
National Patient Safety Agency, London, UK

Bassindale, C
Lancashire Sexual Assault Forensic Examination Centre, Preston, UK

Becker, R F
Chaminade University of Honolulu, Honolulu, HI, USA

Beh, P S L
University of Hong Kong, Hong Kong, China

Bergeron, C E
American Association of Suicidology, Washington, DC, USA

Berman, A L
American Association of Suicidology, Washington, DC, USA

Betz, P
University of Erlangen-Nuremberg, Erlangen, Germany

Black, S M
University of Dundee, Dundee, UK

Blackwell, S A
The University of Melbourne, Melbourne, NSW, and the Victorian Institute of Forensic Medicine, Southbank, VIC, Australia

Blaho-Owens, K
University of Tennessee College of Medicine, Memphis, TN, USA

Blitzer, H L
Institute for Forensic Imaging, Indianapolis, IN, USA

Bock, J H
University of Colorado at Boulder, CO, USA

Bora, B
Tulane University School of Medicine, New Orleans, LA, USA

Briggs, C A
University of Melbourne, Melbourne, VIC, Australia

Brown, T
University of Leicester, Leicester, UK

Buchino, J J
University of Louisville, Louisville, KY, USA

Burbrink II, D F
Louisville Metropolitan Police Department, Louisville, KY, USA

Burke, A
Armed Forces Institute of Pathology, Washington, DC, USA

Burke, M P
Victorian Institute of Forensic Medicine, Southbank, VIC, Australia

Byard, R W
Forensic Science Centre, Adelaide, SA, Australia

Campbell, W B
Royal Devon and Exeter Hospital, Exeter, UK

Carter, J
Sussex Forensic Medical Services, Brighton, UK

Case, M
St. Louis University Health Sciences Center, St. Louis, MO, USA

Casey, E
Stroz Friedberg LLC, Washington, DC, USA

Cerminara, K L
Nova Southeastern University, Fort Lauderdale, FL, USA

Chaturvedi, A K
Civil Aerospace Medical Institute, Oklahoma City, OK, USA

Chiamvimonvat, N
University of California – Davis ACC, Sacramento, CA, USA

Clark, J
University of Glasgow, Glasgow, UK

Clement, J G
Victorian Institute of Forensic Medicine, Southbank, VIC, Australia

Collier, S G
National Drug Recognition Training Unit, Northampton, UK

Cooper, P N
University of Newcastle upon Tyne, Newcastle upon Tyne, UK

Cordner, S
Victorian Institute of Forensic Medicine, Southbank, VIC, Australia

Corey, T S
University of Louisville School of Medicine and Office of the Chief Medical Examiner, Louisville, KY, USA

Couper, F J
Office of the Chief Medical Examiner, Washington, DC, USA

Cox, A R
West Midlands Centre for Adverse Drug Reaction Reporting, Birmingham, UK

Crane, J
Queen's University, Belfast, UK

Czuzak, M H
University of Arizona, Tucson, AZ, USA

D'Arcy, M
Royal Women's Hospital, Carlton, VIC, Australia

Dada, M A
PathCare, Durban, South Africa

Dargan, P I
National Poisons Information Service, London, UK

Davis, D W
Hennepin County Medical Examiner's Office, Minneapolis, MN, USA

Dean, P
Rochford Police Station, Rochford, UK

DeFreitas, K
McMaster University, Hamilton, ON, Canada

Donald, T
Women's and Children's Hospital, North Adelaide, SA, Australia

Downs, J C U
Georgia Bureau of Investigation, Savannah, GA, USA

Drummer, O H
Victorian Institute of Forensic Medicine, Southbank, VIC, Australia

Dworkin, R
Indiana University School of Law, Bloomington, IN, USA

Edelmann, R J
University of Roehampton, London, UK

El-Fawal, H A N
Mercy College, Dobbs Ferry, NY, USA

Ellen, R L
Monash University, Southbank, VIC, Australia

Eriksson, A
Umeå University, Umeå, Sweden

Ernst, M F
St. Louis University School of Medicine, St. Louis, MO, USA

Evans, V
Ilkley, UK

Farrell, M
National Addiction Centre, London, UK

Fegan-Earl, A W
Forensic Pathology Services, London, UK

Ferner, R E
West Midlands Centre for Adverse Drug Reaction Reporting, Birmingham, UK

Fernie, C G M
University of Glasgow, Glasgow, UK

Ferris, J A J
Auckland Hospital, Auckland, New Zealand

Fisher, R P
Florida International University, North Miami, FL, USA

Flannery, W
National Alcohol Unit, London, UK

Flynn, M
Nova Southeastern University, Fort Lauderdale, FL, USA

Foran, D R
Michigan State University, East Lansing, MI, USA

Fornes, P
University of Paris, Paris, France

Fraser, J
University of Strathclyde, Glasgow, UK

Frazer, J
Cleckheaton, UK

Freckelton, I
Monash University, Melbourne, VIC, Australia

Fung, W K
University of Hong Kong, Hong Kong, China

Gaebler, R
Indiana University School of Law, Bloomington, IN, USA

Gaensslen, R E
University of Illinois at Chicago, Chicago, IL, USA

Gaoling, Z
Peking University, Beijing, China

Gatland, D
Southend Hospital NHS Trust, Essex, UK

Gerostamoulos, J
Victorian Institute of Forensic Medicine, Southbank, VIC, Australia

Glatter, K A
University of California – Davis ACC, Sacramento, CA, USA

Goddard, K
National Fish and Wildlife Services, Ashland, OR, USA

Goff, M L
Chaminade University of Honolulu, Honolulu, HI, USA

Goldberger, B A
University of Florida College of Medicine, Gainesville, FL, USA

Golding, S L
University of Utah, Salt Lake City, UT, USA

Goodwin, W
University of Central Lancashire, Preston, UK

Graffy, E A
Michigan State University, East Lansing, MI, USA

Graham, E A M
University of Leicester, Leicester, UK

Gregersen, M
Institute of Forensic Medicine, University of Århus, Århus, Denmark

Gudjonsson, G H
Institute of Psychiatry, London, UK

Gullberg, R G
Washington State Patrol, Seattle, WA, USA

Haglund, W D
Physicians for Human Rights, Washington, DC, USA

Hall, C M
Great Ormond Street Hospital for Children, London, UK

Hayden-Wade, H
Children's Hospital of San Diego, San Diego, CA, USA

Healy, T E J
University of Manchester, Manchester, UK

Henderson, C
Stetson University College of Law, Gulfport, FL, USA

Henry, M M
Chelsea and Westminster Hospital, London, UK

Herkov, M J
University of North Florida, Jacksonville, FL, USA

Hill, A J
Victorian Institute of Forensic Medicine, Southbank, VIC, Australia

Holck, P
University of Oslo, Oslo, Norway

Horswell, J
Forensic Executives, Upper Mt. Gravatt, QLD, Australia

Houck, M M
West Virginia University, Morgantown, WV, USA

Howard, J D
Tacoma, WA, USA

Hu, Y-Q
University of Hong Kong, Hong Kong, China

Hucker, S J
McMaster University, Hamilton, ON, Canada

Hunsaker, D M
University of Louisville School of Medicine, Louisville, KY, USA

Hunsaker III, J C
University of Kentucky College of Medicine, Frankfort, KY, USA

Hunt, N
Forensic Pathology Services, Abingdon, UK

Imwinkelried, E J
University of California at Davis, Davis, CA, USA

Ives, N K
University of Oxford, Oxford, UK

Jackson, R L
Pacific Graduate School of Psychology, Palo Alto, CA, USA

Jawad, R
King's College Hospital, London, UK

Jennett, B
University of Glasgow, Glasgow, UK

Jenny, C
Brown Medical School, Providence, RI, USA

Jones, A L
National Poisons Information Service, London, UK

Jones, A W
University Hospital, Linköping, Sweden

Jones, G R
Office of the Chief Medical Examiner, Edmonton, AB, Canada

Jordan, C E
University of Kentucky, Lexington, KY, USA

Josse, S E
Formerly University of London, London, UK

Jumbelic, M I
Upstate Medical University, Syracuse, NY, USA

Jureidini, J
Women's and Children's Hospital, Adelaide, SA, Australia

Kahana, T
Division of Identification and Forensic Science, Israel
National Police, Israel

Karch, S B
Berkeley, CA, USA

Keeley, S
Women's and Children's Hospital, North Adelaide,
SA, Australia

Kelliher, T P
Niskayuna, NY, USA

Kennedy, R T
New Mexico Court of Appeals, Albuquerque,
NM, USA

Kerrigan, S
Houston, TX, USA

Keyser-Tracqui, C
Institut de Médecine Légale,
Strasbourg, France

Khanna, A
Sandwell General Hospital, West Bromwich, UK

Kibayashi, K
Saga Medical School, Saga, Japan

Kirk, G M
University of KwaZulu Natal, Durban, South Africa

Koehler, S A
Allegheny County Coroner, Pittsburgh, PA, USA

Krous, H F
Children's Hospital and Health Center, San Diego,
CA, USA

Langford, N J
West Midlands Centre for Adverse Drug Reaction
Reporting, Birmingham, UK

Langlois, N E I
Westmead Hospital, Wentworthville, NSW, Australia

Lau, G
Centre for Forensic Medicine, Health Sciences
Authority, Singapore

Lazarus, N G
Path Care, Durban, South Africa

Lee, H C
Connecticut Forensic Science Laboratory, Meriden,
CT, USA

Leslie, L K
Children's Hospital of San Diego, San Diego, CA, USA

Levin, R J
University of Sheffield, Sheffield, UK

Levine, B
Office of the Chief Medical Examiner, Baltimore,
MD, USA

Levinson, J
John Jay College of Criminal Justice, New York,
NY, USA

Lewis, A
McMaster University, Hamilton, ON, Canada

Liang, B A
California Western School of Law, San Diego, CA, USA

Little, D
Westmead Hospital Wentworthville, NSW, Australia

Liu, R H
Fooyin University, Kaohsiung Msien, Taiwan

Loff, B
Victorian Institute of Forensic Medicine, Southbank,
VIC, Australia

Lord, W D
Serial Killer Unit, FBI Academy, Quantico, VA, USA

Ludes, B
Institut de Médecine Légale, Strasbourg, France

Lunetta, P
University of Helsinki, Helsinki, Finland

Luo, B
Sun Yat Sen Medical School, Gungzhou, China

Lynch, M J
Monash University, Southbank, VIC, Australia

Marc, B
Compiegne Hospital, Compiegne, France

Marks, M K
University of Tennessee, Knoxville, TN, USA

Marks, P
The General Infirmary at Leeds, Leeds, UK

Marrero, L
Shands at Vista, a University of Florida Affiliate, Gainesville, FL, USA

Martrille, L
Centre Hospitalier Universitaire de Montpellier, Montpellier, France

May, C P
Criminal Justice Institute, Little Rock, AR, USA

McKelvie, H
Victorian Institute of Forensic Medicine, Southbank, VIC, Australia

McLay, D
Formerly Strathclyde Police, Glasgow, UK

McNamara, J J
Serial Killer Unit, FBI Academy, Quantico, VA, USA

Meadow, R
University of Leeds, Leeds, UK

Mieczkowski, T
University of South Florida, Tampa, FL, USA

Millward, M J
University of Western Australia, Perth, WA, Australia

Milroy, C M
University of Sheffield, Sheffield, UK

Mimasaka, S
Kumamoto University, Kumamoto, Japan

Miyaishi, S
Okayama University Graduate School of Medicine and Dentistry, Okayama, Japan

Moore, K A
Office of the Chief Medical Examiner, Baltimore, MD, USA

Moriya, F
Kochi University, Nankoku, Japan

Morris, G
Plantation, FL, USA

Morton, R J
Serial Killer Unit, FBI Academy, Quantico, VA, USA

Mossman, D
Wright State University School of Medicine, Dayton, OH, USA

Mura, P
Laboratoire Toxicology/Biochimic, France

Murphy, W A
MD Anderson Cancer Center, Houston, TX, USA

Myers, W C
University of Florida, Gainesville, FL, USA

Nadesan, K
University of Malaya, Kuala Lumpur, Malaysia

Naidoo, S R
University of KwaZulu Natal, Durban, South Africa

Nashelsky, M B
University of Iowa Carver College of Medicine, Iowa City, IA, USA

Natarajan, G A
Chief Medical Examiner's Office, Perth Amboy, NJ, USA

Nathan, R
Merseyside Forensic Psychiatry Service, St Helens, UK

Nathanson, M
Compiegne Hospital, Compiegne, France

Negrusz, A
University of Illinois at Chicago, Chicago, IL, USA

Nordby, J J
Final Analysis Forensics, Tacoma, WA, USA

Nordrum, I
Norwegian University of Science and Technology, Trondheim, Norway

Norfolk, G A
Association of Forensic Physicians, Bristol, UK

Norris, D O
University of Colorado at Boulder, CO, USA

Olle, L
Royal Women's Hospital, Carlton, VIC, Australia

Ong, B B
Queensland Health Scientific Services, Brisbane, QLD, Australia

Orlando, F
Nova Southeastern University, Fort Lauderdale, FL, USA

Pagliaro, E M
Connecticut Forensic Science Laboratory, Meriden, CT, USA

Palmbach, T M
University of New Haven, West Haven, CT, USA

Park, G
Addenbrooke's Hospital NHS Trust, Cambridge, UK

Park, J K
University of California – Davis ACC, Sacramento, CA, USA

Parrish, R N
Office of the Guardian ad Litem, Utah, UT, USA

Patel, M F
Royal Berkshire Hospital, Reading, UK

Payne-James, J
Forensic Healthcare Services Ltd, London, UK

Peel, M
Medical Foundation for the Care of Victims of Torture, London, UK

Perlmutter, D
Institute for the Research of Organized and Ritual Violence LLC, Yardley, PA, USA

Pollak, S
University of Freiburg, Freiburg, Germany

Pounder, D J
University of Dundee, Dundee, UK

Prahlow, J A
South Bend Medical Foundation and Indiana University of Medicine – South Bend Center for Medical Education at the University of Notre Dame, South Bend, IN, USA

Provis, A
Mount Hospital, Perth, WA, Australia

Quatrehomme, G
Laboratoire de Médecine Légale et Anthropologie Médico-légale, and Faculté de Médecine, Nice, France

Rabinovich, R
The Hebrew University of Jerusalem, Jerusalem, Israel

Ratcliff, C
Thames Valley Police, UK

Reavis, J A
Relationship Training Institute, San Diego, CA, USA

Rebmann, A J
Connecticut State Police, Kent, WA, USA

Reeves, R
University of Medicine and Dentistry of New Jersey, Newark, NJ, USA

Ren, L
University of Houston Law Center, Houston, TX, USA

Rittscher, J
General Electric, Niskayuna, NY, USA

Rix, K J B
Leeds Mental Health Teaching Trust, Leeds, UK

Robinson, S
Altrincham, UK

Rogers, R
University of North Texas, Denton, TX, USA

Rognum, T O
University of Oslo, Oslo, Norway

Rosner, R
New York University School of Medicine, and the Forensic Psychiatry Clinic of Bellevue Hospital Center, New York, NY, USA

Rutty, G N
Forensic Pathology Unit, Leicester, UK

Rutty, J E
DeMonfort University, Leicester, UK

Sanchez, T L
New Mexico Court of Appeals, Albuquerque, NM, USA

Saukko, P
University of Turku, Turku, Finland

Saunders, C M
QEII Medical Centre, Perth, WA, Australia

Savage, K A
National Forensic Science Technology Center, Largo, FL, USA

Sawaguchi, T
Tokyo Women's Medical University, Tokyo, Japan

Scheuer, L
Royal Free and University College Medical School, London, UK

Schreiber, N
University of Miami, Miami, FL, USA

Schuliar, Y
Institut de Recherche Criminelle de la Gendarmerie Nationale, Rosny-sous-Bois, France

Seals, M
Nova Southeastern University, Fort Lauderdale, FL, USA

Sewell, G J
University of Bath, Bath, UK

Shapiro, L M
Papworth Hospital, Cambridge, UK

Shuttleworth, C
FGI, Ontario, Canada

Simmons, T
University of Central Lancashire, Preston, UK

Simpson, E K
Forensic Science Centre, Adelaide, SA, Australia

Sjøvold, T
Stockholm University, Stockholm, Sweden

Smith, J
Essex, UK

Smock, W S
University of Louisville Hospital, Louisville, KY, USA

Solon, M
Bond Solon, London, UK

Sorg, M H
University of Maine, Orono, ME, USA

Spivack, B S
Office of the Chief Medical Examiner, Louisville, KY, USA

Stark, M M
St. George's Hospital Medical School, Epsom, UK

Sullivan, J E
University of Louisville, Louisville, KY, USA

Swift, B
Forensic Pathology Unit, Leicester, UK

Synstelien, J A
University of Tennessee, Knoxville, TN, USA

Taylor, R
Royal Cornwall Hospital, Truro, UK

Tersigni, M A
University of Tennessee, Knoxville, TN, USA

Thali, M J
University of Bern, Bern, Switzerland

Thatcher, P J
Forensic Science Center, Darwin, NT, Australia

Thid, M
Umeå University, Umeå, Sweden

Thompson, J W
Tulane University School of Medicine, New Orleans, LA, USA

Tsokos, M
University of Hamburg, Hamburg, Germany

Tsunenari, S
Kumamoto University, Kumamoto, Japan

Tu, P
General Electric, Niskayuna, NY, USA

Tully, B
Psychologists at Law Group, London, UK

Tunbridge, R
Transport Research Laboratory, Wokingham, UK

Van der Lugt, C
Dutch National Police Selection and Training Institute, Zutphen, The Netherlands

Vanezis, P
The Forensic Science Service, London, UK

Vayer, J S
University of the Health Sciences, Bethesda, MD, USA

Vege, Å
University of Oslo, Oslo, Norway

Virmani, R
Armed Forces Institute of Pathology, Washington, DC, USA

Vock, P
University of Bern, Bern, Switzerland

Wagner, G
Medical Examiner's Office, San Diego, CA, USA

Walker, A
University of Sheffield, Sheffield, UK

Wall, I
Ruislip, UK

Weakley-Jones, B
Office of the Chief Medical Examiner, Louisville, KY, USA

Wecht, C H
Allegheny County Coroner, Pittsburgh, PA, USA

Welch, J
King's College Hospital, London, UK

Welner, M
NYU School of Medicine, New York, NY, USA

Wetli, C V
Suffolk County Department of Health Services, Hauppauge, NY, USA

White, J
Women's and Children's Hospital, Adelaide, SA, Australia

Wielbo, D
National Forensic Science Technology Center, Largo, FL, USA

Wilets, J D
Nova Southeastern University, Fort Lauderdale, FL, USA

Williams, G S
Northern Illinois University, DeKalb, IL, USA

Wolff, K
Kings College, London, UK

Wolson, T L
Crime Laboratory Bureau, Miami, FL, USA

Wright, M G
London, UK

Wyatt, J
Royal Cornwall Hospital, Truro, UK

Yonemitsu, K
Kumamoto University, Kumamoto, Japan

Yoshida, K-I
University of Tokyo, Tokyo, Japan

Youyi, H
Peking University, Beijing, China

CONTENTS

VOLUME 1

VOLUME 2

H

VOLUME 3

I

N

O

T

V

W

Y

I

IDENTIFICATION

Contents

Prints, Finger and Palm

T P Kelliher, Niskayuna, NY, USA
J Rittscher and P Tu, General Electric, Niskayuna, NY, USA

History of Fingerprints

Finger and palm prints have been of interest to humans for the past 5000 years. This article provides an overview of the development of fingerprinting as a science, followed by a brief introduction to the anatomy that determines print characteristics. The second half of the article discusses forensic aspects of fingerprinting: collection of latent prints, classification of prints, and systems for matching prints. Scientific interest in their properties blossomed in the late nineteenth century. **Table 1** summarizes highlights of the use and study of prints.

Composition of Latent Fingerprints – Friction Skin

Fingertips are not the only part of the body that leave identifiable prints. The palms of the hand and the soles of the feet are also printable in the same fashion. These surfaces are covered with friction skin. Friction skin is covered with papillary ridges that assist in the ability to grasp and hold onto objects. The patterns formed in these ridges are very important since they are determined by the fourth month of gestation and remain fixed throughout life. Only severe mutilation or skin disease can cause them to change. The ridges vary in length and width, starting and stopping on occasion, and branching at points. For the most part they flow along with each other, forming individual patterns. Along the crest of the ridges, sweat pore openings are found. These pores number in the thousands per square centimeter.

Friction skin is formed of many layers. As with all skin, the epidermis is the outer layer and the dermis the inner layer. The composition of the epidermis and dermis is slightly different for friction skin than for other parts of the skin. Starting from the outer surface, the epidermis comprises: stratum corneum, stratum lucidum, stratum granulosum, stratum spinosum, and stratum basale. The top three elements are dead and dying cells while the bottom two are the living layers. These two are also known as the Malpighian layer, after Marcello Malpighi. **Figure 1** shows the basic structure of friction skin.

The glands attached to the pores in the ridges are eccrine glands. These are one of the two types of sweat glands found in humans. The eccrine gland has a coiled, tubular shape at its genesis in the dermis. Rising up through the epidermis is a duct through which secretions travel prior to emission through the pore. Eccrine glands are primarily responsible for regulating body temperature, although those associated with the friction skin are also linked to nervous reactions. Eccrine sweat contains approximately 99% water and 1% solids. The solids include sodium, potassium lactate, urea, ammonia, serine, ornithine, citrulline, aspartic acid, heavy metals, organic compounds, and proteolytic enzymes. These are the components of sweat that are left behind, forming fingerprints.

Table 1 Highlights of the use and study of prints

3000 BC	Masons 'sign' brickwork with finger impressions in their work on projects meant for kings and pharaohs
500 BC	In China and Babylon clay tablets and records of business transactions are imprinted with the author's fingerprints. It is not known if these societies knew of the uniqueness of fingerprints but there was obviously some attachment of identification to the prints
1684	Nehemiah Grew publishes the first written description of fingerprints in the West. Grew, a plant morphologist, was the first to study ridges and pores on the fingers and hands. In addition to writing he also provides detailed drawings of ridge patterns
1686	Marcello Malpighi, a professor of anatomy at the University of Bologna, Italy, publishes *De Externo Tactus Organo*, in which he describes ridges, spirals, and loops in fingerprints. He makes no mention in this work of their value as a tool for individual identification. The "Malpighi" layer of skin is named after him
1823	Joannes Purkinje publishes his thesis *A Commentary on the Physiological Examination of the Organs of Vision and the Cutaneous System*. In this he deals with functions of the ridges, furrows, and pores. He describes and illustrates nine fingerprint patterns. These nine classifications are what Henry will later name arches, tented arches, loops, whorls, and twinned loops
1858	Sir William Herschel, Chief Magistrate in Jungipoor, India, begins using, first, inked palm impressions and later, fingerprints on native contracts as a means of signature. Herschel begins to note that the inked impressions can, indeed, prove or disprove identity. Perhaps Herschel's greater contribution to fingerprint history is in confirming ridge consistency, i.e., friction skin ridge patterns are formed before birth and remain the same throughout life. At times throughout his life, Herschel takes his own fingerprints and notes that no change occurred in them in over 50 years
1870s, 1880	Dr. Henry Faulds, while in Japan, conducts experiments; removing the skin from a patient's fingers after having first fingerprinted them. When the skin grows back he confirms that the pattern is the same. Faulds is credited with identifying fingerprints at crime scenes, which were then compared to suspects who admitted their guilt. Dr. Faulds publishes an article in the scientific journal *Nature*, in which he discusses fingerprints as a means of personal identification, and the use of printer's ink as a method of obtaining such fingerprints. In the article he states: "When bloody finger marks or impression on clay, glass, etc., exist, they may lead to the scientific identification of criminals." His is the first publication to describe fingerprinting as a forensically useful science
1892	Sir Francis Galton, a British anthropologist, publishes *Fingerprints*. The book includes the first classification system for fingerprints. According to his calculations, the odds of two individual fingerprints being the same are 1 in 64 billion. For his classification method, Galton identified the small characteristics by which fingerprints can be identified. These same characteristics (minutiae) are still in use today
1900	Sir Edward Henry develops a classification system that neatly divides 10-print fingerprint cards into 1024 bins. Henry publishes his book *Classification and Uses of Fingerprints*. This system goes on to become the basis for the dominant indexing system in the English-speaking world

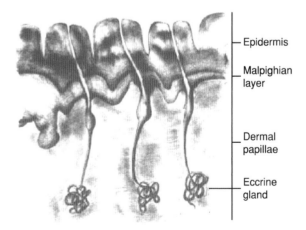

Figure 1 Friction skin: the coiled eccrine glands, located in the dermis, have ducts which rise through the epidermal layers and terminate along the crests of ridge lines. The structure of the dermal papillae gives the fingerprint its characteristic pattern.

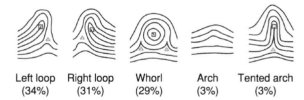

Left loop (34%) Right loop (31%) Whorl (29%) Arch (3%) Tented arch (3%)

Figure 2 Examples of the most common patterns for ridge lines. The five major classes – left loop, right loop, whorl, arch, and tented arch – are used. The approximate frequency of occurrence for each type is stated in brackets. For each type the position of the core is marked with a red square and the delta is marked with a green triangle.

Patterns of Fingerprints

As Purkinje first published and later Henry codified, there are relatively few primary patterns for fingerprints. They are most commonly referred to as loops, whorls, and arches (**Figure 2**). Within the Henry system these basic patterns are classified as: loop (ulnar or radial), tented arch, whorl, twinned loop, central pocket loop, lateral pocket loop, composite, and accidental. In order to interpret the rules for classifying a print into these categories it is first necessary to understand the delta formation and the core. As the name suggests, a delta formation is a triangular arrangement of ridge lines, formed where three separate ridge line flows come together. The core formation is the centermost portion of a ridge flow pattern.

Loop – Ulnar or Radial

Loops constitute between 60 and 70% of the patterns encountered. In a loop pattern, one or more of the ridges enters on either side of the impression, recurves, touches, or crosses the line running from the delta to the core, and terminates or tends to terminate on or in the direction of the side where the ridge or ridges entered. There is one delta. By definition, the existence of a core and one delta makes the pattern a loop. There are two kinds of loop, radial and ulnar, named after the radius and ulna, the two bones in the forearm. The radius joins the hand on the same side as the thumb, and the ulna on the same side as the little finger. To determine whether a loop is ulnar or radial you must know from which hand the print comes. If the ridge lines originate on the thumb side, the loop is radial; origination from the side of the little finger indicates ulnar.

Arch

Arches represent only about 5% of the fingerprint patterns encountered. In arch patterns, the ridges run from one side to the other of the pattern, making no backward turn. Arches come in two types – plain or tented. The difference is that tented arches have a significant upthrust in the middle, while the plain arch does not. Plain arches by definition have no deltas. Tented arches may have a delta at the base of the upthrust.

Whorl

Between 25 and 35% of the patterns encountered consist of whorls. In a whorl, some of the ridges make a turn through at least one circuit. Any fingerprint pattern that contains two or more deltas will be a whorl pattern. If a pattern does contain more than two deltas it will always be an accidental whorl. The technical definition of a plain whorl is a whorl that consists of one or more ridges that make or tend to make a complete circuit, with two deltas, between which an imaginary line is drawn and at least one recurving ridge within the inner pattern area is cut or touched.

Accidental

Under this heading are the relatively small numbers of patterns too irregular in outline to be grouped with central pocket loops and double loops. They have two or more deltas and a combination or fusion of two or more types of patterns, not including the plain, radial, or ulnar arch. This category also includes any pattern or formation that does not conform to any conventional type.

Collection Methods

Prior to classification and identification, fingerprints must first be collected. Fingerprints are typically collected from people using tenprint cards. To use these cards the enrollee's fingers are first inked and then the finger is rolled from side to side on the tenprint card, leaving an impression of the fingerprint. In addition to tenprint cards, fingerprint impressions are actively collected using a variety of scanning techniques for applications such as access control. These scanners use a variety of methods ranging from optical to ultrasound and capacitance to determine the pattern of ridges.

Latent Prints

Latent prints are those that are left behind through interaction of hands, palms, and feet with the environment. Preserving and collecting these prints is important in a forensic context. Occasionally these prints are left cleanly so as to be clearly visible to the unaided eye. It is more often the case that the prints are only partially visible or not visible at all without the use of specialized fingerprint-processing methods and equipment. This equipment has been developed to take advantage of properties of the latent print composition in order to enhance and stabilize the prints. The goal is to differentiate the print from the background surface.

A sequence of techniques is used when processing a crime scene for latent fingerprints. This sequence should always begin with nondestructive techniques before proceeding to potentially destructive ones. Lighting, physical processing, and chemical processing are all used in the development of latent prints. Visible examination of the site is the first line of approach, followed by other optical methods, e.g., diffusion, luminescence, ultraviolet absorption, and/or reflection. After these methods have been exhausted, more intrusive physical and chemical approaches can be considered. These methods will vary depending on the type, coloring, and contamination of the surface to be examined and the time and environmental conditions since the prints were thought to be left. The physical and chemical methods use various approaches to enhance prints by interacting with the secretion from the eccrine and sebaceous glands. The choice of enhancement technique is not always as straightforward as it may seem. Some approaches complement each other while others rule out further processing with what may be a promising alternative.

Lighting

Optical detection methods have the advantage of being nondestructive with respect to the latent fingerprint deposit. As a result, these techniques do not preclude the later application of other fingerprint development procedures. Observation of an object under white light may disclose a visible fingerprint that can be photographed without any further treatment or more complex optical detection methods may reveal otherwise invisible prints that may not be developed by other techniques. Photoluminescence, the emission of light by certain chemicals after exposure to light energy of a given wavelength, has proven to be useful in the detection of latent prints on surfaces such as metal, firearms, human skin, and polystyrene foam. A fingerprint is only visible if its luminescence is more intense or at a different wavelength to that emitted by the background. A similar approach can also be taken using ultraviolet spectrum lighting. Episcopic coaxial illumination is another light-based technique. It works well on normally shiny surfaces such as metal. The technique involves the use of a semitransparent mirror to observe the reflection of light perpendicular to the surface. The light is diffused by the fingerprint deposit but specularly reflected by the surface.

Physical

Dusting a surface with a fine powder of contrasting color is one of the oldest, most common, and most readily available methods for the development of latent prints. Fingerprint powder is applied at the crime scene on smooth, nonabsorbent surfaces and, in general, only to objects that cannot be transported back to a laboratory. The powder adheres to the humid, sticky, or greasy substances in the fingerprint deposit. The application of powder is relatively simple and inexpensive. The ideal powder is one of contrasting color, good adherence properties, and sensitivity, possibly incorporating a luminescent material. Fingerprint-lifting tape is the most common method of collecting fingerprint evidence after powdering. The adhesive tape is placed over the dusted print and smoothed down with the finger. Particles of powder adhere to the sticky surface of the tape and transfer a mirror image of the fingerprint pattern.

Small particle reagent (SPR), a suspension of powder in a surfactant solution, is a method of using powdering in wet applications. The reagent is sensitive to the nonwater-soluble compounds of the latent fingerprint and may be used on a wide range of nonabsorbent surfaces. SPR is effective on surfaces that are wet – a condition that excludes the use of conventional powders or reagents sensitive to the water-soluble components of the print.

Chemical

There are numerous chemical reagents at the disposal of a fingerprint collector. Two of the more widely used are described below. Depending on the surface the print is on, other choices may be more appropriate (Table 2).

Ninhydrin The reaction of amines with ninhydrin to form the colored reaction product known as Ruhemann's purple was discovered by Siegfried Ruhemann in 1910. The value of ninhydrin for the development of latent fingerprints was not realized until 1954, when Odén and von Hofsten suggested its use in criminal investigations. Ninhydrin reacts with the amino acid in the fingerprint deposit (eccrine secretion) to give a dark-purple product. Amino acid-specific agents have particular application for the development of fingerprints on paper. The chemical reactions involved are complex and, as a result, the development conditions need to be controlled if optimum results are to be obtained. Prints developed with ninhydrin may be further treated with a metal salt solution ($ZnCl_2$), which produces a color change to orange. The orange product is strongly photoluminescent when cooled with liquid nitrogen and illuminated with light of a wavelength of around 490 nm. There has been significant research into

Table 2 Applicability of selected reagents to a variety of surfaces commonly encountered in forensic fingerprint examination

Reagent	Surface type									
	Paper	Glossy paper	Currency	Porous	Nonporous	Glass	Plastic	Wet	Metal	Wood
Basic yellow 40		×				×	×		×	
Cyanoacrylate ester		×			×	×	×		×	
Ninhydrin	×			×						×
Iodine fuming				×						×
Physical developer	×		×							
Silver nitrate	×									×
Small particle reagent		×			×	×	×	×	×	

alternative amino acid-specific reagents. Two of the most successful are 1-8 diazofluorenone and a ninhydrin analog, indandione. These reagents produce a photoluminescent product and significantly improve sensitivity of detection compared to ninhydrin.

Cyanoacrylate fuming   Cyanoacrylate esters are colorless, monomeric liquids sold commercially as rapid, high-strength glues, e.g. Superglue®. Cyanoacrylate liquid forms a vapor that reacts with moisture and certain eccrine and sebaceous components in a latent fingerprint. The vapor selectively polymerizes on the fingerprint ridges to form a hard, white polymer known as polycyanoacrylate. Prints with a high sebaceous component appear to be particularly sensitive to cyanoacrylate vapor, although the glue probably also reacts with the moisture and some water-soluble (eccrine) components in the print. The technique is effective on most nonporous surfaces, including metal, glass, and plastic. Originally developed in Japan in the late 1970s, the cyanoacrylate fuming process is now the most widely used fingerprint detection technique for nonporous objects treated in the laboratory.

Fingerprint Matching

Henry Classification System

The basic Henry system assigns a numerical value and an index number to each finger. From right thumb to right little finger, the fingers are indexed 1 through 5, while left thumb to left little finger are indexed 6 through 10. Starting with index 1, the right thumb, the first two fingers are valued 16, the next two 8, the next two 4, the next two 2, and the final two 1. To determine a tenprint's Henry classification, only the fingers with whorl prints are considered. The finger values are summed for every whorl-printed finger indexed with an even number. The same is done for the odd-indexed fingers with whorl prints. Each of these numbers is then increased by 1. The result is expressed as a fraction; the even index value in the numerator, and odd index value in the denominator. This fraction is the Henry classification number.

An example is given in **Table 3**. In practice each of the Henry categories is further refined, in most cases using Galton's details as the next level of indexing.

Automated Fingerprint Identification

The high demand of fingerprint identification services prompted the law enforcement agencies to initiate research into automatic fingerprint identification. The success of fingerprints as a forensic tool for establishing identity led to a much broader use of fingerprints for biometric identification in applications such as access control and passports. These applications require sensors that can quickly and reliably capture an image of a fingerprint. The challenge of automatic fingerprint identification is to transform an art, learnt in time-consuming training, into a precise algorithmic procedure. The following subsections summarize the sensing and enhancement of fingerprints, the representation of digital fingerprints, the classification, and the matching of fingerprints.

Sensing and Enhancement of Fingerprints

Rolled-ink fingerprints, as discussed above, can of course be scanned electronically. However, this acquisition process is slow and requires practice and skill and is therefore both unfeasible and impractical in the operational phase. Fingerprint scanners are used to automate the acquisition process. As opposed to a rolled print, most fingerprint scanners acquire a so-called dab, i.e., the finger is simply pressed on the sensor/paper without rolling it from nail to nail. Obtaining an image of a fingerprint without the intermediate step of getting an impression on paper is termed a live-scan fingerprint. A number of sensing technologies are available to capture live-scan fingerprints: (1) optical frustrated total internal reflection (FTIR); (2) thermal sensing; (3) ultrasonic reflection; (4) differential capacitance; and (5) noncontact two-dimensional and three-dimensional scanning. The FTIR method is one of the most popular concepts.

As opposed to scanning the superficial layers of the surface skin, ultrasound images the internal layers of

Table 3 An example of the Henry classification system. In this example the Henry number is (RR + LM + 1)/(RT + RM +TF + LR + 1). This reduces to (4 + 2 + 1)/(16 + 8 + 2 + 1 + 1) or 7/28 as the Henry index

		RT	1	*RF*	2	*RM*	3	*RR*	4	*RP*	5
Finger	Finger	*16*		16		*8*		8		4	
Name	Index	@				@		@			
		LT	6	*TF*	7	*LM*	8	*LR*	9	*LP*	10
Finger value		4		2		2		1		1	
Whorl				@		@		@			

the friction skin, focusing on the dermal papillae. This method is believed to be capable of acquiring a very clear fingerprint image, although the finger does not have very clear ridge structures. One disadvantage is that it is a relatively expensive sensing technology. Less accurate than FTIR and cheap enough for mass production is the differential capacitance method. In a capacitive sensor the finger acts as one of the plates of a capacitor. The other plate consists of a silicon plate with sensing circuitry. Each pixel is precharged to a reference voltage and discharged by the reference current. The rate of change of the potential on the capacitor plate is proportional to the capacitance seen by the capacitor plate. This technology is used to build single-touch sensors (15 × 13 mm) as well as cheaper sweep sensors (3.6 × 13.5 mm). To date these sensors are capable of producing an image which has a resolution of more than 500 dpi, which is the resolution the US Federal Bureau of Investigation requires for a digital fingerprint.

If necessary, image enhancement methods can be used to improve the quality of fingerprint scans. The most common issues are a significant number of spurious minutiae, and a large percentage of missing or poorly placed genuine minutiae. Commonly image enhancement methods include noise removal or denoising techniques. Sophisticated pattern recognition techniques can be applied to estimate the underlying structure of an image corrupted by noise. In addition, it needs to be taken into account that 2–5% of the total population have poor-quality fingerprints. Often these are older people in whom there is a natural flattening of the dermal papillae with age, people with finger injuries, people living in dry weather conditions, or people with certain genetic attributes.

Representation

In order to establish reliably whether two prints originate from the same finger, the representation of the prints must be invariant to distortion due to the imaging process and the elasticity of the finger, occlusion of a small part of the finger, and orientation of the finger during the capture of the print. Fingerprint features are generally divided into global and local features. Global features are overall attributes of the finger and typically determined by examining the entire finger. The most important global feature of a fingerprint is its classification.

Current automatic fingerprint identification systems use the same classification system as human examiners, as discussed above (**Figure 2**). Additional global features include the ridge thickness, ridge separation, and ridge depth. While global features are used to classify a fingerprint, local features are

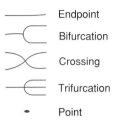

Figure 3 Minutiae types. This figure illustrates the most basic types of minutiae. Human examiners can easily differentiate between 13 different types of minutiae. To date, most automatic fingerprint identification systems do not make use of this information. In practical applications misclassification rates can be very high due to sensor noise and other artifacts.

mainly used for matching. They include ridges, pores on the ridges, and salient features derived from ridges. Typically, standard signal-processing techniques are used to extract the set of ridges. The most frequently used features are the minute details, or minutiae, of the ridges (**Figure 3**). Most automatic fingerprint identification systems use the pattern of the minutiae as a valid representation of the fingerprint. This representation is very compact, hence good for digital storage, and captures a sufficient amount of information about the individual fingerprint. For reasons of robustness, only the most prominent ridge features, the ridge endings, and ridge bifurcations are extracted. The ANSI-NIST (American National Standards Institute – National Institute of Standards and Technology) standard representation of a fingerprint is mainly based on minutiae and includes one or more global features such as orientation of the finger, locations, and fingerprint class.

Matching

Due to deformations, the elastic nature of the finger, the variation caused by the capture of the print, and for partial latent prints, the unknown location and orientation standard pattern recognition methods are insufficient to determine a match between two different prints. In a first step, a print is typically classified with respect to the Henry system. In addition, the ridge count between the core and the delta of the fingerprint is used for broad classification. Once classified, a number of different methods are used to determine a fingerprint match.

A typical latent print contains about 40 minutiae. The location, orientation, and ridge count between any two minutiae are a natural set of features that are used by the different matching methods. For any given minutia, a signature can be computed by considering its local neighborhood. **Figure 4** illustrates two typical choices. It is important to note that any choice of features must be both descriptive

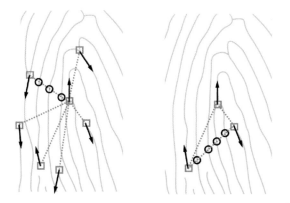

Figure 4 Features for fingerprint matching. A number of different features can be used to characterize minutiae. The graph on the right illustrates how the neighbors of a given minutia can be used. Based on a local coordinate system, the local neighborhood is divided into *N* different sectors. In each of the sectors the minutia closest to the center is used. The resulting signature is composed of the orientation of each minutia, the ridge count (illustrated using black circles) on each edge connecting two minutiae, and relative angles. An alternative to using a local neighborhood system is to use triples of minutiae to form a local signature.

and invariant under transformation. One of the algorithms currently used by the US Federal Bureau of Investigation uses a local signature (**Figure 4**, left) and employs graph-matching techniques to determine a fingerprint match. A commercial system developed by IBM uses features based on minutiae triples. As opposed to directly comparing a pair of prints, an index is computed for each minutiae triple (**Figure 4**, right). The search for a match is then based on the set of indices computed for a given latent print. An alternative to these approaches is adaptive elastic string matching, which explicitly tries to address the problem of large nonlinear distortions of fingerprints.

Although automated fingerprint identification systems are very sophisticated, their performance does not match the precision of human examiners. As the science of fingerprint recognition progresses, one can expect a continuous improvement of such systems.

See Also

Identification: Prints, Challenges To Fingerprints; Prints, Ear; Facial

Further Reading

Beavan C (2001) *Fingerprints: The Origins of Crime Detection and the Murder Case that Launched Forensic Science*. New York: Hyperion.

Cowger J (1983) *Friction Ridge Skin: Comparison and Identification of Fingerprints*. New York: Elsevier.

Cummins H, Midlo C (1961) *Fingerprints, Palms, and Soles; An Introduction to Dermatoglyphics*. New York: Dover.

Jain L, Halici U, Hayashi I, *et al.* (1999) *Intelligent Biometric Techniques in Fingerprint and Face Recognition*. pp. 1–107. Boca Raton, FL: CRC Press.

Lee H, Gaensslen R (2001) *Advances in Fingerprint Technology*, 2nd edn., pp. 1–240. Boca Raton, FL: CRC Press.

Nanavati S, Thieme M, Nanavati R (2002) *Biometrics: Identity Verification in a Networked World*, pp. 45–49. New York: Wiley.

United States, Federal Bureau of Investigation (1982) *FBI Advanced Latent Fingerprint School*. Washington, DC: US Government Printing Office.

United States, Federal Bureau of Investigation (1984) *The Science of Fingerprints: Classification and Uses*. Washington, DC: US Government Printing Office.

Prints, Challenges To Fingerprints

P Tu, T P Kelliher, and J Rittscher, General Electric, Niskayuna, NY, USA

Introduction

For many societies, the reidentification of criminals has been an important aspect of law enforcement. The amputation of a thief's hand marked him for life. The French branded criminals with the fleur de lis. The Romans used tattooing to prevent desertion of mercenary soldiers. Police officers with extraordinary memory were known to identify repeat offenders by sight alone. Photography was used to generate a rogue's gallery.

In addition to having a sound scientific foundation, a biometric identifier needs to survive legal challenges. In 1870, for example, Alphonse Bertillon developed an anthropological system of recorded dimensions such as the length of the femur. These were reduced to a formula that was touted as being unchanging and unique to an individual. However, in 1903 it was determined that a man named Will West was falsely imprisoned after discovering a man named William West with nearly exact Bertillon measurements. Although it has been hypothesized that the two men were identical twins, the Bertillon system never recovered.

Over the last 100 years, fingerprinting has emerged as the biometric of choice for establishing criminal identity. The forensic use of fingerprints goes beyond determining whether or not an individual has a criminal record. Latent prints found at a crime scene have been used both to identify potential suspects and as evidence in the resulting trial.

The credibility of this information has been held in high esteem by the courts. Although convictions have rarely been made on fingerprint evidence alone, it has been a deciding factor in many cases. Today's use of fingerprints is not limited to criminal investigations. The availability of fingerprint readers has made it easy to capture and analyze fingerprints without expert assistance. Hence, they have become a widely accepted biometric for access control and identity authentication.

Fingerprint identification is based on two basic premises: (1) persistence – the basic characteristics of fingerprints do not change with time; and (2) individuality – the fingerprint is unique to an individual. Recently, these assertions have been challenged and the ability to make an identification based on a partial latent print has been questioned.

In this context arguments were raised as to how much information is sufficient to make a decision with certainty. In particular, the 1993 Daubert ruling, which strengthened the requirement for the scientific basis of expert testimony, has resulted in numerous legal challenges to the admissibility of fingerprint evidence. Even though none of these challenges has succeeded, some district attorneys are now for the first time "plea bargaining" when the whole case hinges on a fingerprint, in order to avoid the cost and risk associated with such legal actions.

The study of fingerprints was initially an anatomical inquiry. Their value as a biometric identifier was discovered later. With the emergence of fingerprint analysis as a law enforcement tool, various terms and methods of operation have been defined. After the 1993 Daubert ruling, a number of challenges to the admissibility of fingerprint evidence have been made. Many of these legal arguments revolve around the belief that a scientific basis for fingerprint analysis requires a probabilistic paradigm. However, at a philosophical level, the statistical approach is at odds with the assertion of individuality. This article concludes with an exposition of this conflict.

Naturally, a discussion of these issues cannot avoid controversy. Historical and scientific developments are reviewed so that opposing points of view can be presented in context without passing judgment on the merit or motivation behind them. The author does not claim to speak on behalf of any institution or governing body.

History

In ancient China, thumbprints were found on clay tablets. As early as the third century BC inked fingerprints were used on various official documents. Whether or not these prints were used for identification or just ceremonial purposes is not known.

Grew in 1684 first wrote about the anatomical nature of the surface of the skin. Malpighi in 1686 focused on the substructures of the skin and described fingerprint patterns in terms of ridges, spirals, and loops. Neither recognized the uniqueness of fingerprints. The first to theorize that the arrangement of fingerprint ridges might be unique was Mayer in 1798.

Purkinji published a thesis in 1823 discussing nine fingerprint patterns. These descriptions are the predecessors for the fingerprint pattern classes of arch, tented arch, whorl, and twined loop. Herschel (1856) had local businessmen impress their fingerprints on contracts. Initially this was done on a whim, but as his collection of fingerprints grew, he realized that fingerprints could be used to prove or disprove identity. He observed that his own fingerprints as well as those of various prisoners did not change over the years.

After noticing fingerprints on ancient Japanese pottery, Faulds in 1880 realized their potential use for identification and developed a system of classification. He conjectured that they did not change over time and that they were highly variable. He also observed that "latent" prints, which are prints found at a crime scene, could be used for the scientific identification of criminals. He presented his findings to Charles Darwin who passed them on to his cousin Francis Galton.

Thompson in 1882 used his own fingerprint to prevent forgery. This was the first use of fingerprints in the USA. In 1883 Mark Twain's book *Life on the Mississippi*, a fictional court used fingerprints to solve a murder.

Galton in 1888 published his book *Fingerprints* where he established the concepts of fingerprint individuality and permanence. He presented his own classification system and defined the characteristics known as minutiae or Galton's details which are the main features by which fingerprints are identified today.

In Argentina, Vucetich in 1891 developed a classification system based on Galton pattern types and in 1892 he made the first criminal identification of a woman named Francisca Rojas. She murdered her two sons but accused a neighboring ranch worker of the crime. Her bloody print was found on a doorpost, thus exonerating the worker and implicating Ms. Rojas.

Henry in 1901 established the Henry classification system, which persists today in most English-speaking countries. Such a system provides a method for sorting fingerprints based on type. When a comparison of a reference print against a set of candidate prints is performed, the classification system is used so that the majority of prints can be ruled out without requiring direct comparison.

The first systematic use of fingerprints in the USA was headed by DeForrests in 1902. Locard wrote in 1918 that a correspondence of 12 Galton details between two prints was enough to establish identity.

In 1924 the Federal Bureau of Investigation (FBI) consolidated what are now the FBI fingerprint files. By 1946 the FBI had processed 100 million fingerprint cards, and as of 1971 the collection had grown to 200 million. In 1980 the FBI created a computerized fingerprint file system and by 1989 most fingerprint match requests were performed automatically, although all final individualizations were still reviewed by expert examiners.

In 1993 the Daubert ruling strengthened the requirements for establishing the reliability of experts. The first of many legal challenges to fingerprint admissibility under Daubert was made in 1999.

Definitions

"Classification systems" are methods by which fingerprints are ordered based on fingerprint pattern type.

"Latent" prints are fingerprints found at a crime scene that may not be directly visible to the naked eye. In the UK, they are called "marks."

"Tenprints" are a record of all 10 fingerprints of an individual taken under controlled conditions.

"Identification or individualization" is the conclusion of an expert that two fingerprints show sufficient information in agreement with no principal differences. This leads to the conclusion that the same donor has generated them.

"Level 1 detail" is the overall pattern configuration of a fingerprint. Examples of these pattern types are arches, loops, and whorls.

"Galton level 2 detail" can be described as minutiae and other ridge formations. A minutia is an event that occurs in a regular flow of papillary ridges. The event is a natural disturbance to the normal parallel system of the ridges such as ridge termination and bifurcation.

"Level 3 details" are small shapes on the ridge (edgeoscopy). This includes ridge unit thickness, thinness, and relative pore location (poroscopy). Third-level detail is always used in agreement with second-level detail.

"Points of agreement" are corresponding points between two prints that are deemed to be sufficiently similar.

"AFIS" is an automatic fingerprint identification system that generally relies on level 1 and level 2 features.

Methodology

In this section the various principles for establishing a fingerprint identification are reviewed.

Galton first defined minutiae as the principal features by which two fingerprints are to be compared. Locard established the first rules for the minimum number of minutiae necessary for identification.

Locard was a student of Bertillon, the founder of the anthropometric system of identification. Locard argued that a fingerprint match must use details such as ridge shape and pore location and not just rely on the correspondence of minutiae. Locard is known as the father of poreoscopy, edgeoscopy, and ridgeology. Locard in 1914 developed the tripartite rule, summarized as follows.

If more than 12 concurring points are present and the fingerprint is sharp, the certainty of identity is beyond debate. If 8–12 concurring points are involved, then the case is borderline and the certainty of identity will depend on the sharpness of the fingerprints; the rarity of its type; the presence of the center of the figure (core) and the triangle (delta) in the exploitable part of the print; the presence of pores (poreoscopy); the perfect and obvious identity regarding the width of the papillary ridges and valleys, the direction of the lines, and the angular value of the bifurcations (ridgeology/edgeoscopy).

Locard also stated the value and the importance of qualified conclusions to the identification process. He said, "if a limited number of characteristic points are present, the fingerprints cannot provide certainty for an identification, but only a presumption proportional to the number of points available and their clarity."

In 1973 the International Association for Identification (IAI) standardization committee stated that: "No valid basis exists at this time for requiring that a pre-determined minimum number of friction ridge characteristics must be present in two impressions in order to establish positive identification." Because of this ruling, countries such as the USA have no minimum threshold for feature correspondence. The remainder of the report dealt with the development of minimum standards with regard to the training and experience needed to testify.

In 1980 the IAI issued what is now referred to as resolution V, establishing the types of conclusion that can be drawn from a fingerprint examination. A direct interpretation of this resolution is that an examiner must state that there is either sufficient information to make an absolute identification or the print is of no value. This implies that no statements regarding the probability of identification should be made. It has been argued that this interpretation can be harmful in that it prohibits the expression of conclusions such as "there is enough information to rule out certain segments of the population but not enough to make an exact identification." Although not conclusive, such information could be useful for investigative purposes. As will be seen, this policy has also been targeted by a number of Daubert challenges.

In 1998, The Interpol European Expert Group on Fingerprint Identification (IEEGFI) explored the feasibility of determining a common European method for fingerprint identification. Two methods were defined: the holistic quality approach and the empirical standard approach.

In the holistic approach, the examiner compares all three levels of fingerprint detail. These details are considered in totality in order to arrive at a conclusion. It is assumed that biological uniqueness exists or does not exist. Uniqueness cannot sometimes be partial and at other times not partial. Any portion of a fingerprint, no matter how large or small, has only one source. However, it is accepted that the content in a given latent print may prove to be insufficient to establish uniqueness.

The empirical standard method advocates a numerical approach to identification. Points of agreement are annotated so that the matching process can be documented and compared. Like the holistic approach, it is assumed that uniqueness either exists or it does not. As a safeguard many European countries set a minimum number of points of agreement needed to ensure uniqueness. This is usually between 12 and 16.

In *United States* v. *Harvard* (2001), an expert witness described the manual comparison of a latent print with an exemplar as a three-stage process. This is described as follows: initially the examiner compares the general level 1 ridge patterns of the two prints. The orientation of the latent print is determined. At this point there is not enough information to individualize but many exemplars can be excluded. Second, the relationship between each ridge and the remaining ridges for both prints is determined. The totality of ridge location, type, direction, and relationships are considered. Some degree of individualization can occur at this point. Finally correspondence of individual ridges between the latent and the exemplar are checked. This is based on level 3 details such as the location of sweat pores. Typically, decisions are confirmed via peer review.

Legal Challenges

In the USA, fingerprint testimony has been generally admitted as evidence based on the concept of "general acceptance" established in *United States* v. *Frye* (1923). However, in 1993 the Daubert ruling (*Daubert* v. *Merrell Dow Pharmaceuticals*) strengthened the requirements for establishing the reliability of expert testimony. The criteria for establishing reliability were defined based on the following factors: (1) whether the particular technique or methodology in question has been subject to statistical hypothesis testing; (2) whether its error rate has been established; (3) whether standards controlling the technique's operations exist and have been maintained; (4) whether it has been peer-reviewed, and published; and (5) whether it has a general widespread acceptance.

The first challenge to fingerprint identification under Daubert was in *United States* v. *Mitchell* (1999) using the argument that the premise for fingerprint identification has not been tested and that the error rates are not known. The motion to exclude fingerprint evidence was denied. Since then there have been numerous challenges under Daubert. The following is a review of significant rulings.

State of Georgia v. McGee (2000)

The defense argued that latent print examination is not a science because statistical probabilities are not used to establish a minimum number of points needed to individualize. The court concluded that, despite numerous challenges, fingerprint identification is reliable evidence.

State of California v. Ake (2001)

The judge ruled that Daubert is not applicable in California and, since fingerprint analysis is neither new nor novel, expert testimony is admissible.

United States v. Harvard (2001)

The defense argued that the government has not established the scientific reliability of fingerprint comparisons so as to render such evidence admissible. The ruling stated that claims of uniqueness and permanence are scientific because those assertions can be falsified and that much of the comparison process is objective. Also, 100 years of adversarial testing make up for any lack of publications.

United States v. Plaza (2002)

The court allowed experts to present fingerprints, describe how they were collected, and point out various similarities. However, the experts were not allowed to present their opinion that a given latent print is in fact the print of a particular person. On appeal the decision to prohibit opinion-based testimony was reversed.

United States v. Crisp (2003)

Lawyers attempted to dismiss fingerprint testimony on the basis that the premise for fingerprint analysis had not been tested and that operators work without uniform and objective standards. The challenge was defeated with a two to one majority. The following is a summary of the dissenting opinion. It was argued that general acceptance of fingerprint identification does not establish reliability. Persistence of the technique for 100 years under the judicial adversarial system does not imply scientific acceptance, because defendants do not have sufficient access to scientific and financial resources. The judge was not presented with studies that show how likely it is that prints taken from a crime scene will be a match for only one set of fingerprints in the world. He argued that the testing of examiners does not always reflect real-world conditions. He questioned the peer review process for fingerprint publications. He stated that the government had ignored error rates of examiners and referred to tests where examiners are unable to correctly identify matches and eliminate nonmatches. He stated that the subjectivity of the examination process allows the examiner to explain away differences rather than discount the match. He criticized the field for a lack of universal standards and a refusal to hedge testimony in terms of probability. He noted that different examiners come to different conclusions regarding the certainty of identity. Finally, acceptance of the field in the scientific community was questioned. The dissenting judge did not say that fingerprint analysis could not satisfy the Daubert criteria but in his opinion the government has up to now failed to do so.

One of the main issues behind this dissenting decision is the contention that the uniqueness assertion does not necessarily imply reliable matching. The argument is that latent prints are distorted impressions of a fingerprint and skill levels vary from examiner to examiner. It has never been claimed that examiners are infallible and, admittedly, mistakes can be and have been made. That being noted, the FBI performs numerous identifications on a daily basis and to date no challenge has ever overturned an FBI identity decision. Since the quality of both examiners and latent prints varies, these types of challenges may have to be handled on a case-by-case basis.

A more fundamental concern is centered on the fact that many examiners insist on absolute certainty of their identifications and they resist attempts to present fingerprint analysis in a probabilistic framework. In order to understand this issue better, the various probabilistic approaches that have been developed for the purposes of establishing uniqueness of a fingerprint have been reviewed. This will be followed by a discussion of the philosophical issues associated with the statistical paradigm.

Modeling Uniqueness

Over the years scientists have developed a number of statistical models for the purpose of analyzing fingerprints. Initially configuration-based approaches were devised so as to estimate the potential size of the fingerprint population. This was followed by attempts to predict the probability that a given print will have a certain degree of commonality with a print selected at random from the population. Attempts have been made to take into account the variability associated with deformations between multiple impressions of the same fingerprint as well as distortions associated with a latent print.

The first attempts to establish a probabilistic model for uniqueness were to hypothesize that there are a limited number of distinguishable fingerprints. Assuming that all prints are equally probable, the uniqueness of a given print is then proportional to the number of distinguishable prints. To make this estimate, authors such as Galton in 1892 associated a grid with the fingerprint. For a given square in the grid it was argued that there are q possible states or configurations. Based on this logic, the number of possible fingerprints is estimated to be proportional to q^N where N is the number of squares in the grid.

Henry estimated, in 1900, the probability p of observing a minutia at a given location. If a fingerprint has n minutiae, then the probability of observing a fingerprint selected at random from the population with corresponding minutiae would be a function of p^n.

In 1977, Ostenburg took a more refined view of minutia type. He argued that each 1×1 mm region of a fingerprint could be classified by either being empty or having one of 12 different types of minutiae. By computing the probability of each of these states, the probability of two prints matching over a given area can be estimated.

It is argued that probabilistic models must take into account the fact that what takes place in one part of the print is not independent of what takes place in another part of the print. In 1979, Scolve investigated the correlation between neighboring cells of Ostenberg's scheme, which resulted in slightly lower estimates of uniqueness. In 1989, Stoney developed a model of pairwise minutia dependencies.

In the 1999 Daubert trial, attempts were made to assess the intrinsic uniqueness of fingerprints via the results attained from processing 50 000 reference prints using an AFIS system. The scores of the best false matches were compared with the scores associated with the reference print matched against itself. This experiment was criticized because it did not take into account the fact that there is a significant deformation between multiple impressions taken from the same finger. This phenomenon is known as intraclass variation.

Trauring, in 1988, was the first to look at intraclass deviations. He estimated that corresponding features could be displaced by up to 1.5 times the interridge distance between the features. In 2000, Pankanti modeled fingerprint identification as a form of template matching. He used an AFIS system and a model for intraclass variation to compute the probability that two fingerprints with n and m minutiae will have r correspondences.

In 2000, Tu developed a similar template-matching scheme based on a set of Bernoulli trials with the aim of addressing feature correlation. Instead of defining an explicit model for interfeature relationships, measurements based on group statistics were used to compensate for dependencies.

Philosophical Issues

In the statistical frameworks that have been proposed for measuring fingerprint uniqueness, every possible outcome has a distinct nonzero probability of occurring. Even if it is concluded that the probability of observing two identical fingerprints from different individuals is miniscule, the fact that this probability is by definition nonzero flies in the face of the individuality assertion.

At the root of the probabilistic approach is a paradigm based on discrete events. Either a minutia is at a specific location or it is not. A given cell can only be in one of q different states. The criteria in which events are differentiated can be viewed as a type of formulaic thresholding.

Various members of the fingerprint communities would contend that to date no proposed formulaic criteria can match an examiner's ability to determine whether or not two ridges or two points of interest are in correspondence. This is based on the argument that the fingerprint contains a theoretically infinite spectrum of complex detail that cannot be fully characterized in mathematical terms. If this argument is taken to its extreme, an examiner could in theory make an identification based on a single ridge, assuming the mechanisms by which the impressions are captured have sufficient fidelity.

This argument leads to the assertion that the granularity of a probabilistic framework cannot match the fidelity of a human examiner and hence estimates of uniqueness can only be viewed as a lower bound. This is in stark contrast to DNA matching, which is fundamentally discrete in nature and must therefore submit to the conclusions that can be drawn from statistical analysis.

From the point of view of the scientific method, fingerprint individuality represents a hypothesis that has yet to be contradicted. In 1963, Popper had argued that the strength of a hypothesis is proportional to the ease with which it can be falsified. Thus, the individuality hypothesis must be viewed as extremely strong since it could be shown to be invalid with just a single counterexample. To support this argument, in 1990 the Los Angeles fingerprint agency performed 127 732 reference fingerprint searches using a standard AFIS system. This resulted in over 2.5 trillion comparisons. For each search print the top 10 closest false mates were manually compared with the reference print. All were found to be distinguishable from the reference prints.

The debate regarding the justification of the individuality assertion may be academically interesting but fundamentally intractable. An alternative point of view is that all systems benefit from a statistical understanding of their workings. At some point where there is an extremely low degree of probability, in human endeavors that point becomes indistinguishable from certainty. The vast amount of daily fingerprint identification is generally accepted to fall into this category. Most of the current activity is engaged in setting the borders for extreme cases where the information content is much harder to use.

Clearly the courts demand answers to these complicated issues. Whether or not a satisfactory resolution can be achieved will depend on the wisdom and understanding of the judiciary, the defense bar, scientists, law enforcement officials, and practitioners of fingerprint identification. The importance of this outcome cannot be overstated since both lives and society's right to receive justice are at stake.

See Also

Identification: Prints, Finger and Palm; Prints, Ear; Facial

Further Reading

Beavan C (2001) *Fingerprints: The Origins of Crime Detection and the Murder Case that Launched Forensic Science*. New York: Hyperion.

Cowger J (1983) *Friction Ridge Skin: Comparison and Identification of Fingerprints*. New York: Elsevier.

Drake AW (1967) *Fundamentals of Applied Probability Theory*. New York: McGraw-Hill.

Jain L (1999) *Intelligent Biometric Techniques in Fingerprint and Face Recognition*. Boca Raton, FL: CRC Press.

Kinnison RR (1985) *Applied Extreme Value Statistics*. New York: MacMillan.

Lee H, Gaensslen R (2001) *Advances in Fingerprint Technology*, 2nd edn. Boca Raton, FL: CRC Press.

Popper K (1963) *Conjectures and Refutations*. London: Routledge and Keagan.

United States Federal Bureau of Investigation (1982) *FBI Advanced Latent Fingerprint School*. Washington, DC: US Government Printing Office.

United States Federal Bureau of Investigation (1984) *The Science of Fingerprints: Classification and Uses*. Washington, DC: US Government Printing Office.

Prints, Footprints

T Brown, University of Leicester, Leicester, UK
G N Rutty, Forensic Pathology Unit, Leicester, UK

Introduction

Forensic podiatry is an emergent discipline, defined in 1999 by Vernon and McCourt as "the application of sound and researched podiatric knowledge in the context of forensic and mass disaster investigations." From this definition forensic podiatry may concern issues related to human identification, linking a suspect with a crime scene or resolving legal issues concerned with the function of the foot. It may be used to associate or eliminate a suspect from a crime scene by direct comparison of a footmark left at the scene with a suspects' feet. The field encompasses footprints and barefoot impressions but excludes footwear analysis. Thus, within the topic of forensic podiatry are impressions made by bare feet that retain skin ridge patterns (footprints); impressions made by bare feet devoid of skin ridge patterns; and impressions made by sock-clad feet. In many cases, excellent morphological features are deposited and retained on a variety of substrates or media. This could include impressions made into soil, sand, or snow, blood-stained impressions on to hard surfaces, or residue impressions. On a two-dimensional surface the bare human foot is known to leave relatively consistent foot impressions with little effect due to slippage or distortion, although

these latter problems are encountered in foot impressions made into three-dimensional substrates such as sand. The importance of such evidence should not be overlooked, although such impressions may occur less frequently in western countries compared to other areas of the world, for example in India, where footwear is less frequently worn. The purpose of this article is to provide the reader with an overview of the methods employed in the field of forensic podiatry and to consider other areas that may be of value, such as dermatoglyphic or chiropody studies.

Historical Review

The analysis of footprint evidence and its use in criminal procedures is not new to forensic science or popular crime fiction. Records of the use of plantar footprint identification in criminal trials date back to the Le Dru case of 1888, with gait analysis of footmark evidence left at scenes, for example used to follow criminals to hideouts, dating to the 1920s, although this specific area had been published in 1887 within the Sherlock Holmes novel entitled *A Study in Scarlet*. The Falkirk burglar case demonstrated how offender identification from footmarks left inside shoes could be achieved. In 1935 the Ruxton case, where Dr. Ruxton killed and dismembered his wife and housemaid, illustrated the use of foot casts to assist in the identification of the mutilated body parts. When the feet of the victims were discovered, casts were made of them which were subsequently shown to fit the missing women's shoes. In 1938, the Supreme Judicial Court of Massachusetts in the case of *Commonwealth* v. *Bartolini* upheld a blood-stained footprint comparison. Within the UK, three cases in the 1950s made use of plantar print evidence left at scenes of crime, although since then the use of forensic podiatry remains infrequent. It is therefore not surprising that, from a forensic viewpoint, there are few published data regarding the uniqueness of barefoot impressions. The main area of research has been within shoe mark analysis, within the industry, army, and forensic world with few small studies into footmark analysis. The growing belief is that feet are unique and the evidence used to support this claim is central to the validity of such evidence.

The Individuality of Human Feet

As with other features of the human body, for example, fingerprints, ears, or facial details, feet are assumed to be highly individualized in shape, size, and form, and it is these features that the forensic podiatrist uses to identify an indizvidual. The nature of each foot is influenced by congenital and acquired influences which may be genetic, racial, ethnic, environmental, physiological, biomechanical, or pathological, be it naturally acquired disease of any component of the foot or as the result of an injury to the foot, leg, or pelvis. It is these influences that lead to a person's individuality. Other factors that will affect the print are the substrate on to which the foot is pressed and the method of locomotion, i.e., standing, walking, running, or jumping.

Forensic Podiatry

The actual forensic examination compares the shape, size, and relationship of individual parts of the foot, such as the toes (singularly or together), ball, arch, and heel to each other. This provides the ability to discriminate an individual from larger populations, but assumes an inherent degree of variability within barefoot impressions. To this can be added the presence and site of natural diseases such as corns and verrucas, and the examination of plantar ridge detail. At present there are only a few forensic studies that provide quantitative evidence toward the uniqueness of barefoot morphology. Although the individuality of human feet is acknowledged, the methods lack the necessary degree of objectivity to be compatible with a forensic approach. Forensic studies have used a range of methods to investigate "uniqueness," although to date there is no standardized system to analyze barefoot impressions. However, the methods can be summarized into three main categories: (1) quantitative methods; (2) dermatoglyphics; and (3) chiropody.

Quantitative Methods of Footmark Analysis

To date there are three published quantitative manual methods for footmark analysis, which can be used on their own or in combination: (1) linear axis method; (2) linear measurement method; and (3) optical center method.

Linear Axis Method

The linear axis method of footmark analysis was first published by Robbins in 1976. He described both a quantitative and qualitative method of footmark analysis. Taking a footmark, he divided the foot into 10 sections which comprised morphological features such as the toes, ball, arch, and heel, as well as shape contours. He then placed a centimeter grid over the print such that the zero point was positioned at the medial posterior point of the heel and the zero line parallel to the longitudinal axis of the foot. The grid was then used to identify points on the toes where the curvature occurred as well as how much curvature was present. Standard linear measurements were also taken, such as width of the big toe, ball, arch, and heel.

Barker and Scheuer later provided a quantitative method of plantar footprint analysis for the purpose of individual forensic identification building upon the method of Robbins. Measurements were obtained from the walking and standing footprints of 105 adult volunteers. Standard construction lines were made on each print according to a series of predetermined rules (**Figure 1**). The construction lines were secondary to a central "linear axis" that passed through the footprint between the first and second

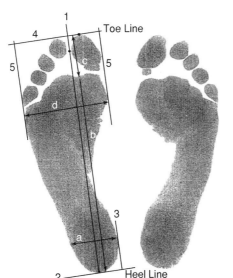

1. Linear axis: From the apex of the heel through arch and ball regions, passing through a point equidistant between the first and second toes.

2. Heel line: Drawn perpendicular to the linear axis, to pass through a tangent of the heel print.

3. A perpendicular construction line is drawn from the heel line through a tangent of the medial aspect of the heel print. "Heel width" can then be measured perpendicularly from the intercept to the lateral border of the print (a).

4. Toe line: Drawn perpendicular to the linear axis, to pass through a tangent to the most distal point of the footprint.
   Print length is measured along the linear axis from the heel line to the toe line (b). "Big toe length" is the distance from the toe line to the ball intersection with the ballprint (c).

5. Perpendicular construction lines are dropped from the toe line to pass through tangents to the ball print both medially and laterally. The "ball width" (d) is measured between these perpendiculars along the toe line.

Figure 1 Linear axis method of footmark analysis.

toes. In theory, therefore, this method ensures reproducible measurements from barefoot impressions. The measurements obtained were not used to highlight the individuality of barefoot impressions, but instead were used to establish the predictive value of associating a footprint with specific subpopulations. For example, the footprints showed a normal distribution in both sexes but, not surprisingly, male footprint length was found to be greater than female footprint length for any given height.

Linear Measurement Method

The next advancement in methodology for footmark analysis was made by Qamra et al., who published a method for footmark analysis in 1980 that utilized linear measurements from predefined landmarks of the plantar footprint (**Figure 2**). This method was applied to two-dimensional ink-stained prints taken from the feet of 725 healthy subjects. The dimensions of the toes, ball, arch, and heel of the footprint were converted into length–width indices to minimize the effect of intrapersonal and intraobserver errors. This can occur when the same person elicits different footprints due to the foot becoming fatigued or when different substrates are used during registration of the print, for example in dust, wet mud, paint, or cement. Using these interdependent indices a range of probabilities for a positive chance match were identified. Qamra also identified the potential value of "humps" (protruding curvatures in the ball line) to distinguish footprints. Although these data were only treated empirically,

one, two, or three humps were found to be more common than no humps or four or five humps (the maximum number identified). Qamra noted that the number of humps on each foot of an individual may not be the same, although this particular feature of footmarks may be difficult to confirm or may be absent under scene-of-crime conditions. Finally, he also made reference to foot creases which tend to occur on the inner margin of the instep, radiating toward the toes or outer margin of the foot. Creases were found to be more prevalent in females than males and in flat feet rather than normal feet, although no further observations were made in relation to the potential use for identification purposes by the authors.

This method was later expanded upon in 1988 by Laskowski and Kyle, who not only used a linear measurement method with index nomenclature but also introduced additional measurements to the system measurements, such as the angle between the great toe and the medial site of the foot. They investigated the use of a "well index" as well as the "well impression," revisited the notion of the analysis of "humps" (up to seven in their series) and proposed the consideration of both racial and cultural aspects of foot morphology, although ultimately agreed with the findings and methods of Robbins and Qamra.

The Optical Center Method

Since 1989 a database of approximately 4000 footprints has been compiled by the Royal Canadian Mounted Police to study the uniqueness of barefoot

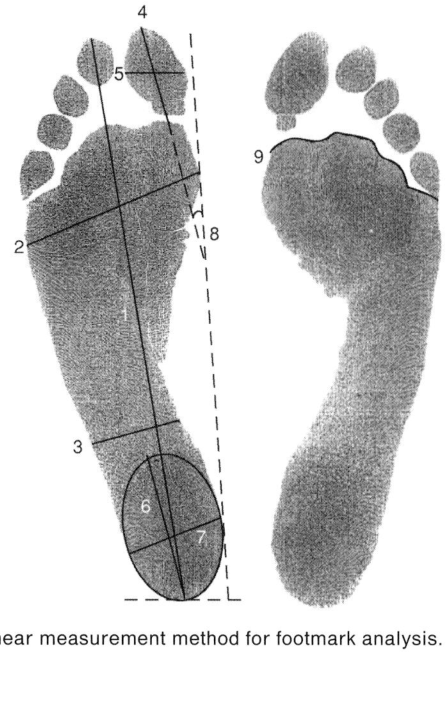

1. Foot length
   Base of heel – tip of the longest toe.

2. Maximum foot width
   Width at the ball of the foot across the 1st–5th metatarsal heads.

3. Minimum foot width
   Minimum width measured across arch of the foot.

4. Toe length
   Maximum length of big toe: tip prominence–ball line.

5. Toe width
   Maximum width of the big toe.

6. Heel length
   Maximum length of the heel portion.

7. Heel width
   Maximum width of the heel measured across encircled area.

8. Great toe angle
   Measured from the intersecting vertices passing through the center if the great toe and along the medial site of the foot.

9. Metatarsal humps
   Number of protuberances, i.e., peaks and dips projecting from the ball line.

Figure 2   Linear measurement method for footmark analysis.

morphology. Inked two-dimensional impressions were taken from volunteers and 38 measurements were entered into a computerized database along with a tracing of each barefoot impression. The optical center of the toes and heel were introduced as landmarks to obtain a greater range of barefoot dimensions.

The method published by Kennedy illustrated the use of the optical center of the heel to ensure reproducibility for foot measurements. He used a simple concentric circle template to identify the optical center of the heel and then took measurements to the optical center of the toes as well as to points on the metatarsal ridge and finally, as with other methods, peripheral point measurements (**Figure 3**). A computer database was used to store and compare the measurements from each barefoot impression. As each new set of impressions was obtained the data were entered into the system and compared with the features of previously entered impressions. The results obtained from this study have shown that a significant degree of individuality can be established for barefoot impressions. To date, there are no two impressions that share the same characteristics. Kennedy also found that only three to five input measurements were required to eliminate all other impressions from the search. To increase the chances of a positive chance match, a ±5 mm error range was arbitrarily given to each measurement. Even with this variance, all the other impressions were eliminated using no more than 15 input measurements. Blind searches were also used where the inked impression may or may not have been present in the database. In each case, the impression was correctly identified or eliminated from the database search.

Combined Methods

Studies by the Federal Bureau of Investigation have combined a linear axis method similar to that described by Robbins, but instead the metric grid is aligned using a longitudinal axis that passes through the optical center of the heel and the second toe. The grid is used to fix the most medial and lateral points of the metatarsal areas and the impression is entered into a computer. Software is used for the comparison of numerous attributes or measurements on each of the left and right feet. The results were similar to those found by Kennedy in that, of a limited database of 500 footprints, only three to five of the most general characteristics were required either to identify or discriminate these footprints from all others in the study.

Plantar Dermatoglyphics

Dermatoglyphics is the study of ridge patterns in the skin. To date, in the case of fingerprints, these ridge patterns are unique and so confer individual identification regardless of the size of the population database. Fingerprints are often used to make formal identifications and are still a primary source of evidence in linking a suspect to a particular crime

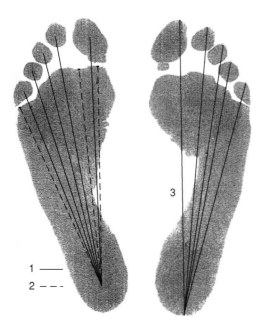

Foot length
Base of heel–tip of the longest toe.

Maximum foot width
Width at the ball of the foot across the 1st–5th metatarsal head.

Minimum foot width
Minimum width measured across arch of the foot.

1   Optical center of heel to optical center of toes.
     (illustrated on left footprint)

2   Metatarsal measurements
     Optical center of heel to three predefined metatarsal
     ridge points
     (illustrated on left footprint)

3   Edge of heel to edge of toes
     Apex of heel to the most distal point on each toe.
     (illustrated on right footprint)

Figure 3 Optical center method for footmark analysis.

scene, although nowadays the role of DNA is rapidly overtaking traditional policing methods. Despite the value of fingerprints in forensic investigations, relatively little study has been carried out into plantar dermatoglyphics.

Historically, the earliest research into plantar dermatoglyphics was undertaken by Wilder in 1902, when he compared the sole prints of humans with quadripedal mammals. Over the next 23 years he made many observations in relation to sole pattern, including both interracial observations and analysis of the patterns of twins. Although interest in this area continued intermittently throughout the twentieth century, fingerprints became the main subject of interest with little work continuing in Caucasians on the sole, especially the toes.

This lack of research into plantar dermatoglyphics in part is due to the difficulty in taking sole and toe print impressions. Recovered barefoot impressions rarely show ridge detail because either the substrate smudges the print or the individual is wearing socks. There have, however, been instances in the UK where the use of plantar dermatoglyphic evidence has been crucial in resolving forensic investigations. Footprint identification via papillary ridge detail is regarded as being no less valuable, where available, than identification by fingerprints: it is equally infallible and admissible. If plantar friction ridge detail is observed, then a positive identification can be made in exactly the same way as fingerprint identification.

Fox and Plato undertook a study of American Caucasian plantar dermatoglyphics. They considered both the toes and the soles in their study and found that epidermal ridge detail produces specific patterns of arches, loops, and whorls that are found on both the distal toe pads and the plantar surfaces (which have eight dermatoglyphic areas) of the feet. They concluded that areas of the toes and sole containing important details are difficult to print and thus these details may be lost. They also found that plantar dermatoglyphics differ from palmar dermatoglyphics and that toe patterns differ from fingerprints in distribution, location, and pattern type. There appeared to be no interpopulation polymorphism in toe pattern frequencies and no racial differences that were attributed to the later embryological development of the foot compared to the hand. However, further work remains to be undertaken within this area.

Chiropody

The last area of potential interest to the forensic podiatrist is the much underutilized area of forensic chiropody. Originally described by Doney and Harris in 1984, this field makes use of acquired diseases of the foot which may necessitate the visit of the individual to a chiropodist. The subsequent records made at the clinical consultation can be used for comparative identification of deceased

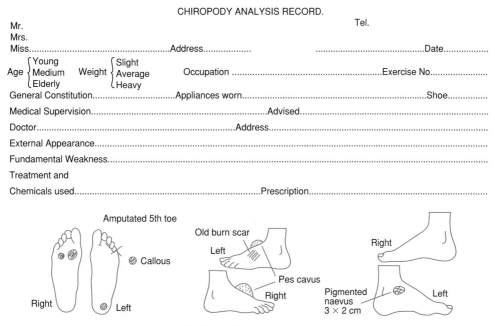

Figure 4 An example of a chiropody analysis sheet with a fictitious patient.

individuals, for example in a mass-disaster arena (**Figure 4**). Such charting of the feet is undertaken, for example, of American naval crews as often, in cases of death due to fire, the thick boots worn by the crew protect the feet resulting in the feet being the last body part to be destroyed and thus potentially the only part available for use for identification purposes. Later work by Vernon has shown that the use of chiropody notes may lead to a positive identification of an individual in up to 86% of cases.

See Also

Identification: Prints, Finger and Palm; Prints, Challenges To Fingerprints; Prints, Ear

Further Reading

Barker SL, Scheuer JL (1998) Predictive value of human footprints in a forensic context. *Medicine Science and Law* 38: 341–346.

Bodziak WJ (1999) The examination of barefoot evidence. In: *Proceedings of the First International Conference of Forensic Human Identification*. London.

Doney IE, Harris PH (1984) Mass disaster identification – can chiropodists help? *Police Surgeon* 25: 15–20.

Fox KM, Chris CP (1987) Toe and plantar dermatoglyphics in adult American Caucasians. *American Journal of Physical Anthropology* 74: 55–64.

Kennedy RB (1996) Preliminary study on the uniqueness of barefoot impressions. *Canadian Society of Forensic Science* 29: 233–238.

Kennedy RB (1996) Uniqueness of bare feet and its use as a means of identification. *Forensic Science International* 82: 81–87.

Kerr WG (2000) Seen at the scene – plantar dermatoglyphic use in identification and detection. *British Journal of Podiatry* 3: 57–60.

Laskowski GE, Vernon KL (1988) Barefoot impressions – a preliminary study of identification characteristics and population frequency of their morphological features. *Journal of Forensic Sciences* 33: 378–388.

Nesbitt J (1962) Prisoner of the night. *Reader's Digest* July: 28–30.

Qamra SR, Sharma BR, Kaila P (1980) Naked foot marks – a preliminary study of identification factors. *Forensic Science International* 16: 145–152.

Robbins LM (1978) The individuality of human footprints. *Journal of Forensic Sciences* 23: 778–785.

Vernon W (1994) The use of chiropody/podiatry records in forensic and mass disaster identification. *Journal of Forensic Identification* 44: 26.

Vernon DW, McCourt FJ (1999) Forensic podiatry – a review and definition. *British Journal of Podiatry* 2: 45–48.

Prints, Ear

C Van der Lugt, Dutch National Police Selection and Training Institute, Zutphen, The Netherlands

History

The ear has always been considered as one of the most important organs of man. In the days of Aristotle for instance, the length of the earlobe was considered to be a sign of precision of memory. Also, in some Southeast Asian regions, long earlobes were considered to be a sign of great wisdom. During the Renaissance, when the doctrine of physiognomy was introduced, which stated that the face is a reflection of all qualities of intelligence in a human being, much attention was paid to the shape of the ear.

Darwin attracted scientific attention to the ear, during his studies on primates, by defining the ear as one of the elementary organs. He regarded the bulge in the middle of the helix (auricular tubercle) as the proof for this assumption, pointing out that this could be nothing other than a corner of the primitive ear reducing. Scientifically, this reducing of the corner has been recognized, and this part of the ear has been assigned the name "tubercle of Darwin." Schwalbe was one of the first scientists to invent a method for measuring the external ear and was able to prove Darwin's theory. He was also the first to describe the racial peculiarities of ear structure.

The Belgian statistician Quételet (1796–1874) initiated the first scientific steps for positive identification of individuals, by theorizing that no two members of the population were exactly alike. The French statistician Bertillon continued work in this area and formulated in 1882, his results, which came to be known as the Bertillon system.

Many research projects were carried out by various medical scientists to study whether the ear could be utilized to establish identity. A survey by Imhofer states that the ear can indeed be very important in establishing identity: a comparison of 500 pictures of ears established that a combination of any three features of ear appears only in two cases; a combination of four features is enough to establish the identity.

In 1959 Iannarelli described an identification method on the basis of ear structure based on a survey carried out over the previous 14 years. No attention was paid to earprints in this article. However, a reprinted and revised edition of *The Iannarelli System of Ear Identification* in 1989 introduced methods of recovery and comparison of latent earprints.

Research on development of the ear of newborns, where pictures of infants were taken over a period of time, showed that the ear remained constant whilst other features of the face changed. A study was conducted to include a series of photographs of the right and left ears from a group of infants, taken daily from the day of birth to the day of discharge from the hospital. These photographs were taken to document the minute changes that took place in the growing ear during each 24-h period and to document the gross morphological changes during the period between birth and the day of departure from the hospital. It was concluded that the described photographic procedure has thus met all of the requirements of a reliable and standardized identification technique: individuality, continuity, and immutability.

In connection with a 1965 burglary case in Bienne (Switzerland) earprints were reported to have been found. A comparison of these prints was carried out by studying individual characteristics, as well as using an overlay technique. The earprints of left and right ears could be identified. The study reported work done regarding the position where the earprint was found and the height of the perpetrator.

In a report from the 61st Annual Meeting of the German Society of Forensic Medicine, a paragraph is dedicated to the use of earprints as a means of identification. In this report, Händel quotes Trube-Becker, who pointed out that there are no absolutely identical ears, but only similar ears. Even two ears of an individual are not identical. This is also true for identical twins. Händel warns that the properties of ears can change, for example, as they are pressed against a wall or a door.

Another early report dealt with earprints found after a series of burglaries at Freiburg (Germany). Two girls were seen close to the scene of the burglaries and were suspected of having listened at the door. The girls were arrested for identification purposes. During the investigation, prints of their left ears were taken. Three girls in Stuttgart were arrested for the same type of burglary. Investigations showed very quickly that the girls from Stuttgart – according to the left earprints – could not be excluded from being suspects in the burglaries in Freiburg. A fingerprint expert in Baden–Württemberg identified one of the girls. Hammer and Neubert have also stressed that earprints can be a useful tool in identification.

The first Dutch case in which an earprint led to a conviction by a Dutch District Court of Law was published in 1988. During the investigation, a forensic odontologist and an ear, nose, and throat specialist were consulted. The District Court accepted the earprint as evidence and convicted the suspect. The Court of Appeals subsequently accepted the earprint only as supporting evidence and based its conviction on other evidence in the case.

The Concerns of US and UK Courts with Ear Print Evidence

Earprint evidence has been used in courts in various countries around the world. Earprints have been used as evidence or supporting evidence in various cases and have contributed in the conviction of perpetrators of crimes. Nevertheless, concerns about the reliability of earprints have been expressed. It must be stated that earprints have not been fully accepted by the relevant scientific community. Apart from the fact that an earprint itself is hardly ever directly connected to the crime (it only indicates the fact that a person has been on or near the crime scene at a certain time) the "science" of earprints is still in its infancy.

In the US a District Court admitted this type of evidence during a Frye hearing, with the restriction that a positive conclusion for that reason could not be accepted. The Court of Appeal allowed the use of an earprint in the same case, but limited the conclusion once again. The experts were to limit their opinion in stating that a person could either be included or excluded as being the donor of the print. The case ended in a mistrial, and the suspect was not prosecuted again on the assumption that evidence connecting the suspect to the crime "beyond reasonable doubt" could not be provided.

More or less the same applied to a case in the UK. In a *voir dire* the judge admitted the evidence, but contrary to the US case, did not limit the experts' opinion. The Court of Appeal in this case accepted the earprint evidence and allowed its use in a retrial. During the preparations for the trial, the prosecution decided to drop the charges against the suspect because of the fact that evidence "beyond reasonable doubt" could not be provided.

Morphology of the Ear

The external ears (auricles and pinna) are found on both sides of the skull. The opening in the middle of the ear leads to the auditory canal, at the end of which is the eardrum. The function of the external ear is to receive incoming sound, amplify it, and direct it to the middle ear (**Figure 1A**).

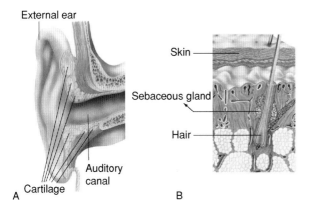

Figure 1 Morphology of ear: (A) external ear and (B) subcutaneous tissue.

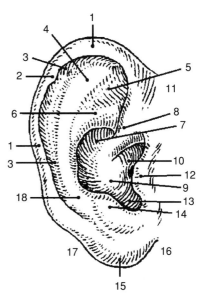

Figure 2 Drawing of the anatomical features of a human ear (right). 1 crux of the helix, 2 helix, 3 auricular tubercle (knob of Darwin), 4 anterior notch, 5 anterior knob, 6 tragus, 7 intertragic notch, 8 antitragus, 9 posterior auricular furrow, 10 anthelix, 11 lower crux of the anthelix, 12 upper crux of the anthelix, 13 lobule, 14 triangular fossa, 15 scaphoid fossa, and 16 concha.

The skeleton of the ear (pinna) consists of cartilage. The cartilage is elastic and makes the ear flexible but prevents it from adopting a different shape permanently. The cartilage is covered with skin and contains hairs, sebaceous glands, and earwax-producing glands (**Figure 1B**).

The development of a human form starts soon after conception. At first, it can hardly be seen, but by the 38th day, various parts of the ear can be recognized, among them the helix and the lobe. In this early stage, the ear is not yet in its right place. The ear acquires its 'normal' place on about the 56th day after conception. At that point, features of the ear, such as the helix, anthelix or antihelix, concha, and earlobe, are clearly discernible. After the 70th day, the growth of the human ear speeds up, without major changes in the configuration taking place.

In some cases, the ear growth is disturbed because of the fetus's position or movements, and this will affect the unattached anatomical form of the ear. After birth, however, the ear can proceed with its free and natural configuration without disturbance.

The proportions of the skull bones of children differ from those of adults. For instance, the inner ear (auris interna), consisting of the hearing (cochlea) and the balance organ (labyrinth), and the ossicles of the middle ear (auris media), the hammer (malleus), the anvil (incus) and the stirrup (stapes), already have their final size at birth. The surrounding bones develop into their final size much later in life, and in addition their proportions change.

At birth, the pinna has a length of about 30 mm. However, it does not yet have its final shape. Shortly after birth, the auricle grows rapidly, about 4 mm, thereby reaching its finite and unique shape; this occurs after approximately 1 month. At the end of the first year, it is of about 45–50 mm in length.

During the next 2 years, it grows evenly, reaching a length of 53 mm at age 3. At 10 years of age, the ear is 55 mm, and at 15 its final length is reached, which is slightly less than 70 mm (50–82 mm) in the normal West European male. The female ear is about 3.5 mm smaller.

The human ear has various anatomical features. These features are shown in **Figure 2**.

Ears can be categorized into four basic shapes: oval, round, rectangular, and triangular (**Figure 3**). Ears of all shapes and sizes occur in every race, but the distribution of different shapes within races differ. The difference between shapes of ears is only a class characteristic. The same applies for sizes of ears and differences between male and female ears. Ear shape and size do not identify an individual's race.

Anatomical Ear Features and their Appearance

In addition to their own anatomical names, each of the ear features also has its own appearance when an ear is pressed against a surface and leaves an impression. These appearances will be briefly discussed.

The crux of the helix (**Figure 4**) is the starting point of the rolled up edge of the helix and originates from the upper part of the concha. For identification purposes, this point is referred to as an area. The crux

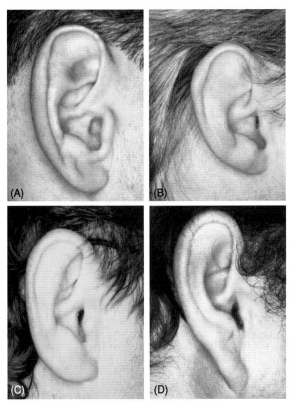

Figure 3 Photograph of an oval ear (A), round ear (B), rectangular ear (C), and triangular ear (D).

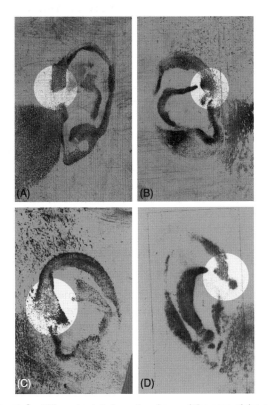

Figure 4 Different prints from the shape of the area of the crux of the helix. The white circle indicates this area.

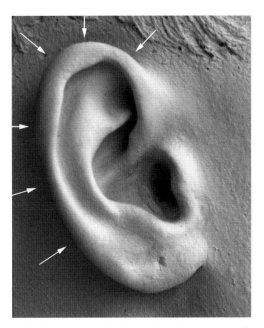

Figure 5 The helix; the whole rim – from the start near the crux of the helix to the lobule section – is pointed out by arrows.

of the helix is a folded type of rim and the cartilage is rather thick at this point, which is why this crux of the helix area often leaves prints when an ear is pressed against a surface. It leaves prints in many different shapes, some of which are shown here.

The helix (**Figure 5**) is the outer rim or frame of the ear. The whole rim consists of cartilage with covered skin and basically defines the shape of the ear. The helix starts at the crux of the helix and ends near the lobule (earlobe). The helix is a rolled-up edge near the crux of the helix and "unrolls" on its way to the lobule. This folded or rolled helix rim has many variations. The extent to which the helix is folded or rolled is different in each ear. Even the ears of one individual can show different helix rims, with differences in positions where the unrolling starts and ends.

In addition to the characteristics of folding of the helix, we also have to deal with the inside line of the helix (the inside edge) when it leaves prints. This edge can be very typical. It often shows different pressure points and can even be "double," which means that the helix prints its inside and outside edge but not the skin in between. This type of helix has great identification value. In prints, the top part of the helix will usually be visible. Depending on the shape and elevation of the helix and the anthelix, more parts will be visible.

The next feature of a human ear that can be found is the auricular tubercle (**Figure 6**) or "knob of Darwin."

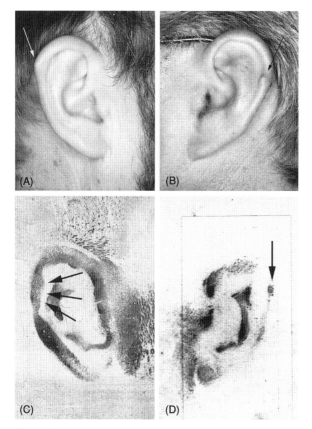

Figure 6 Different types of the auricular tubercle (see arrows).

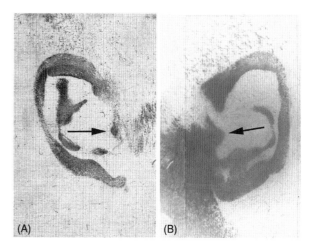

Figure 7 Prints of different types of the tragus (arrow).

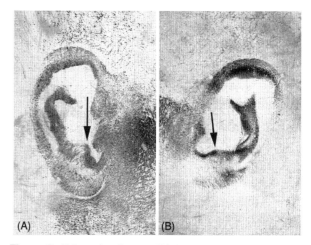

Figure 8 Prints of antitragus: (A) dominant (arrow), (B) hardly visible (arrow).

This feature is not present in all ears. In one individual it may be present in one ear and absent in the other; or it may be very prominent in one ear and hardly recognizable in the other. The auricular tubercle comes in various shapes. It is located on the helix rim around the 2-o'clock site, or the 10-o'clock site, depending on whether it is the left or the right ear. The auricular tubercle can be located on the inside of the helix rim, but also on the outside. But the auricular tubercle may be hardly recognizable as well and may not be visible instantly when it is located on the rim itself. There may even be two knobs on the inside or outside, or on both sides.

The fourth characteristic anatomical feature is the anterior notch, which is located – if visible – between the crux of the helix and the tragus or the anterior knob. In a way, the shape of the anterior notch is affected by the presence of an anterior knob. The anterior knob is located above the tragus and is sometimes very hard to discern on a picture of the ear. Viewing it from a different angle however, the knob may suddenly be very well recognizable. If the knob is present and there is a protruding tragus, it will certainly print and leave a distinct characteristic.

The tragus (**Figure 7**) is a built-in protective device for the auditory canal; if something hits the head on the side, the tragus covers the canal. The tragus consists of rather thick cartilage and is usually protruding and, therefore, almost always visible in prints. Because the tragus point is so close to the head, it hardly moves, even when pressed hard, and so it is one of the most important features that can be used for comparison. Also, the tragus comes in different shapes. Because it is usually protruding, it is visible in impressions as a dominant feature. The shape of the tragus is affected by the presence or absence of the anterior knob. Examples of the various different shapes are given in **Figure 7**. Opposite the tragus is the antitragus (**Figure 8**). It can be very dominant or hardly visible.

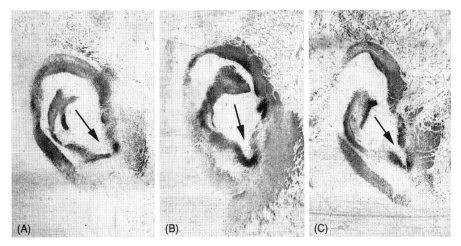

Figure 9   Three types of an intertragic notch: round (A); horseshoe-shaped (B); V-shaped (C). See arrows.

Between the antitragus and the tragus is the intertragic notch. Depending on the shapes of the tragus and antitragus, this notch can have three different types of appearances (**Figure 9**).

The next and very important feature of the ear is the anthelix. This Y-shaped ridge can either form a straight vertical line (anthelix superior) or bend in the direction of the face (anthelix anterior). The upper parts of this Y-shaped anthelix are the lower crux of the anthelix (crux inferior) and the upper crux of the anthelix (crux superior). In rare cases there is a third crux, usually pointing backwards (to the rear side of the head; crux posterior). The lower crux of the anthelix usually points in the direction of the face (anterior). The upper crux of the anthelix can either point in the same direction, point upwards (superior) or, in rare cases, backwards (posterior). In most ears, the anthelix leaves prints when the ear is pressed against a surface. There are ears, however, that have an anthelix situated much deeper than the helix. In these cases, the anthelix and often the lower crux of the anthelix will not leave a print.

Between the antitragus and the anthelix, sometimes another feature appears: the posterior auricular furrow. This feature is not present in every ear and, if it is, it may be hardly recognizable. When present, the furrow can be very superficial and not visible in prints left by hard pressure. Deep furrows usually leave a characteristic print. The furrow will point to the back of the head (posterior) in most cases. The lowest part of the ear is called the lobule or earlobe. Earlobes can have various shapes, which can be categorized into four groups: round, triangular, square, or lobed. All features of the ear that – under normal circumstances – can leave a mark

when an ear is pressed against a surface have been covered. Nevertheless, there are some features left with clear anatomical names but that will not leave a mark. Those features usually are located in a deeper area of the ear. Sometimes, however, when surrounding features leave a clear print, the shape or contours of these features can become visible and add very characteristic information to the impression.

The first of these features is the triangular fossa. The shape of the triangular fossa will be visible when the helix, including a part of the crux of the helix, and the lower and upper cruxes of the anthelix leave their mark on the surface. The shape of the fossa is usually triangular, as its name suggests. In most cases, the shape of the triangular fossa is not clear or visible at all, because one of the surrounding features – most often the upper crux of the anthelix – does not leave a print.

The second feature that can only be found if other parts leave prints, is the scaphoid fossa. If the helix and anthelix leave a clear mark, the shape of the scaphoid fossa is clearly recognizable. This shape can be very characteristic, and often shows great detail. The last, but not the least, important feature that can be recognized is the concha. The concha is the deep inner part of the auricle, leading to the auditory canal. The full shape of the concha can only be found in an earprint when many other parts leave their characteristic marks.

Peculiarities of the Ear

As discussed before, apart from the natural features of ears, there may be some peculiar ones as well.

These features are not present in all ears. Some of them are "natural" in the way that they exist throughout life, others can develop at different times in life. They can be categorized, for instance, into:

- birthmarks – important because of an elevation of the skin and possible different skin texture;
- knobs – on the auricle itself or more often in the pre-auricular area;
- scars – usually caused by accidents involving the ear;
- ear "defects" – ear defects or injuries often originate from specific kinds of sports, like boxing, judo, and rugby. The ears are usually referred to as cauliflower ears;
- missing parts of the ear – this may be caused by an accident. The newly arisen shape will be very characteristic and, without treatment, will stay the same for the rest of its existence.

Medical Treatment, Ear Surgery, and Plastic Surgery

There are many reasons for ears to become the object of medical treatment or plastic surgery; it would take too long to discuss all the possibilities. If for any reason the auricle is missing and an artificial ear is made that has great resemblance to the other ear (if still present), the artificial ear does not contain sebaceous glands and therefore hardly ever leaves a mark. In cases of defects on ears, because of a disease or accident, reconstruction of the ear is often carried out. These methods all aim to give the auricle a shape that is very much like the original or like the other ear.

With respect to our goal to identify people from the print of their ear, it is important to realize that the intended medical treatment does change the ear characteristics. Depending on the scope of the reconstruction, this impact will be substantial or only minor, affecting a small part of the ear. If the texture of the skin is used for identification, one must realize that in certain types of reconstruction a different skin is used to repair the defect, and will, therefore, leave different prints. In addition, in cases of reconstruction of the ear because of missing parts – perhaps even since birth – the size and shape of the ear can change.

Hereditary Factor Effect on Ear Configuration

These are divided opinions about whether hereditary factors affect ear configuration.

Ever since World War I, much research has been done, especially in Germany, that shows that some elements in the human ear could have been inherited from parents: at least they justified a strong suspicion or belief. Some new studies, however, using modern DNA techniques, show that these conclusions have not always been right.

To the author's knowledge, there has been no scientific research in this respect with regards to earprints. It will however be obvious that the ear prints of related people will differ because their ears do. It would be hard to believe that the same two-dimensional print could originate from two different three-dimensional objects.

Ears of Twins and Triplets, etc.

Like fingerprints and like the right and left ears of one individual, ears of identical twins differ. In fingerprints one can often observe similar features like whorls, loops, etc, occurring in the same finger of two individuals. In ears, a similar effect can be observed. The overall shapes of the ears, as well as some features of the ears, often look the same. By close observation, one can find the differences, e.g., in size, but differences can also be found in specific features, like the helix rim, the tragus and antitragus, and the shape of the anthelix. Sometimes, these differences are hard to observe, and require special skill and equipment. If prints of both ears are available, offering the opportunity to overlay one with a transparency of another, the differences will show instantly.

The Area around the Ear

Finally, useful information can be obtained not from the ear itself, but from the area around the ear. Often a part of the cheek, called the preauricular area, located immediately in front of the ear, leaves a print. The print will show the texture of the skin and often contains creases. These can be of great help because, in almost all prints of the same person, they should be more or less the same. Of course, the amount of pressure applied will influence the appearance, but in most cases a person listens with more or less the same pressure. Other areas that could often be present in earprints are the areas above and behind the ear. Usually, there is hair, and one might be able to observe the hair texture. Although a visit to the hairdresser may change this, prints of these areas can be very useful when, for example, the hair texture is obviously that of

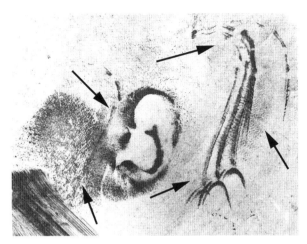

Figure 10   Print of an ear, found at a crime scene, with clearly visible dreadlocks (arrows).

dreadlocks (see **Figure 10**), which is often very simple to recognize.

Distortion of Earprints by Pressure and Rotation

Because of the variation in pressure, earprints recovered from a crime scene are never identical, in all aspects, to standard ones taken from a suspect. This is due to the fact that the exact pressure exerted at the crime scene is unknown and, therefore, cannot be reproduced. Likewise, the direction from which the pressure was applied cannot be duplicated exactly. The amount of pressure applied by a person is very much dependent on the configuration of the ear. In general, an ear creates a kind of vacuum, a closed area in the concha region; one tries to eliminate other sounds by closing off the concha area. Too little pressure will not only result in a bad earprint, but the person listening will not hear much or anything at all. Because the ear is a flexible, three-dimensional object, with features in different shapes which protrude to some degree, the pressure that each individual will need to apply differs. Experienced listeners usually have found the right pressure to apply; they are "experienced" in that respect, and the print of their ear is almost always exactly the same.

Research on Pressure Distortion

Several papers have been published on the effects of pressure upon the ear. It is generally agreed, that no two ears are completely similar in this respect. In addition to pressure, the effect of rotation has to be considered. In the act of listening, most individuals adopt a comfortable stance, with the head slightly bent forward from its normal upright position. This type of distortion has an influence on the type of print obtained. Depending on the angle with the surface, increased pressure might be applied to the top of the helix rim, to the back part of the helix, or to the lobule or lower parts of the auricle. It might even be the case that a comparison with standards taken from a suspect in a normal upright position is very difficult to make. At first sight, the prints may look different, but certain key features lead the investigator in the right direction.

When and Where to Find Earprints

In numerous cases (e.g., burglaries and homicides), perpetrators listen at doors and windows before entering the premises. However, it may not be at the door or window where entry was gained. Perpetrators may have listened at several premises along a street, or several windows in one house. In the Netherlands, the majority of earprints are found on doors in blocks of apartments with porticos. They are found at different heights, depending on the perpetrator's habits or the local circumstances. In most cases, earprints are found at a normal standing height, usually between 130 and 180 cm from the floor. Commonly, they are found in the middle of the door or window. Most people listen by pulling back one shoulder and placing the side of the head against the surface. By doing so, one usually bends forward slightly. The area to be searched for earprints will be from the middle of the door (vertically) to the top. There is also a group of people who bend over, when listening. Their earprints will be found approximately at the same height as the doorknob. The tragus point of the ear will be visible on the bottom of the print, whereas the helix rim will be on the top. Earprints can sometimes be located at a height of ~30 cm from the floor. These prints occur on doors of houses with porticos, next to a staircase.

Recovery and Lifting of Earprints

There are a variety of methods for the enhancement and subsequent recovery of earprints left at a crime scene. The method to be employed will depend on the availability of products and the nature of the surface on which the earprint is found. Commonly, the same techniques will be applied as for fingerprints. In most cases, a fingerprint powder is used in combination with photography or lifting of the marks found.

An additional tool, useful in relation to earprints, is the calculation of a person's stature from the height where the earprint is found. Based on a study by Hirschi, the author noted that a formula could be found for calculating the average distance that people bent forward while listening, combined with the average distance between the top of the skull and the middle of the auditory canal and added to the height of an earprint above the floor. This height needs to be measured from the tragus point in the earprint.

Preparing a Comparison

For an actual comparison of earprints, several methods are in use:

1. *Measurement.* The different features of the ear are measured from the print. Data on overall sizes of the parts and distances between them are obtained. Often, arrows are used to indicate special shapes of various parts. A problem with this method can be caused by differences in pressure or rotation of the ear. Measuring outlines, either on the inside or outside of a feature, is very difficult, as is trying to find the middle of a feature. Therefore, this method is not advisable.
2. *Overlay technique.* One of the available earprints (either the known or the unknown one) is copied onto a transparent sheet. The other print will usually be copied on a nontransparent sheet and put one on top of the other and fixed on one side. The transparency can now be lifted, in order to make the prints visible separately.
3. *Quartering technique.* In this technique, the prints are divided into four separate parts and put together, two by two (known and unknown), to get a full print again.

In order to copy the earprints, one needs to photograph or digitize them. For earprints on a gelatine foil or lifter, a flatbed scanner is very suitable. The advantage of using a scanner is the fact that the result will always be a 1:1 image of the original, unless different settings are used. The scanning resolution should be at least 600 dpi. A three-color scan (RGB) has proven to give better detail and possibilities for optimum quality. To economize the storage requirement, the color information can be removed.

Obtaining Earprints from Suspects

Legal methods for obtaining earprints from suspects differ between countries around the world. This will not be discussed here. Most documented methods for obtaining standards include photographing the ear, in addition to any other technique employed. The most useful method to get earprints is to ask the suspect to listen several times at a glass pane or at a very flat (and clean) surface. Usually, three prints per ear are sufficient. The first print should be a "functional" pressure print. The suspect needs to listen to a sound and if possible memorize what he has heard. After obtaining the first print in this way, a second one with gentle, obviously less pressure, and a third print, should be taken with considerably more pressure (see **Figure 11**). The prints must be recovered and lifted in the same way as for fingerprints.

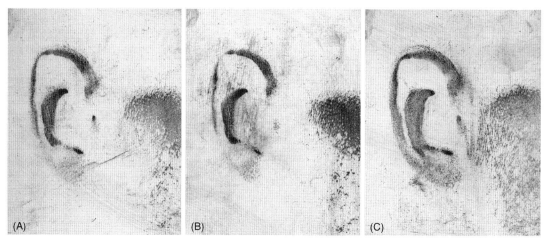

Figure 11   Earprint taken with functional (A), gentle (B), and hard pressure (C).

In all cases, a photograph of the right and the left ear should be taken, with the camera at an angle of 90°, corresponding to the head. From noncooperative suspects and those who offer passive resistance, five prints per ear should be taken, placing a glass or a synthetic plate with varying pressure on each ear, preventing one part of the ear (upper, lower, front, or back side) from being pressed more firmly than another.

It is often preferable to attempt to recreate the crime scene conditions so that height, rotation, and pressure can be accounted for.

The Process of Comparison

After collecting the traces as well as the reference prints from suspects and/or witnesses, the earprint traces need to be individualized. This is achieved by finding agreement of corresponding individual characteristics of such number and significance as to preclude the possibility (or probability) of their having occurred by mere coincidence, and establishing that there are no differences that cannot be accounted for. "Agreement of corresponding individual characteristics" means that the characteristics used for comparison must be found to agree in shape or appearance and in position and orientation. These corresponding characteristics must be of "such number and significance as to preclude the possibility (or probability) of their having occurred by mere coincidence." It does not say how many need to be found, because there is no fixed number! Particularly in earprint comparisons, the required number depends on the assessment of the significance of each characteristic. It is important to establish that there are no differences that cannot be accounted for. Since earprints can differ because of pressure and rotation, at least three prints, made with different pressures, are needed to be able to see how the (flexible) ear reacts when put against a surface. Further procedure is divided in three major steps: analysis, comparison, and evaluation (ACE).

Analysis

The process of analysis consists of two steps. First the unknown earprint must be examined carefully. It is important to start with the unknown print, before getting into the details of the known earprint of a suspect. The general and specific information about the print needs to be precisely documented including the morphology and anatomy of the earprint. Often a small drawing will help. After observing the earprint in full detail, it is possible to answer a very important question: is the information sufficient for comparison with a known print? The characteristics that can be used to individualize an impression fall into two categories:

1. Class characteristics, i.e., "characteristics which are common to several objects." The examples are size, general shape, or even the presence or absence of a feature. This type of characteristic has no value in the process of individualization: it can, however, be used as a preliminary screening technique.
2. Individual characteristics, i.e., "characteristics that are unique." A general appreciation of the origin of individual characteristics is useful in their recognition. They are basically attributable to natural variation.

The second step is to describe the known prints (the standards taken from a suspect) along the lines of the same procedure as followed for the sample collected.

Comparison

In this step, a comparison is made between the characteristics found on the unknown earprint and the characteristics of the known earprint. All the similarities and dissimilarities of the characteristics observed must be documented. To show the similarities and dissimilarities, the overlay and quartering techniques can be used.

Evaluation

Evaluation which is the critical step where one must decide the terms of the opinion to be offered. The scope of the opinion can vary: positive (certainty), highly probable (strong belief), probable possible (consistent with; may be), or no basis for comparison.

Positive opinion A positive opinion can be given when the examiner is certain beyond a reasonable doubt that the trace matches with the reference standards. Enough information on class and individual characteristics are present to lead to his/her unique conclusion. There is no possibility of the similarities having occurred by coincidence on two different objects and there are no differences, except those that can be accounted for.

Probable opinion Highly probable and "probable" are both probabilitistic opinions. Their judgment on the match between the traces and the standards lies somewhere between impossible and certain. Most often it is very difficult to decide which opinion to offer, probable or highly probable.

Possible opinion   The use of the word "possible" in this perspective would mean that there are some class characteristics available but do not have any significant individual characteristic.

No basis for comparison   This category of conclusions is very close to the category "possible." In fact, quite a number of features are missing, which means that a positive identification will not be possible. However, this print, though worthless for individualization might be suitable for exclusion.

Negative opinion   All conclusions explained here can also be used in the negative. The strongest in this category, of course, is an exclusion. On the basis of the earprint found at the scene and the standards taken from the suspect, especially if many features are present, one can conclude in the negative. "This earprint, found on the outside of the front door was not made by this suspect."

Further Reading

Bertillon A (1995) *Identification Anthropométrique, Instructions signalétiques.* Melun, Imprimerie administrative.

Dabois N (1988) Oren near hebben. *Technisch Informatie Bulletin* 1: 7–22.

Fields C, Falls HC, Warren CP, Zimberof M (1960) The ear of the newborn as an identification constant. *Obstetrics and Gynecology* 16: 98–102.

Gerasimov MM (1949) The ear. In: *Osnovy Vosstanovlienniia Litsapo Cherapu*, pp. 47–50.

Hammer H-J (1986) The identification of earprints secured at the scene of the crime. In: *Fingerprint Whorls*, pp. 49–51. Leipzig: Proceedings of the Institute for Forensic Medicine of the Karl Marx University.

Händel K (1983) Streiflichter. *Kriminalistik* 183: 53–56.

Hirschi F (1970) Identifizierung von Ohrabdrücken. *Kriminalistik* 24: 75–79.

Iannarelli AV (1989) *Ear Identification.* New York: Paramount.

Imnofer T (1906) Die bedeutung der Ohrmuschel für die Feststellung der Identität. *Archiv für Kriminologie* 26: 150–163.

Lugt C van der (1997) Determining a person's height based upon the vertical distance of a located earprint. *Journal of Forensic Identification* 47: 406–419.

Lugt C van der (2001) *Earprint Identification.* Amsterdam: Elsevier.

Meyer K (1984) Identifizierung van Tatveraächtigen anhand von Ohrabdrücken. *Kriminalistik* 12: 84–519.

Saddler K (1997) *Earprints.* MSc thesis, Strathclyde University, Glasgow, UK.

Schwalbe G (1897) Das äussere Ohr. In: *Handbuch der Anatomie*, pp. 112–190.

Facial

G Quatrehomme, Laboratoire de Médecine Légale et Anthropologie Médico-légale, and Faculté de Médecine, Nice, France

Introduction

The identification of human remains is a major issue for forensic systems. A number of people disappear every year; others are buried anonymously. Furthermore, mass murders are committed worldwide. Identification may be very difficult, either because the body is in a poor condition, or because of a lack of identification records (dental charts, X-rays, or DNA databases). Therefore, the identification strategy depends on the available evidence, the thoroughness of the police investigation, and the presence (or absence) of antemortem records. Sometimes the only possible form of identification is through facial reconstruction. There are several means of facial reconstruction: (1) video or photographic comparison (comparison of a video image or photo with the actual face, video, or photo of a suspect); (2) superimposition (overlaying a facial image, i.e., a portrait, a photo, or video footage, on a skull); (3) facial restoration, or craniofacial restoration (when sufficient soft tissues persist on the head: the aim is to restore the head to its original appearance); (4) facial reconstruction or craniofacial reconstruction (when no tissue remains on the skull); and (5) aging the face of a missing child or adult.

These methods are very sophisticated, and are used in current forensic cases, with a certain amount of success, even if the techniques have not been scientifically validated. They are based on the relationship between the bony frame (the bony face and skull), and the corresponding soft-tissue points.

Superimposition

Superimposition compares the skull with a photo of the missing person. This technique is complex, either directly superimposing questioned skull photos with a photo of the missing person, or comparing the skull and the photo using video or a computer-assisted process. The distance, magnification, orientation, distortion, and depth of field must be carefully checked. It is important to establish the number and quality of criteria necessary to determine if the identity can be ascertained (probably very difficult), excluded, or simply included.

Video or Photographic Comparisons

In this process an image of the suspect (video image or photo) is compared with the actual face of the suspect, or with a video or photo of him/her. This is an increasingly popular method, due to the widespread use of video in public places, and in sensitive locations such as banks, airports, and stores. These comparisons are both qualitative and quantitative. Quantification is based on horizontal, vertical, or oblique measurements; however, the distance, orientation, and magnification of the images must be thoroughly checked, avoiding any distortion.

Facial Reconstruction

Facial reconstruction is an important tool in the identification of unknown remains. It is based on the relationship between anthropological (bony) points and the soft-tissue points to which they are connected. Average soft-tissue thicknesses are known in relation to some bony points. Unfortunately, the skull does not provide all the clues to enable a perfect reconstruction to be made. As a result, facial reconstruction can be only an approximation that helps to stimulate the eyes or brain of the next of kin, and it is followed by other comparative methods. There are many types of facial reconstruction: two- or three-dimensional, manual, and computer-assisted.

Two-dimensional methods include the lateral craniographic George's method, which creates a profile of the subject by connecting points drawn in relation to radiographic points; and a sketch of the face, drawn by a forensic artist, directed by a forensic anthropologist or scientist.

The most popular three-dimensional method is probably the manual (or plastic, or sculptural) three-dimensional one. This is carried out by a forensic pathologist, anthropologist, odontologist, scientist, or artist. It starts with a thorough osteological examination, assessing skull morphology, taking anthropological measurements, and paying particular attention to classical anthropological items (age, sex, race, stature), as well as the size and shape of the skull and face, and its own particular features. The study is completed by a cephalometric (radiographic) analysis, which allows detailed study of skeletal abnormalities, such as skeletal balance and dental occlusion. Then, average soft-tissue thickness is translated into clay or clay-like material and placed on specific anthropological landmarks. The space between these points is filled in, and gradually the face is reconstructed. Areas such as the ears, eyes, nose, mouth, lips, and chin are difficult to place correctly and to check, despite comprehensive studies published in the literature. Scientific validation of the method is scarce, and includes only isolated forensic cases and controlled blind reconstruction in small series. Computerized methods are very sophisticated, rendering the results in either two or three dimensions. The advantages of computerized methods are speed and the possibility of editing several versions of the reconstruction.

Aging a face on a photo is a complex process that can be performed by an artist and, rarely, using a computer-assisted method. The size, shape, and features of the faces of both parents are usually taken into account, and used as predictors of possible changes in the facial features of the missing child. However, these methods are not scientifically validated.

Facial Restoration

Facial restoration deals with a face that is altered by decomposition, fire, or trauma. The idea of restoring the body comes from the common use of this technique in the forensic context to obtain fingerprints. Water or a saline solution is injected under the pulp of the fingers, in order to swell the tip of the decomposed finger. This permits the forensic pathologist to take the fingerprints, which may identify the deceased, even before the autopsy is completed. Furthermore, the face and hands of the deceased are commonly improved, or even restored, by morticians, before the decedent is presented to the next of kin.

The aim of facial restoration is to improve recognition of the face, in order to generate leads to identification. Nevertheless, in a forensic context, facial restoration is rarely reported in the literature. Dérobert has described individuals with faces that were badly altered by trauma whose facial restoration permitted a spectacular improvement, allowing their photograph to be published or shown to the family for identification. Spitz and Fisher have presented the photograph of a decomposed face, which was restored, sketched, and then broadcast. Ubelaker has shown sketches from decomposed faces, which were released for identification purpose. Pötsch and colleagues worked on mutilated faces, restored them, and issued the results in the media, as sketches or photographs, depending on the quality of the results.

There are three steps to the process: (1) restoration; (2) restitution; and (3) appropriation. Restoration is achieved by surgery or with the embalming process. Surgical techniques are used whenever the face is badly altered by trauma; the stitching can be perfect stitches, and skin losses are covered by various surgical techniques, such as grafts or rotation flaps. These techniques may lead to a high-quality restoration, even if the face is severely damaged and is missing some parts.

The embalming process is commonly performed by morticians. Formaldehyde solutions are injected into the body, and the facial outlook can be improved by the injection of specific products under the skin. This process is primarily used for decomposed bodies and faces. The embalming products make it possible to sustain the soft tissues, remodel emaciated parts of the face, and give some tonicity to the eyeballs. These techniques must be used after autopsy, and after samples have been taken for toxicology, histopathology, and DNA analysis.

Presentation of the result is the second step, and this can be achieved with various methods. The simplest is to take a photograph of the restored face: this has the advantages of speed, ease, and cost-effectiveness. However, there are some obvious drawbacks; the most significant is the ethical issue, because the result is not always suitable for viewing by the media or the next of kin.

The second process is sketching the restored face. The advantage is that the sketch can always be viewed by the family, and can be shown to the media. The drawback is that it must be performed by a forensic artist (raising the cost), and the possible subjectivity, since the artist is asked to humanize the result of a crude restoration. In one way, this last point may be an advantage, because a more human aspect of the face would stimulate the cognitive processes of the next of kin.

The third method is to cast the restored face. Quatrehomme and coworkers discussed two cases where the face was severely damaged, one by decomposition and one by trauma. In both cases, publishing the photograph of the face either before or after restoration was inconceivable.

In the first case (decomposition), the gases were released at the time of autopsy by making incisions along the frontal area and the mandibular arch. Then the face looked dehydrated and badly emaciated. Subcutaneous injections were used, filling out the sunken temples and eyes, plumping up the nose tip, the lips, and the forehead. A second product was used to remodel the facial contours. This material looks like wax, but is soft enough to be injected, molded, and handled. The interest of this restoration is multiple. First, it aims to give the face a human appearance; second, it is excellent preparation for use before the casting step, bearing in mind that this material (used by any mortician) is able to hold the tissues firm in any position, and stick to them, even if they are wet.

The casting process is quite easy, once one has some experience in this field. It requires polyurethane elastomer, which ensures flexibility and faithful reproduction. The elastomer is spread on to the face, and several hours later a plaster cover is laid on top. The cast is removed 24 h later, and consolidated by subsequent layers of plaster. Eventually, the cast is done, representing a "negative" of the face. The positive printing is achieved with either a polyester resin or a plain plaster. The interest of this technique is to give a three-dimensional representation of the head of the missing person that can be given to the judge, and photographed in any orientation. In the specific case described by Quatrehomme and colleagues, the individual was immediately recognized from a television program.

In the second case (trauma), the state of the head was worse, because the individual committed suicide by standing between the rails of a train track, waiting for the collision. Flesh and bone fragments were found up to 100 m away from the scene. The face was extremely damaged, and most of the bones of the skull were absent; only small fragments of the occipital bone and a few teeth were still present. The process of restoration was very difficult, but gradually the face was rebuilt, using surgical techniques. Then a cast was made and a three-dimensional representation of the head was created. In this case, the results were unsatisfactory because the face was too thick. From the autopsy results we knew that the subject was very thin. This "overthickness" was explained by the fact that the weight of the cast on the face of the cadaver was excessive, and had a gravitational effect, spreading the face badly. Furthermore restoration of the nose was almost impossible, due to the absence of the nasal bones.

The advantages of casting a face are numerous. The result of the work is very objective, and three-dimensional, so more realistic. The elastomer is able to retain the slightest facial details, such as wrinkles, and the proportions of the face are globally accurate, which is key to recognition by the family. The main advantage is that the casting can always be communicated to the media, and shown to the next of kin, even when the restoration could not have been. The drawbacks are the complexity of this time-consuming method.

To conclude, in the future it will be interesting to carry out computer sketching or computer modification from the restored (or unrestored) face.

Recognition and Identification

The last step is recognition of the face by the family or friends. In the end, as in facial reconstruction, it is probably impossible to achieve a perfect copy of the missing person's face. At least, facial restoration aims at making identification possible, if the family can see a resemblance to the missing relative. Comparative methods of identification should then be used, in order to prove positive identification beyond reasonable doubt.

Figure 1 shows an example of restoration in a case of advanced decomposition, where the head was autopsied. It was badly decomposed and damaged, but some soft tissue remained, so we decided to attempt a restoration process (**Figure 2**). This

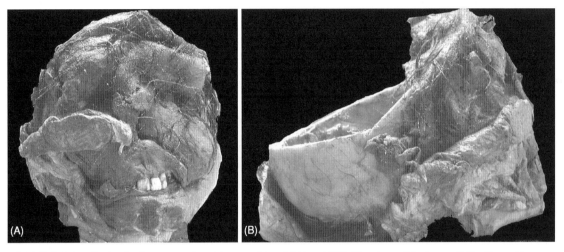

Figure 1 Initial status: the badly decomposed and damaged head ((A) and (B)). (Courtesy of Professor Didier Gosset.)

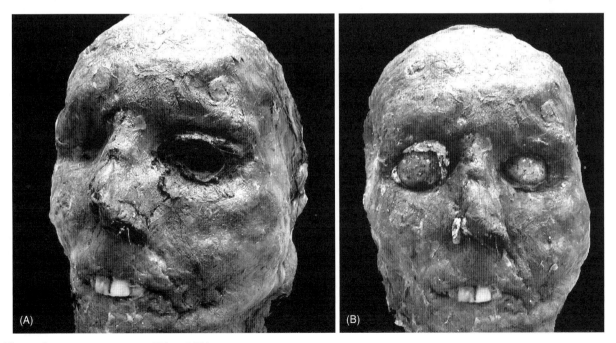

Figure 2 Restoration process ((A) and (B)).

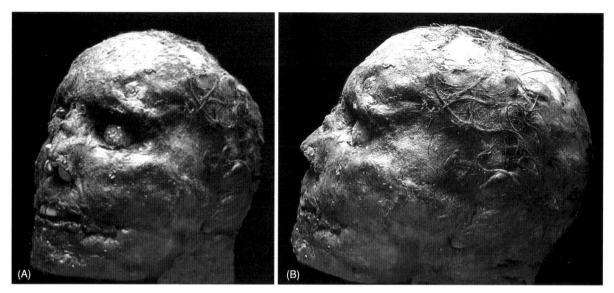

Figure 3   Results of the restoration of the face ((A) and (B)).

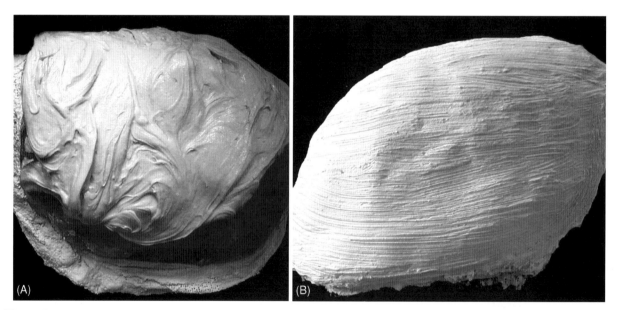

Figure 4   Casting process ((A) and (B)).

restoration was extremely complex and time-consuming. The result of the restoration is shown in **Figure 3**. Despite lengthy restoration, the result could not be made public. Therefore, we tried two solutions: casting and drawing. The casting process is partly shown in **Figure 4**. The result of the three-dimensional casting is demonstrated in **Figure 5** (full profile), and **Figure 6** (oblique views). These pictures show that the cast can always be shown to the next of kin, and then released to the media. Nevertheless, the problem of casting is that the result often gives quite a "ghostly appearance" (**Figures 5** and **6**). This is why only the sketches of the results are presented. **Figure 7** shows sketches of the restored head, and **Figure 8** shows a sketch of the casting of the restored head. The artist is able to draw versions with closed or open eyes, or with closed or half-open mouth (**Figure 7**). Usually, it is easier to draw from the three-dimensional casting (**Figure 8**) than from photographs of the restored face (even with full-face, profile, and oblique views), because the three-dimensional casting allows the artist to get an excellent perception of the volumes and proportions. Obviously, in the case presented here, the sketch gives a more "human" appearance

to the result, and, in our opinion, will probably be of more assistance to the family.

The indications for restoration are numerous. In our department, we use it in cases ranging from decomposition and drowning to burning; wherever sufficient soft tissues remain on the skull, even if the quality of these soft tissues is poor. The results, in terms of possibility of recognition by the next of kin, are good, and often very fast. This rapidity of recognition was underlined by Pötsch and coworkers. The explanation is that the general shape of the face persists, despite the dramatic alteration of the soft tissues, and that the proportion between various parts of the face persists (especially what we call the "noble parts" of the face, including eyes, nose, lips, chin, and ears). In the case we have presented above, the soft tissues were dramatically altered, but the whole shape and proportions of the face were preserved; the only important issue in this case was that part of the nose tip was absent, due to animal activity. However one side of the nose tip was sufficiently preserved to reconstruct the other side, and give a correct result.

In conclusion, this method is of interest in difficult forensic identification cases. Once the autopsy has been carried out and samples have been taken, restoring the face is a good technique to stimulate the cognitive functions of the family or friends, in order to get a lead toward a positive identification. This method is preferred to facial reconstruction, whenever possible, because facial reconstruction is far more difficult (in terms of a resemblance) than facial

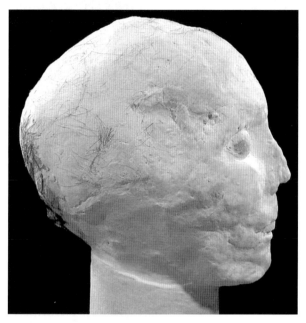

Figure 5 Result of the casting process: full profile.

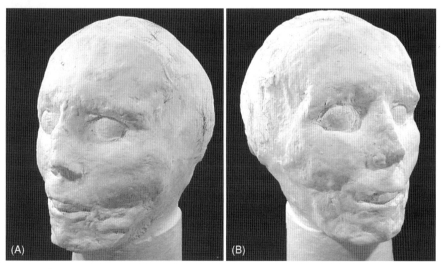

Figure 6 Result of the casting process: oblique views ((A) and (B)).

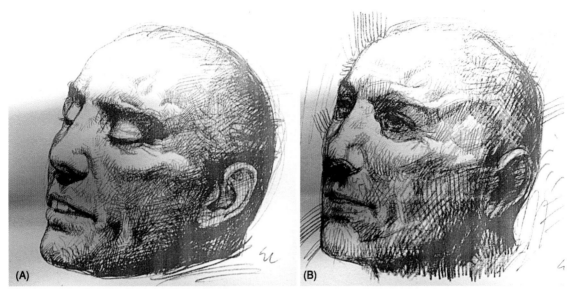

Figure 7   Sketches of the restored head ((A) and (B)). (Courtesy of Giovanni Civardi.)

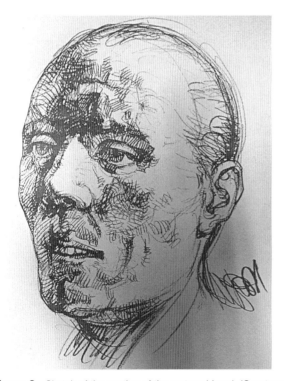

Figure 8   Sketch of the casting of the restored head. (Courtesy of Giovanni Civardi.)

restoration. Furthermore, facial reconstruction can always be done, even after an attempt at facial restoration, since facial reconstruction works on the skulls when no soft tissue is left.

See Also

Anthropology: Overview; Stature Estimation from the Skeleton

Further Reading

Dérobert L (1974) *Médecine Légale*. Paris: Flammarion Médecine-Sciences.

George RM (1987) The lateral craniographic method of facial reconstruction. *Journal of Forensic Science* 32: 1305–1330.

Helmer RP, Röhricht S, Petersen D, Möhr F (1993) Assessment of the reliability of facial reconstruction. In: İşcan MY, Helmer RP (eds.) *Forensic Analysis of the Skull*, pp. 229–246. New York: Wiley-Liss.

Pötsch L, Herz U, Leithoff H, Urban R, Rittner Ch (1994) Zur postmortalen Gesichtsrekonstruktion. Arbeitskonzept einer schnellen Identifizierungsmöglichkeit. *Rechtsmedizin* 4: 61–68.

Quatrehomme G (2000) *Reconstruction Faciale: Intérêt Anthropologique et Médico-Légal.* PhD thesis. Bordeaux, France: Université de Bordeaux.

Quatrehomme G, İşcan MY (2000) Computerized facial reconstruction. In: Siegel JA, Saukko PJ, Knupfer GC (eds.) *Encyclopedia of Forensic Sciences*, pp. 773–779. San Diego, CA: Academic Press.

Quatrehomme G, Garidel Y, Grévin G, *et al.* (1995) Method for identifying putrefied corpses by facial casting. *Forensic Science International* 74: 1–2, 115–124.

Quatrehomme G, Garidel Y, Grévin G, *et al.* (1996) Facial casting as a method to help identify severely disfigured corpses. *Journal of Forensic Science* 41: 518–520.

Quatrehomme G, Cotin S, Subsol G, *et al.* (1997) A fully three-dimensional method for facial reconstruction based on deformable models. *Journal of Forensic Science* 42: 647–650.

Spitz WU, Fisher R (1980) *Medicolegal Investigation of Death*. Springfield, IL: Charles C Thomas.

Ubelaker DH (1991) Human skeletal remains. In: Sadler LL (ed.) *Manuals of Archaeology*, 2nd edn., p. 124. Taraxacum, WA: Library of Congress.

IMAGING

Contents

Photography

H L Blitzer, Institute for Forensic Imaging,
Indianapolis, IN, USA

Introduction

Purposes

In general, photography is used to provide a view of a scene or object that a viewer can see later, or in a different location, and understand what was at the original scene. This means that the devices used to capture the image of the original scene must be able to respond in a way that will enable the production of a replica that a person can view and understand. In essence, the photographic process is a surrogate eye. However, in investigative work, the issues are more complex because the objective is not limited to "seeing." There are three main reasons for using photography in forensic medicine (**Table 1**) and it is useful for the photographer to be aware of the intended purpose for each photo taken. This is because each photo will be optimized differently in each case.

Tools

Just a few years ago the tools of photography were films, cameras, and lights for use in the field. In the laboratory there were enlargers, chemicals, and optical and mechanical devices. Today the toolkit is expanded to include digital cameras and scanners for image capture, software tools for image enhancement and analysis, and a variety of output devices for making prints, displaying images, and storing image information. The photographer's capabilities are greatly expanded. In general, film-based photography is highly flexible, highly accurate, and easy to use. Digital techniques offer faster response and greatly expanded analytical capability.

Measures of Performance

In the early days, photographic quality was measured in terms of the ability to make "pleasing renditions."

As the use of photography expanded into scientific investigation, new metrics were formulated, but these are largely specific to the purposes of each type of use. At this point in time, there is not a generally accepted set of measures of performance for forensic medicine. This lack of standards has been discussed by the scientific working group on imaging technology (SWGIT), organized by the US Federal Bureau of Investigation, but no action has been taken yet.

Comparisons: Human Visual System Versus Photography

It is often said that people see with their eyes. In reality, they see in their brains. The eyes capture data and only start processing it. The actual image is not retinal, but cortical. Eyes dart about, focusing on various locations within the scene in front of the viewer. As they do, they adapt to localized conditions and acquire a portion of the overall scene. The adaptations include adjustments in focus, exposure, colors, and resolution. The bits and pieces are put together by the brain and given meaning. It is the processed result that is "seen." Photographic systems are not nearly as versatile. Thus what the observer at the scene "sees" is not necessarily what the photograph will show and the photographer must consider the intended purpose for the photo and how best to portray that aspect (**Table 2**).

Definitions

The Nature of Light

It is not necessary to delve deeply into physics to understand the key photographic issues. First of all, light can be thought of as composed of small, massless particles called photons. These travel in straight lines unless their paths are bent by reflection (as off a mirror) or by refraction (as passing through a lens), or by diffraction (as by passing close to the edge of an obstacle). The paths that photons follow are called rays. Light can also be described as an electromagnetic wave. Each photon has a particular wavelength or

Table 1 Purposes for photography

Reason	Future reference	Measurement and analysis	Communication
Purpose	Record for review by the investigator of a perishable or large sample	A model of a sample that is suitable for certain analytical procedures	A surrogate of a sample that helps another person visualize a key point being made by the investigator
Objective	A representation that reminds one of the original situation	Accurate and rendered in a form suitable to the specific analytical procedure	Shows the key aspects of the original sample without evoking inappropriate emotional issues

Table 2 Differences between photo and visual processes

Issue	Human vision	Photography
Focus and depth of focus	Everything seems in sharp focus, from near to far	Only a limited portion of the image is in focus – the subject and short distances in front of and beyond the subject
Dynamic range	Detail in both bright highlight areas and deep shadow areas can be seen. Brightness range of about one million to one	With color negative films, a range of 20 000 to one is possible. With slide films, about 2000 to one; with digital cameras, less than 2000 to one
Sharpness	Retinal image processing enhances edges, providing higher than expected sharpness	Edge enhancement can be applied, but care must be used to avoid the creation of artifacts that can impair analyses and create misleading interpretation during communications with others
Color	The brain applies color names that we use to define our world. Some are based upon the wavelength of the incoming light (e.g., red). Others are based upon mixtures and have no physical wavelength basis (e.g., brown)	The system applies coloration according to the manufacturing parameters. There is the ability to adjust the settings. People tend to see reproduced colors differently than they see natural objects because of contextual interpretation differences
Adaptation	Our visual system can adapt in a matter of seconds from very dark environments (tens of photons) to very bright ones (tens of millions of photons)	Manual intervention is usually required. For example, change the film, apply a filter, change a camera setting, or, with digital cameras, use a different camera

frequency. Wavelength is what controls what is seen as color, and it also controls the energy the photon can impart to particles with which it might collide. Some of the measurements of light are key to making photographs, and these are described in **Table 3**.

Taking Pictures

The overall setup for taking a picture is as follows.

1. Ambient light is incident upon a scene containing a subject of interest.
2. Some of the light is reflected off the elements in the scene and moves toward the camera.
3. Some of that light is admitted into the camera through the lens. The amount of light actually entering the camera will depend upon the lens aperture and the exposure time.
4. The lens will project a real image on the image sensor.

5. Responses of the sensor to the light projected on it are used to form an image, which is representative of the original scene.

The photographer must compose the image to show the subject according to some photographic mission. Then the aperture, as determined by the f/stop (**Table 4**), and exposure time are adjusted based on the sensitivity of the sensor and the reflected light to ensure that the key features of the subject fall within the responsive portion of the sensor's dynamic range. When there is not sufficient ambient light, the photographer will employ additional lighting.

Most of the newer cameras have light meters built into the cameras and achieve "though-the-lens" measurement of light levels. In general, these are quite reliable and can accommodate a wide range of photographic situations, often including the use of electronic flash. The photographer can set the light metering system either to concentrate on the overall

Table 3   Descriptions of common terms

Term	Description	Measurement	Photon basis
Luminous intensity	An indication of the brightness of a light source	Candela (cd)	Total number of photons per unit time from a light source
Luminance	The brightness of a surface at a point	Candela meter^{-2} (cd m^{-2})	Photons per unit time per unit of area on the surface of a source
Luminous flux	The amount of light emitted into space	Lumen (lm) (cd sterradian^{-1})	Photons per unit time emitted into a solid angle of space from a source
Illuminance	Amount of light falling per unit area	Lux (lx)	Photons per unit time per square meter on a receiving surface
Exposure	The amount of light reaching a sensor	Lux seconds (lx s)	Photons per unit area on a receiving surface

Table 4   Exposure terminology

Measure	Description	Controls
Focal length	The distance between the center of the lens and the point behind it where it forms an image of a distant object, usually measured in millimeters	Image magnification
Aperture	The opening through which light can pass through a lens, normally the diameter of the limiting opening, measured in millimeters. Most lenses have an internal device called an iris, or diaphragm, which sets the aperture. In most camera lenses, this is adjustable	Illuminance on the sensor surface for the given lens
f/stop	A dimensionless number defined as the ratio of the focal length of a lens divided by its aperture. An indicator of the illuminance falling on the image sensor for any lens, no matter what its focal length	Illuminance on the sensor surface
Shutter	A device inside a camera that controls the exposure time	The time that the light impinges on the surface of the sensor. Determines the range of relative movement speeds that can be ''stopped''
ISO	A measure of the sensitivity of a sensor used in a camera. Defined by the International Standards Organization (ISO) and proportional to the reciprocal of the amount of exposure needed to achieve a threshold of sensor response. A film with an ISO of 400 requires only half of the light of an ISO 200 to achieve the same degree of response. ISO is often referred to as ''speed'' and a 400-speed film is twice as sensitive as a 200-speed film, and half as sensitive as an ISO 800 film	Sensor sensitivity
Depth of field	The range of distances in front of the lens at which scene details are rendered sharply. Adjusted by the f/stop setting	Range of subject to camera distances capable of sharp focus

frame, or on portions of it. Central weighting will give greater attention to the more central portions, while spot metering will concentrate on a very small portion of the center. In situations where the subject is not in the center of the frame, there is usually the means to lock in a reading by pointing at the subject first, then, while holding that reading, move the camera and take the photo. Instructions for accomplishing all of these are generally included in the camera manufacturer's user manual.

There are always special occasions where the photographer must manually override the automatic exposure controls. For small deviations, there is usually an adjustment knob on the camera, while for significantly unusual situations, such as "painting with light," the process can be fairly complex. Fortunately, most medical applications can be accommodated with the automatic metering capabilities of modern cameras.

Most automatic cameras will accommodate three exposure control modes. These are:

1. Program mode, in which the camera automatically sets both the aperture and the exposure time. This is quite suitable for most assignments and is usually the default setting on the camera.
2. Aperture priority mode, in which the photographer sets the aperture and the camera automatically chooses the exposure time. This is used when subject motion is not an issue, and the photographer wants to control depth of field. For example, if the photographer wants to have the subject in sharp focus and the foreground and background less well focused, a wide aperture, or low f/stop number, would be chosen. Conversely, if it were important to have as much of the foreground and background in focus as possible, a small aperture or large f/stop number would be chosen.
3. Shutter priority mode, in which the photographer chooses the shutter speed, and the camera selects the proper f/stop. Typically this is used when the subject is moving and the photographer needs to "stop action" by using a very short shutter time. This is also often needed when using a telephoto lens. The focal length of the lens is an indicator of the exposure time for a handheld camera. For example with a 300-mm lens, the slowest shutter time that should be used is 1/300 s.

It should be noted that, when electronic flash is used, it normally controls the exposure time. Typically, these have a very short flash duration, and so the mechanical shutter time is not an issue unless it is very short as well.

There are several well-known techniques used by photographers to deal with special assignments. A list of some of these is shown in **Table 5**. These techniques are well described in the literature given in the further reading section.

Composition

There are a few cardinal rules that one should follow when engaged in investigatory photography. They are as follows:

1. Crop in the camera. It is often the case that the really significant aspects of a photo are contained in only a small portion of an overall picture. While this is acceptable in amateur photography, it is not appropriate in professional work. The investigative photographer is expected to be aware of the true subject of a photo before the picture is taken. Accordingly, the photographer should move in on the subject either physically or by lens selection and frame the picture closely around the subject. The closely cropped photo should be augmented by "positioning" or "establishment" photos, which show the subject in relation to the broader frame of reference.

Both film and digital photography sensors have finite resolving capability. This means they are capable of resolving only so many details across a frame. If the frame is dedicated to the subject, then the highest ability to render the subject is preserved. If the frame also covers a lot of non-crucial material, then some of the resolving power of the medium is used to reproduce background. The crop in the camera therefore provides the highest quality possible for the key subject matter. The positioning shots are exhibits that are used when communicating with others afterwards.

2. Insert a measuring instrument. In order to preserve the ability to make measurements of aspects of a photo at a later time, it is important to place a reference in the image itself. This is conveniently done by placing a ruler in the photo, close to the part of the image that will be measured. There are several rulers available for this purpose. Some, in addition to distance scales, include other markings such as squares, circles, and color patches. It is good practice to have several such rulers on hand and use them regularly. Many investigators will take two photos of certain key elements, one without the ruler and another, a repeat of the first shot, but with the ruler inserted. It is important that the ruler be located in the plane of the object to be measured.
3. Perpendicular to subject. In most investigative photos, there is a key subject that the photographer wishes to depict. If that subject has a flat surface, or a major dimension, the camera should be held perpendicular to that surface or dimension. This will greatly simplify subsequent measurement and analysis. In addition, the photographer should avoid extreme configurations that can complicate analysis. Examples of such configurations would include the use of very-wide-angle lenses (fisheye), very-narrow-angle lenses (long telephoto), and compositions that place the key subject near the edge of the frame instead of near the center.
4. Normal lenses for positioning shots. When the focal length of the lens is roughly equal to the diagonal of the image sensor frame, the angle of view and the depiction of perspective will closely resemble that of the human visual system. The lens is called the "normal lens" in this situation. Lenses with longer focal lengths (telephoto) will compress distances by comparison, and lenses with shorter focal lengths (wide-angle) will expand distances.
5. Subject failure. Over the years, engineers have developed all sorts of devices to take the guesswork

Table 5 Photographic techniques of note

Technique	Objective	Basic description
Painting with light	Record a large scene in very dim light	Place the camera on a fixed mount, leave the shutter open, walk around the scene, lighting each segment individually with a handheld flash attachment
Macrophotography	Produce close-up images of small objects, generating images that are the same size as the object or larger	Use of specially designed ''macro'' lenses
Alternative light source	Record images of special substances without confusion due to substrate patterns	In situations where there is a pattern on a substrate that either fluoresces or phosphoresces. Exposures are made at short wavelengths to excite the response and the image is recorded at a longer wavelength
Three-point lighting	Standard portrait studio lighting arrangement that controls contrast, provides some shading on the subject, and separates the subject from the background	Uses three lights. The first is in front and to one side of the subject; the second is in front, on the other side from the first and at a lower intensity. The third light is above the subject, highlighting the forehead and filling in background shadows. Sometimes a fourth light is used, shining from below and behind the subject to help separate the subject from the background
Direct flash	A convenient means of adding light with a handheld and frequently moved camera	Since the flash attachment is mounted on the camera, and is pointed at the subject, the light comes from roughly the point of image capture. The front of the subject will be brightly illuminated and the rest will be considerably darker. Scene contrast is high and shadows are pronounced
Diffused direct flash	To soften the harsh lighting associated with direct flash	A diffuser, such as a translucent sheet of plastic or cloth, is placed over the flash attachment
Bounce lighting flash	Retains the convenience of on-camera flash but reduces the harsh shadows that normally result	A flash attachment is used but it is aimed at a diffuse white surface such as a large card, a wall, or the ceiling
Ring light	In close-up work, this reduces sensitivity to surface roughness	Utilizes a camera-mounted flash attachment in the form of a ring that encircles the lens
45–90 illumination	A lighting arrangement meant to minimize front surface reflections	Typically used on copy stands, the axes of the lights are set to 45° relative to the object's main surface and the camera is set to 90° (normal to the surface). This is the standard for measuring instruments such as reflection densitometers as well
Perspective grid	To determine three-dimensional information from normal photographs	Typically used at crime scenes and accident scenes, a flat square of known size is placed in the scene, usually on the floor or ground in front of the camera and used to extrapolate to vanishing points and establish a basis for making measurements
Infrared photography	To see by means of heat instead of visible light. Also, to determine temperatures	Special films or digital sensors are used that have high sensitivity to long wavelength (infrared) light. Visible light is blocked. Special arrangements must be made to focus the camera
Zone system	A process for determining exposure levels in order to maximize the impact of a scene's dynamic range	The brightness levels of key parts of a scene are categorized into zones, then the exposure is set to locate these key parts on the usable exposure range of the film or sensor
Component panorama	A process of making a photographic representation of a very wide scene	Several photos are taken, each at a different angle from a single point. Care must be taken to ensure that the images overlap enough to be properly joined or ''stitched'' together to create a single image
Push processing	A process for taking photos in very low light using silver halide film	The film is deliberately underexposed by a fixed amount and then the film processing is modified to compensate. Often has contrast and grain consequences
Bracketing	A means to help assure getting a good exposure under conditions that are difficult to measure	For each object or scene, a few shots are made instead of just one. With each shot the exposure level is increased from below what is expected to be correct to above. One of the photos should be well exposed

Continued

Table 5 Continued

Technique	Objective	Basic description
Lens translation	A process for obtaining photos with the 90° perspective when there is an obstacle preventing the camera being held directly above an object	Using a flexible bellows device, the camera lens is moved laterally off to the side with its axis still normal to the object's principal surface
Polarized light	A process for reduction of front surface glare	A special polarizing filter is placed over the camera lens and rotated until front surface glare is minimized
Contrast filtering	A means for increasing or decreasing contrast for object elements of selected colors	Colored contrast filters are used over the camera lens to change the contrast of certain items in the scene selectively. Contrast in items of the same color of the filter will be decreased and those of opposite color will be increased. This is generally limited to black and white photography
Stereo photography	A means for showing depth in photography	One uses either two cameras or a single camera with two lenses. The lenses are slightly separated (as are a person's two eyes). The means is provided to show one of the images to one eye and the second image to the other eye. This can be done with polarizers, color filters, or stereo viewers
Three-dimensional scanning	A means for recording a three-dimensional photograph of an object with a single device. The resulting image is a computer model of the object	A special camera which takes both a normal photograph and also records spots that correspond from a location where a laser scanner intersects the subject surface. The laser points at an oblique angle to the object and its beam progresses along the object in preset steps. The device then computes a three-dimensional model of the object and attaches the normal photo to render the object's surface markings
Photomicrography	The capturing of images at very high magnification	A special adapter is placed on a microscope to allow a camera to receive the enlarged image
Fisheye photography	The capture of very-wide-angle photographs. These are distorted compared to normal vision, because the eye cannot capture such a wide angle	Fisheye photography depends upon the use of a specially designed lens. Fisheye lenses have very short focal lengths compared to ''normal'' and cover a view considerably greater than the 40° view of humans
Telephotography	The capture of detailed images of distant objects. Lenses with about twice the normal focal length are often used for portrait photography	Telephotography depends upon the use of a specially designed lens. Telephoto lenses have long focal lengths compared to ''normal'' and cover a small angle of view compared to normal human vision
Fill flash	A process for reducing harsh shadows resulting from existing light	A flash attachment is used to illuminate portions of a scene that are not well lit by existing light
Off-camera flash	A process for using a flash attachment to light an object at an oblique angle. It is used to show surface textures	A normal flash attachment is used along with an extension cable that allows the flash attachment to be held somewhere off to the side of the camera
Exposure compensation	Overriding the camera's automatic exposure control system or a light meter-based setting because of unusual contents of a specific scene	Using the camera's controls, purposely deviate from the indicated level of exposure to bring out needed detail in a subject where the metering system is responding too strongly to background light levels. Sometimes referred to as correcting for ''subject failure,'' examples include a dark subject against a light background, or a light subject against a dark background

out of photography. These include light meters, automatic exposure controllers, automatic printers, image analyzers, in-camera white balance devices, auto focus, to name a few. These are wonderful devices that usually allow the photographer to concentrate on the composition of the photo instead of the setting of the camera or printer. However, all of these devices assume a "normal" scene. For the investigative photographer most scenes are quite different from the normal vacation photos. For example, in a normal scene, one can generally assume that the average reflectance from the scene is close to that of a gray card that reflects 18% of the light. This can be used to set the exposure properly. In the case of a digital camera, it can read the overall red and blue light levels and determine the color temperature or basic coloration of the light source and balance accordingly (white balance). It can also generally be assumed that the subject of the photo is near the center and that the rest is background. The camera can thereby set correct focus. However, if a pathologist is taking a close-up photo of a red (blood) wound on dark-brown skin, the scene is not normal. The autofocus will probably work well enough, and the autoexposure will be fairly close, white balance will be greatly in error, and manual adjustment will be helpful (inserting a gray ruler in the image will help with subsequent color balancing). Engineers regard the nonnormal aspects of a scene as "subject failure," but nomenclature notwithstanding, the investigative photographer must know when he or she is taking a nonnormal photo and must take steps to make manual overrides. Some of the appropriate photographic techniques are listed in **Table 5** and some of the more common postimage capture-processing techniques are listed in **Table 6**.

Film Versus Digital

With recent improvements in digital-imaging technology, digital approaches and the traditional silver halide film methods have begun to complement each other well. However, there is no longer much of a difference in areas such as sensitivity and resolution. Film still has a better dynamic range though, and it is more flexible (one can change the film and not have to exchange the whole camera). When considering the developing and printing of all images, silver halide technology is slightly cheaper. The big advantage to digital photography is the immediacy of the result. It allows the photographer to see the pictures immediately, and if not fully satisfied with the result, make changes and take the photo again.

It is becoming quite common that the best overall approaches involve hybrid systems. Films are used for certain photography assignments, and digital cameras and scanners are used for others. Film scanners can be used to convert film images into digital images for analysis. Digital printers that print to photographic papers are a low-cost output option. Moving files among media is becoming easier each year.

Image Processing

Photographers, over decades of darkroom work, have developed a large array of techniques to enhance (and modify) images to achieve special results. The publishers of digital image-editing software have now captured the essence of all of these using mathematics and computer algorithms. These allow one to apply complex and arcane techniques with ease on a wide range of photos, and it is recommended that the investigative photographer adopt this technology and learn to use it. There are protocols which help facilitate legitimate image enhancement and avoid questionable manipulation. These are available from the SWGIT *Guidelines*. SWGIT coordinates with counterparts in several other countries, and its findings are therefore quite robust.

As with photographic techniques, it is impossible to review all of the options in this article, so a listing of the more commonly used techniques is provided in **Table 6**.

Outputs

Hard-copy Prints

Paper-based reflection prints are what one most commonly takes to be the output from a photographic process. In traditional silver halide photography, negatives are printed directly on to photographic paper and the result is a paper print. Forensic pathologists have a history of using slide films in their cameras to create transparencies. Now, with the advent of digital technology, one is quite likely to use a digital camera or to use a film camera and scan the negatives to create a digital image. It is then easy to enhance the images, store them, and make prints using a digital printer of some sort. If the source of the image was a digital camera or a flat bed scanner, digital-printing technology is clearly a requirement. Digital printers are available in four distinct varieties. These are summarized in **Table 7**.

Projection

Increasingly, investigators are making computer presentations to both colleagues and courts since this allows them to show a wider range of photos and to intersperse video clips and animations. Frequently there are hard-copy versions of key images for members of the audience to study closely. Transforming all images to digital format greatly facilitates these options.

In a courtroom setting, the recommended arrangement is to have monitors on the lawyers' desks as well as one on the desk of the judge. This allows those people to preview images before they are shown to a jury. It is best to have the main screen near the witness so that the jury can see the witness and the presentation in a single view. Some courtrooms have installed

Table 6 Image enhancement techniques

Technique class	Specific techniques	Objective	Summary description
Size adjustment	Cropping, interpolation, sizing	To create a new image of a different size	Cropping is the process of cutting off sections of an image either to reduce its size or to concentrate on only parts of the image. Sizing refers to taking the existing image content and either spreading it over a larger area or concentrating it into a smaller area. Interpolation is a process for accomplishing sizing with digital images
Selection	Similarity outline, exclusion masking	To define areas of an image that will be subjected to further processing	Outlining involves drawing a line around the area(s) to be selected. Similarity tools allow one to identify a small area and use it to define a basis for seeking other similar areas. Exclusion tools allow one to identify a portion, and then select everything else. Once initially identified, masking tools allow one to cover an area and then process either the covered or noncovered areas
Tone scale adjustment	Brightness contrast curve adjust dodge burn equalization	To adjust the relative darkness, brightness, and rate of change of brightness within an image	Increasing the brightness makes the lighter portions lighter while contrast adjustments change the relative levels of bright areas relative to dark ones. Curve adjustment tools allow one to apply different amounts of adjustment to various portions of the tonal scale. One can increase the contrast in the bright areas and at the same time decrease the contrast in the mid-scale areas. The dodge and burn tools allow one to apply these adjustments to a geometric area instead of a tonal range
Color adjustment	Correction change copying	To change the coloration of either a full image or parts of an image	In color correction there are indicators of what the original coloration should have been, or the photographer is making adjustments to render colors of familiar objects in a color so that it can be recognized how those items should appear. Sometimes it is desirable purposely to change colors to highlight certain features of an image and there are several tools for accomplishing this, including the means to copy, directly change, or compute new colors based on image content. Any adjustments beyond simple color correction will require description and justification
Edge adjustments	Sharpening, blurring	To render the edges of objects in an image either more clear or more diffuse	There are a wide range of tools for both sharpening and diffusing images, but, as a general rule, they all involve changes in contrast only along edges. If edge contrast is increased, the edges appear sharper and, if the contrast is decreased, they are more diffused. These tools are useful up to a point, and then there is noticeable indication of image manipulation. Also, it is not possible to reconstruct what was never there in the first place

Table 6 Continued

Technique class	Specific techniques	Objective	Summary description
Defect removal	Cloning redeye, despeckle writing airbrush	To correct for known accidental image defects such as dust spots and redeye effect	Cloning copies image values from one area and writes them into another. It is a tool to be avoided in investigatory work since it begs questioning of the degree to which one altered an image. This is the tool one would use to add or remove items from a crime scene, put a person's face on another's body, etc. Redeye, despeckling tools are less inclined to support gross alteration. Writing involves the direct addition of information to an image that is not part of the original scene and the tool should only be used with clear need and clear description
Frequency filtering	Fourier spectral, other	To accentuate or remove patterns from an image	An image is nothing but a series of changes of brightness over space on a surface. As such they can be represented by a sum of sine and cosine waves of brightness with distance. In this way, all of the mathematically based frequency filtering techniques can be used selectively to enhance or remove patterns from images
Area and shape adjustments	Transforms perspective	Change the apparent shape of an object in an image. In the case where it was not possible to take the original photo perpendicular to the object, these tools can be used to change the apparent perspective	The area of the image containing the shape that needs to be repaired is selected and the tool is applied. These tools utilize basic geometric rules and interpolate as needed to complete local sizing

Table 7 Digital printers

Type	Modes	Description	Pros and cons
Inkjet	Paper transparency	Small drops of ink are applied to the surface of a receiver sheet. Several such drops are required to render a picture element, or pixel	Inexpensive; printer inks are moderately expensive. Can write to plain paper as well as to glossy, photolike paper. Does not make high-quality transparencies since inks scatter light. Printing speeds tend to be relatively low. Image stability can vary
Dye sublimation	Paper transparency	Dye is fumed off a coated ribbon and applied to the surface of the receiver sheet. The amount of dye applied in each location can be adjusted so that the number of dots and the number of pixels are the same	Devices are somewhat expensive, as are the materials. It makes high-quality paper prints and transparencies. Printing speeds are relatively high. Image stability is very good
Photographic paper	Paper	Laser beams are used to expose regular photographic paper. Usually the printing device is attached to a mini lab paper processor such that the same device can be used to process traditional silver halide photos as well	The device is somewhat expensive, but the paper is relatively inexpensive. Printing speed is fairly high. Image quality is very high and image stability is quite good
Photographic film	Negative or transparency film	Laser beams expose normal slide or negative films. The film is then processed normally to produce either negatives, or, more commonly, slides	The device is somewhat expensive. The image quality and stability are both excellent

smaller monitors in the jury area so that jurors have access to a personal, close-up view. The key factors in choosing a projector are brightness, resolution, and contrast ratio. Common today are projectors with at least 1500 lumens or more, and screen resolution of 1024 × 768 pixels. Contrast ratios of 200 to 1 are relatively easy to find. Almost all of the better projectors will also accept video signals and play audio.

Data Storage

When using photographic film, the film itself is the storage medium. To assure long-term stability of the images, they should be stored in a cool, dry, dark location. It is also important that the films are properly processed. Failure to remove certain chemicals from the film can lead to degradation during storage. A reliable filing index system must be developed so that a future user can find an old piece of film.

Storage of digital images involves additional and different issues. There are three main concerns: file format, storage medium, and filing system.

Digital images reside in computer files, and these files must adhere to a strict file format for them to be readable in the future. When presented on a screen or sent to a printer, an image has a certain number of pixels, and each pixel is defined by three numbers (for a color image). Consider an image with 6 million pixels, laid out in 2000 rows of 3000 pixels. If this is a color image, then each pixel has three numbers. Thus, the content of the file comprises 18 million numbers (there is additional header and trailer information also associated with each image file). This is a large file, and if one were to store a significant number of these files, the storage requirement for the overall system would become quite large.

Experimenters have found that there is a substantial amount of redundant information in the typical image and that steps can be taken to remove the redundancy. This is known as compression. If it is done without losing any essential information, the process is called "lossless compression." On average, one can achieve lossless compressions of as much as 2 to 1. Thus, the 18 million numbers (18-Mb) file can be reduced to 9 million without loss of information. When the file is opened to show the image, all of the original information will be intact. The most common such file format is called TIFF (tagged image file format).

In addition to lossless compression methods, there are "lossy compression" methods. These utilize complex mathematical relationships and are able selectively to eliminate information that is very unlikely to be important to the substance of the image. The most common such method is called JPEG (joint photographic experts group) and it has the advantage of being variable. The investigator can adjust the amount of compression that is applied. It is important to note that higher compression results in increased amounts of lost information. In addition to losing information, JPEG compression creates and inserts artifacts in the image. Again, the greater the degree of compression, the greater the insertion of artifacts. Modest levels of JPEG compression, achieving compression ratios of 5 to 1 or less, are generally quite satisfactory. There are several file formats and some of these are listed in **Table 8**.

Once the format issue has been resolved, one needs to choose a medium for storage. Some systems rely on servers that are backed up and protected as the means of archival storage. Others write the files to be archived to stable, write-once media such as WORM (write once, read many) CDs. The server approach is convenient for the end-user and, if properly maintained, is quite satisfactory. It has a downside, however. In forensic work, material must often be kept for decades, and there is a very low likelihood of calling any of this material up after the first few years. The result is that very large amounts of live storage space are dedicated to materials that may never be retrieved. The utilization of separate CDs, on the other hand, provides reliable long-term storage capability, but it does not require large amounts of active storage. The problem with CD storage is that of updating old records as technology evolves. For example, if DVD technology starts to replace CD technology significantly, then it would be necessary to call up large numbers of CDs and rewrite them on to DVDs. In practice, both approaches are being followed successfully today.

Summary and Conclusions

The evolution of new digital photographic technology has had a significant impact on all applications of photography, including forensic medical work. The trend will not stop any time soon. The result has been to expand greatly the capabilities of the investigator to document and analyze evidentiary material. Fortunately, there are organizations that are working to evaluate technology, recommend practices, and provide training. These include government-based organizations such as SWGIT, which is sponsored by the US Federal Bureau of Investigation. There are similar efforts in other countries and these can be found through national police forces. In addition, there are specialized organizations such as the Institute for Forensic Imaging, which is affiliated with Indiana University and is located in Indianapolis, Indiana, USA. Book and magazine publishers have developed good reference literature supporting this

Table 8 Common file formats

Format	Type	Compression	Comments
TIFF	NC	None	A robust and widespread format that does not compress the image. Often recommended for archiving
TIFF-LZW	LLC	2:1	Based upon the standard TIFF format but adds lossless compression
JPEG	LC	2:1 5:1 >10:1	A widespread file format that utilizes lossy compression. The user can adjust the amount of compression that is actually applied. At low levels, it is almost impossible to detect the losses. As the level of compression is increased, the losses increase, becoming quite noticeable beyond 10:1. Along with losses, this format inserts artifacts into images
PICT	Optional	Optional	Primarily designed for use on Apple Macintosh computers. Compression is optional and different routines, including JPEG, can be chosen
EPS	NC	None	Specific to the Adobe PhotoShop software
RAW	NC	None	Several professional digital cameras offer a RAW image file format. Each camera has its own version. These generally preserve more image details but require special techniques. They are primarily used by professional photographers and graphic artists
PCD	VLC	4:1	One of the earlier image file formats was Photo CD, developed by Eastman Kodak for home use. While this format is lossy, it preserves the image information that people can see, hence the term "visually lossless." This format is no longer in widespread use
GIF	NC	none	Originally designed for use in web pages, it allows for transparent pixels. It suffers from a limited range of colors and is losing popularity
JPEG 2000	LC	<100:1	A very-high-quality compression is achieved, that will allow reductions of up to 100:1 or so with minimal image degradation. It is not available as "freeware" and so is not yet in widespread use
Fractal	LC		Very-high-quality system, but difficult to use

NC, no compression; LLC, lossless compression; LC, lossy compression; VLC, visually lossless compression.

evolution. Some of the literature is primarily scientific and describes the principles and how technology is implemented. Other writings are designed to help the practitioner learn how to apply the tools and techniques to advantage.

See Also

Crime-scene Investigation and Examination: Collection and Chain of Evidence

Further Reading

Blitzer H, Jacobia J (2002) *Forensic Digital Imaging and Photography.* London: Academic Press.

Burdick H (1997) *Digital Imaging Theory and Applications.* New York: McGraw-Hill.

Clark S, Ernst M, Haglund W, Jentzen J (1996) *Medicolegal Death Investigator.* Big Rapids, MI: Occupational Research and Assessment.

Giorgianni E, Madden T (1998) *Digital Color Management.* Reading, MA: Addison Wesley.

Hinkle D (1990) *Mug Shots.* Boulder, CO: Paladin Press.

Jacobson R, Ray S, Attridge G, Axford N (2000) *The Manual of Photography,* 8th edn. Oxford, UK: Focal Press.

Langford M (1985) *Advanced Photography,* 5th edn. Oxford, UK: Focal Press.

Meyer-Arendt J (1995) *Introduction to Classical and Modern Optics,* 4th edn. Englewood Cliffs, NJ: Prentice Hall.

Miller L (1998) *Police Photography,* 4th edn. Cincinnati, OH: Anderson.

Pedrotti F, Pedrotti L (1993) *Introduction to Optics,* 2nd edn. Upper Saddle River, NJ: Prentice Hall.

Redsicker D (1994) *The Practical Methodology of Forensic Photography.* Boca Raton, FL: CRC Press.

Russ J (1995) *The Image Processing Handbook,* 2nd edn. Boca Raton, FL: CRC Press.

Russ J (2001) *Forensic Uses of Digital Imaging.* Boca Raton, FL: CRC Press.

Radiology, Overview

W A Murphy, MD Anderson Cancer Center, Houston, TX, USA

Scope

Medical examiners and coroners are responsible for investigating all instances of human death by homicide, suicide, accident, injury, hazardous substance, or during custody, or if unattended by a physician, or if otherwise sudden or suspicious. Since such circumstances encompass the full range of human behavior and biology, broad expertise is necessary to unravel the facts of each death, to assure the greatest quality in the assessment, to interpret those facts in their proper context, and to present the facts and conclusions in a logical and effective manner. As a result, many scientific disciplines engage in death investigation.

Forensic radiology is the portion of science that deals with the relation and application of medical imaging facts to legal problems. It contributes to death investigation, medical malpractice, paleopathology, and examination of inanimate antiquities such as pottery, paintings, and musical instruments. This article only examines forensic radiology in relationship to death investigation.

Regarding death investigation, forensic radiology is a method that documents the anatomical features of the individual who died. It is based upon detailed knowledge of human anatomy, of the medical conditions that affect people, and of the imaging methods that display normal and pathological anatomy. Diagnostic radiologists are clinical experts who apply radiological methods to document anatomic features present at death. There are no subspecialty training programs that produce forensic radiologists. Such experts arise after clinical specialty training and certification when individual diagnostic radiologists develop a personal interest in forensic matters and learn by experience. Some medical examiner and coroner jurisdictions have attracted such interested radiologists. Working with volunteer diagnostic radiologists, forensic pathologists provide on-the-job training in death investigation. In return, diagnostic radiologists contribute their specialized expertise.

Team Effort

Forensic radiology is not practiced in a vacuum. Team effort is required for maximal success. Death investigation is initiated by police officers who are the first professionals to arrive on the scene. This officer or a professional death investigator is responsible for the integrity of the scene and the gathering of information regarding the circumstances surrounding the death. Once the body is removed from the scene, the forensic pathologist assumes responsibility for the scientific facts regarding the remains, including laboratory tests, imaging tests, and an autopsy.

A radiological technologist works under the supervision of the forensic pathologist to obtain the best possible images at the appropriate stage of the investigation without alteration of the remains. Since images are best interpreted within the standard conventions of clinical medical imaging, the technologist must adhere to these requirements even when inconvenient due to the condition of the remains.

The forensic radiologist should freely communicate with the death investigator, the imaging technologist, and the forensic pathologist to be certain that the correct facts are available. This ensures that interpretation of the images is in a proper context and presented in a logical and professional fashion. The characteristics that define a worthy forensic radiologist include inquisitiveness, dedication to public service, integrity and objectivity, and a willingness to testify in court. The forensic radiologist should define him- or herself as a cooperative partner and be willing to delve deeply into the complexities of the forensic sciences. The accuracy and success of future legal proceedings depend upon excellence of the team effort.

History

While studying the properties of cathode rays in a vacuum tube, the German physicist Wilhelm Conrad Röntgen (1845–1923) discovered the X-ray on November 8, 1895. On December 22, 1895, using his wife's hand he obtained the first human X-ray image. He mailed this image to colleagues in Europe on New Year's Day 1896 and an international sensation ensued. The ability to see through objects and within the human body fascinated the world. From this serendipitous beginning, the specialty of diagnostic imaging emerged. Today, imaging has subspecialties, certifications at several levels of expertise, new technologies every decade, and daily refinements.

During 1896, the first year following the discovery, X-ray pictures were used as evidence in a spectrum of legal matters. Cases in Canada, the UK, France, and the USA included X-ray evidence of gunshot wounds, negligence, malpractice, worker's compensation, and public transportation injury. These experiences set the foundation for the intensive use of imaging evidence that is so common in modern legal proceedings.

To achieve appropriate recognition, status, and acceptance in court, the court had to consider the accuracy and trustworthiness of X-rays. This happened quickly and generally followed the principles previously determined for photography. Of the several court cases in 1896, one in the USA became an accepted landmark regarding admissibility of the X-ray as scientific evidence. A young law student in Denver fell and sustained a hip injury. Upon examination, the treating surgeon found no evidence of fracture and recommended treatment for a contusion. Later, other surgeons diagnosed a femoral neck fracture and disagreed with the initial therapy. Thus, a malpractice action was initiated against the first surgeon. Before trial in December 1896, X-ray pictures of the hip were obtained. The defense argued that since the actual bone could not be seen, there was no proof that the X-ray actually represented truth. A defense expert witness explained how impossible it was to obtain images of complex hip anatomy. The plaintiff attorney displayed X-ray images of the injured hip alongside a normal hip. Following the theatrics, Judge Own LeFevre ruled:

> Modern science has made it possible to look beneath the tissues of the human body, and has aided surgery in telling of the hidden mysteries. We believe it to be our duty in this case to be the first ... in admitting in evidence a process known and acknowledged as a determinate science.

As with photographs, court cases tested the correctness of the content of X-ray images. The validity of photographs had been found to require certain skills, in particular the expert skill of the person taking or developing the photograph. Likewise, X-ray images were found to require expert verification and interpretation. Finally, X-ray images were determined to be secondary evidence. They could not stand alone, but were to be used by the expert to illustrate and clarify the expert's opinion.

Resulting from a series of judicial decisions in many countries, today X-ray images are admissible in courts of law, are accepted as scientific evidence, and provide a factual basis in support of expert opinion. The two major forensic applications of radiology are identification of human remains and documentation of injury.

Identification

Commonly, relatives or other persons visually identify the deceased with support by circumstantial evidence such as location where found (home, business, automobile), clothing worn, and forms of identification present (such as photoidentification cards). Unfortunately, simple visual identification with additional circumstantial corroboration is not possible with human remains that are decomposed, incinerated, dismembered, or skeletonized. In these situations, other methods of identification are utilized, but each has shortcomings. Forensic odontology is ineffective when teeth are absent or when no previous records exist. Fingerprints only provide identification when postmortem prints can be gathered and when matching prints are on record. DNA typing is only effective when other appropriate DNA is available for matching.

Identification by medical X-ray is effective for two major reasons. First, citizens of industrialized countries often obtain medical X-ray examinations. In the USA, the number of X-ray examinations per 100 citizens per year has steadily risen. In 1964, just over 30 examinations per 100 persons per year were obtained. By 1980, that number reached just under 60 examinations. Today, the number is estimated at 80 examinations. Records are the brackets that frame people's lives. Medical documents are important and maintained for long periods of time. Some X-ray files are maintained for 5 years, others for 10 years, and still others for the lifetime of the patient. Therefore, medical X-ray images exist for the vast majority of citizens and are readily available.

Second, each person's bone structure is unique. Just as DNA is individually unique, the anatomy (facial features, fingerprints, and bone structure) it codes is also unique. Bone is structured as a cortical sheath with internal trabeculae. Bone slowly replaces itself over many years; it is faithful to its structure. The minute details of cortical and trabecular patterns are specific for the individual and durable over long timeframes.

Moreover, bone resists destruction. Putrefaction may destroy soft tissues through enzymatic liquefaction, but the bone remains unaffected. Fire may burn away the soft tissues and char the surface of the bone, but the fundamental structure of the cortical and trabecular bone remains (**Figure 1**). Adipocere formation may alter the appearance of all soft tissues, but bone is totally spared (**Figure 2**). When a body is dismembered, bones remain. Bone is always available unless it has been mechanically destroyed in a deliberate manner – an exceedingly rare situation.

The magnitude of problem identifications is between 1.5% and 2.0% of the cases processed in forensic jurisdictions. Thus, for an office that accrues 2000 cases a year, the number requiring scientific identification is 30–40 cases. Identification is important to: (1) satisfy relatives that the unrecognizable remains are indeed their loved one; (2) prove death for financial matters, primarily survivor benefit; and (3) prove that a victim exists for legal action. These reasons persuade the medical examiner or coroner to provide a sound scientific identity in as short a time as possible. Dependent upon the resources available, DNA, fingerprint, dental, or medical X-ray comparisons may alone or together provide the scientific identification.

Availability of antemortem images is the fundamental requirement for scientific identification. Scientific identification by forensic radiology is only as successful as the death investigation is at establishing presumptive identity(s). Once possible identities are determined, relatives, friends, or acquaintances are interviewed to define a past medical history. Typically the investigator learns of hospitalizations, emergency room visits, or episodes of medical care, any of which

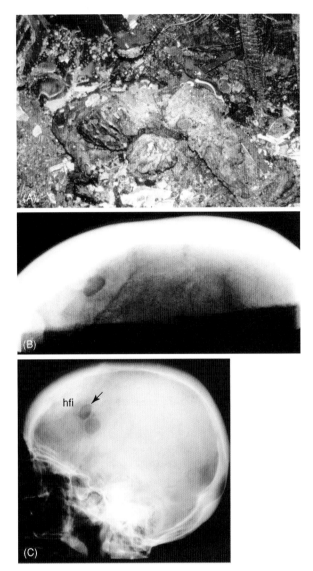

Figure 1   Identification of incinerated remains. (A) Photograph of scene in vacant structure shows a body burned beyond recognition; the skull is toward the upper left and the knee toward the lower right. (B) Radiograph of skullcap was obtained after autopsy but before presumptive identity was determined. (C) Antemortem skull film shows hyperostosis frontalis interna (HFI), a normal variant, and a surgical burr hole (arrow), features that exactly match the postmortem image. Scientific identification was successful. (B) and (C) reprinted with permission from Murphy WA, Spruill FG, Gantner GE (1980) Radiologic identification of unknown human remains. From *Journal of Forensic Science* 1980; 25(4): 731. Copyright ASTM INTERNATIONAL. Reprinted with permission.

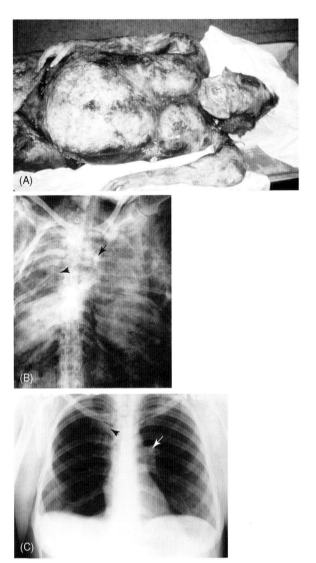

Figure 2   Identification of remains recovered from a river. (A) Photograph of recovered body shows adipocere formation and facial deformity preventing visual identification. (B) Postmortem radiograph shows gas throughout tissue caused by putrefaction, presence of a left hilar calcified granuloma (arrow), and a partially absent rib from a prior thoracotomy (arrowhead). All the left ribs are fractured due to trauma while in the river. (C) Antemortem 100 mm survey chest radiograph shows concordant features (arrow, granuloma; arrowhead, missing rib). Scientific identification was successful.

may provide medical X-ray images. The large amount of medical care provided increases the likelihood that one or more antemortem images of a person will be available.

Successful comparison of antemortem and postmortem images depends on their technical similarity. Therefore, the radiologic technologist must approach imaging human remains as if the images were being obtained in a routine clinical fashion. The technologist should attempt to replicate an ideal clinical antemortem examination when imaging the postmortem remains of the unidentified person.

The goal of the forensic radiologist is to confirm or exclude identity with scientific certainty. The task compares the images of unidentified remains with the retrieved antemortem images of the person selected as the best possible presumptive identity. The forensic radiologist screens the images and searches for concordant and discordant anatomic features. Concordance begins with detection of any major or obvious anatomic feature(s), such as presence of a specific anatomic variation that most other persons do not have. Presence of the major feature on both antemortem and postmortem images is indicative of eventual scientific identification. Other major unique features might include specific results of disease, presence of healed fractures, evidence of surgery, or presence of devices or unique calcifications. Once major features are detected and compared, general features (size, shape, and other general anatomic features of the visualized bones) are reviewed. Then minor anatomic details are surveyed, including local trabecular patterns, small cortical irregularities, or any other small details. No magic number of identical features exists that determines an exact match of antemortem and postmortem images. Usually, the evident features are simply concordant or they are discordant. If images are of standard quality, very seldom is there an in-between situation where the decision as to a match is unresolvable.

Discordance between antemortem and postmortem features occurs in several circumstances. First, when none of the antemortem and postmortem anatomic features match. The comparison excludes the proposed identity. Second, a transient discordance is encountered when an event occurred between the times when antemortem and postmortem images were obtained, e.g., all anatomic features match except for a certain explainable subset. An example would be intercurrent trauma. As long as a history of the trauma was documented, evidence of the trauma would not exclude the identity. All discordances must be adequately explained. Third, children may be difficult to identify when interval growth occurs and bones are no longer alike (**Figure 3**). Fourth, while not exactly discordant, poor-quality images may prevent confident analysis. In these instances the interpretation may be classified as indeterminate.

With skeletons, the tasks are more complicated. Bones must be radiographed as similar to a standard clinical image as possible. This may require several attempts with sequential repositioning of the part and adjustment of the exposure factors. At times, it helps to reassemble anatomic regions. At other times, it is more beneficial to examine bones individually. If unavoidable, random positioning with a mixture of bones still provides much useful information (**Figure 4**).

As skeletonized remains are often a serious challenge for the death investigator who may have few leads to identity, examination of the remains by a forensic anthropologist may provide useful information such as gender, estimated age, and stature. The anthropologist may also contribute information regarding prior health status and cause of death. The

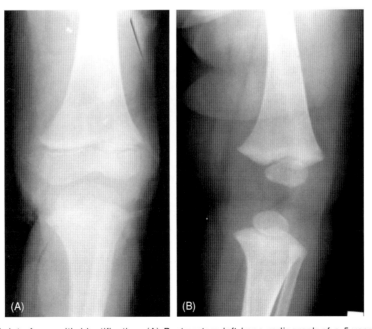

Figure 3 Interval growth interferes with identification. (A) Postmortem left knee radiograph of a 5-year-old child burned beyond recognition. Image shows burned soft tissues with bone structures normal for age. (B) The only antemortem image was from age 1. The differences between (A) and (B) are entirely due to interval normal growth. The discordant features prevented scientific identification by forensic radiology. Other forensic methods confirmed identity.

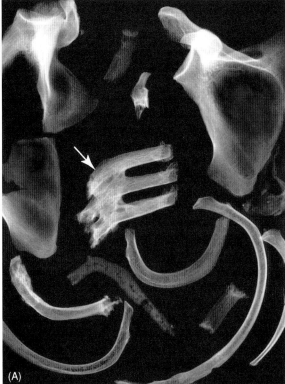

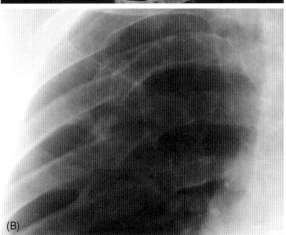

Figure 4 Identification of skeletonized remains. (A) Postmortem radiograph of random bones from skeletonized remains. Among the bones is a fragmentary set of ribs (arrow) fused together due to an injury years before death. (B) Coned-down image from antemortem chest film shows a concordant set of fused ribs. This unique feature was among many that contributed to successful scientific identification. Reprinted with permission from Murphy WA, Gantner GE (1982) Radiologic evaluation of anatomic parts and skeletonized remains. Adapted from *Journal of Forensic Science* 1982; 27(1):14. Copyright ASTM INTERNATIONAL. Reprinted with permission.

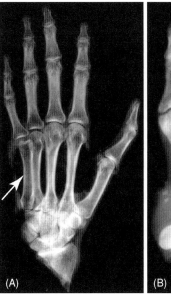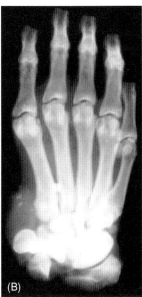

Figure 5 Determination of species by forensic radiology. (A) A desiccated "hand" was found by workers on a roof. Radiograph shows unmistakable human features, even though the fifth metacarpal had fallen out and been reinserted upside-down (arrow). The source of the human hand was never determined. (B) A "hand" was found by children playing in a park. A radiograph shows the unmistakable features of a bear paw. No additional investigation was required. (A) Reprinted with permission from Murphy WA, Gantner GE (1982) Radiologic evaluation of anatomic parts and skeletonized remains. From *Journal of Forensic Science* 1982; 27(1):10. Copyright ASTM INTERNATIONAL. Reprinted with permission.

Effective death investigation then recovers the antemortem images. With appropriate postmortem images the forensic radiologist confirms or excludes identity based upon careful comparison.

When anatomic parts or single bones are recovered and taken to the police, the first task is to determine whether they are human (**Figure 5**). Generally, it is very simple for a forensic radiologist to differentiate animal anatomy from human anatomy. The forensic radiologist then examines the images to provide as much useful prior medical information about the person as possible. Any anatomic part may be sufficient for scientific comparison. Among the most well-studied anatomic sites are the paranasal sinuses. The frontal sinus displays so much variability that comparison is simple (**Figure 6**). Patterns of rib calcifications also provide targets for scientific comparison. The list of individual anatomic features useful for radiologic comparison is nearly infinite. Even single bones or bone fragments may be sufficient to establish a solid identity providing the quality of the antemortem and postmortem images is excellent and assuming due care is exercised by the radiologist (**Figure 7**).

forensic radiologist can provide similar estimates. The combined information gathered by the team effort of anthropologist and radiologist may help the death investigator develop and narrow leads until a most likely presumptive identity is established.

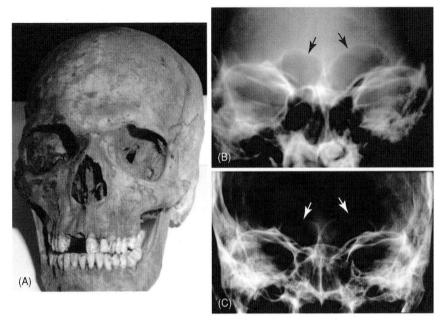

Figure 6 Identification of skeletonized remains through frontal sinus comparison. (A) Photograph of skeletonized skull. (B) Antemortem skull film obtained from medical record. (C) Postmortem skull image obtained by careful match of clinical position. The concordant sinus anatomy (arrows) established scientific identification. (B) and (C) Reprinted with permission from Murphy WA, Gantner GE (1982) Radiologic evaluation of anatomic parts and skeletonized remains. From *Journal of Forensic Science* 1982; 27(1):15. Copyright ASTM INTERNATIONAL. Reprinted with permission.

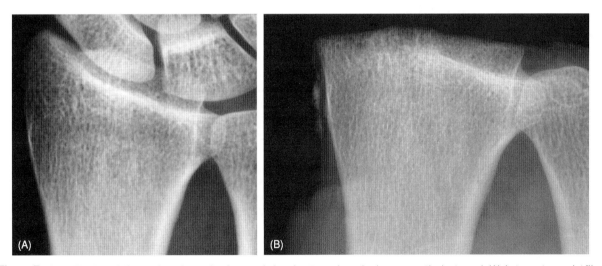

Figure 7 Identification of dismembered remains from a victim of torture whose body was mostly destroyed. (A) Antemortem wrist film. (B) Postmortem wrist image obtained with precise position and exposure shows that all details of bone size, shape, cortical contour, and trabecular pattern are concordant, yielding scientific identification.

Postmortem Artifacts Created by Scavengers

Scavengers alter and scatter human remains. These activities confound attempts to investigate the death and identify the individual because antemortem features may be destroyed or lost from the scene. Likewise, important perimortem skeletal trauma may be obscured or destroyed. The two major scavengers are rodents and canids.

Rodents create nearly all their damage with their incisors. This results in characteristic regular parallel groves of uniform pitch extending from the inner surface of a bone to its outer surface. Rodents rarely scatter human remains but on occasion transport the small tubular bones of the hands and feet.

In contrast to rodents, canids cause considerable damage. In general, the longer the interval between death and discovery, the greater the amount of damage done by canid scavengers. The magnitude of the damage depends upon tooth morphology, jaw mechanics, and the size and strength of the particular canid. Canids first deflesh the head, neck, and upper thorax, after which the upper extremities are dismembered and transported. Later the abdomen, pelvis, and thighs are consumed, with the lower extremities disarticulated and transported.

Bones are heavily damaged by gnawing, beginning with the softer cancellous articular regions (**Figure 8**) and flat bones, moving to the more resistant shafts of long bones and skull. Carnivore tooth marks include punctures through thin bones, pits, or indentations when penetration did not occur, scoring from teeth dragging across the bone, and furrows from molars scraping the bone. Spiral fractures of long bones occur with strong-jawed larger canids. Canid activity leaves tell-tale tooth marks and crushed, splintered bone ends (**Figure 9**).

Radiologically, bone alterations created by scavengers must be recognized as artifacts and not misinterpreted as features associated with the cause of death or confused with other antemortem trauma. Once recognized, the scavenger-induced skeletal changes may be correctly classified and the search for other features of importance in the death investigation may proceed. Cooperation between the radiologist, anthropologist, and pathologist resolves uncertainties.

When unidentified remains are discovered, even with extensive scavenger damage, an opportunity to complete a scientific identification by comparison of antemortem and postmortem radiography still exists. At times, a search for additional scattered remains is necessary to recover missing parts of the skeleton needed to complete the confident identification.

Mass Casualties

In instances of mass casualty, the complexity of the identification effort depends on the number of casualties and the type of disaster. A multicar vehicular accident with a dozen casualties is much less complicated than an airline crash with 500 deaths. Disasters with mass casualties are challenging because the damage to bodies tends to be more (often incinerated and dismembered), the deceased are found in unfamiliar surroundings, often without personal belongings, and the remains may be commingled. The goal is to identify as many persons as possible, to the greatest surety achievable in the shortest amount of time attainable. The standard is to recover

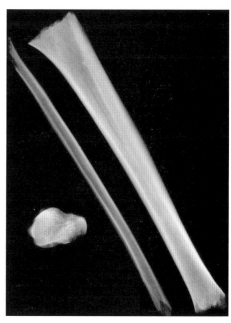

Figure 8 Canid gnawing of long bones. Radiograph of tibia, fibula, and talus that a dog brought into its owner's backyard. The image showed unmistakably human bones. Note that the ends of the bones are gnawed away. Later, the remainder of the body of this homicide victim was recovered. Reprinted with permission from Murphy WA, Gantner GE (1982) Radiologic evaluation of anatomic parts and skeletonized remains. From *Journal of Forensic Science* 1982; 27(1):11. Copyright ASTM INTERNATIONAL. Reprinted with permission.

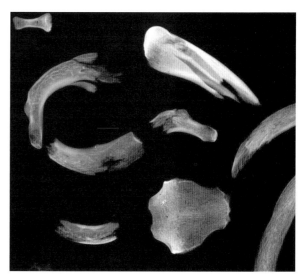

Figure 9 Canid fragmentation of small flat bones. Radiograph of assorted bones from scattered skeletonized remains shows perforated, crushed, and irregularly splintered margins of portions of ribs and clavicle.

all remains with as much circumstantial documentation as is available. Then the remains should be tested with all applicable methods of identification. The combined results optimize the number of individuals eventually identified as well as the surety of those conclusions.

In 1949, forensic radiology was first tried in a disaster when the steamship Noronic burned at a dock in Toronto, Canada, and 119 passengers died, many with severe burns. Antemortem radiographs were recovered for 35 of the deceased and confident identifications were developed for 24 (70%). Also confirmed were the principles that any anatomy could be used for comparison and that a variety of skeletal features proved effective. Uniqueness of skeletal anatomy was firmly established. Since then, forensic radiology has helped identify human remains in many disasters. Well-documented examples include the March 1977 collision of two Boeing 747 jets in the Canary Islands with the loss of 576 lives, the December 1985 crash of an airliner in Gander, Newfoundland, with the loss of 256 lives, and the April 1995 bombing of the Alfred P. Murrah Federal Building in Oklahoma City, Oklahoma, with the loss of 168 lives. In each instance, multiple identification methods were employed and forensic radiology either confirmed the results of other methods or provided the unique identification.

Disasters with mass casualties have special requirements and considerations. Compulsive screening of all remains, tracking of features, and matching of findings are intense and complicated. Detailed organization, special data collection diagrams, computer programs to manage huge amounts of data, and task-oriented teams of investigators are required. Fatigue and emotional responses must be recognized and sensitively managed.

Beyond the urgency of human identification, disasters provide opportunities to study injury patterns. For an individual, the injury pattern provides hints about the mechanism of injury, the interaction with surrounding environmental structures, and perhaps the cause of death. For groups, injury patterns may shed light upon mechanisms of injury, factors that prevented survival, and similar injury patterns from previous situations. The ultimate goal is to learn enough to reengineer the physical features of a vehicle or building to improve safety and prevent future deaths and disasters.

Body Packing

Illegal transportation of drugs within human beings is common because it is simple to accomplish and lucrative. Body packers are persons who smuggle drugs from one country to another by filling balloons or condoms with drugs and then swallowing the sausage-shaped packets. If timing is accurate, the packets are transported in the alimentary canal and excreted

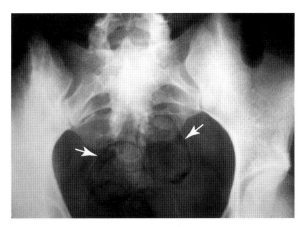

Figure 10 Body packer. Frontal view of pelvis shows packets (arrows) of drugs in rectum outlined by trapped gas.

at the target destination. If transportation is delayed or if bowel transit time quickens, the packets may pass through the intestines before the destination is reached, perhaps while still in transit. If the smuggler is unlucky, the packets may cause a bowel obstruction secondary to torsion, intussusception, or impaction. The resulting pain leads to medical attention and radiographs detect the packets. If the smuggler is particularly unlucky, one or more packets leak or rupture while in the intestine, leading to drug overdose and sometimes death. Postmortem imaging detects these packets because air trapped inside the packet or surrounding the packet outlines the shape. Travelers who are suspected of smuggling packets may be imaged upon arrival at international airports (**Figure 10**). Both conventional radiography and computed tomography (CT) successfully detect the drug-filled packets. Administration of an oral contrast agent may render the packets more conspicuous.

Documentation of Injury

Forensic imaging has another major application: documentation of injury. Many physical forces accidentally kill people and there are many motivations for causing nonaccidental injury. Among accidental injuries, motor vehicle and industrial accidents are common. Among nonaccidental injuries, gunshot wounds, knife wounds, and various forms of physical abuse are most common. Bombings are deliberate acts of aggression perpetrated for many reasons.

Physical trauma results in fractures and soft-tissue injuries. Traditionally, orthopedic surgery and medical imaging define how the fractures are detected, characterized, and categorized. To detect traumatic soft-tissue injuries in confined spaces such as the skull (e.g., epidural and subdural hematomas) or the abdomen (e.g., ruptured liver and spleen), CT is sometimes used. Recently, some forensic scientists have recommended whole-body CT as a routine screening tool to detect fractures, soft-tissue injuries, and foreign bodies. As yet, CT has not been widely adopted for this function because the technology is expensive. Conventional radiography remains the imaging method of choice.

Postmortem imaging of vehicular deaths is valuable. Victims include occupants of the vehicles, pedestrians, or riders of two-wheeled conveyances struck by vehicles. Experience and academic studies documented the high frequency of injury to the skull, spine, chest, pelvis, and long bones. Studies show that the class and severity of these skeletal injuries were dependent upon the mechanisms and force of the injury. In the mid-1960s, vehicle occupants had high prevalences of skull fracture, cervical spine fracture, and craniocervical dislocation (**Figure 11**). Documentation of these injury patterns and their mechanisms contributed to engineering and legislation that resulted in seatbelts, front compartment airbags, and specialized child restraints. The forensic team worked to define a problem and effect corrective action.

Other injury patterns result from pedestrian–vehicular accidents. A tibia-fibular fracture occurs where an automobile bumper contacts the leg of a pedestrian. A boot-top fracture occurs in similar circumstances but with the booted foot firmly planted on the pavement. The force from the bumper is dissipated at the boot top where the leg is no longer protected instead of at the point of bumper contact.

Many industrial injury patterns have been detected and documented radiographically. Efforts by forensic scientists led to many improvements and reduced the number of victims and the severity of their injuries.

Gunshot Wounds

Forensic pathologists routinely employ radiographs to locate and document bullets, fragments, and other projectiles. Because this use of imaging is so routine and well established, it is unusual for a forensic radiologist to be involved. There are pitfalls to assessment of bullet caliber or shotgun range from radiologic features. Usually, radiologists do not have expertise in ballistics and casual analysis is hazardous.

Description of skull fractures caused by gunshot wounds is challenging. The fractures initiated by a bullet as it enters the skull travel rapidly until they reach an open suture or another terminus such as the foramen magnum, at which point they stop. By the time the bullet exits the skull, the entrance wound fractures have completed their course, and the new set of fractures initiated at the exit wound stop when they reach the already existing entrance fractures. Secondary fractures do not cross the existing fractures. Second bullet fractures stop when they reach fractures created by prior bullets. With carefully obtained radiographs and cautious interpretation, entrance and exit wounds may be determined and later bullets may be differentiated from the initial bullet.

Bombings

Bombs are detonated to intimidate or eliminate people. Individuals target relatives; organized criminals select rivals; drug dealers pick persons who place them at risk or fail to pay debts, and terrorists maim and kill for political ends. Most bomb-makers have particular construction styles or use certain components. Therefore, bombs tend to have personalized aspects to their construction.

Conventional radiographs are used to survey survivors or human remains following a bombing to detect bomb components (**Figure 12**). Three types of imbedded trace evidence (radiolucent and radiopaque materials and explosive residues) are recovered from victims. Repeated images may be required to recover all possible bomb fragments. The goal is to locate and recover as much trace evidence as possible for reconstruction of the particular bomb. In this manner,

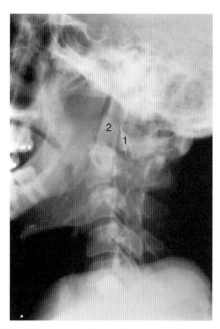

Figure 11   Vehicular accident with cervical dislocation causing death. The C1 vertebra (1) is posteriorly dislocated with respect to the C2 (2) vertebra, a finding best demonstrated with a lateral film of the cervical spine, like this one.

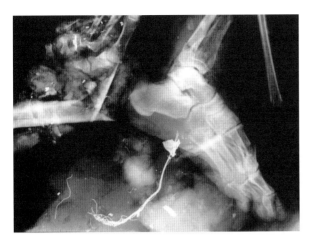

Figure 12 Bombing victim. Radiograph of fragmented lower legs and feet shows many metallic objects, some of which are trace evidence of the bomb.

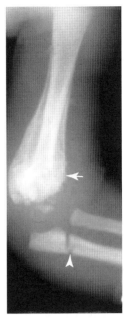

Figure 13 Nonaccidental childhood injury. Radiograph of arm shows diaphyseal fractures of humerus (healing) (arrow) and ulna (fresh: arrowhead) indicative of at least two episodes of trauma, a characteristic of child abuse. These probably occurred when the arm was grabbed and the child thrown on more than one occasion.

patterns of construction are identified that help to identify the bomb-maker and associate that individual with other similar bombings.

With undetonated bombs, radiographs of the device or package will show the details of construction yielding information about the detonation system, containment of the explosive, electronics that control the device, and an energy source.

Nonaccidental Injury

Abuse comes in many forms (e.g., child, spouse, elderly), occurs in many venues (e.g., homes, schools, hospitals, chronic care facilities), and takes place for many reasons (e.g., drug dependence, anger, mental illness). Forensic radiology plays a documentary role through detection and characterization of skeletal and visceral trauma. The results are particularly valuable in the courtroom. Discussion of abuse is beyond the scope of this article, with the exception of child abuse.

Child abuse is a combination of neglect, battery, and sexual molestation perpetrated on very young children. It is the fourth largest cause of childhood death under age 5 with a prevalence of about two million cases per year in the USA. At least 2000 children die each year. In 1946, John Caffey, one of the foremost pediatric radiologists, described the association of subdural hematomas and long-bone injuries in young children. Imaging has since become the primary method to identify, classify, and document the anatomic features of child abuse.

Imaging identifies sites of injury, documents patterns consistent with abuse, and helps establish a sequence of events and timeframe. A skeletal survey is used to detect fractures. Since the injuries may be

very subtle, the highest-quality images are preferred. CT is the method of choice to assess blunt abdominal trauma. Either CT or magnetic resonance imaging is effective to document, localize, and classify intracranial injury. Since many abused children spend time in an emergency room or hospital, imaging examinations may be obtained from these sources.

Diaphyseal fracture is the most common skeletal injury, but it is not specific. Femora and humeri are frequently affected, but fractures of other long bones also occur. When multiple bones are involved and when various stages of fracture healing are present, these findings indicate more than a single episode of trauma (**Figure 13**). Transverse fractures correlate with direct blows. Spiral fractures correlate with torsional forces. Typically, interviews with caregivers indicate a history of trauma that is disproportionately small as compared with the magnitude of detected fracture.

Metaphyseal fractures are less common than diaphyseal fractures, but are more specific for child abuse (**Figure 14**). These fractures occur at the corners of metaphyses, where the periosteal attachments are very strong and the bone is weakest. Sudden traction or twisting causes the corners of the metaphyses adjacent to the physeal plates to break free. Such "corner" fractures are most common about the knee joints.

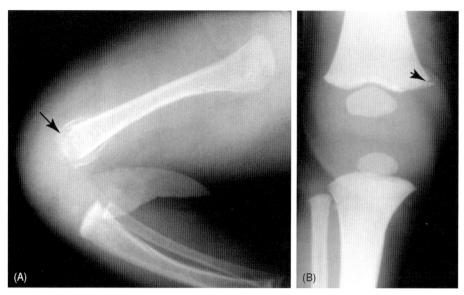

Figure 14   Nonaccidental childhood injury. (A) Radiograph of knee shows transmetaphyseal fracture (arrow) with periosteal healing indicating a subacute injury. (B) Radiograph of knee from another child shows metaphyseal "corner" fracture (arrowhead). Both examples are specific features of child abuse. These probably occurred when the legs were held and quickly twisted.

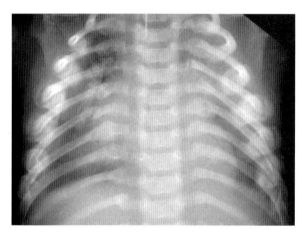

Figure 15   Nonaccidental childhood injury. Chest radiograph shows bilateral healing rib fractures. These probably occurred when the child's chest was held tightly with two hands as the child was shaken. Two sets of fractures (posterior and lateral) are present bilaterally.

Rib fractures, the third most frequent fractures in child abuse, are caused by squeezing the thorax during episodes of shaking (**Figure 15**). Sudden compression causes the ribs to break. Rib fractures tend to be multiple and in similar locations in a series of adjacent ribs.

Visceral injuries include duodenal and mesenteric hemorrhage, laceration of liver and spleen, and contusion of kidneys, bladder, and colon. Major chest trauma produces pulmonary contusion, pleural effusion, and cardiac injury. Direct blunt force, such as a kick, is causative.

A common cause of death, particularly for young victims, is cerebral injury due to direct blunt trauma, violent shaking, or both. Subdural hematomas, brain contusions and lacerations, and cerebral edema are all common injuries.

The forensic radiologist must be prepared to supervise the radiographic examination to ensure optimum positioning, spatial resolution, and exposure factors. Otherwise minute corner fractures or other subtle injuries may escape detection. The forensic radiologist must be certain the detected injury patterns are consistent with abuse and cannot be attributed to some other situation or condition. He/she must be prepared to go to court to present and defend the opinion in an evidence-based scientific manner.

Summary

For many reasons, medical examiners and coroners may not have established partnerships with radiologists. When the facilities in which each work are geographically separate, cooperative efforts are inconvenient. Possibly, medical examiners and coroners do much imaging themselves and feel comfortable being alone. Perhaps, utilization of imaging facilities or engagement of a radiologist is too expensive. Maybe radiologists are too busy, uninterested, or wary of involvement in legal matters or with a system they do not understand. Whatever the reason, failure to build a team effort with an interested radiologist is a lost opportunity. Combined professional expertise and perspective enhance results. To a great degree, the outcomes of forensic radiology are only limited by the willingness of professionals to act as a team, to follow natural investigative curiosity, and to use combined imagination to solve human anatomic problems.

See Also

Head Trauma: Pediatric and Adult, Clinical Aspects; Neuropathology; **Imaging:** Radiology, Pediatric, Scintigraphy and Child Abuse; **Injury, Transportation:** Motor Vehicle; **Mass Disasters:** Role of Forensic Pathologists

Further Reading

Alker GJ, Young SO, Leslie EV, *et al.* (1975) Postmortem radiology of head and neck injuries in fatal traffic accidents. *Radiology* 114: 611–617.

Brogdon BG (1998) *Forensic Radiology.* Boca Raton, FL: CRC Press.

Gill JR, Graham SM (2002) Ten years of "body packers" in New York City: 50 deaths. *Journal of Forensic Sciences* 47: 843–846.

Haglund WD (1992) Contribution of rodents to postmortem artifacts of bone and soft tissue. *Journal of Forensic Sciences* 37: 1459–1465.

Kahana T, Hiss J, Smith P (1998) Quantitative assessment of trabecular bone pattern identification. *Journal of Forensic Sciences* 43: 1144–1147.

Kirk NJ, Wood RE, Goldstein M (2002) Skeletal identification using the frontal sinus region: a retrospective study of 39 cases. *Journal of Forensic Sciences* 47: 318–323.

Kleinman PK, Blackbourne BD, Marks SC, Karellas A, Belanger PL (1989) Radiologic contributions to the investigation and prosecution of cases of fatal infant abuse. *New England Journal of Medicine* 320: 507–511.

Kuehn CM, Taylor KM, Mann FA, Wilson AJ, Harruff RC (2002) Validation of chest X-ray comparisons for unknown decedent identification. *Journal of Forensic Sciences* 47: 725–729.

Lichtenstein JE (1996) Forensic radiology. In: Gagliardi RA, McClennan BL (eds.) *A History of the Radiological Sciences Diagnosis,* pp. 579–605. Reston: Radiology Centennial.

Lichtenstein JE, Madewell JE, McMeekin RR, Feigin DS, Wolcott JH (1980) Role of radiology in aviation accident investigation. *Aviation Space and Environmental Medicine* 51: 1004–1014.

Messmer JM, Fierro MF (1986) Radiologic forensic investigation of fatal gunshot wounds. *RadioGraphics* 6: 457–473.

Mulligan ME, McCarthy MJ, Wippold FJ, Lichtenstein JE, Wagner GN (1988) Radiologic evaluation of mass casualty victims: lessons from the Gander, Newfoundland, accident. *Radiology* 168: 229–233.

Nye PJ, Tytle TL, Jarman RN, Eaton BG (1996) The role of radiology in the Oklahoma city bombing. *Radiology* 200: 541–543.

Owsley DW, Mann RW, Chapman RE, Moore E, Cox WA (1993) Positive identification in a case of intentional extreme fragmentation. *Journal of Forensic Sciences* 38: 985–996.

Puerini S, Spruill FG, Puerini A (1977) Forensic odontology: identification problems in Rhode Island. *Rhode Island Dental Journal* 10: 5–7.

Quatrehomme G, İşcan Y (1999) Characteristics of gunshot wounds in the skull. *Journal of Forensic Sciences* 44: 568–576.

Singleton AC (1951) The roentgenological identification of victims of the "Noronic" disaster. *American Journal of Radiology* 66: 375–384.

Stewart JH, McCormick WF (1981) A sex- and age-limited ossification pattern in human costal cartilages. *American Journal of Clinical Pathology* 81: 755–759.

Radiology, Non-Invasive Autopsies

M J Thali and P Vock, University of Bern, Bern, Switzerland

Introduction

In recent times, radiology has been one of the few fields in medicine that have witnessed impressive progress: digital data acquisition and postprocessing of images have revolutionized the practice of radiology and have brought about a growing interest in this field on the part of other medical professionals. The application of imaging methods for documentation and analysis of relevant noninvasive forensic findings in living and dead persons has lagged behind the enormous technical development of imaging methods. There are only a few textbooks dealing with forensic radiology, most of which concentrate on classical roentgenographic methods and hardly cover the newer sectional imaging techniques of computed tomography (CT) and magnetic resonance imaging (MRI) in detail.

Forensic radiology, including all techniques and their many uses for forensic purpose, now is a rapidly growing interdisciplinary subspecialty of both forensic medicine and radiology.

Imaging Techniques and Historical Development

In 1895 Conrad Roentgen obtained the first radiograph of a human being: the hand of his wife. He called the new kind of rays "X-rays." Shortly after the detection of X-rays, the new noninvasive technique was used for forensic documentation purposes.

Since the 1970s, there have been several impressive new developments in radiology: ultrasonography, CT, MRI and magnetic resonance spectroscopy were developed and soon utilized for medical applications. The introduction of true tomography, increased contrast, and resolution opened absolutely new possibilities of two- and three-dimensional visualization. Diagnostic imaging is still underutilized in forensics, because its potential is less well known and also because of the cost. There is also limited access to and training for newer cross-section modalities, such as CT and MRI.

Computed Tomography

Computed tomography was introduced by Hounsfield and Cormack in the early 1970s, for which they won the Nobel Prize in 1979. CT was also called computed axial tomography (CAT), and the examinations, thus, were named CAT scans. CT uses the same technique as radiography to produce X-rays. However, to obtain transverse (axial) images of body sections, the tube rotates around the longitudinal (z-) axis of the body, transmitting radiation from many angular positions through the body. Within the human body, X-rays are absorbed according to the radiographic density of tissues; those not absorbed reach the detector system beyond the patient, contributing to the absorption profile of one specific tube angle. The many profiles measured during one rotation are used by the computer to calculate a density map of the body section with discrete absolute density values of all image elements (voxels). Density is expressed in Hounsfield units (HU): −1000 HU corresponds to gas, around −50 HU to −200 HU to fat, around −10 to 20 HU to fluid, 20–70 HU to solid tissue, whereas >100 HU usually means calcification; metal objects can reach very high densities, far more than 1000 HU, and may then cause streak artifacts. Historically, the first CT scanner was specifically engineered to image the brain; the total scan time was approximately 25 min. Although imaging time for one slice has been reduced to less than 1 s in the meantime, these CT scanners, now referred to as conventional CT scanners, involved alternating patient exposure and patient translation. A major advance in CT technology occurred with the development and implementation of helical or spiral CT in 1989. CT became very fast, and instead of one slice previously measured during one rotation of the tube and the detectors, a spiral (or helical) scanning technique, combining tube rotation with longitudinal

transportation of the patient, allowed for acquisition of a complete volumetric data set of a body region. The most recent advance in CT technology has brought multidetector row helical CT, multiplying the measurement capacity by acquiring 4–16 or more slices during each tube rotation. As a result, CT data can be obtained faster, with thinner slice collimation and/or over a larger volume than with single-slice helical CT. With the development of "multislice CT" and current imaging workstations, the examiner is no longer restricted to axial slice review. Isotropic voxels, that is, image volume elements of identical dimension in all three directions of the space, are an ideal basis for image postprocessing using multiplanar reformation to obtain images in sagittal, coronal, oblique, or curved planes; similarly, three-dimensional presentation methods allow for specific views of the entire volume. Multislice CT offers many advantages over single-slice CT and has become the standard for CT imaging.

Magnetic Resonance Imaging

In MRI, because of the dependence of resonance frequency on local magnetic field strength, it is possible to encode spatial information by using a magnetic gradient in the slice direction. Although a large number of nuclei offer the magnetic characteristics required for magnetic resonance, medical MRI nearly exclusively uses hydrogen nuclei (^{1}H). A strong magnetic field is primarily produced by a supraconducting magnet, and gradients are temporarily superposed to minimally change the field strength during the measurement in order to encode the topographic position of specific nuclei. Radiofrequency waves of the specific wavelength matching the field strength of protons in one specific position are then used to stimulate the tissue; energy introduced into the body will be emitted again as radiowaves of identical wavelength. Their intensity depends on the delay period and characterizes the chemical neighborhood of the protons. A coil or antenna is needed for sending and receiving these radiofrequency waves. The unique advantage of MRI is its flexibility in producing variable contrast, reflecting different tissue characteristics, just by modifying the sequence (this term means the specific combination of radiofrequency waves and magnetic field gradients used to acquire a number of usually parallel images). For instance, MRI can produce separate images of the protons bound to water and of those chemically bound to lipids of the same plane of tissue. In routine practice, the majority of the MRI sequences now in use are two-dimensional techniques, producing a number of separate parallel images, whereas three-dimensional sequences produce a three-dimensional data set, similar to spiral CT.

Furthermore, a modification of the method called magnetic resonance spectroscopy (MRS) concentrates on differentiating molecules based on the minimal modification of the resonance frequency by the chemical neighborhood of ^{1}H or other nuclei. This nondestructive chemical analysis has recently gained wide clinical interest, and it has the potential to become an important forensic tool despite its low spatial resolution.

Postprocessing: Two- and Three-Dimensional Visualization

Postprocessing, particularly three-dimensional reconstruction of cross-sectional images satisfies an esthetic requirement and also has become a tool useful for representing complex anatomical structures and for the understanding of relevant forensic pathological changes and traumatic findings. Surface rendering (surface shaded display, SSD) and volume rendering (VR) displays represent the most important techniques used for three-dimensional visualization.

SSD represents a visualization technique which is well established for three-dimensional imaging of skin and bone surfaces. The key idea of surface-based rendering methods is to extract an intermediate surface description of the relevant objects from the volume data. The SSD method basically involves construction of polygonal surfaces in the data sets, whereas VR assigns a color and an opacity value to each voxel of the data set and projects the elements directly onto the image plane without the use of polygons. VR is a popular and basically more powerful technique than SSD to represent and analyze volume data. In volume rendering, images are created directly from the volume data, and no intermediate geometry is extracted; however, the volume of data to be handled is much larger than for the pure surface extraction of SSD.

History of Forensic Application of CT

The first forensic application of CT was a description of the pattern of a gunshot injury to the head. In the early years of CT application, due to limited image quality, resolution, and postprocessing techniques, only a few studies correlated pathologic findings of full-body postmortem CT to forensic autopsy. Even the introduction of spiral CT, which opened the door to three-dimensional data acquisition and processing, did not significantly increase the interest of forensic science in this new modality. In contrast, nondestructive analysis by CT has been used

for many years in paleoimaging, e.g., for examining mummies.

History of Forensic Application of MRI

Full-body postmortem MRI in nonforensic cases has been described by different groups for the detection of gross cranial, thoracic, and abdominal pathology.

The Swiss Virtual Autopsy Project (VIRTOPSY)

The Institute of Forensic Medicine, with the Institute of Diagnostic Radiology, the University of Bern, Switzerland, started a research project in 2000, hypothesizing that noninvasive imaging might predict autopsy findings and perhaps give additional information. In this joint project called "VIRTOPSY" the newest generation of multidetector row CT (MSCT) and a 1.5 T MR scanner were used. Nearly 100 forensic cases have since received a full-body examination by CT and MRI before autopsy. The results of CT and MRI were correlated with the findings of autopsy.

Based on this experience, CT is the superior tool for two- and three-dimensional documentation and analysis of fracture systems, pathologic gas collections (whether air embolism, subcutaneous emphysema after trauma, hyperbaric trauma, or decomposition effects) and it also shows gross tissue injury (**Figures 1–3**). The scan times are short, around 1–10 min, depending on the slice thickness and the volume to be covered. Postprocessing with three-dimensional SSD and VR can provide useful visualization for use in court (**Figures 1** and **2**). For example, in gunshot cases, the determination of entrance and exit wounds is possible based on the characteristic fracture pattern with inward or outward beveling of the bone, respectively. CT and MRI are excellent tools for visualizing bullet tracks with hemorrhage. Metal artifacts from the bullet can appear on CT images; these effects will be reduced in the near future by metal artifact reduction algorithms. As compared to clinical imaging in trauma or forensic victims, the major drawback of postmortem CT is the lack of availability of intravenous contrast enhancement after circulatory arrest, which makes analysis of parenchymal and vascular injury much more difficult, less sensitive, and less specific.

MRI, compared to CT, clearly has a higher sensitivity, specificity, and accuracy in demonstrating soft tissue injury, neurological and nonneurological organ trauma, and nontraumatic pathology (**Figures 4–7**). Studies of child abuse victims confirm the sensitivity of postmortem MRI for contusion, shearing injuries, and subdural hematoma. Differences in morphology and signal characteristics between antemortem and

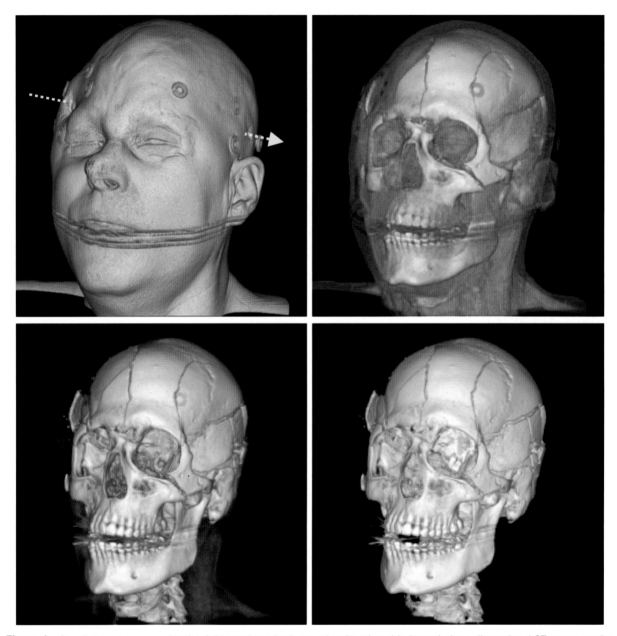

Figure 1   Gunshot entrance wound at the right temple and exit wound at the other side (arrow): three-dimensional CT reconstruction (VR and SSD) showing skin defect and fracture system. (Radiological ring landmarks are used for orientation purposes.)

postmortem MRI do exist; however, they have not yet been studied systematically. If the results of clinical MRI can be transferred to postmortem analysis, there is a great future for nondestructive analysis of visceral pathology, such as cardiac (including coronary), pulmonary, and hepatic disease.

Finally, MRS, combined with MRI, has a great potential in documenting preterminal and postmortem metabolite concentrations in tissues. Since decomposition continuously changes the concentration of chemical compounds, postmortem MRS might be helpful in determining the time of death.

Forensic Application of Radiological Microimaging: Virtual Histology

In many cases, the resolution of clinical scanners is not sufficient to answer questions relevant to forensic medicine nondestructively. This favors the idea of using microimaging methods with their much higher resolution to visualize forensic specimens. We have used micro-CT of a knife blade inside cortical and trabecular bone to determine the injury pattern and the weapon involved. In forensic soft tissue injury, retinal hemorrhage and electric injury to the skin

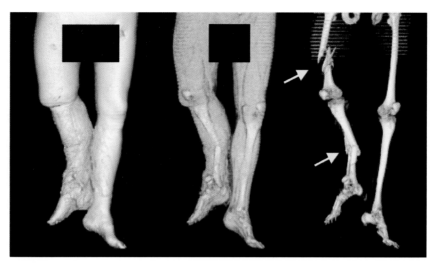

Figure 2 Three-dimensional CT reconstruction (VR) of a right leg fracture.

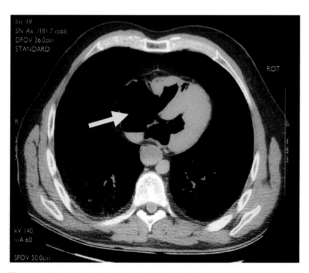

Figure 3 CT showing intracardial air embolism in heart chamber (arrow).

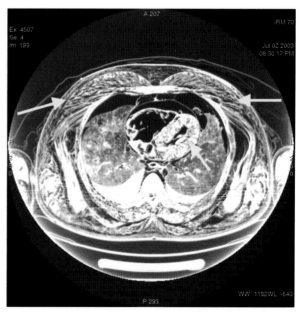

Figure 4 Decomposed body: CT showing typical signs of soft-tissue decomposition with decomposition gas in muscle and heart tissue (arrows).

were studied by micro-MR (MR microscopy). We expect these new radiological cross-sectional micro-imaging methods to have a comparable impact on (forensic) histopathology, leading to virtual histology.

Outlook

Evidently imaging techniques are excellent tools for forensic medicine. Although these are similar to inspection and photography, with imaging techniques it is possible to freeze the findings at the moment of investigation without causing any damage. Freezing means permanent (analog or digital) preservation as a document of proof, whether the victim is dead and undergoing postmortem decay or surviving and losing evidence due to healing. Causing no damage is an essential prerequisite in a living person, which is

indisputably fulfilled by these techniques. Even in the case of dead persons, nondestructive documentation is important for two reasons. First, it brings the information without precluding any other conservative or destructive forensic investigation. Second, it can be used in cultures and situations where autopsy is not tolerated by religion or is rejected by family members. Whether and to what degree radiological minimally invasive "virtual autopsy" will replace the classical dissection technique in well-defined situations will be decided in the near future.

Two innovative forensic documentation methods will soon be available: the combination of sectional

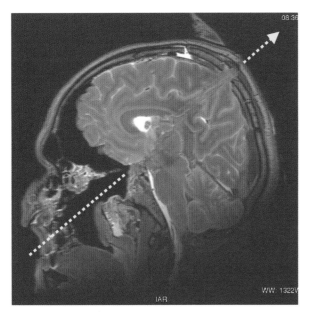

Figure 5 Gunshot through the mouth: sagittal MR image showing the bullet track (arrow) through the brain. Note the typical configuration of the exit lesion of the skull (arrowhead).

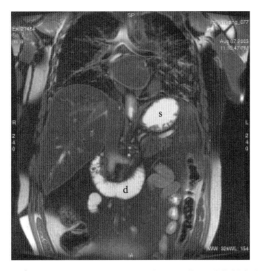

Figure 6 Coronal MR image showing swallowed fluid in both the stomach (s) and the duodenum (d) in a case of drowning. This finding is a forensically relevant feature, the so-called "vital reaction sign," in drowning cases.

imaging with surface documentation methods, such as photogrammetry and three-dimensional optical scanning and the combination of noninvasive imaging with minimally invasive image-guided tissue sampling from any body location needed. Tissue samples can be used for cytologic, histologic, chemical, and microbiological analysis. Radiologic virtual autopsy offers other advantages, such as easy examination of bodies contaminated by infection, toxic

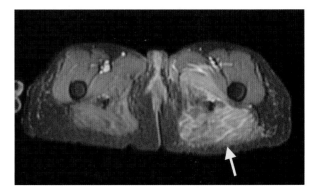

Figure 7 Axial MR image of the pelvic area showing contusion and hematoma of the left musculus gluteus maximus (arrow) after blunt force impact by a motor vehicle.

substances, radionuclides, or other biohazards. Two- and three-dimensional postprocessing helps in visualizing the findings by people not present during the examination, e.g., in court. Complete, easily retrievable digital archives will support the process of quality improvement.

Imaging technology is developing fast, and new technical solutions will be introduced soon, such as area-detector CT, high-field MRI, or moving-table whole-body MRI. They will be supported by improved two- and three-dimensional sequences and user-friendly postprocessing two- and three-dimensional software with a significant impact on forensic sciences. The cost of high-tech imaging systems, although currently often a hurdle that is slowing their routine forensic application, will decrease in the near future.

In conclusion, imaging has already proved to be a reliable tool in modern forensic medicine to answer a number of questions. It is currently limited where color is important and where *in vivo* imaging uses contrast agents distributed by the circulation and accumulated locally by a tissue leak or metabolism. In these and other situations, upcoming approaches have to undergo validation by correlation with classical autopsy before their value can be assessed. Further technical developments in radiology are likely to enhance the forensic applications of imaging.

See Also

Imaging: Radiology, Overview; Radiology, Pediatric, Scintigraphy and Child Abuse

Further Reading

Brogdon BG (1998) *Forensic Radiology.* Boca Raton: CRC Press.
Hart BL, Dudley MH, Zumwalt RE (1996) Postmortem cranial MRI and autopsy correlation in suspected child

abuse. *American Journal of Forensic Medicine and Pathology* 17(3): 217–224.

Institute of Forensic Medicine and Institute of Diagnostic Radiology, Berne University (2001) "VIRTOPSY" project. Available online: www.virtopsy.com

Thali M, Braun M, Kneubuehl B, *et al.* (2000) Improved vision in forensic documentation: forensic, 3D/CAD-supported photogrammetry of bodily injury external surfaces, combined with volumetric radiologic scanning of bodily injury internal structures to provide more leads and stronger forensic evidence. In: Oliver W (ed.) 3D Visualisation for Data Exploration and Decision Making. *SPIE*, 2000, pp. 213–221.

Thali M, Taubenreuther U, Braun M, *et al.* (2001) *Micro-CT and Forensic Pathology.* Proceedings of the 80th Annual Congress of the German Forensic Society 2001. Germany: Rostock.

Thali M, Dirnhofer R, Potter K (2003) *Forensic MR Microscopy: Analysis of Blunt Forces Trauma in Skin and Subcutanous Fat Tissue.* Proceedings of the International Society for Magnetic Resonance in Medicine 2003. Canada: Toronto.

Thali M, Potter K, Dirnhofer R (2003) *From Virtopsy to Micro-Virtopsy: Virtual Forensic Histology.* Proceedings of the 81th Annual Congress of the German Forensic Society. Germany: Rostock.

Thali M, Braun M, Dirnhofer R (2003) Optical 3D surface digitizing in forensic medicine: 3D documentation of skin and bone injuries. *Forensic Science International* 137: 203–208.

Thali M, Braun M, Wirth J, Vock P, Dirnhofer R (2003) 3D surface and 3D body documentation in forensic medicine: 3D/CAD photogrammetry merged with 3D radiological scanning. *Journal of Forensic Science* 48(6): 1356–1365.

Thali MJ, Yen K, Schweitzer W, *et al.* (2003) Virtopsy, a new imaging horizon in forensic pathology: virtual autopsy by postmortem multislice computed tomography (MSCT) and magnetic resonance imaging (MRI) – a feasibility study. *Journal of Forensic Science* 48(2): 386–403.

Radiology, Pediatric, Scintigraphy and Child Abuse

C M Hall, Great Ormond Street Hospital for Children, London, UK

Introduction

Nonaccidental injury or physical abuse is most commonly seen in nonambulant, totally dependent infants. It accounts for 22% of all forms of child abuse, the most common being that of neglect. The number of reported cases of physical abuse has been rising steadily over the years, partly as a result of increased recognition of the problem by clinicians, healthcare workers, and social workers, and partly because of an increasing incidence attributable to poverty, family stresses, and a general breakdown of family stability, structure, and support. Whilst abuse is most common in deprived, lower-social-class families, often with a history of substance abuse and themselves having been the subject of physical abuse in childhood, it occurs in all strata of society and across all ethnic groups.

Clinical presentation is often as a result of the superficial evidence of bruising, burns, or bleeding from an orifice or torn frenulum. It may also be as a result of a major fracture, the effects of which cannot be ignored by the regular carers, or by an acute collapse from intracerebral trauma or a ruptured abdominal viscus. Whenever physical abuse is suspected social services should be informed and it is imperative that a skeletal survey and a computed tomographic (CT) head scan should be performed. This is because many of the fractures caused by abuse are clinically silent in that they are not associated with overlying swelling or bruising, and in a similar way subdural bleeding following shaking may be occult.

Imaging Strategy

The skeletal survey should be performed in normal working hours after explaining the reasons for it to the carers. Two healthcare professionals (radiographer or nurse) should remain with the baby throughout the examination and initial each film. The skeletal survey should include:

- skull – anteroposterior (AP) and lateral
- spine – lateral
- chest – AP
- upper and lower limbs – AP
- pelvis – AP
- both hands – posteroanterior (PA)
- both feet – dorsoplantar (DP).

Additional views may be necessary. These may include oblique views of the chest to identify rib fractures, coned views of the metaphyseal regions when these are not clearly seen on the limb views, lateral long-bone views when a fracture has been identified to evaluate displacement, and a Townes view when an occipital fracture is suspected.

Delayed images after a few days or weeks may help in identifying previously unrecognized acute rib fractures and in dating fractures. Early new bone formation (periosteal reaction) at the site of a fracture is first seen 7 days after the injury and then gradually increases in size (soft callus) and consolidates (hard callus), before remodeling takes place. When the fracture is relatively undisplaced, remodeling of rib and long-bone fractures has occurred by about 12 weeks. The fracture line usually disappears between 6 and 8 weeks after the fracture has been sustained.

If fractures are identified, then other children under the age of 2 years with the same carers should be examined clinically and have a skeletal survey performed to identify clinically occult fractures. Children over this age would be expected to be able to communicate painful areas and do not require a full skeletal survey.

A radioisotope bone scan is not a routine investigation and should not replace the skeletal survey, but as an adjunct it may identify unrecognized injuries, in particular those involving the spine and ribs, which may be missed on conventional radiography. Scintigraphy, however, fails to demonstrate certain fractures. Skull fractures show no evidence of increased uptake of isotope and because normal infants' metaphyses show increased uptake, metaphyseal fractures may be missed.

A CT head scan is recommended as part of the initial investigation whenever physical abuse is suspected, even when there are no neurological signs, to identify occult and old subdural hematomas. This should also be performed on bone window settings for further evaluation of any fractures, but should not replace the skull views on the skeletal survey. Sometimes skull fractures may not be demonstrated on the CT scan when they lie in the same plane as the plane of the scan.

When the infant presents with an acute head injury, the initial CT head scan should be followed by magnetic resonance imaging (MRI) head scans for clinical management and for more accurate dating.

Cerebral ultrasound, in experienced hands, may be a useful adjunct to the CT scan in the acute phase but is not a routine part of the investigation.

If visceral injury is suspected, ultrasound is the initial imaging modality of choice, followed by a CT scan of the abdomen or a contrast study of the gastrointestinal tract.

This imaging strategy is broadly recommended by the UK Royal College of Radiologists, but certain local protocols may differ depending on specific expertise and timely availability of equipment.

The role of the radiologist is to supervise the films being performed, both their number and quality, to identify all the bony injuries and soft-tissue changes,

and to give an age range for each fracture and indicate potential mechanisms of causation. Any explanations for the injuries occurring as a result of accidents should be fully explored and evaluated. The skeletal survey should be carefully examined for the radiological changes of any medical condition that might predispose to fracturing. Knowledge of normal variant findings, which may be present in the infant's developing skeleton, is essential and generally requires consultation with a specialist pediatric radiologist. A full report should be issued immediately and the findings communicated to the relevant consultant pediatrician. This process should not be delayed, even if a further opinion from a specialist pediatric radiologist is being obtained. The radiologist should recommend delayed views when appropriate for more accurate dating of specific fractures. The radiologist may be the first person to identify specific injuries associated with nonaccidental injury, for example, rib fractures on a chest radiograph performed for a chest infection, and should be personally responsible for ensuring that the relevant agencies are informed and the child is safely placed in a nonabusing environment.

Diaphyseal Fractures

The commonest presenting fracture is of a diaphyseal long-bone fracture, most commonly affecting the humerus. The fracture may be spiral, caused by an applied twisting force below the site of the fracture, or occurring when the infant is rapidly lifted by one limb, with the counter forces of gravity and the weight of the infant resulting in the body twisting. Alternatively, the fracture may be transverse (oblique), caused either by a direct blow at the site of the fracture or by an applied levering force with the pivot or fulcrum at the site of the fracture. Diaphyseal fractures are not specific for nonaccidental injury but there would need to be an appropriate accidental explanation of a significant incident to account for such a fracture in an infant. The specificity would increase if an additional injury is present, there is an inappropriate history, or if there has been delay in presentation for medical attention. Deformity may be immediately apparent if there is angulation of the broken ends of the bone to each other. Diaphyseal fractures are usually associated with overlying soft-tissue swelling from edema, which may extend up and down the injured limb, gradually developing over the course of the first 2 days. The presence of bruising will depend on the mechanism of causation of the fracture. Forces applied by adult hands cover a relatively large surface area and are usually not associated with superficial bruising. Fractures resulting from a direct blow however are more likely to have bruising. The infant experiences pain when the fracture occurs and whenever the limb is handled

and on movement of the injured limb, resulting in a reluctance or inability to move it, with the limb appearing floppy. The pain is demonstrated as soon as the fracture occurs and is ongoing on being handled for about 1 week (**Figures 1–3**).

Metaphyseal Fractures

Metaphyseal fractures occur at the ends (the metaphyses) of the long bones, commonly above and below the knees, and consist of a thin rim of bone detached from the adjacent metaphysis. Depending on their angulation relative to the X-ray beam they may have a "bucket-handle" appearance or appear as "corner" fractures. They are considered to be highly specific for nonaccidental injury as they are caused by applied gripping, twisting, and pulling forces applied to the ends of the bones. Rarely they are caused by shaking when the limbs flail around and are subject to torsional forces. The amount of force required to cause them is entirely inappropriate for the normal handling of an infant and they do not occur as a result of heavy-handedness, playful handling, or inexperience. They are difficult to date as they may heal without callus formation, gradually consolidating to the adjacent metaphysis. An estimate of the age of the injury may be made from the clarity or otherwise of the fracture line. When it becomes indistinct the fracture is in the process of healing and is at least 7 days old. Unless

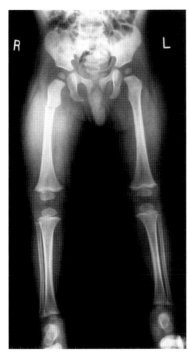

Figure 1 There is a transverse fracture of the upper shaft of the right femur with surrounding soft tissue swelling and loss of definition of the soft tissue planes due to edema.

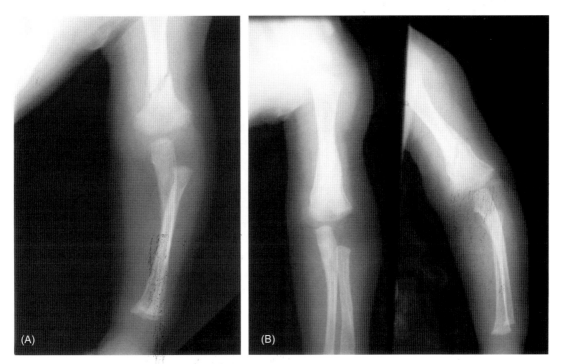

Figure 2 (A) An oblique fracture of the lower shaft of the left humerus showing a very early healing reaction. (B) The same fracture three weeks later shows a good healing response with callus formation. The fracture line is still visible.

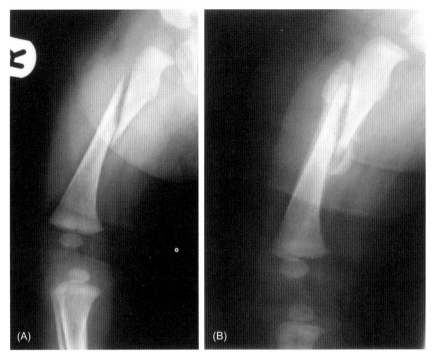

Figure 3   (A) Acute oblique fracture of the upper right femur. (B) The fracture two weeks later shows soft callus formation.

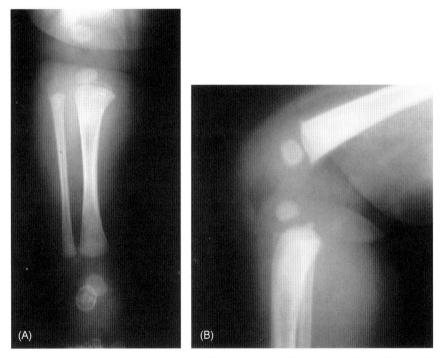

Figure 4   (A) There is a fracture separation of a right upper tibial metaphyseal fracture together with the adjacent epiphysis. The metaphyseal fracture is seen as a rim of bone giving a 'bucket handle' appearance on this frontal projection. (B) The same fracture on a lateral projection has an appearance of 'corner' fractures.

they are widely displaced from the adjacent shaft of the bone, metaphyseal fractures have completely healed by 4 weeks. They are rarely associated with overlying soft-tissue swelling or bruising and therefore are not apparent on clinical examination. Metaphyseal fractures result in tenderness on direct palpation of the injured area for a few days (**Figures 4** and 5).

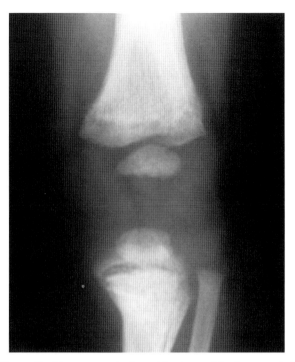

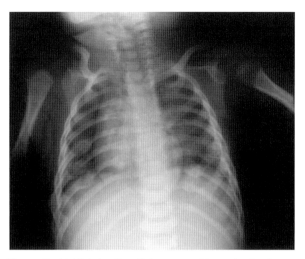

Figure 6 Multiple healing rib fractures with good callus formation are present at the posterior ends of the ribs, along the posterior arcs of the ribs and in the mid axillary line at the side of the infant.

Figure 5 There are metaphyseal fractures of the lower end of the left femur and the upper end of the left tibia. These are both in the process of healing with consolidation to the adjacent bone and loss of definition of the fracture lines. They are therefore more than one week but less than four weeks old.

Rib Fractures

Rib fractures are caused by severe compressive or squeezing forces to the chest and may occur at any point along the ribs, although posterior fractures adjacent to the spine are thought to be more specific for nonaccidental injury. The amount of force required to produce them is considerable, for example, they hardly ever occur as a result of cardiac resuscitation when the chest needs to be compressed by one-third of its depth to be effective. In the absence of an underlying medical condition rib fractures are highly specific for nonaccidental injury. They are not usually associated with superficial changes in the form of swelling or bruising at the sites of the fractures, although rarely there may be evidence of fingertip bruising in the position of the applied squeezing force. Occasionally the carers identify a crackling sensation, felt when the infant is picked up: this signifies a rib fracture. Rib fractures result in immediate pain and there is ongoing pain when the infant is picked up for a period of a few days. One effect of the pain from rib fractures is for the infant to breathe more rapidly and shallowly than usual and this may lead to the development of a lower respiratory chest infection. Occasionally underlying lung contusion or hemothorax may occur as a direct consequence of the

chest trauma. Rib fractures may not be identified until healing periosteal new bone is seen some 7 days after they have occurred. This is because only those fractures in the same line as the X-ray beam can be identified in the acute phase (first 7 days). Oblique views of the chest help to reduce the number of acute fractures that are missed. The squeezing force causing rib fractures may sometimes be associated with a shaking action, resulting in subdural hemorrhages. If the infant dies, acute rib fractures are readily identified at postmortem examination because of bleeding, but the pathologist may not readily identify older fractures where the callus has almost remodeled (**Figure 6**). Specimen high-resolution radiographs performed postmortem provide more information on the number of rib fractures and other subtle fractures (metaphyseal) (**Figure 7**).

Costochondral Junction Fractures

Costochondral junction fractures at the very anterior ends of the ribs are difficult to identify and commonly missed. They behave like metaphyseal fractures in that they usually heal by gradually consolidating to the adjacent rib without developing callus; this makes them difficult to date with any accuracy. Whilst they may be caused by a squeezing force to the chest, they may also result from a direct blow or punch to the epigastrium. This latter mechanism is more common in young, actively mobile children, rather than in infants. There is a significant association between costochondral junction fractures and abdominal visceral injuries.

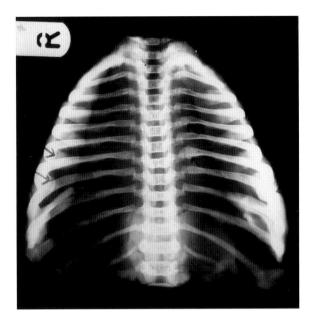

Figure 7 High-resolution specimen radiograph following dissection of the thorax at postmortem. Arrows identify anterior rib fractures which would have been difficult to identify before the postmortem.

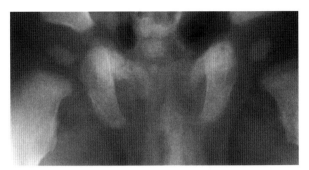

Figure 8 The coned view of the hips shows a healing fracture of the right pubic ramus.

Periosteal reactions along the shafts of long bones may occur from gripping and twisting shearing forces around the limbs. They are the healing response to damage to the superficial periosteum around the surface of the bone. Those resulting from trauma usually extend down to the metaphyses, and may be asymmetric or layered like an onion skin. To be visible on the radiograph they must be at least 7 days old. They gradually consolidate to the adjacent bone. They need to be differentiated from normal physiological periosteal reactions, which are the result of rapid bone growth and are seen in about 40% of infants under the age of 4 months. They are usually symmetrical and affect only the mid-diaphyses.

Unusual Fractures

Unusual fractures in infants are considered to be highly specific for nonaccidental injury. These include fractures of the acromion processes, first ribs, short tubular bones of the hands and feet, pubic rami, vertebrae, and long-bone epiphyseal separation fractures. Because they are unusual it is difficult to be certain of their precise mechanisms of causation. A fracture of the acromion process of the scapula is thought to be caused by forcefully swinging the infant by one arm. Fractures involving the hands and feet occur from crushing, bending, or stamping actions. Pubic rami fractures occur as a result of direct forces on the front of the pelvis. Vertebral body crush fractures are thought to occur when the

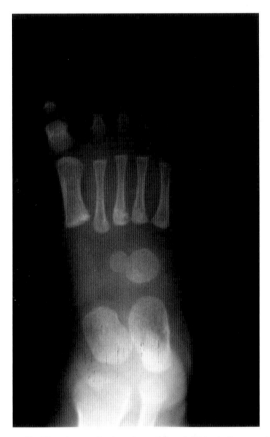

Figure 9 The dorso-plantar view of the right foot shows subtle healing fractures of the bases of the third and fourth metatarsals.

infant's body is forcefully flexed or when forces are transmitted along the spine, for example, from a blow to the top of the head. Long-bone epiphyseal separation fractures occur when the limbs are forcefully pulled, pushed, and twisted (**Figures 8–11**).

Skull Fractures

Skull fractures may occur as a result of accidental or nonaccidental injury and presentation may be because of an overlying soft, boggy swelling. The

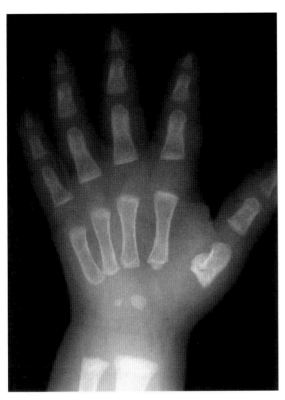

Figure 10 There is a healing fracture of the base of the first metacarpal in this young infant.

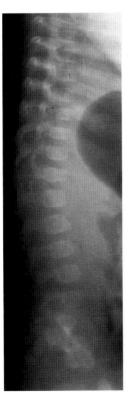

Figure 11 The lateral spine shows several crush fractures with loss of height of the affected vertebral bodies in the lower thoracic region.

commonest pattern is that of a single, linear, hairline, parietal fracture, which may be seen as a result of either accidental or nonaccidental injury. Accidental skull fractures need an appropriate history of a significant incident, usually of a fall from at least a meter on to a firm or hard surface, to account for them. Even these significant domestic falls rarely result in any fracture, the incidence being of the order of 2%. Fractures resulting from accidental domestic falls are rarely associated with intracranial injuries. Patterns of skull fractures which indicate that forces greater than those normally occurring as a result of simple domestic falls of between 1 and 2 m are recognized. Each one is suggestive, but not diagnostic, of nonaccidental injury and include wide fractures (5 mm or more), fractures affecting more than one bone in the skull, multiple fractures, those crossing sutures, those which are fissured or branching, those affecting the occipital bone, or those which are depressed. Skull fractures do not heal by developing callus. They may remain visible for weeks and even months and cannot be dated from the radiographic appearances. If soft-tissue swelling is present overlying the fracture it is likely to have occurred within the previous 7 days (**Figures 12** and **13**).

Any isolated fracture occurring in a nonambulant infant, without an appropriate incident to account for it, should be regarded as being the result of nonaccidental injury. It should be remembered however that sometimes an accident has occurred which the carer is unable to admit and the whole family and social circumstances should be evaluated. Medically it is important to exclude any skeletal disorder which may predispose to fractures, such as osteogenesis imperfecta, a metabolic bone disease, or underlying neurological disorder. When more than one fracture is present, or there is evidence of other forms of abuse, and when they have occurred on more than one occasion without appropriate explanations, then the diagnosis of nonaccidental injury becomes more certain. Inevitably a multidisciplinary approach is required.

Differential Diagnosis

Infants who present with multiple fractures need full evaluation for possible medical causes of undue bone fragility. In general, by the time the infant is sustaining fractures from an underlying medical condition, there will be some evidence of specific and diagnostic findings on the radiographs. These need to be evaluated in conjunction with clinical and biochemical findings and with the family history. Osteopathy of prematurity is seen in a small proportion of neonates of 32 weeks' gestation or less who have not had

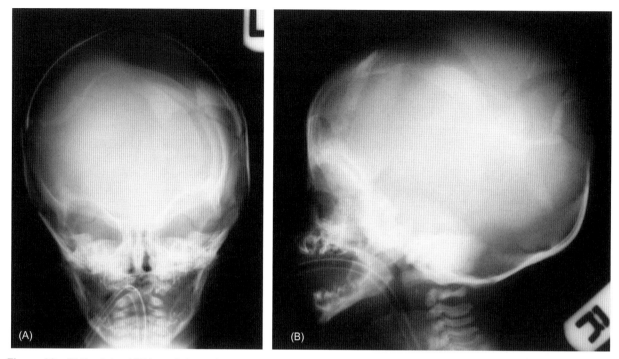

Figure 12   (A) Frontal and (B) lateral views of the skull showing multiple, depressed, wide fractures affecting serval bones in the skull, all fractures suggesting significant impacts.

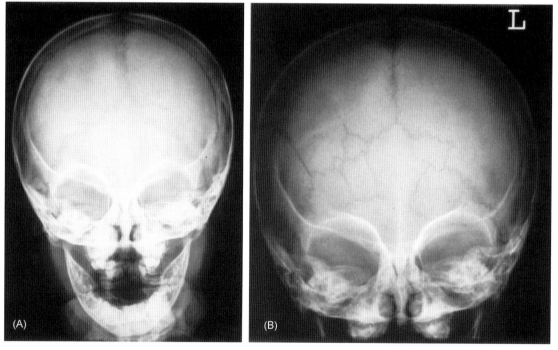

Figure 13   (A) A normal frontal skull radiograph showing a single wormian (sutural) bone in the left limb of the lambdoid suture. (B) The same patient three months later showing multiple occipital and right parietal fractures. The occipital fractures were mistakenly identified as multiple wormian bones.

appropriate phosphate supplements. Fractures may occur under 6 months of age and radiologically there is osteopenia with coarsening of the trabecular pattern and some irregularity and fraying of the

metaphyses (**Figure 14**). Similar radiological changes occur in older infants suffering from rickets, resulting from various causes. Copper deficiency may predispose to fractures, but by the time fractures occur,

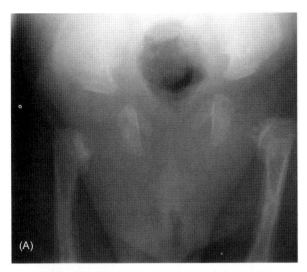

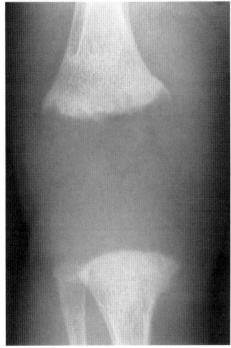

Figure 14 (A) This premature infant shows the typical findings of osteopathy of prematurity with irregular femoral necks and periosteal reactions. (B) The same infant has irregularity of metaphyses adjacent to the knees and absent (delayed) ossification of the epiphyses at the knees. They should be ossified by about 32 weeks gestation.

there is osteopenia with changes at the metaphyses in the form of sickle-shaped spurs. This is rarely seen, and only in small neonates who have required prolonged intravenous feeding and in which the parenteral fluids are deficient in copper. Scurvy, resulting from vitamin C deficiency, is hardly ever seen in developed countries nowadays. Radiologically there is osteopenia with a "pencil" outline of epiphyses,

"pelcan" spurs at the metaphyses, and extensive sub-periosteal bleeding with calcification and subsequent ossification. Clinically there is bleeding from gums and easy bruising. The milder forms of osteogenesis imperfecta (types I and IV) show the radiological features of osteopenia, slender long bones and ribs, and wormian bones. These are small discrete islands of bone seen within the sutures of the skull. Wormian bones are present in about 80% of patients suffering from osteogenesis imperfecta. There should be more than 10 in a mosaic distribution to differentiate them from those that are few, small, and discrete, present as a normal variant in about 10% of the normal population. Clinically, patients with osteogenesis imperfecta often have blue sclerae, although many normal infants also have this finding. A positive family history may help to establish the diagnosis. The vast majority of patients with osteogenesis imperfecta may be diagnosed from the combination of radiological, clinical, and family history findings. In difficult cases, testing for mutations in type 1 collagen from a skin biopsy and fibroblast culture may assist. However, this is still a research tool and only about 85% of patients who have been clearly diagnosed with osteogenesis imperfecta will demonstrate an abnormality of collagen or procollagen. In addition, it is not known what proportion of the normal population may have minor abnormalities of collagen, but never present with fractures. Another genetic disorder presenting with fractures is Menke's syndrome, in which there is an abnormality of copper metabolism resulting in a neurodegenerative disorder. Radiologically there is osteopenia and multiple wormian bones in the skull.

Normal Variants

Misinterpretation of normal variants may result in overdiagnosis of nonaccidental injury when interpreted as fractures, or in underdiagnosis when fractures are attributed to normal findings (**Figure 15**).

Intracranial Injuries

These are the commonest cause of death as a result of nonaccidental injury. Typically they result from shaking or an impact injury or a combination of the two. A shaking injury may be associated with rib fractures and retinal hemorrhages. Subdural hemorrhage results from tearing of bridging veins over the cerebral convexities during a shaking episode and also is typically seen in the interhemispheric fissure. Hypoxic–ischemic changes result in swelling of the brain and separation of the sutures and may

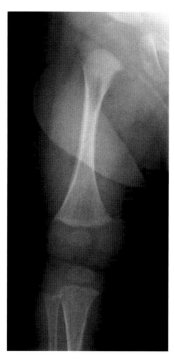

Figure 15 Small spurs are present at the metaphyses of the lower femur and upper tibia. These are normal variants seen in a small proportion of normal infants.

result in the "reversal sign" on the CT scan, in which there is low attenuation of the cerebral cortex and high attenuation of the white matter and basal ganglia. These changes have a poor prognosis. Shearing injuries in the form of small tears may also be seen in the brain substance. Localized contusion or bruising of the brain may be seen underlying a skull fracture following a direct impact, as may a localized subarachnoid or subdural hemorrhage. In addition, contrecoup injuries may be seen on the opposite side of the brain to the site of impact.

There is a wide range of presentation as a result of intracranial injury. The infant may be irritable, vomiting, not feeding, or may show major neurological signs in the form of seizures or loss of consciousness. When presentation is as a result of an acute collapse with loss of consciousness, the injury has occurred shortly before. An estimate of dating subdural hemorrhage may also be made from the initial CT scan. High attenuation (white) indicates recent bleeding, occurring within a week of the scan. There is a gradual reduction in attenuation from gray to black with increasing age of the subdural hemorrhage. Bleeding older than about 1 month appears black and is the same attenuation as normal cerebrospinal fluid. In practice, the age of an intracranial

injury is assessed from a combination of the history, clinical findings, and CT scan.

Visceral Injuries

Intraabdominal injuries are relatively uncommon, found in between 2% and 3% of all cases of nonaccidental injury. They arise mainly from blunt trauma resulting in contusion, laceration, or rupture of solid or hollow organs such as liver, spleen, kidneys, pancreas, and bowel and bladder. Small-bowel hematomas, mesenteric tears, and vascular injuries may also occur.

Oral and pharyngeal injuries occur when objects are forced into the mouth, causing mucosal tears. These may be complicated by perforations resulting in mediastinal air and mediastinitis, pneumothorax with lung collapse, and surgical emphysema.

Conclusions

The safety and welfare of the child are paramount and generally this results in the baby being moved to a place of safety and care proceedings being instituted through the civil courts. Occasionally, and when there is some acknowledgment of responsibility for the injuries, or of a failure to protect, it is possible to work with the family to address the problems and with appropriate safeguards the child may eventually be returned to the family. This would seem to be the most desirable outcome. In other cases the child may be placed with the extended family or with foster parents and then placed for adoption. Depending on the extent and severity of the injuries the perpetrator may be charged with criminal offenses through the criminal courts and undergo a custodial sentence.

The pediatric radiologist as an expert witness should be familiar with the radiological aspects of nonaccidental injury, both the standard texts and the peer-reviewed literature. There should be an awareness of the relative significance of isolated case reports. There should be knowledge of the normal skeletal findings in infants and of normal variants, together with the skeletal findings associated with accidental trauma. This means that significant experience of pediatric casualty radiology is necessary. Specialist knowledge of skeletal changes associated with skeletal dysplasias, such as osteogenesis imperfecta and metabolic bone diseases, and deficiency disorders, such as rickets or renal osteodystrophy, and neurological changes from cerebral palsy is also required. In addition to identifying the injuries, their ages, and mechanisms of causation, the report should indicate the anticipated clinical findings such as swelling and bruising and evaluate the explanations which have been put forward and the effect of the individual injuries on the baby. This again requires an understanding of normal babies and how they respond to pain, both from pediatric casualty work and from experience of performing painful (but necessary) procedures on neonates and infants, such as intravenous injections and catheter placements. Sometimes levels of probability for each injury occurring by a particular mechanism are helpful. The report, participation in experts' meetings, and oral evidence given in court should be confined to the professional limitations of the individual expert. It is important that the court is aware of the areas of expertise of individual expert witnesses and that undue weight is not given to nonexpert medical opinions. The evidence should be independent of all the parties involved and provided to assist the court.

See Also

Children: Legal Protection and Rights of Children; Physical Abuse; Sudden Natural Infant and Childhood Death; **Expert Witness:** Qualifications, Testimony and Malpractice

Further Reading

Hall C (1994) Non-accidental injury. In: Carty H, Shaw D, Brunelle F, Kendall B (eds.) *Imaging Children*, pp. 1188–1202. Edinburgh, UK: Churchill Livingstone.
Kleinman PK (1998) *Diagnostic Imaging of Child Abuse*, 2nd edn. St Louis, MO: Mosby.

IMMUNOASSAYS, FORENSIC APPLICATIONS

S Miyaishi, Okayama University Graduate School of Medicine and Dentistry, Okayama, Japan
F Moriya, Kochi University, Nankoku, Japan

This article is adapted from 'Immunoassays, Applications: Forensic' in *Encyclopedia of Analytical Science*, Volume 4 pp. 339–335, © 2005, Elsevier Ltd.

Introduction

Forensic pathological diagnosis often requires the knowledge and techniques of its related sciences: death from poisoning could not be diagnosed without determining the chemical compounds/natural toxin; personal identification of an unidentified autopsied body requires the genetic analysis of the material obtained from the corpse. In this sense forensic sciences should be included in forensic medicine in the broad sense and it could be divided into the following three main fields: (1) forensic pathology; (2) forensic biology; and (3) forensic toxicology.

The medical term immunoassay commonly means quantitative analysis of a substance using immunoreactions. However, the original meaning of the word "assay," to test metal, is not restricted in the quantitative analysis and enzyme-linked immunosorbent assay (ELISA) has been developed in the area of histology as a method of qualitative investigation to identify the existence/localization of antigens (immunohistochemistry). Immunohistochemical findings are also often quantitatively analyzed when their significance is evaluated. Therefore in this article we deal with the term immunoassay in the broader sense, including both quantitative and qualitative/semiquantitative analysis using immunoreactions, and describe its application in the above-mentioned three fields.

Forensic Medicine and Immunoassay

Determination of substances with pharmacological or poisonous effects on humans in autopsy materials is important in forensic toxicological practice. The detection of drugs of abuse in the urine or blood of living subjects is frequently required in this field. Some immunoassays are also used to detect common drugs of abuse in hair, which assists in monitoring past drug history.

When detailed qualitative and precise quantitative analyses of drugs are required, we must choose instrument-based testing without immunoreaction, because it cannot discriminate the parent drug from its metabolites/derivatives and chemicals that have similar structures. For example, putrefactive amines, such as phenethylamine, frequently give false-positive results for amphetamines, and dihydrocodeine gives positive results for opiates. However, immunoassay kits for chemical compounds are still useful, especially in screening.

The role of immunoassay in forensic toxicology is different from other fields of forensic medicine. In forensic pathology and biology, immunoassay is a tool for diagnosing and determining the target substance, but it is not the final purpose of analysis. For example, a precipitation test for human IgG is a method of forensic species identification, but the essential purpose is not to detect IgG itself, but rather to identify human origin, and there may be other more useful immunoassays for new substances such as human hemoglobin. In contrast, the result obtained by immunoassay is the specific purpose of forensic toxicology. Tests have been developed and investigated as a methodology in this field. In the following section we describe the present situation of immunoassays distributed in the market for forensic or clinical toxicology with their characteristics and principles.

Forensic biology encompasses both anthropological and genetic aspects. The analysis of genetic markers is indispensable for paternity testing and the personal identification of stains or unidentified bodies. In these circumstances, examination of genetic markers is the most frequent and important aspect of forensic biological practice.

Up to the mid-1990s, blood types were examined using immunoreactions as important genetic markers and many immunoassays have been developed to determine their phenotypes. The situation of immunoassays in this field, however, has greatly changed in recent years. According to the development of DNA technology, blood cell/serum protein types as the tool for personal identification/paternity test were substituted for short tandem repeats (STRs) or single nucleotide polymorphisms (SNPs), and the need for examining classical genetic markers was remarkably reduced. Nevertheless, immunoassay will still be necessary in forensic biology in the future, because some examinations required in this field are not suitable for DNA analysis (e.g., identification of semen).

Some commercially available immunoassay kits are also useful in forensic biological analysis for a different purpose and using different material. For example, an immunoassay kit for detecting prostate-specific antigen (PSA) in serum as a marker of prostate cancer can also be used to identify semen using the extract obtained from a suspected dried body fluid stain.

Forensic pathology is the main field of forensic medicine and involves the diagnosis of the cause of death, determination of time of death, estimation of degree/properties of injuries and so on. Analysis of morphological changes and pathogenesis induced by the external factors or internal diseases are also important issues in this field. However, it is sometimes very difficult to solve such problems by autopsy

findings alone and it has been attempted to develop useful examinations for forensic pathological diagnosis. For this purpose proteins/hormones as clinically useful markers have been noticed in this field and many authors have determined such substances in autopsy materials quantitatively using commercially available immunoassay kits and discussed the meaning of the results obtained.

However, the nature of autopsy materials is quite different from that used in clinical medicine. A blood sample obtained at autopsy is sometimes markedly hemolyzed and its supernatant is neither serum nor plasma, because postmortem intensive fibrinolysis following blood coagulation had already occurred in the corpse at autopsy. Body fluids other than blood and urine or extract of tissue homogenate cannot be considered of clinical use. The most important factor is that many kinds of proteins are contained in huge amounts in autopsy material; this would not be expected in clinical laboratory medicine at all. Such samples with too many antigen molecules can cause strong suppression of immunoreactions that are necessary in the assay system established for clinical use. These facts mean that the determined values may not be able to be compared if different immunoassay kits are used, even if the same protein is assayed. Besides, the determined value of the postmortem sample may be false, if its assay is left to the clinical laboratory where nobody knows the particular nature of the autopsy material. This may be the reason why some conclusions obtained from different studies on the same substance differ from one another, although the attempted quantitative analysis has been described as useful in most studies.

Many morphological studies have also been reported where several antigens are stained by immunohistochemistry and the diagnostic value of findings are evaluated according to the issues such as cause of death, nature of injury, postmortem interval, or other viewpoints. In these studies commercially available antibodies have been used.

The above-mentioned situation of immunoassay in forensic pathology means that none has become a common examination as a useful tool for autopsy diagnosis. In the following section we introduce the hitherto reported approaches to forensic pathological diagnosis using immunoassays and some are described in **Table 1**.

Immunoassays in Forensic Practice

Applications in Forensic Toxicology

Immunoassays are used in forensic toxicology for routine screening and quantifying compounds.

Table 1 Approaches to forensic pathological diagnosis using immunoassays

Issue analyzed/identified	Material	Type of assay	Representative antigen(s) noticed
Diagnosis of cause of death			
Sudden cardiac death	Blood, pericardial fluid	Qt	Myosin, troponin, myoglobin
	Heart	IH	C5b-9, fibronectin, troponin
Drowning	Blood	Qt	Pulmonary surfactant
	Lung	IH	Pulmonary surfactant
Asphyxia by neck compression	Blood	Qt	Thyroglobulin
	Soft tissue of the neck	IH	Myoglobin, fibronectin, glycophorin-A
Sudden infantile death	Lung or other organs	IH	Milk components, S-100, insulin
Diagnosis of nature of injury			
Wound age	Skin	IH	Collagen, fibronectin, cytokeratin, interleukins
	Brain	IH	GFAP (glial fibrillary acidic protein), thrombomodulin
Vital reaction	Skin	Qt	FDP-D dimer
	Hematoma	IH	Glycophorin-A, CD62
Diagnosis of postmortem interval	Some organs	Qt	Vascular endothelial growth factor
	Pancreas	IH	Insulin, glucagon
	Thyroid gland	IH	Thyroglobulin
	Heart	IH	Myoglobin

Qt, quantitative analysis; IH, immunohistochemistry.

They have excellent sensitivity and specificity, and can be completed in a short period. Many immunoassays are available for testing common poisons in both urine and serum. The most common immunoassays used in forensic toxicology are: (1) radioimmunoassay (RIA); (2) enzyme-multiplied immunoassay technique (EMIT: Behring Diagnostics); (3) fluorescence polarization immunoassay (FPIA); (4) cloned enzyme donor immunoassay (CEDIA: Roche Diagnostics/Boehringer Mannheim); (5) kinetic interaction of microparticles in solution (KIMS: Roche Diagnostics); and (6) ELISA. The substances most commonly measured are amphetamines, barbiturates, benzodiazepines, cannabinoids, cocaine, methadone, opiates, phencyclidine, propoxyphene, and tricyclic antidepressants.

Radioimmunoassays RIAs are preferred for postmortem samples due to their resistance to matrix effects. Most other techniques are difficult to apply to these specimens. Postmortem samples are homogenized in a deproteinizing medium, such as acetonitrile or a mixture of zinc sulfate, sulfosalicylic acid, and methanol. As a result of their sensitivity and low matrix effect, RIAs can detect low levels of lysergic acid diethylamide (LSD) in urine, ricin in tissues, and tetrahydrocannabinol (THC) in hair. Although RIAs have many analytical advantages, and ^{125}I has been used instead of ^{131}I to label drugs in most current RIA methods because of its longer half-life, there are problems in disposing of radioactive waste and using an isotope with a short shelf-life (approximately 60 days). These shortcomings have reduced the demand for RIA and manufacturers no longer make kits for common drugs.

EMIT EMIT is a homogeneous assay that uses an enzyme-labeled (glucose-6-phosphate dehydrogenase) drug to compete with unlabeled drug for a specific antibody. If the labeled drug is free from the antibody, the enzyme oxidizes glucose-6-phosphate and reduces NAD to NADH, which is measured at 340 nm with a spectrophotometer. Automated analyzers are available for these immunoassays, and hundreds of samples can be processed in an hour. While the EMIT assay was developed for drugs in urine, it has also been applied to aqueous extracts from other biological samples (e.g., meconium). If a clear and nearly neutral solution can be obtained from a sample, then the sample can be assayed by EMIT.

FPIA FPIA methods use a fluorescein-labeled drug to compete with the unlabeled drug for an antibody. If the fluorescein-labeled drug combines with the antibody, emitted light remains polarized when the incoming light is polarized. As the concentrations of drug in the sample increase, free fluorescein-labeled drug molecules also increase in number. Since the unbound fluorescein-labeled drug molecule rotates freely, the polarized light emitted is reduced. Automated analyzers, such as TDx, ADx, and Axysm (Abbott Laboratories), are used to measure these reactions. Drugs are more accurately measured by FPIA than EMIT because sample matrices have less effect on changes in fluorescein polarization.

CEDIA CEDIA is a relatively new technique that uses two genetically engineered fragments of *Escherichia coli* β-galactosidase as an enzyme label. The activity of the enzyme requires assembly of the two fragments, termed enzyme donor and enzyme acceptor fragments. The enzyme donor fragment is bound to a drug. The enzyme donor fragment-labeled drug competes with the drug existing in urine samples for a specific antibody. When the enzyme donor fragment-labeled drug combines with the antibody, the fragment does not associate with the enzyme acceptor fragment and enzyme activity does not develop. When the enzyme donor fragment-labeled drug associates with enzyme acceptor fragment, it becomes active and hydrolyzes chlorophenolred-β-galactoside to chlorophenolred and galactose. Production of chlorophenolred is measured at 570 nm with a spectrophotometer. The concentration of the drug of interest is directly proportional to the change in absorbance and automated analyzers are commercially available for toxicology laboratories.

KIMS KIMS assay (Abuscreen Online®: Roche Diagnostics®) uses microparticles labeled with several drug molecules. The drugs on the microparticles compete with the drug in urine for a specific antibody. Reaction of the drug molecules on the microparticle with several antibody molecules forms a large aggregate that increases absorbance. Thus, the concentration of the drug is inversely related to the change in absorbance. Since microparticle drug conjugates are more stable than enzyme drug conjugates, these kits have a long shelf-life.

ELISA ELISA is a sensitive and specific method that has been used for many years to detect body components and pathogenic microorganisms. However, its application to drug testing is relatively new. Since ELISA is a heterogeneous assay, it is not as sensitive to matrix effects. Thus, this technique is easily applied to postmortem fluid samples. A commercially available kit (MTA-8, Venture Labs) can simultaneously test for eight drugs of abuse on one microtiter plate. Micro-Plate forensic enzyme immunoassay kits (OraSure Technologies®) are also marketed.

Many immunoassay kits that do not require special instrumentation are commercially available. They do not require a formal laboratory and are used for on-site testing, such as cases of driving under the influence, workplace drug testing, and emergency room settings. These kits are also used in toxicology laboratories to test a relatively small number of samples at low cost. On-site drug-testing devices use competitive immunoassay and the results are visualized as red bands of immunoreacted colloidal gold-labeled antibodies or drugs. The kits available for forensic on-site testing of urine are summarized in **Table 2**. Triage DOA (drugs of abuse) has been successfully applied to postmortem blood samples if they are properly pretreated. For testing drugs of abuse in saliva, Cozart's RapiScan (Cozart Biosciences®) is the only device currently available.

Detecting agricultural chemicals in biological samples is important in forensic toxicology. A forensic toxicologist can use enzyme immunoassay kits (Rapid Assay®, Ohmicron Environmental Diagnostics) that were originally developed to monitor environmental chemicals, such as organophosphates, carbamates, organochlorines, and paraqaut, to measure these compounds in biological samples. These assays use an antibody bound to magnetic particles and the final color development is measured with a spectrophotometer. Since this method is a heterogeneous immunoassay, matrix effects are minimal.

Table 2 Descriptions of noninstrumental immunoassay kits for qualitative on-site drug testing

Test	Analytes	Testing time required (min)	Sample volume required
Abscreen Ontrak	AMP, BAR, BZO, THC, COC, MTD, OPI, PCP	5–7	0.011 ml
Accusign	AMP, BAR, BZO, THC, COC, MTD, OPI, PCP, TCA	3–5	3 drops
EZ-Screen	AMP, BAR, THC, COC, OPI	3–5	6 drops
Frontline	AMP, BZO, THC, COC, OPI	3–10	Test strip immersed
InstraCheck	AMP, BAR, BZO, THC, COC, MTD, OPI, PCP	3–8	4–5 drops
Ontrak TesTcup	AMP, BAR, BZO, THC, COC, OPI, PCP	3–5	At least 30 ml
Ontrak TesTstik	AMP, BZO, THC, COC, OPI	3–5	Test strip immersed
Syva RapidTest	AMP, BAR, BZO, THC, COC, MTD, OPI, PCP, TCA	3–10	3 drops
Triage	AMP, BAR, BZO, THC, COC, MTD, OPI, PCP, TCA	11–15	0.14 ml
Visualine II	AMP, BZO, THC, COC, OPI	3–5	3 drops

AMP, amphetamines; BAR, barbiturates; BZO, benzodiazepines; THC, cannabinoids; COC, cocaine metabolite; MTD, methadone; OPI, opiates; PCP, phencyclidine; TCA, tricyclic antidepressants.

Applications in Forensic Biology

In the field of forensic biology, many kinds of immunoassay have been used to examine blood groups. A hemagglutination test using antisera is the classical method of determining red blood cell types: ABO, Rh, MNSs and so on. Human leukocyte antigen types have been determined using a complement fixation test. Some serum protein polymorphisms have been examined using an immunoblotting or immunofixation technique following isoelectric focusing.

Although these examinations of blood types were substituted for DNA analyses, especially STRs and SNPs, because STRs/SNPs are much more polymorphic than classic blood types, they have a great advantage in forensic biological practices. Besides, polymerase chain reaction used for DNA analysis is very sensitive.

However, blood group determination may be required in cases other than personal identification or paternity tests, for example, in incompatible blood transfusion. A recipient's ABO blood group may quickly be identified if a distinct mosaic pattern with both agglutinated and nonagglutinated red blood cells is observed by hemagglutination test. A saliva absorption test may assist in identifying a receipient's blood group. Though immunostaining of ABO blood group antigen using autopsy material is also useful for this purpose, DNA analysis is more commonly used nowadays.

Absorption and absorption–elution tests are conventional methods that have been used to determine ABO blood group from stains. The immunohistochemistry technique can be applied to some stains and autopsy material. Absorption tests of body fluid stain can identify whether the individual is a secretor or nonsecretor. Many ELISAs to detect or quantify ABO or Lewis blood group antigen have also been reported. Although ELISAs had satisfactory specificity and sensitivity, absorption/absorption–elution tests were not replaced by them, and in recent years ABO blood grouping by DNA analysis has become routinely used. ELISAs using monoclonal antibody, however, may still be useful, because some can determine the ABO blood group of a specific component in a mixed stain, e.g., ABO blood grouping of vaginal secretion mixed with semen.

Immunoassays have also been applied to species identification of stains. A precipitation test of the extract from the suspected stain against antihuman serum or antihuman immunoglobulin G (IgG) is a classical method for this purpose. Immunological detection of human hemoglobin is now a popular method for species identification of blood stains. This method has the advantage of not only identifying human origin but also confirming blood at the same time, comparing the methods for detecting other human components. Recently, commercially available immunoassay kits for clinical laboratory investigations to detect occult blood in feces have been applied to forensic human identification of blood stains, because the antibodies used reveal excellent specificity for humans. In the last decade, a highly sensitive immunochromatography device has been introduced to the market. It can be applied to species identification of stains from body fluids other than blood, if they are only minutely contaminated with hemoglobin. However, highly sensitive DNA analysis methods for this purpose have also been developed.

It should be noted that DNA analysis is unsuitable for some kinds of forensic biological examinations and immunological analysis is required. Identification of semen is a typical and important issue from this viewpoint. PSA is a well-known semen-specific substance and its detection by ELISA is the most common method of identifying semen from body fluid stain or vaginal content. Since it is an important clinical marker for prostate carcinoma, devices for detecting serum PSA using immunochromatography are marketed worldwide. Although the prepared sample is not serum in a forensic biological examination, such a device is useful for detecting and identifying semen in cases of sexual assault. γ-Seminoprotein is also a good marker for this purpose and it is said to be the same substance as PSA. ELISAs for β-microseminoprotein, semenogelin, and other substances were developed for the identification of semen.

In blood stain analysis there are also problems for which DNA analysis can give no solution. For example, in cases of murder or injury of a menstruating woman, the offender sometimes claims that the blood stain at the scene originates from menstrual blood. In such cases, the immunological determination of FDP is useful, as it is contained in large quantities in menstrual blood. There are more examples in which immunoassay can be a useful tool for analysis. The detection of human chorionic gonadotropin permits identification of the blood of a pregnant woman. Myoglobin is contained in large volumes in the blood of a corpse and determination of its content is useful for discriminating between antemortem and postmortem blood.

Identification of an injured organ or tissue from a blood stain also requires immunological analysis, and ELISAs for the following proteins have been developed: S-100 protein (specific for brain), β-enolase (specific for skeletal muscle), elastase III (specific

Table 3 Forensic biological analysis requiring immunoassay

Material	Issue analyzed/identified	Representative antigen(s) determined
Blood stain	Blood of pregnant woman	Human chorionic gonadotropin
	Menstrual blood	FDP
	Postmortem blood	Myoglobin
	Injury of skeletal muscle	β-enolase
	Injury of brain	S-100 protein
	Injury of liver	Liver-specific antigen
Body fluid stain/vaginal content	Semen	Prostate-specific antigen, γ-Sm, semenogelin
Body fluid stain/tissue fragment	Human origin	Human hemoglobin, human immunoglobulin G
Tissue fragment	Brain	Myosin, neurofilament
	Skin	SCC (squamous cell carcinoma-related antigen)
	Skeletal muscle	Myoglobin

for pancreas), and Tamm–Horsfall protein (specific for kidney). Liver-specific antigen was originally isolated and ELISA of this protein was also developed for the investigation of liver injury. Identifying an organ or tissue from a fragment left at the scene is also an important issue in forensic stain analysis and some ELISAs for myosin or neurofilament for identifying brain tissue, myoglobin for identifying skeletal muscle, and SCC (squamous cell carcinoma-related antigen) for identifying skin have been reported. Some ELISAs for organ- or tissue-specific substances reveal good specificity for humans. Representative analyses requiring immunoassay in forensic biology are shown in **Table 3**.

Applications in Forensic Pathology

The main issue in which qualitative immunoassay is used in forensic pathology is in diagnosing the cause of death. The most frequent approach is to diagnose sudden cardiac death (SCD)/myocardial infarction/ischemic damage of myocardium by determining the proteins in myocardium such as myosin, myoglobin, and troponin I in blood and/or pericardial fluid. Determination of the content, not activity, of CK-MB by immunoassay has also been attempted. Other approaches analyzing the relationship between the concentration of a protein in blood and the cause and/or pathogenesis of death were: asphyxia by neck compression and thyroglobulin, drowning and SP-A or -D (pulmonary surfactant), electric death and myoglobin, and so on. Some authors took note not of the particular cause of death but of a special substance, e.g. SP-A in blood, CRP (C-reactive protein) in blood, or myoglobin in urine, and analyzed the relationship between the substance and causes of death in general.

Quantitative or semiquantitative immunoassays are also applied to analyze the nature of injury. Attempts have been made to estimate the grade and analysis of

pathogenesis of brain injury by determining NSE (neuro-specific enolase) and tumor necrosis factor-α (TNF-α) in cerebrospinal fluid. Concerning skin wounds, it has been said that the FDP-D dimer can be used as a marker of vital reaction and that the content of interleukin-6 (IL-6), IL-1β, and TNF-α in the tissue is useful for estimating wound age. To discriminate subcutaneous hemorrhage from exuded hemoglobin due to putrefaction, assay of glycophorin-A was recommended.

Some examples of other studies using quantitative immunoassays in forensic pathology are vascular endothelial growth factor (VEGF) contents in brain and some other organs for the diagnosis of postmortem interval/time of death, melatonin concentrations in blood, urine, and pineal gland for the same purpose, and serum tryptase concentration for the diagnosis of heroin-related death.

Immunohistochemistry is the most widely used method as qualitative immunoassay in the field of forensic pathology. The most frequent approach using this technique is to diagnose the cause of death, especially SCD. C5b-9, fibronectin, cardiac troponin, and other proteins have been stained for this purpose and the usefulness of their staining has been discussed. Many studies on sudden infant death syndrome or infantile sudden death using immunostaining have also been reported. In these studies S-100 protein, hypophysial hormones, insulin, GFAP (glial fibrillary acidic protein), calcitonin, CD4, SP-A, and other proteins/hormones were stained in various organs/tissues and the meaning of such staining was evaluated from a forensic pathological viewpoint. An interesting approach to diagnose the cause of infantile sudden death was the immunostaining of the components of human and cow milk in the lung. Other applications of immunohistochemistry to the diagnosis of cause of death were investigations of the relationship between SP-A in lung and drowning, adult respiratory distress syndrome, or death due to fire, pulmonary mast cell tryptase and amniotic fluid embolism, glycophorin A, myoglobin, or fibronectin in muscle and asphyxia by neck compression and so on.

There have also been many immunohistochemical studies on injury. To estimate the age of a skin wound many substances were stained and their usefulness discussed. The stained proteins used were fibronectin, collagen, laminin, cytokeratin, CD54, IL-6, IL-1β, TNF-α and so on. In order to confirm the vital reaction in skin wound immunostaining of α_1-antichymotrypsin, α_2-microglobulin, fibronectin, and other substances were reported to be useful. In the analysis of brain injury using immunostaining the following combination of proteins with purposes were described to be useful: NSE for demonstrating vital reactions and diffuse axonal injury; collagen IV, thrombomodulin, GFAP, and some other proteins for estimating wound age; HSP (heat shock protein) 70, GFAP and other proteins for the analysis of hypoxic/ischemic brain damage; beta-amyloid precursor protein for evaluating traumatic brain damage, and so on. For discrimination of antemortem bleeding from postmortem hemoglobin diffusion, immunostaining of glycophorin A is also used. In another report it was described that immuno-electron microscopical staining of CD62 and other antigens on platelet could distinguish intravital from postmortem hematoma.

Other analyses using qualitative immunoassays in forensic pathology are as follows: insulin and glucagon in the pancreas, myoglobin in the heart, thyroglobulin in the thyroid gland, S-100, cytokeratin, and other substances in the sweat gland, and other tests to diagnose the postmortem interval/time of death, thyrosin-phosphorylated proteins in thymus to demonstrate child abuse, β-amyloid, GFAP, and Tau protein in the brain for postmortem diagnosis of Alzheimer's disease, leukotoxin in the lung for analysis of the pathogenesis of paraquat poisoning/hyperoxic condition and so on.

There have been some advances in the area between pathology and biology or toxicology. An example is the method used to identify a weapon used in cases of injury or homicide by detecting the organ-specific antigen. If the specific antigen of an injured organ is detected from a stain on the suspected weapon, it could be identified as the used weapon. Although identifying the weapon used is an essential issue in forensic pathological diagnosis, stain analysis principally belongs to forensic biology. Another example is the analysis of cause and/or pathogenesis of death in cases of poisoning or death under the effects of a drug or poison. Although this kind of analysis is an issue of diagnosis required at forensic autopsy, it also depends on forensic toxicological analysis of drug-related pathological changes, including the immunohistochemical detection of a drug or poison distributed in the body and the quantitative determination of drug/poison in autopsy materials.

See Also

Autopsy, Findings: Postmortem Drug Sampling and Redistribution; **Postmortem Changes:** Electrolyte Disturbances; **Serology:** Blood Identification; Bloodstain Pattern Analysis

Further Reading

Betz P (1995) Immunohistochemical parameters for the age estimation of human skin wounds: a review. *American Journal of Forensic Medicine and Pathology* 16: 203–209.

Coe JI (1993) Postmortem chemistry update: emphasis on forensic application. *American Journal of Forensic Medicine and Pathology* 14: 91–117.

Jenkins AJ, Goldberger BA (2002) *On-Site Drug Testing*. Totowa, Canada: Humana Press.

Smith ML (1999) Immunoassay. In: Levine B (ed.) *Principles of Forensic Toxicology*, pp. 130–152. Washington, DC: AACC Press.

Takahama K (1996) Forensic application of organ-specific antigens. *Forensic Science International* 80: 63–69.

INJURY, FATAL AND NONFATAL

Contents
Documentation
Blunt Injury
Burns and Scalds
Explosive Injury
Firearm Injuries
Sharp and Cutting-Edge Wounds

Documentation

J Payne-James, Forensic Healthcare Services Ltd, London, UK

Introduction

The need for medical practitioners to keep objective factual records of consultations and contact with individuals whom they see in the course of professional work is a principle that is generally accepted in most jurisdictions. The need for such records becomes much more apparent in issues where medicine may be interrelated with various legal processes – of which criminal matters and medical negligence are key examples. In both cases the medical practitioner's records will be scrutinized by a number of lay persons and medical and legal professionals, and failure to have kept appropriate records can lead to criticism of a practitioner's competence, or fitness to practice. It is therefore in the interest of every medical professional to take great care in the contemporaneous documenting and recording of notes. It is not just in the interest of the forensic medical professional. This article focuses on appropriate documentation of injuries in the living injured person, although the broad principles apply to the deceased and have been covered in other articles.

Need for Documentation of Injuries

Documentation of injuries presenting to medical practitioners in the community or in hospital is generally poor. In many cases documentation is appropriate for the therapeutic management of the injured person, but is rarely of the quality required subsequently to assist in issues such as causation or timing of an injury. Such issues may still be difficult to determine even where documentation has been good, but it is in the interests of the injured person, those alleged to have caused the injury, and justice in general to ensure that as much information as possible is available. The purpose of assessment and documentation of injury is, as far as possible, to define the type of injury caused, to assist in establishing how such a wound or injury was caused, and to determine how consistent the varying accounts of causation are with those that may have been given. Terms such as injury, assault, and wound may have specific applications dependent on jurisdiction, and it may not be for the medical practitioner to assign those definitions within a case, but merely to assist the court in making the determination. For example, in England and Wales the term "wound" has specific meaning relating to whether the skin or mucosa is completely breached. This article will use the term "injury" in the following sense: "damage to any part of the body due to the deliberate or accidental application of mechanical or other traumatic agent." All forensic practitioners should be aware of the definitions in the jurisdiction in which they work. It is appropriate for those documenting injuries to ensure that they have documented the account of causation, and the nature of the injury, accurately in detail and unambiguously so that the courts or other bodies interpreting the findings can make the decision as to the most appropriate judicial interpretation of the injury or injuries described and their specific relevance to the case in question. The examination may be of victims, of perpetrators, or those where cross-allegations and the early stage of the investigation may make it unclear who is the aggrieved individual. Therefore, it is of the absolute essence that any documentation reinforces the principles of independence and fairness, so that courts or other legal bodies can make judgments based on the best possible factual information.

Examination and Documentation of Injury

Examination and documentation of injury and its interpretation follow broad general medical principles. It is dependent on establishing a good history of how injury occurred (from the injured person or others if not possible or if they can add to the history), a more general medical history exploring other matters that may affect the nature or interpretation of the injury and undertaking a physical examination appropriate to the injury and documenting the findings clearly and unambiguously. An examination should always be done with the best possible lighting conditions available, and if necessary moving the person being examined to better light or bringing additional light sources in. A hand magnification lens may be useful to look at details such as wound edges and patterns, and to establish the direction of force in scratches and skin lifts. It must always be borne in mind by the examining doctor that each interpretation and each set of notes and records may subsequently be reviewed by other medical professionals, legal advisers, and interested parties, and the courts or other legal bodies. Consent for the assessment including for the taking of the history, the examination, the taking of samples, and for subsequent production of a medical report should be sought from the individual being examined, with a clear explanation made as to the possible extent of circulation of any reports or notes. An individual may give a limited consent to certain aspects of such consent, and if so its limitations and potential problems must be explained to the examinee and documented in the notes. It should also be borne in mind that vexatious or frivolous accusations of assault can be made, and examiners should place themselves in the best position to establish the veracity of any accounts, as false allegations and counterallegations frequently occur, by ensuring the completeness of the assessment.

Specific Factors

A number of factors can be relevant when assessing injury in the living person (Table 1) and all should be considered when a history is taken. It is important to reinforce that it may also be very important to document relevant negatives in certain cases, for example the absence of preexisting skin disorder, or the absence of bleeding diatheses.

Not each of the factors in Table 1 will be applicable or relevant for every individual. A general health background is as important to establish as preexisting illnesses and this may include the use of regular prescribed medication (e.g., steroids, anticoagulants) or intermittent or pharmacy-bought preparations (e.g., aspirin) which may cause systemic effects that may alter or change the appearance of an injury. Misinterpretation of disease processes for injury is not uncommon and can sometimes result in inappropriate criminal charges. Figures 1 and 2 show two examples where a more detailed history and assessment may have prevented the misdiagnosis. Figure 1 illustrates a patchy psoriasis by the elbow which was interpreted as a series of abrasions by a junior doctor and Figure 2 shows a 2-day-old burn (which had been deliberately inflicted due to unpaid debt) in which the primary care physician accepted the account of a fall to concrete causing abrasion 2 h earlier.

Participation in certain contact sports may result in the presence of injury unrelated to any alleged assault. It is very important to document for each injury the time or dates at which the injury was said to have occurred. Most injuries heal and thus the appearance of an injury following assault is time-dependent. In

Table 1 Some factors that may be relevant from a history

Factor	Additional comments
Time of injury or injuries	With multiple injuries, ensure that accounts of timings and causation are relevant for each
Has the injury been treated?	If so, how, when, and where? Be aware that there may be a different history given which may conflict with the one obtained at this examination
Preexisting illness	Particularly those that can mimic or be misinterpreted as injury
Regular physical activity	Particularly issues such as contact sports where injury unrelated to any allegation of assault is common
Employment	Is the employment likely to result in injury, even of a minor nature (e.g., burns to hands of a chef)?
Regular medication	Any prescribed or nonprescribed medication which may predispose to worsening appearance of an injury, e.g., anticoagulants, steroids. Establish how well the treatment regimen is complied with. Antiepilepsy medication may indicate fits which themselves may result in sites of injury
Handedness of victim and suspect	May be relevant when comparing accounts of how a particular injury was sustained
Use of drugs and/or alcohol	Acute or chronic drug or alcohol intoxication may affect injury assessment in a number of ways, including: (1) memory for incident; (2) misinterpretation of factors related to drug use, e.g., intravenous sites, being interpreted as an assault injury. Chronic alcoholics commonly have multiple different ages of bruises and scars related to accidental injury whilst intoxicated
Type of weapon or implement used	Knowledge of type of implement may allow matching up of particular patterns of assault, e.g., imprint bruises
Clothing worn	Clothing might have affected result of assault: many layers may reduce effect. Occasionally may have account of clothing and mechanism of injury that are not consistent, e.g., stab wound through clothing with no disruption or cut in fabric

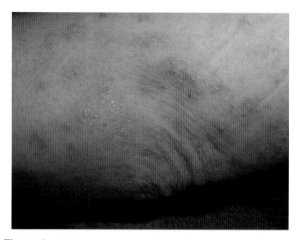

Figure 1 Patchy psoriasis on elbow – the emergency physician interpreted these lesions as abrasions. Reproduced with permission from J Payne-James, "Assault and Injury in the Living", from Jason Payne-James, Anthony Busuttil, William Smock, *Forensic Medicine: Clinical and Pathological Aspects*, 2003. Greenwich Medical Media, now published by Cambridge University Press.

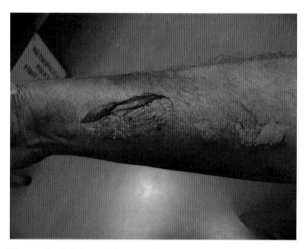

Figure 2 A 2-day-old burn to the arm, passed off and accepted as a 2-h-old graze. Reproduced with permission from J Payne-James, "Assault and Injury in the Living", from Jason Payne-James, Anthony Busuttil, William Smock, *Forensic Medicine: Clinical and Pathological Aspects*, 2003. Greenwich Medical Media, now published by Cambridge University Press.

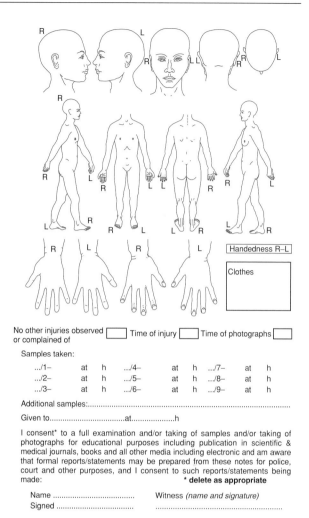

Figure 3 Example of a recording system for injuries and taking of samples.

many cases assaults may be reported days or weeks afterwards. There may be a number of injuries from different incidents. The same principles apply to injuries that may be sustained as a result of the individual's type of employment. Specific times should be sought for each. Similarly, the type of assault (e.g., baseball bat, kicks, fists, knives, scissors) must be documented, and if more than one type of assault has occurred clear records must be made of which injury was accounted for by which implement. Document the handedness (left- or right-, or both) of both victim and assailant if known, as this may affect the interpretation of injury causation. The size (weight and height) of victim or assailant may have relevance and if this information is available it

should be documented. It is often the case that widely diverging accounts are given by different witnesses – it is the forensic physician's role to assist the court in determining the true account. These differing accounts may also be influenced by the effect of drugs and/or alcohol and it is appropriate to assess the influence that these may have in each case. An assessment of the state of intoxication (or lack of) at the time of examination is important and this should also be related to what the likely state was at the time injury was sustained. Knowledge of the type of weapon used can be very important when assessing injury: particular implements (e.g., batons, serrated-edged knives) give characteristic identifiable injuries. The type of clothing worn (e.g., long-sleeved shirts, armless vests) should be noted. It is not unusual for individuals to make claims about how an injury (e.g., knife wound, bite) occurred despite the presence of clothing which would have precluded that particular mechanism of injury. When examining any individual for injury all these features should at least be considered to see whether they may have relevance

Table 2 Possible characteristics which may be relevant for each injury (optional and dependent on history)

Characteristic	Additional comments
Location	The site of an injury may have relevance with regard to whether it is feasible for such an injury to have been created in the way alleged. If there are a number of injuries, then documentation of the precise site can be assisted by precise anatomical distance measurement from fixed anatomical landmarks (e.g., olecranon or greater trochanter). Does it overlie significant anatomical landmarks?
Pain	The site of pain should be documented, as this may subsequently be the only documented evidence of injury
Tenderness	Similarly, the location and size of the area of tenderness (determined by manual palpation and inquiry of the injured person) may be the only documented evidence of injury
Limitation of range of movement	Which joints are involved? How much is the limitation? Is there a possibility of fracture?
Type	What type of injuries are represented, e.g., bruise, laceration, incised wound, fracture? When examining, consider what alternative mechanisms may account for what is seen, and whether the account given is itself consistent
Size	Use uniform systems of measurement, preferably metric. Estimates are not appropriate or accurate – always use a ruler. Accurate measurements may become important, for example, when attempting to establish the size of a weapon, e.g., knife, used in an assault
Shape	Describe or draw as clearly as possible the shape. Does it have any patterning characteristics?
Surface	Is there a palpable swelling or deformity, or other abnormal feature?
Color	Important to describe but be aware of substantial inter- and intraobserved variation. Where possible, if color may be significant, e.g., in certain aspects of bruise aging, get photographs with color bars
Orientation	May be significant in terms of causation
Age	Note the age of the injury as indicated by the individual. Is it consistent with the account given? If not, ask for clarification and document account given
Causation	Do the accounts of injury vary? If so, which ones seem consistent and which ones don't?
Handedness	Is the person right- or left-handed, or ambidextrous?
Time	Note the time for which each injury is said to occur. Is it consistent? If not, seek clarification
Transientness (of injury)	The appearance of injury, particularly reddening or bruising after blunt impact, can be subject to quite marked change, even after a few hours, in the living. Do the accounts and the appearance appear consistent at the time of examination? Is there any need to suggest further reassessment of additional documentation such as photography or video?

to the case; others may become relevant as the examination progresses or as other accounts of any assault are given.

Documentation of injuries can be in a variety of formats, including hand-drawn notes, annotated pro forma diagrams, photographic, and video. **Figure 3** illustrates one form of body chart and note system. However, more detailed body charts may be required where multiple or complex injuries are apparent.

Table 2 lists some of the key characteristics that may be needed to document each injury appropriately.

Digital and print-on-paper photographic images are an acceptable means of documenting injury in some jurisdictions but in each case the image evidence should be supported by contemporaneous written and hand-drawn notes. Storage and chain of custody of such images can represent problems in terms of admissibility of evidence and disclosure of images. If photographs are being taken by a photographer ensure that he/she is aware what is to be photographed and to include color charts and rules in each photograph. It is best to form an opinion at the time of examination as to whether injury or injuries are new or old, and whether they have specific characteristics of particular types of injury (e.g., self-inflicted, defense-type). Ensure at the time of examination that

each injury is accounted for by the account given. If an injury appears not to be consistent with the account given, question it at the time. In many cases individuals who have been involved in fights or violent incidents are simply unaware of the causation of many sites of injury. It is often appropriate (particularly with blunt injury) to reexamine injuries 24–48 h later to see how injuries evolve and whether bruises have appeared or other sites of injury noted. Pre- and posttreatment examination and photography may be very useful. Those injured should always be advised to document any visible or symptomatic evidence of injury that later becomes apparent.

Other Issues for Nonforensic Healthcare Professionals

Anyone assessing injury in the living also has a duty to ensure that appropriate treatment has been undertaken or further investigations of management advised. It is helpful when referring an injured person to another professional for further review to advise on the nature of findings and the account that the person has given for the injuries obtained.

In a number of cases of the more seriously injured, the individual may pass straight to specialists – e.g., emergency medicine, surgeons, or intensivists – for life-saving treatment. Colleagues outside the forensic setting should be aware that even on the operating table or in the resuscitation room, attention should be paid to documenting the injury – once stability of health status has been achieved, this early documentation of injury is more likely to be useful in later legal proceedings. In particular, the size, shape, and form of stab or other cutting injuries are useful if documented before exploration and suture or repair. Additionally, the apparent depth of penetration of an injury is also an issue that frequently arises in assault cases and can be assisted by good medical documentation. A photograph of a healed wound several weeks after the assault combined with medical notes that simply report "stab to abdomen" and an operation note that simply reports "stab wound to abdomen explored at laparotomy" may be the only evidence on which to try and interpret depth of penetration and causation – an impossible task. The presence or absence of other materials, e.g., from firearms, or materials carried into a wound, should be documented. It would be good practice for all such departments, which may see victims of assault and other violent crime, to have standard protocols for the secure documentation of injury appearance and collection of potentially forensically relevant material. In some jurisdictions, forensic medical specialists can make themselves available to document injury and supervise evidence collection, whilst those primarily responsible for the medical care can focus on the treatment of the individual.

Conclusion

The appropriate documentation of injury is crucial in order to assist courts with consistency of accounts and causation. Generally such documentation is poorly done. Proper attention using the general medical principles of history-taking and examination applied to the documentation of injuries, taking into account the particular aspects of general health and injury, will allow appropriate assessment and interpretation of injuries sustained by individuals, and therefore assist the legal and forensic process for which it is undertaken. Those not directly involved in forensic medicine may find it of use to seek forensic advice at an early stage when treating or investigating those involved in assaults or violence causing injury.

See Also

Injury, Fatal and Nonfatal: Blunt Injury; Burns and Scalds; Explosive Injury; Firearm Injuries; Sharp and Cutting-Edge Wounds

Further Reading

Langlouis WEI, Gresham GA (1991) The ageing of bruises: a review and study of the colour changes with time. *Forensic Science International* 50: 227–238.

McLean I, Anderson CM, White C (2003) The accuracy of guestimates. *Journal of the Royal Society of Medicine* 96: 497–498.

Munany LA, Bernard PA, Mok JYQ (2002) Lack of agreement on colour description between clinicians examining childhood injury. *Journal of Clinical Forensic Medicine* 9: 171–176.

Palmer RN (2000) Fundamental principles. In: Stark MM (ed.) *A Physician's Guide to Clinical Forensic Medicine*, pp. 15–37. New Jersey: Humana Press.

Payne-Jones JJ (2002) Assault and injury in the living. In: Payne-Jones JJ, Busuttil A, Smock W (eds.) *Forensic Medicine: Clinical and Pathological Aspects*, pp. 543–563. London: Greenwich Medical Media.

Payne-James J, Dean P, Wall I (2004) *MedicoLegal Essentials in Healthcare*, 2nd edn. London: Greenwich Medical Media.

Peel M, Iacopino M (2002) *The Medical Documentation of Torture*. London: Greenwich Medical Media.

Stephenson T, Bralas V (1996) Estimation of age of injury. *Archives of Diseases in Childhood* 74: 53–55.

Blunt Injury

T S Corey, University of Louisville School of Medicine and Office of the Chief Medical Examiner, Louisville, KY, USA

Introduction

Blunt impact to the human body is arguably the most common type of injury sustained by humans – all of us regularly incur bumps and bruises in our activities of daily life. Blunt-force injury also represents a common cause of serious injury and death. Motor vehicle collisions are one of the leading causes of death in all countries, whether industrialized or nonindustrialized. Additionally, many severe injuries occurring in accidental or assaultive situations at home or work are blunt-force injuries. These have a high cost to society, as they often result in loss of productivity or life.

Often, small injuries may have extreme forensic importance. Many times such injuries are so minor or superficial that they are completely overlooked or ignored by medical caregivers, who are interested in injuries requiring treatment and medical intervention. But it is often these same injuries that show patterns or configurations that can help elucidate the factors involved in the traumatic incident. Such injuries may allow the examiner to interpret many factors surrounding their production, such as the instrument involved, the direction and duration of impact, and the minimum number of impacts. A clear understanding of blunt-force injuries and their formation allows the medical professional to understand better and interpret the forces and events that cause them.

Anatomic Regionalization

Various anatomic regions of the body possess unique compositions and characteristics that affect the injury patterns resulting from the application of blunt force. Whenever injury patterns are assessed, the examiner must consider the substrate – the nature and composition of the tissue involved in the impact. Skin trapped between underlying bony prominences and impacting surfaces may display injuries such as abrasions, contusions, and even lacerations, as the skin and intervening soft tissue are crushed between the impacting object and the underlying rigid skeleton. These injuries may appear very different from cutaneous injuries in other areas of the body in which there is abundant subcutaneous tissue, or no immediately underlying bone.

The head is arguably a unique region, as the relatively soft gelatinous brain is encased in a tough fibrous protective layer (the dura mater), which in turn is encased within the rigid bony skull. The skull is then covered by a relatively small amount of soft tissue with a rich vascular supply (the scalp). Added to this is the unique anatomic location of the head, able to move and rotate in many directions, atop the neck. Because of these physical properties, the head and its intracranial contents manifest different reactions to the application of blunt force, and therefore are considered elsewhere in this encyclopedia.

The torso of the human body, composed of skin and soft tissue external to a discontinuous axial skeleton which protects and supports the visceral organs, may suffered marked, even lethal internal injuries while the external skin surface appears relatively pristine. This may occur due to the pliability of the external soft tissues, such that forces are transmitted through the more superficial tissues to damage the deeper vital organs. Blunt forces impacting the torso will cause varied injury responses, depending on many factors, including, but not necessarily limited to, the angle of force, the angle of impact in relationship to the anatomic configuration (longitudinal loading versus side impact), and the composition of the body at the impact site. For example, impacts identical in duration, amount of force, and direction

may create different injury patterns depending on whether the impact occurs on the skin overlying the vertebral column and/or ribs, or the midportion of the anterior abdomen, with its insulating adipose tissue and lack of rigid bony structures. In injuries over the bony prominences of the torso, cutaneous abrasions, lacerations, and contusions, with or without underlying osseous fractures, are likely resulting injuries. In contrast, blunt impacts to the soft pliable abdominal wall may result in serious injury to vital organs with relatively little external evidence of injury (**Figures 1** and **2**).

Blunt forces acting upon the extremities will cause varied injury responses as well, depending on the

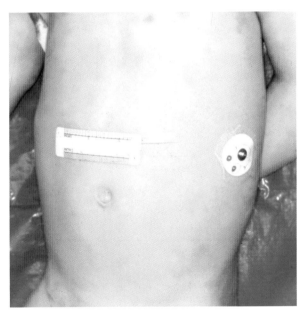

Figure 1 External skin surface of a child dying of blunt abdominal trauma. Note the absence of significant injury on skin surface of the abdomen.

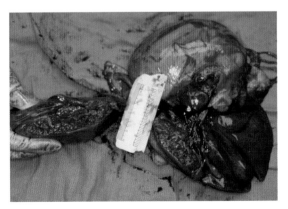

Figure 2 Internal findings of the child depicted in **Figure 1**. Massive hepatic lacerations resulting in complete transection caused by blunt-force injury.

many factors elucidated above. Again, the composition of the tissue at the impact site affects the appearance of the wound pattern as much as the type, force, and duration of impact. The same type and force of blunt impact may create different injury patterns depending on whether the impact occurs on the skin overlying the lateral malleolus of the ankle (with relatively little in the way of soft tissue between the skin surface and the bony protuberance), or the upper one-third of the thigh, with its more abundant adipose tissue and heavy musculature encasing the shaft of the femur.

In this article, the injuries will be artificially separated into various types. First, injuries to the skin and soft tissues will be considered, followed by osseous injuries, and last by blunt-impact injuries to internal viscera. In reality, a single impact may cause injury to all three structure types within a given anatomic location. Additionally, the reader is urged to refer to other articles dealing specifically with blunt impacts to various anatomic locations for more detailed accounts of the effects of such trauma to the internal viscera.

Blunt Injuries to the Skin and Subcutaneous Tissues

Blunt-force injuries to the skin and subcutaneous tissues usually fall into one of three broad categories: (1) abrasion; (2) laceration; and (3) contusion.

An abrasion is often the most superficial and minor of these three injury types. It commonly happens as an impacting object moves over the skin surface with an angle of impact of less than $90°$ (**Figure 3**). A scraped or skinned knee on a child sustained in a bicycle mishap is an example of a superficial abrasion. Often the abrasions are located over bony prominences. More often than not, the pattern and shape are nonspecific. In fact, the pattern and shape may be more reflective of the underlying anatomic structures than the actual impacting object (**Figure 4**). Even so, there are indeed instances in which it is possible to determine information regarding the causation. An abrasion may demonstrate an impact "rolled edge" of skin along one side of the abrasion, allowing the examiner to determine the direction of force, or the injury itself may display a pattern or periodicity reflective of the impacting object (**Figure 5**).

A laceration occurs when the skin tears open in response to a blunt impact. Various areas of the body, such as those in close proximity to underlying bone, may be more likely to lacerate in response to an impact. Classically, lacerations exhibit two characteristics that allow differentiation from sharp-force injuries: (1) wound margin abrasions; and (2) wound bed tissue bridges.

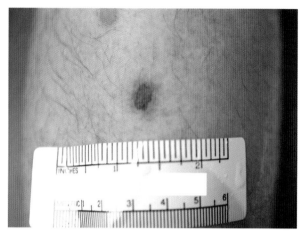

Figure 3   Healing superficial abrasion.

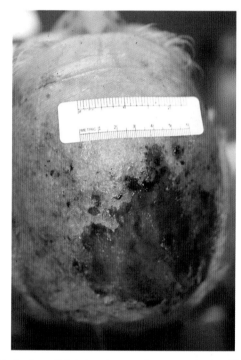

Figure 4   Superficial abrasion over bony prominence. The injury configuration is dictated by the contour and composition of the body (rounded osseous tissue immediately deep to cutaneous surface) rather than by the impacting object.

First, the wound margins of a laceration often display abrasions which were formed at the time of impact, as the tissues are crushed by the impacting object (**Figure 6**). Second, the wound bed displays tissue bridges. The subcutaneous tissues have many different types of tissue of varying strengths and angles of orientation in relation to the angle of impact. Therefore, some tissues may tear while others remain intact. This creates varying amounts of "bridging" of tissues within the wound bed itself (**Figure 7**).

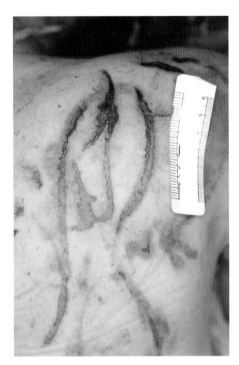

Figure 5 Pattern abrasions and contusions mirroring the basic shape of the impacting object. The victim in this case was beaten with a crutch – the pattern mirrors a surface of the impacting instrument.

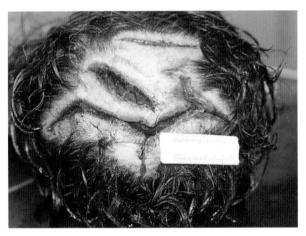

Figure 6 Lacerations with abrasions along the wound margins.

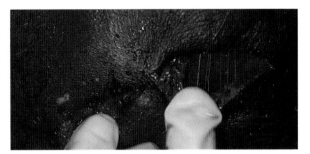

Figure 7 Laceration with tissue bridging of the wound bed.

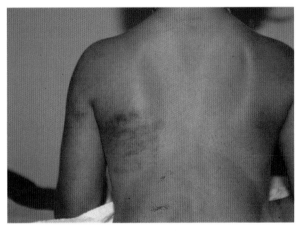

Figure 8 Pattern contusion "outlining" the impacting object. The impacting object in this case was a hand.

A contusion may be defined as an area of bleeding beneath the intact skin at the site of impact. It is commonly referred to as a bruise. Contusions are usually nonspecific in shape. At times, however, pattern contusions may be present. A pattern contusion may be defined as a contusion in which the size and shape mirror a portion of the object which created it, a contour of the body, or a combination thereof.

A rapid impact with a relatively lightweight object may create a contusion in the shape of the outline of the object. Cylindrical objects will thus create patterns consisting of two parallel linear contusions with central sparing. This occurs because the tissues that are deformed and damaged the most are those along the edges of the object (**Figure 8**). With heavier impacts or objects, the tissues beneath the impacting object are crushed as well, and the contusion pattern is solid rather than outlined (**Figure 9**).

The terms contusion, ecchymosis, and hematoma should not be used interchangeably, but when used must be used with an understanding of each term. As stated earlier, a cutaneous contusion is bleeding beneath the intact skin at the site of impact. In contrast, an ecchymosis represents a collection of blood that has dissected through fascial planes from one site to another. An ecchymosis may be associated with blunt trauma, or it may be associated with other forms of injury. The source of blood in ecchymosis often involves an osseous fracture. Blood dissects from the site of origin through fascial planes to a subcutaneous location where it is observed as an area of discoloration. Perhaps the most common ecchymosis observed in forensic pathology is the periorbital ecchymosis associated with a fracture of

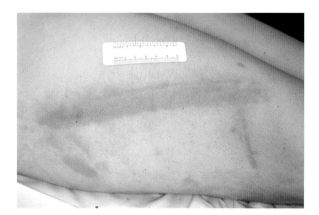

Figure 9 Pattern contusion caused by impact with a large wooden instrument with intervening clothing. The tissue underlying the impacting object was crushed, and therefore the injury appears as a solid pattern.

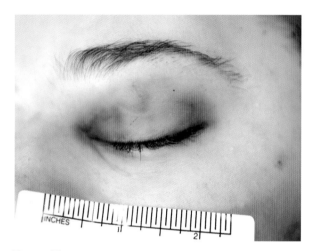

Figure 10 Periorbital ecchymosis associated with a gunshot wound.

the anterior fossa (orbital plate) of the base of the skull (**Figure 10**). This is often seen in conjunction with contact gunshot wounds of the head. Other commonly encountered ecchymoses include discoloration over the mastoid process in association with the basilar skull fracture, and discoloration over the flank in association with a pelvic fracture. Hematoma is an additional term that should be differentiated from the term contusion. The term hematoma simply refers to a collection of extravasated blood either within the tissue parenchyma or within a potential space. Examples include subcapsular hematomas of the liver, and intracranial subdural hematomas. Hematomas may occur in the absence of impact, and must be interpreted in the context of the individual case. The mere presence of a hematoma in a given case does not allow the examiner to conclude automatically that blunt impact has occurred.

Osseous Injuries

A fracture may be defined as an interruption in the structure of a bone. There are various types of fractures, as described in more detail in other articles in this encyclopedia. Regarding fractures associated with blunt trauma, a bone will usually fracture at leverage point, as this represents the point of maximum tension. Assessment of the distribution and nature of fractures may help to elucidate the causative events. Precise determination of fracture location may be important in cases such as pedestrian injuries and assessment of driver versus passenger in motor vehicle collisions. In the living patient, fractures may be documented by radiographic methods. In the deceased patient, fractures may be documented through radiographs and/or autopsy examination. Some fractures occur as a result of direct blunt impact, while others occur for a variety of reasons and in a variety of biomechanical scenarios. It should not be assumed that the presence of a fracture necessarily indicates blunt-force trauma at the fracture site.

Visceral Blunt Injuries

Blunt forces applied to the torso may result in injuries to the visceral organs. As stated previously, the head represents a unique structure and is considered elsewhere. Blunt-force injuries to the visceral organs of the thorax and abdomen may include contusions or lacerations of the organ itself, or avulsion of the organ from its pedicle or supporting structures. Mortality and morbidity of blunt traumatic injuries depend on many factors, including the organs involved, the degree of trauma, and access to medical treatment. The degree of injury evident on the external skin cannot be used to assess the degree of damage to the internal organs. This is particularly true in injuries to the abdomen where it is not uncommon to find severe – even fatal – internal injuries while the external skin surface appears atraumatic.

Visceral blunt trauma associated with death often involves lacerations of either the heart or the liver. In lacerations of the heart, if the pericardial sac remains intact, then a hemopericardium with cardiac tamponade may result in death within minutes. Depending on the nature of the trauma, this injury may be solely causative or may be found with other lesser, but contributing injuries, such as pulmonary contusions and/or lacerations arising from motor vehicle collisions.

Compared to other visceral organs, the liver is relatively friable, has little elastic tissue, and is very vascular. While clinicians may rate lacerations on a numeric scale to describe severity, forensic pathologists usually assess the anatomic location and general size of the traumatic lesion. Large complex hepatic lacerations may cause internal exsanguination within relatively short order (minutes).

Blunt traumatic injuries of other solid visceral organs may, on some occasions, be the sole cause of death, but are more commonly seen as contributing factors in multiple blunt traumatic injuries. These organs may include the spleen, the pancreas, the lungs, and the kidneys. When the latter two are involved as the sole cause of death, the injury pattern often involves disruption of the large vessels supporting these organs.

Dating of Injuries

Forensic physicians are frequently asked by investigators to assess the age of a blunt-force injury. The injury in question may be any of the four main types previously discussed (abrasion, laceration, contusion, or fracture). Commonly, a forensic physician will be asked to assess the age of cutaneous contusions. Various medical texts display charts on the dating of contusions based on color. It is strongly advised that such charts be used only as a very rough guide, as many factors affect contusion color and the evolution thereof. Factors affecting contusion colors include: (1) depth of bleeding; (2) amount of bleeding; (3) environmental lighting; and (4) overlying skin color.

Experimental animal studies have confirmed the variability of the evolution of color and contusions. Indeed, in one prospective study involving sheep, only one consistent statement could be made regarding injury duration and color change: contusions displaying yellow color had been present for at least 18 h. In deceased individuals, tissue samples submitted for microscopy may assist in age estimation based upon the breakdown of red blood cells and the succession of inflammatory cells responding to an injury site. Recent research has involved investigation of various immunohistochemical markers in an attempt to narrow the time window further; however, no specific marker has emerged to date. Even with microscopy, individual variation exists. In summary, dating of injuries in general, and contusions in particular, remains an imprecise science. Although general comments and subjective terms may be of use, precise timing of injury duration is not possible with our current state of knowledge.

Summary

With the "bumps and scrapes" of everyday life, blunt injuries are undoubtedly the most common type of trauma sustained by humans. More severe blunt traumatic injuries are significant causes of morbidity and mortality, resulting in substantial loss of both productivity and life.

Blunt trauma should be assessed in several ways. Individual injuries are examined regarding size, shape, and color. The anatomic location of the injury is noted. Patterns are assessed for consistency with external objects and/or body contours. The injury is examined in relation to, and in the context of, the overall injury pattern. Historical information of the causative event is then compared to the injury for assessment of consistency with the size, shape, severity, and distribution of the injury pattern. Documentation of specific information regarding blunt injuries allows reassessment at later times and/or independent assessment by other parties. This documentation may include reports, diagrams, and photographs.

Written documentation of blunt injuries includes a description of injuries' size, shape, color, pattern, and anatomic location. Preparation of a "wound diagram" consists of noting the location of injuries or other notable external findings on a standard diagram of the human form or a particular anatomic region.

Photographic documentation provides a permanent representation of the injury in question. Ideally, photographic documentation includes distant images and close-ups. Distant images document the injury in relation to the body as a whole, and also in relation to other injuries. Close photographs allow documentation of injury pattern details. Photos are obtained in a plane of focus perpendicular to the injury. A measurement scale in the plane of injury allows both assessment of injury size and the potential to develop computer-generated comparisons of possible causative instruments at a later date.

In certain cases, it is often the small blunt injuries to the external surface that provide more information to the forensic investigator than the larger, lethal internal injuries. Such small subtle injuries may help elucidate the events leading to, or involved in, the death. Proper appreciation of the importance of such injuries improves the quality of forensic investigations. Adequate documentation of a pattern injury allows the injury to "speak for itself" when the examiner is called upon to defend his/her conclusions and opinions.

See Also

Children: Physical Abuse; **Computer Crime and Digital Evidence; Deaths:** Trauma, Head and Spine; Trauma, Thorax; Trauma, Abdominal Cavity; Trauma, Musculo-skeletal System; Trauma, Vascular System;

Imaging: Photography; **Injury, Fatal and Nonfatal:** Firearm Injuries; Sharp and Cutting-Edge Wounds; **Injury, Transportation:** Motor Vehicle

Further Reading

DiMaio VJ, DiMaio D (2001) *Forensic Pathology*, 2nd edn. New York: CRC Press.

Froede RC (ed.) (2003) *Handbook of Forensic Pathology*, 2nd edn. Northfield, IL: College of American Pathologists.

Knight B (1991) *Forensic Pathology*. New York: Oxford University Press.

Langlois NE, Gresham GA (1991) The aging of bruises: a review and study of the colour changes with time. *Forensic Science International* 50: 227–238.

Reese RM (ed.) (1994) *Child Abuse: Medical Diagnosis and Management*. London: Lea & Febiger.

Burns and Scalds

B B Ong, Queensland Health Scientific Services, Brisbane, QLD, Australia

Introduction

Burns are a commonly encountered forensic problem. Even though the majority of cases presenting with burns are accidental, the forensic practitioner is often required to rule out abuse. A body pulled from a fire may not necessarily have died from burns or smoke inhalation. The fire may be used to destroy evidence and deter identification. Postmortem burns have to be differentiated from those caused before death. Artifacts caused by burns have to be recognized.

Burns are defined as tissue reaction to injury due to heat, chemicals, or radiation. It causes disruption of the metabolic processes of cells that ultimately ends in tissue death. The main cellular manifestation is coagulation necrosis.

This article describes clinical classification, type of burns encountered, causation of burns, and the medicolegal aspects.

Classification of Burns

Burns may vary from simple erythema (e.g., sunburn) to soft-tissue burns to deep charring. In clinical practice, burns are classified according to the depth: superficial, partial-thickness, and full-thickness. In another classification, the depth is categorized as first-, second-, and third-degree burns (**Table 1**).

The mildest skin damage is simple erythema. The most common cause is sunburn. It involves only the epidermis and manifests clinically as erythema and pain. Mild blistering may occur and, in most instances, there will be peeling of the damaged skin after a few days and healing without any scarring.

In partial-thickness burns, the epidermis is destroyed together with part of the dermis. Partial-thickness burns are further divided into superficial or deep. There is usually preservation of the appendages of the skin in a superficial partial-thickness burn. Pain sensation is preserved. Blisters may occur. The wound usually heals without scarring. A deep partial-thickness burn is also known as a deep dermal burn. Most appendages are destroyed. The clinical appearance is not unlike full-thickness burns with little or no pain. Scarring will occur if left to heal naturally.

In full-thickness burns, the entire layers of epidermis and dermis are destroyed. There is destruction of blood vessels and nerve endings, rendering the area avascular and painless. The clinical appearance is white or leathery brown due to blood vessel damage. Healing occurs through epithelialization from the edges, and will produce scarring unless skin grafting is performed.

In most cases, patients will present with burns of different depth in different regions of the body, often next to each other. Clinically it may be difficult to diagnose the depth accurately. It may become clearer after a few days and a repeat examination may be needed for accurate assessment. Doppler or thermographic imaging has been used to assess the depth of burns but does not seem any better than clinical assessment.

An important clinical assessment is to estimate the extent of burns on the body surface. The surface area involved has a direct effect on the morbidity and mortality. The assessment can be made roughly by using the rule of nines. This is where various body parts are given certain percentages of total body surface (9% for head and each upper limb, 18% for each lower limb, front and back of trunk) (**Figure 1**). A more accurate assessment can be made by using the Lund and Browder chart, which is available in most hospitals.

In addition to body surfaces, inhalation injuries and burns in the gastrointestinal tract can occur. The proportion of inhalation injuries in burn victims is known to be quite high and found in about 20% of admissions to burn centers. Dry heat does not penetrate easily and is limited to the oropharynx and upper airway. On the other hand, steam penetrates further (4000 times better) and thermal injury may be seen beyond the larynx. Apart from heat, chemicals in smoke may cause bronchospasm and mucous

Table 1 Classification and brief clinical presentation of burns

Classification	Depth and appearance	Clinical	Healing
Superficial	Epidermis only. Dilation of vessels	Erythema, mild discomfort	Skin peeling within 5–10 days without scarring
Partial-thickness: Superficial (first-degree)	Epidermis with part of dermis. Skin appendages preserved	Erythema with blisters formation. Painful	Heal within 10–14 days without scarring
Deep (second-degree)	Entire epidermis with part of dermis. Most skin appendages destroyed	Usually no blisters. May or not have pain sensation	Heal slowly (months) with dense scarring
Full-thickness (third-degree)	Entire epidermis and dermis. All skin appendages including blood vessels destroyed	White to brown leathery appearance. No pain sensation. May have charring or carbonization	Heal slowly (months) with dense scarring

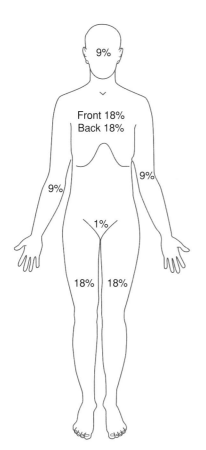

Figure 1 Rules of nines for estimating extent of surface burns.

Table 2 Summary of contact time with temperature in causing partial-thickness burns[a]

Temperature (°C)	45	50	55	60	65
Time taken	3 h	4 min	30 s	5 s	1 s

[a]Data modified from: Moritz AR, Henriques FC (1947) Studies of thermal injury. II. The relative importance of time and surface temperature in the causation of cutaneous burns. *American Journal of Pathology* 23: 695–720; Department of Health and Social Security (1977) Safe temperature for heated surfaces and hot water. Quoted in: Hobbs CJ, Hanks HGI, Wynne JM (1999) *Child Abuse and Neglect. A Clinician's Handbook,* 2nd edn, Chapter 5. London: Churchill Livingstone.

membrane ulceration, including damage to the cilia and edema.

Gastrointestinal burns may occur when hot food or liquids are ingested. They may occur accidentally, in the setting of abuse, or in suicidal attempts such as ingestion of corrosive and caustic chemicals.

Mechanism of Injury

Thermal injury occurs when energy is transferred from a heat source to the body, causing an increase in the temperature of local tissue. When tissue temperature rises above a certain threshold, irreversible cellular injury will occur, with interruption of metabolic processes. Experiments by Moritz and Henriques, as far back as 1947, revealed that burns will not occur if the temperature is below 44 °C. Once heat applied is 44 °C or above, tissue injury will occur, although it requires at least 6 h. Above 44 °C but below 51 °C at the skin surface, the rate of thermal injury doubles with each degree increase in temperature. Temperature above 51 °C will cause almost immediate destruction of the epidermis. Above 70 °C, full-thickness tissue destruction occurs in seconds. An estimation of thermal injury according to time and temperature is given in **Table 2**.

Using this table and charts in similar studies, a deduction of the severity of burns can be made. However, due to limitation of the experiment (e.g., based on certain parts of the body and exposure of temperature with a heated metal pipe), it is at best an estimate rather than a clinical certainty. Other variables such as variation in thickness of skin at different sites of the body, circulation of blood, and influence of clothing also play a vital role in influencing the outcome.

Clinical Effects of Burns

The clinical effects of burns are dependent on a few important factors:

- percentage of body surface involved
- depth of burns
- location of burns
- presence of inhalation or gastrointestinal burns.

Other important factors influencing severity of burns include age of patient and presence of associated injury or disease.

Any burns exceeding more than 50% of body surface are regarded as potentially fatal, regardless of the depth. The most important complication in the early stages is loss of body fluid, which may result in hypovolemic shock if not corrected promptly. The loss of fluid is further exacerbated by tissue edema.

Infection is also a common and serious complication. Devitalized tissue provides an ideal site for bacterial colonization leading to septicemia. Another source of infection is from the lungs. Sepsis with multiple organ failure is probably the most common cause of death encountered by forensic pathologists in burnt patients with a period of survival. Fatal infections are often caused by virulent opportunistic organisms such as *Pseudomonas aeruginosa*, methicillin-resistant *Staphylococcus aureus*, and fungi.

Another important effect is an increase in metabolic rate necessitating nutritional support. Failure to correct the hypermetabolic state may lead to loss of protein and eventual starvation. There is excessive heat production, which may lead to eventual heat loss.

Source of Burns

Burns can be caused by a variety of means: physical, electrical, chemical, and radiation are among the known causes.

Physical Burns

Transfer of heat to the skin results in burns. There are two main types of physical burns: those caused by dry heat and liquid (scalds).

Dry heat   Dry heat causes burns by direct conduction or radiation to the skin. In flame burns, there is direct contact with flame. Contact burns involve physical contact of body with a hot object. Radiant burns are caused by exposure to a heat source. The most common radiant-heat injury is due to sunburn. A special type of burn is due to flash fire. Here, one normally sees singeing of hair with partial-thickness burns due to brief but intense exposure to heat.

Depending on the severity of the heat and time of exposure, the burns can be partial or full-thickness. If left exposed longer, charring and carbonization may occur; this involves deeper tissues or even bones, as commonly seen in bodies recovered in a fire.

Scalds   Scalds result from hot liquids. The source is usually water but hot oils, other liquids, and even steam can cause scalds.

A scald caused by water does not cause charring or singeing of hair since the temperature is not high enough (**Table 3**). It is usually well demarcated. If caused by immersion, patients will present with a horizontal fluid level commonly known as a "tidemark." If hot fluid has been tipped over the body, there will be a trickle pattern with the part of initial exposure being the most severe. As the fluid flows down the body, the width will be narrower due to the mechanics of flow and rapid cooling at the edges. Splash burns may be seen in association with such burns.

In addition to surface burns caused by steam, inhalation burns may occur due to its greater penetration capacity.

Electrical Burns

These are specific burns, which are usually deep and may involve extensive tissue damage. Thermal injury occurs when electrical energy is converted to heat, causing local damage. The thermal effects and picture are dependent on the type of current (domestic or industrial), time of exposure, and resistance of tissues. Electrical burns can occur at both entry and exit points.

The typical electrical burn consists of a depressed leathery area of tissue necrosis, occasionally with a blister. There may be a faint rim of erythema. Metallization may occur.

Table 3   Differences between dry heat and scalds

	Dry heat	Scald
Source	Contact or flame burns	Hot liquid, usually water or steam
Clinical appearance	May be partial- or full-thickness	Red base with blisters. Usually partial-thickness
	May have charring or carbonization	No charring or carbonization
	Hair may be singed	Hair not singed
	Variable borders	Usually sharply demarcated. May have splash marks
Uniformity of burns	Usually not uniform	Usually uniform depth

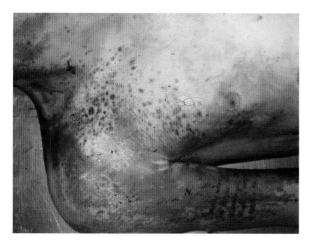

Figure 2 "Crocodile skin" due to burns resulting from high-voltage electrocution.

A specific severe burn is caused by the application of high-voltage electricity. In addition to the contact mark, further thermal injuries are caused by arcing. Presentation may show spotty areas of burns, sometimes described as "crocodile skin" (**Figure 2**).

Lightning causes a specific type of burn. Exposure is usually brief, with the current passing over the body with a flashover effect. It causes streaks of interrupted linear burns, which reflect its passage downwards to the ground. There is usually partial charring and singeing of hair. There may be arborescent fern-like markings known as Lichtenburg figures or filigree burns. Histology of the lesion shows extravasated red blood cells in the subcutaneous fat with intact epidermis and dermis. Burns due to heating and melting of metallic objects worn by the deceased may be seen.

Chemical Burns

The extent of burns is dependent on the concentration, area of exposure, duration of contact, and type of chemical. Burns can also occur in the gastrointestinal tract in both accidental and suicidal ingestion. Inhalation of fumes can cause respiratory damage. Systemic toxicity due to absorption of the chemicals through skin can be more serious than the burns.

A common type of chemical burn is due to acids and alkalis, followed by a range of other increasingly complex chemicals (**Table 4**).

The chemical will continue to cause tissue damage as long as it is present and will cease when neutralized by tissue or other means. Tissue damage is dependent on the following factors:

1. type of chemical
2. concentration
3. quantity
4. duration of contact
5. presence of exothermic reaction.

Table 4 Summary of chemicals capable of causing burns

Acids	Exothermic reaction in addition to corrosive injury. Results in coagulation necrosis. Further penetration is inhibited
Hydrofluoric acid	Similar to other acids. Fluoride ion binds with tissue Ca and Mg ions, resulting in cell death. Causes intense pain
Alkali	Saponification of fat-forming soluble proteinates, resulting in liquefactive necrosis. Tendency to penetrate deep to cause deep burns
Phenols	Weak acid. The burn may be painless because it causes demyelination of nerve fibers and destruction of nerve endings. Due to easy absorptivity of phenols, systemic toxicity may occur
Petroleum products	Defattening. Usually results in irritation unless there is prolonged exposure
Mustard gas	Mustard gas causes blisters leading to sloughing of skin. May cause inhalation injuries

Acids The mechanism is usually direct corrosion (via its hydrogen ion) and heat (exothermic) reaction. It causes coagulation necrosis, which prevents deeper tissue from being exposed to the chemical. It acts quite rapidly, causing superficial burns after only 5 s of contact and full-thickness burns after 30 s.

An important exception is hydrofluoric acid. Apart from its corrosive effect, it exerts further destruction effect via the fluoride ion. The ion can penetrate deeply into the tissue, combining with intracellular calcium and magnesium and causing cell death.

Alkalis The main mechanism of the hydroxyl ion is saponification of fat and alkali proteinates to cause liquefaction necrosis. Although they do not act as rapidly as acids, alkalis have the ability to penetrate much deeper into the tissue, exerting their effects longer.

Other chemicals There is an ever-increasing number of organic and inorganic compounds. Traditional ones include organic solvents and phenols. Chemicals of warfare, including mustard gas (vesicants) and lewisite, can cause blistering of skin similar to burns.

Radiation

The incidence of radiation burns is low. In principle, long-wavelength radiation causes direct damage by producing heat. Short-wavelength radiation on the other hand causes severe burns due to ionization of tissue in addition to local production of heat. **Table 5** summarizes different types of radiation.

A specific type of radiation burn is caused by microwave ovens which use nonionizing radiation.

Table 5 Types of radiation

Nonionizing radiation	Radiowave, microwave, infrared light, ultraviolet light
Ionizing radiation	X-rays, gamma-rays

The microwave oven heats food from within, unlike conventional ovens, by creating molecular agitation of polarized molecules such as water. Thus, tissue with high water content produces more heat than tissue with low water content. Typically, it produces sandwich-type burns involving skin and muscle with relative sparing of the subcutaneous fat.

Histology

The effect of heat is to cause coagulation necrosis of the cells. The cellular features will appear indistinct and become more intense with histological stains.

In the skin, blister formation will occur by subepidermal separation of epithelium. The vesicles may contain occasional inflammatory cells. The cells at the periphery of the blisters become elongated and show streaming which is parallel with the basement membrane. There is a decrease in the thickness of the epidermis with a compact homogeneous dermis without empty spaces between collagen bundles. It is postulated that the epidermis has been compacted by the dermis swollen by heat, resulting in horizontal stretching of the cells. These findings are similar to those seen in electrocution marks on the skin.

Thermal injury to the airway will cause destruction of respiratory epithelium with sparing of areas protected by mucosal folds and ducts of mucous glands. The necrotic epithelium may be fused together to form a pseudomembrane or form casts within the airway. There is submucosal edema and capillary congestion. It may be accompanied by inflammation when there is adequate survival time.

Forensic Aspects

There are numerous settings where the forensic practitioner will see persons with burns. Burns can deliberately be induced to maim, kill, or torture. Fire has been used to commit suicide. It has also been used as a means of committing offenses (e.g., arson). Suspected cases of abuse must be differentiated from accidental causes. An autopsy has to be performed on a body recovered in a fire not only to find out the cause of death but also to confirm how it occurred. Additional forensic pathology issues such as artifactual injuries, identification and differentiation between antemortem or postmortem burns are also essential assessment during autopsy.

Accidental Burns

Most burns and scalds are accidental. Only a small proportion is deliberate. Accidental burns can occur due to neglect.

Accidental burns occur in extreme age groups. In younger children, burns and scalds are common. The peak age of accidental burns is usually 1–2 years old, when they acquire mobility to explore but insufficient dexterity to avoid accidents. Most elderly burn victims have some form of motor impairment. Another group who are prone to burns are epileptics. Usually, the burns are full-thickness type and may involve the bones and joints. Persons who are intoxicated are also more susceptible to burns.

Spill injuries resulting in scalds are common. Children tend to pull cups, saucepans, and other utensils. The flex of an electrical kettle can be pulled. Similar accidents can occur to the elderly and infirm. Tapwater scalds are not uncommon. A hot water tap may be turned on accidentally to wash hands without appreciating the dangers, both by children and those who are mentally impaired. Accidental immersion of hands into the sink containing hot water is not unknown.

Contact burns can be found especially with heaters, irons, or hair dryers.

Flame burns can occur when children start playing with fire using matches or cigarette lighters. Clothes may catch fire accidentally, causing serious burns. In countries that use kerosene or wood/charcoal stoves such as India, accidental ignition of clothes has been reported. The severe burns are usually found in the front of the body. Burns on hands, particularly the dominant one, can occur due to attempts to put out the flames.

Another potential hazard is chemical burns. Household chemicals with corrosive potential include bleach and hydrocarbons. Accidental burn caused by bathing a child in bleach solution due to ignorance on the part of the carer has occurred before.

Abuse

The commonest setting of burns is in child abuse but it can be seen in all forms of abuse, including domestic and elderly abuse. It must not be forgotten that burns can occur due to criminal neglect.

In physical child abuse, burns and scalds occur in about 10% of cases, usually in conjunction with some other form of trauma. About 10–25% of burns in children are deliberate. The mortality rate is significantly higher when compared to accidental burns (30% compared to 2%). Burns in child abuse may be impulsive but more often than not are premeditated.

A common injury is exposure to hot tapwater. Children are punished by exposing their limbs, frequently their hands, to hot water, causing scalds limited to that part of body.

Another frequent injury is forced immersion in hot water. It may affect hands, feet, and buttocks but sometimes almost the whole body (**Figure 3**). Depending on the position the child is immersed in the water, a clear demarcation between scalded and unburnt skin is noted. The usual position is a child being forced on to a basin of hot water, causing scalds to the hands, feet, and buttocks. There will be a glove-and-stocking distribution with sparing of the soles and part of buttocks if held firmly against the cooler base. There will be minimal splash marks associated with accidental fall into the bath.

Another form of scalding is due to splashes from deliberate spilling or throwing a bucket or bowl of hot water. The margins are irregular, influenced by gravity, and characterized by nonuniform depth of injury. One would find flow marks and "satellite" scalds due to splashes. The mark will typically narrow inferiorly following the flow pattern. The findings may be modified by clothing. Clothing can either protect the child from further injury or retain hot water (heat) to cause more severe scalds.

Another common injury is cigarette burns (**Table 6**). Cigarette burns can occur not only in the setting of child abuse but also in domestic and elderly abuse. They appear as full-thickness burns with craters. It is important to differentiate accidental burns from intentional acts. Accidental cigarette burn is usually due to brief brush contact. Care must be taken to exclude skin conditions (e.g., impetigo) with a similar appearance.

Contact burns using hot objects can sometimes be seen. Usually domestic objects are used. For example, a child may be forced to sit on a hot plate. An iron may be used. Usually, the burns take a similar shape as the offending object (**Figure 4**). A careful history has to be taken to differentiate accidental burns.

Other forms of burns may be due to force-feeding of hot food into the mouth, resulting in burns around the lips and cheek. Other atypical types of abusive burns include corrosive and electrical burns. Deep burns due to placing the infant/child inside a microwave oven have been reported. A summary of the types of burn seen in abuse is given in **Table 7**.

Presentation in abuse cases may be acute, chronic, or when complications arise, for example, secondary infection. Suspicion may be aroused when there is a delay in taking the victim for medical treatment, the presence of other injuries, evidence of neglect, or discrepancy in history (**Table 8**).

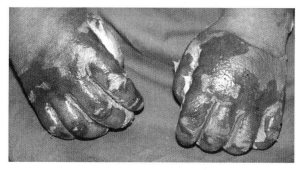

Figure 3   Glove distribution of scalds on hands of child due to forced immersion into basin of hot water. Courtesy of Dr. Bhupinder Singh.

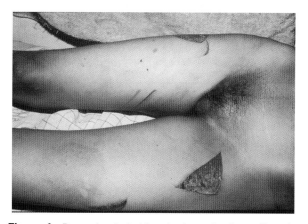

Figure 4   Burns due to hot iron in domestic abuse. Note the shape of the burns.

Table 6   Differential diagnosis of cigarette burns

Abuse	Deep and cratered, full-thickness, may be on unusual sites not associated with accidental injury, e.g., soles of feet. Usually healed by scarring. Old cigarette burn scars may be present
Accidental	Area of reddening, sometimes with a tail or elliptical in shape, signifying an accidental brushed contact
Bullous impetigo	Usually clustered together. Healed without scarring, usually centrally

Table 7   Types of burn found in abuse

Scalds	Immersion burns
	Spill burns
	Tap burns
Flame burns	Fire/matchstick
	Cigarette burns
Contact burns	Hot plates
	Domestic objects such as iron, hair dryer, heater grills
Miscellaneous	Forcibly feeding hot food/liquids
	Use of caustic/corrosive liquid
	Electrical burns
	Microwaves

Table 8 Features suspicious of abuse

- Inconsistent history
- Physical features of burns not in keeping with the history
- Burns not compatible with psychomotor ability
- Delay in treatment or treatment when complications arose
- Presence of old burns and/or other injuries
- Features of neglect and/or sexual abuse
- Burns/scalds typical of abuse (e.g., glove-and-stocking distribution, clear tidal marks, atypical sites – buttocks, back of body, genitalia, back of hands, soles of feet)
- Signs of abuse in siblings (for child abuse)

A particular type of abuse encountered in South Asian communities is dowry death. Here the young bride is tortured or burned to death by the husband or in-laws due to poor expectation of dowry or other reasons. Death may be initially reported as accidental (e.g., while cooking). In most instances, kerosene, which is the most common accelerant used, may be detected on the body or clothing. Information on the type of stove (kerosene or otherwise) would be important to rule out accidental death. There may be the presence of both antemortem and postmortem burns (e.g., heat contractures and fractures), which indicates burning even after death. Information of burns in other members of the family may be useful as it indicates an attempt to douse the fire.

Punishment by Causing Hurt

Unlike blunt and sharp injuries, thermal injury is not common as a form of assault.

In Asian society, corrosives are well known as a weapon to cause hurt and injury. The typical situation is that of a spurned jealous lover who deliberately uses a corrosive in order to scar his partner. The corrosive is usually aimed at the face in order to cause maximum deleterious effect.

The usual corrosive is concentrated acids rather than alkalis. This may be due to the public perception of the rapid action of acids. The findings are usually coagulation burns with flow marks due to gravity. They may be modified by the clothes and rapidity of treatment (washing). The eyes may be affected. Unfortunately, the injuries heal by scarring. Occasionally death can occur, especially when inhalation occurs, causing chemical pneumonitis or when complications arise (e.g., secondary infection).

Torture

Among the reported methods of torture that cause thermal injury are use of hot implements (branding), molten liquids, cigarette burns, and electrical injury. There is usually variation depending on local culture. A common problem is the long delay between injury and time of examination. Consequently, the victim presents with scars or keloids as manifestation of previous burns.

Self-Infliction

Suicidal death by burning is known as immolation. The frequency is dependent on culture. It is a common method of suicide in South Asia but uncommon in the west. Immolation has been used as a method of political protest.

It can occur within the confines of a house or vehicle, which is deliberately set on fire. More commonly, the victims douse themselves with an accelerant, commonly petrol or kerosene. There are usually extensive burns more prominent on the front of the body with sparing of skin folds.

Swallowing of corrosives is a known method of suicide. Severe damage may occur in the upper gastrointestinal tract, leading to erosion and healing by stricture formation.

Occasionally, burns are self-inflicted for the motive of gain or spite, e.g. through the use of an iron. The usual characteristics of self-inflicted injuries are applicable (similar depth, usually superficial, clustering).

Examination of Deaths due to Burns

If death occurs immediately or soon after the incident, the victim usually presents with severe burns. Inhalation of smoke is frequently attributed as a cause of death. In house fires, the body may be charred. Additional issues such as identification of severely charred body, whether the person was alive before the fire, reconstruction of circumstances, and postmortem induced artifact may be a problem.

In deaths occurring after a period of survival, it is important to document the burns, evidence of medical intervention (e.g., skin grafting, escharotomy), inhalation injuries, and presence of medical complications. Known complications include shock due to burns, secondary infections, including septicemia and pneumonia, pulmonary embolism, small intestinal ulceration (Curling ulcer), renal failure, and other miscellaneous causes such as pancreatitis and fat embolism.

Other Situations

Occasionally the forensic physician may be asked to examine a suspected arsonist, especially when the alleged person has ignited the fire directly. Liquid accelerants can evaporate easily, forming an explosive mixture with air. Inexperienced offenders risk an explosion when attempting to ignite the accelerants, sustaining burns as a result.

According to Bohnert and coworkers, the explosion causes typical heat changes and injuries to the exposed person. There may be singeing of exposed hair (frontal head hair, facial hair, and hair on exposed body) and skin burns of varying degree (back of hand, face). These features, especially singed hair, may be seen weeks after an alleged offense. Toxicology analyses of the blood for accelerants and evidence of inhalation of smoke (carbon monoxide levels) may be useful if the assailant is apprehended soon after the offense.

Natural Disease Mimicking Burns

Certain natural disease, especially dermatology conditions, can mimic burns. Bullous disease like porphyria and erythema multiforme can present with blisters, which are similar in appearance to burns. Impetigo and chickenpox can be mistaken for cigarette burns. Other conditions capable of an appearance similar to burns include allergic conditions (allergic dermatitis, urticaria) and insect bites.

Approach to Investigations

A few considerations may be undertaken to ascertain if the circumstances are consistent with appearance of burns:

1. A full and detailed history. More often than not, the injuries inflicted may not be consistent with the history. This is true not only in child abuse but in other types of domestic abuse as well. Persons who are abused may not reveal the truth for fear of further reprisals or to protect the abuser.
2. Scene visit may be important. This may include examination of the alleged appliances used, assessment of the water temperature and the position in which the body is found.
3. Full examination, including careful charting of burns.
4. Often in abuse cases there may be other associated injuries. Therefore, it is imperative that a detailed examination is carried out, partly to rule out sexual abuse.
5. Assess if the manifestation of burns is consistent with the circumstances. This includes taking into account the history, scene examination, and time period exposed to the heat source.

In addition, there are several other considerations in a postmortem examination:

1. Was the person alive before the fire? The standard technique is to look for evidence of smoke inhalation in the airway and the presence of agents of combustion (e.g., carbon monoxide) in the blood.
2. Cause of death, for example, smoke inhalation or directly to thermal injury. If death occurs after a

period of time, complications of burns may be responsible for death.
3. Look for antemortem injuries, which may be masked by destruction of body. Conversely, assess whether any of the injuries present are artifactual.
4. Issues of identification if the body is badly disfigured. An X-ray of the body may be useful for identification purposes. It can also assist in ruling out other forms of injury, which may be masked (e.g., gunshot wounds) by the disfigurement.
5. Collection of trace evidence (e.g., clothes for evidence of accelerants) and toxicology to look for products of combustion (e.g., carbon monoxide) and contributing factors such as drugs and alcohol.

See Also

Autopsy, Findings: Fire; **Children:** Physical Abuse; **Drug-Induced Injury, Accidental and Iatrogenic**; **Drugs, Prescribed:** Licencing and Registration; Product Liability; **Electric Shocks and Electrocution, Clinical Effects and Pathology**; **Torture:** Physical Findings

Further Reading

Bohnert M, Ropohl D, Pollak S (1999) Clinical findings in the medico-legal investigation of arsonists. *Journal of Clinical Forensic Medicine* 6: 145–150.
Cooper PN (2003) Injuries and death caused by heat and electricity. In: Payne-James J, Busuttil A, Smock W (eds.) *Forensic Medicine: Clinical and Pathological Aspects*, pp. 181–200. San Francisco, CA: Greenwich Medical Media.
Demling RH (1985) Burns. *New England Journal of Medicine* 313: 1389–1398.
DiMaio VJ, DiMaio D (2001) Fire deaths. In: *Forensic Pathology*, 2nd edn., pp. 367–387. Boca Raton, FL: CRC Press.
Gee D (1984) Death from physical and chemical injury, starvation and neglect. In: Mant AK (ed.) *Taylor's Principle and Practice of Medical Jurisprudence*, 13th edn., pp. 249–281. Edinburgh, UK: Churchill Livingstone.
Hettiaratchy S, Dziewulski P (2004) ABC of burns. Pathophysiology and types of burns. *British Medical Journal* 328: 1427–1429.
Hobbs CJ, Hanks HGI, Wynne J (eds.) (1999) Burns and scalds. In: *Child Abuse and Neglect. A Clincian's Handbook*, 2nd edn., pp. 105–121. London: Churchill Livingstone.
Janssen W (ed.) (1984) Injuries caused by heat and cold. In: *Forensic Histopathology*, pp. 234–260. Berlin: Springer-Verlag.
Kumar V, Tripathi CB (2004) Burnt wives: a study of homicides. *Medicine, Science and the Law* 44: 55–60.
Moritz AR, Henriques FC (1947) Studies on thermal injury II. The relative importance of time and surface temperature in the causation of cutaneous burns. *American Journal of Pathology* 23: 695–720.

Saukko P, Knight B (eds.) (2004) Burns and scalds. In: *Knight's Forensic Pathology,* 3rd edn., pp. 312–325. London: Arnold.

Settle JAD (ed.) (1996) *Principles and Practice of Burns Management.* New York: Churchill Livingstone.

Settle JAD (2000) Burns. In: Mason JK, Purdue BN (eds.) *The Pathology of Trauma,* 3rd edn., pp. 211–229. London: Arnold.

Explosive Injury

J Crane, Queen's University, Belfast, UK

Introduction

Terrorist activity in many parts of the world is associated with the use of a variety of explosive devices, and the doctors treating live casualties from bomb explosions as well as pathologists dealing with the dead need to have knowledge of the types of injury explosion can cause. Pathologists in particular may find themselves dealing with large numbers of bodies requiring identification and examination to establish the cause of death. In addition, a careful examination of the victims and in particular the nature and distribution of their injuries may help in reconstructing the circumstances in which the death occurred.

It is important to appreciate that terrorists use bombs for different reasons against a variety of targets, which may range from simple crudely constructed home-made devices using "low-order" explosives to sophisticated bombs using powerful military plastic explosive materials and incorporating elaborate radio-controlled detonators and antihandling devices. Pathologists and others must be aware of the use of "suicide" bombers and should therefore bear in mind that amongst the casualties/fatalities there may be those who have actually instigated the incident by detonating a device attached to their body.

An understanding of what happens during an explosion is important in order to appreciate the types of injuries seen in victims. When an explosion occurs, the explosive material is suddenly converted into a large volume of gas with the release of tremendous amounts of energy. Pressures of up to 150 000 atm can be generated, and the temperature of the explosive gases can rise to 3000 °C. Exposure to an explosion produces a well-defined pattern of injury from:

- direct transmission of a detonation shock wave, manifested principally as blast lung, bowel contusion, and tympanic membrane rupture

- secondary injury caused by fragments and other missiles
- injury resulting from displacement of the victim's body as a whole by the complex pressure loads imposed upon it (any injury caused by collapse of buildings or nearby structures is included in this category).

Thus individuals in the vicinity of an explosion can experience a number of effects:

1. If they are very close to the seat of the explosion, they may be blown to pieces and scattered by the force of the explosion gases.
2. If they are near enough for the skin to be in contact with the explosion flame, they may sustain flame burns, whilst at greater distances, exposure to the momentary heat radiation causes "flash" burns.
3. They may be injured by the shock wave, which spreads concentrically from the blast center. This pressure wave is followed by a postblast wind, which also does damage.
4. They may be struck by flying missiles propelled by the explosion.
5. They may be injured or crushed by falling debris and masonry, usually of buildings demolished by the explosion.
6. They may be overcome by fumes formed as a result of the explosion or from the effects of fire (burns and smoke inhalation) if a secondary fire develops, for example, following fracture of a gas main.

Types of Injury

The injuries seen in victims of explosion can be separated into six categories:

1. complete disruption
2. explosive injury
3. flying-missile injury
4. injury from falling masonry
5. burns
6. blast.

Complete Disruption

When individuals are in the immediate vicinity of an explosion there may be complete disruption of the body. The victim may be literally blown to bits and the parts scattered over an area of 200 m radius. This is relatively uncommon but may occur in current terrorist situations when someone is carrying a large bomb that explodes or when a victim is blown up by a landmine. It is also to be expected in suicide bombers who strap explosives to their bodies.

When collected, washed, and examined, the identifiable remains are typically seen to comprise pieces of scalp and skin, portions of spine, major limb joints, and lumps of muscle. Usually most of the internal organs are missing (**Figure 1**). Nonhuman tissue is often found amongst the material submitted for examination and must be identified and discarded. In one explosion in a fish market, the terrorist as well as nine victims were killed. Amongst the material submitted for examination there was a variety of different types of fish and crustaceans.

Explosive Injury

Perhaps surprisingly, most individuals close to the seat of an explosion remain, by and large, relatively intact. Those within a couple of meters of the explosion may have parts of their limbs blown off (traumatic amputation) and sustain severe mangling of other parts of the body, often with breaching of the chest or abdominal cavities, but they usually remain sufficiently intact for a detailed autopsy to be carried out (**Figure 2**). A detailed study of the mechanism of traumatic amputation by bomb blast in victims in Northern Ireland concluded that flailing of the limbs is not the cause but instead direct coupling of explosive shock waves causes fractures and preferential amputation through the shafts rather than the joints of the long bones (**Figure 3**).

Those injured or killed following a bomb explosion usually exhibit wounds, not from the effects of blast,

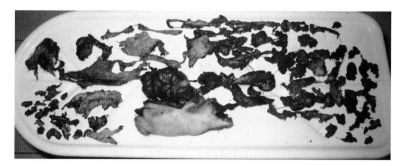

Figure 1 Complete disruption of the body caused by a terrorist bomb. The remains were scattered over a large area and consisted of pieces of scalp and skin, lumps of muscle, and a few of the major limb joints. The severity of the injuries indicate that the victim must have been in contact with the bomb when it exploded. He was in fact a terrorist blown up when the bomb he was loading into a vehicle exploded prematurely.

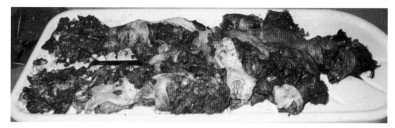

Figure 2 Explosive injury. There is severe mangling of the head, trunk, and limbs but the body has remained relatively intact. The arms and feet were blown off. The victim was a terrorist killed by his own bomb which exploded prematurely. Identification required comparison of his teeth with dental records.

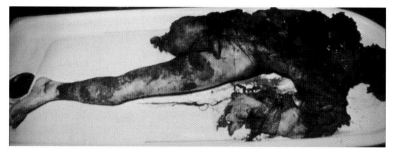

Figure 3 Traumatic amputation of right lower limb and left forearm following a bomb explosion. Note the fragment of patterned clothing on the left forearm, which gave a clue to the identity of the deceased.

but because of the effects of material propelled in all directions from the seat of the explosion, possibly shrapnel deliberately placed around the device or frequently, in the terrorist situation, from fragments of a car filled with explosive. Other kinds of solid material propelled by the explosion consist of the remains of the explosive mixture itself and debris from the surroundings, for example, brick, plaster, and wood, varying from reasonably large fragments to dust. In general, the larger the fragment, the deeper it will penetrate the body and the more lethal it is likely to be.

The characteristic type of injury due to fragments propelled by an explosion is a triad of small bruises, punctate abrasions, and irregular puncture lacerations (**Figure 4**). The triad of injuries may be so confluent as to give the skin a purple discoloration. The bruises and abrasions tend to be quite small, up to 1 cm in diameter, whilst the lacerations, which may vary between 1 and 3 cm in diameter, may contain small fragments of metal or wood derived from the bomb or its container. Superimposed on this triad of small lesions, larger lacerations may be present due to the penetration of fragments of greater size (**Figure 5**).

Dust or minute fragments of dirt will also be propelled by the explosion and, when there is a large amount, it can be driven into the skin to cause fairly uniform tattooing and a dusky purple discoloration of the skin. This discoloration provides a background for the triad of small bruises, abrasions, and puncture lacerations. Whereas the fragments that cause the triad of injuries have sufficient momentum to perforate clothing, the dust/dirt tattooing is typically only seen on exposed skin (**Figure 6**).

Flying-Missile Injury

The triad of bruises, abrasions, and puncture lacerations is due to the violent impact of small particles and the victim usually has to be within a range of a few meters of the explosion to be struck by debris of this size. Beyond this distance the peppering injuries disappear but serious injury and death can occasionally result from the impact of larger separate fragments, usually of metal (**Figure 7**).

It is difficult for those with no firsthand experience of explosions to appreciate the penetrating force of a

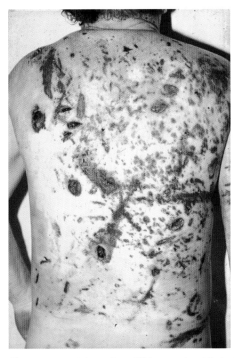

Figure 5 Explosive injury. In addition to the triad of small bruises, abrasions, and puncture lacerations there are larger irregular lacerated wounds due to penetration by larger fragments.

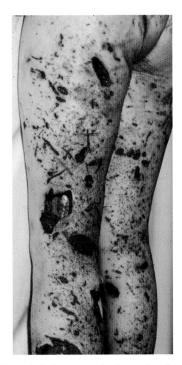

Figure 4 The triad of punctate bruises, abrasions, and puncture lacerations typical of bomb explosions. This victim was several meters away from the bomb when it exploded.

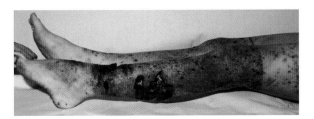

Figure 6 Dust tattooing of the lower limbs following a bomb explosion. Note how the feet have been protected by footwear and the thighs by clothing.

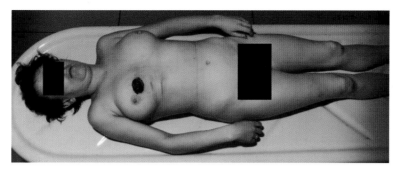

Figure 7 Flying missile injury. This victim was struck by a solitary fragment of metal from a window frame. The fragment penetrated the underlying chest causing fatal hemorrhage. She sustained no other injuries.

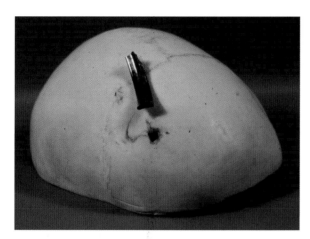

Figure 8 Penetration of the skull by a fragment of door handle from a car which was packed with explosives. The victim was over 100 m away from the vehicle when it blew up.

relatively small explosion fragment. These fragments can penetrate the soft tissues of the body quite deeply, even traversing bone, their momentum being obtained not from their mass but from their velocity (**Figure 8**).

Injury from Falling Masonry

Many of the victims inside or adjacent to a building demolished by an explosion are buried under the rubble. They can receive serious or even fatal impact injuries from the collapse of heavy structural components or may suffer crush asphyxia; on many occasions these injuries are the only effects of the explosion on the body.

When removed from the rubble the body and its clothing are soiled by dust from brick, cement, or plaster, and the extent and nature of the injuries are only revealed when the clothing has been removed and the body thoroughly washed (**Figure 9**). The injuries, which do not differ materially from those seen in people killed in "ordinary" accidents, are often found to be sufficient to account for death.

If death is due to crush (traumatic) asphyxia, the signs are usually quite clear – purple discoloration of the upper parts of the body with petechial hemorrhages in the skin and conjunctivae and perhaps some congestive hemorrhage from the nose and ears.

Burns

When a bomb explodes, the temperature of the explosive gases can rise to 3000 °C. Contact with the momentary flame causes burns but individuals close to the seat of the explosion usually sustain severe disruptive injuries and the burns are a minor component, if any at all, in the fatal outcome (**Figure 10**). Individuals outside this range can be burned by the radiant heat but the effects decrease rapidly from the seat of the explosion and protection from heat radiation of this intensity is afforded by solid objects and even clothing.

Severe burns are usually the result of any later fire started by the bomb either because of the incorporation of incendiary materials into the device or as a result of disruption of a source of flammable material, for example, liquefied petroleum gas tanks. Severe burns may present difficulties in respect of identification and obliteration of surface injuries (**Figure 11**).

Flash burns may also be seen when bomb-making chemicals ignite. The ignition is associated with a momentary flash of very high temperature and those exposed can have their outer clothing burned off and sustain extensive uniform-thickness cutaneous burns. Tight clothing such as a bra, underwear, and footwear may protect the underlying skin (**Figure 12**).

Blast

An explosion is associated with a narrow wave of very high pressure, which expands concentrically from the seat of the explosion and temporarily engulfs a person in its path. The pressure is exceptionally high at the front of the wave but decreases toward its rear and becomes a slight negative pressure, or partial vacuum, before the wave is complete. The total duration of the

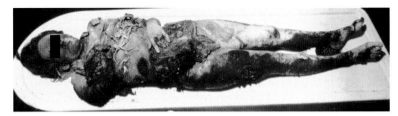

Figure 9 Injury from falling masonry. A body recovered from a building demolished by a bomb explosion. The exposed skin and clothing are heavily soiled by dust, plaster, and cement. Death was due to crush injuries of the trunk.

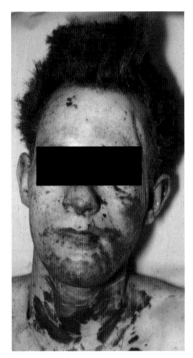

Figure 10 Burns. Singeing of the hair and scorching of the skin of the face and neck in an individual close to the seat of an explosion. Note also the presence of explosive injuries.

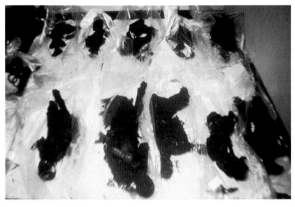

Figure 11 Burns. These victims were inside a building which went on fire after an explosive device, incorporating cans of petrol, exploded on an outside wall. Twelve badly charred bodies were recovered from the scene.

shock wave is brief; the pressure component lasts perhaps 5 ms for a relatively modest explosive device whilst the negative suction component may be 30 ms. As the distance from the explosion is increased, the pressure component lasts longer because the front of the wave where the pressure is highest always travels faster than the tail of the wave where the pressure is much lower. The blast wave can knock a person down, move objects, and demolish buildings – these effects are usually due to the impact of the steep pressure wavefront (**Figure 13**).

It was previously thought that lung damage resulting from blast was due either to a wave of pressure traveling down the trachea or to the suction component of the wave acting also through the trachea. These mechanisms have now been discredited. Whilst the mechanism of blast lung is still not fully understood, the three favored hypotheses as summarized by Maynard and coworkers are:

1. damage to epithelial surfaces within the lungs as a result of a stress wave passing through the parenchyma and encountering interfaces of different density
2. transmission of pressure pulses and subsequent flow of blood from the great vessels of the abdomen to the pulmonary vessels leading to rupture of pulmonary capillaries
3. compression and subsequent violent reexpansion of small air spaces in the lungs as a result of the passage of the shock wave.

Blast lung is the term used to describe the direct damage to the lung produced by the interaction with the body of the blast wave generated by an explosion. Macroscopically it is apparent as areas of blotchy purple-black areas of subpleural hemorrhage. Usually these are scattered at random but occasionally may be seen as parallel bands of bruising related to the overlying ribs (**Figure 14**). Sectioning the lungs reveals more discrete areas of hemorrhage scattered in the tissue, often with a tendency to be more central than peripheral. The rest of the tissue is patchily edematous. The overall weight of the damaged lung is increased due to both hemorrhage and edema.

Microscopically there is intraalveolar hemorrhage, sometimes confined to within intact alveoli but also

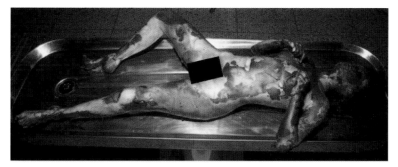

Figure 12   Flash burns associated with the ignition of bomb-making chemicals.

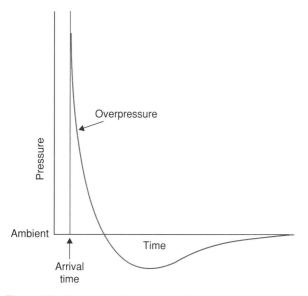

Figure 13   Illustration of blast wave, with steep pressure wave-front.

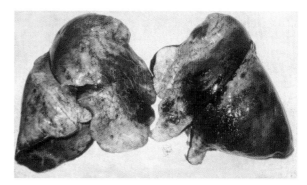

Figure 14   Blast lung. There are extensive areas of blotchy purple-black subpleural hemorrhage on the surfaces of both lungs.

larger areas of confluent hemorrhage may be identified with disruption of alveolar walls. Hemorrhage extends into the bronchioles in places and there is a variable amount of edema fluid in the alveoli. Emphysematous dilatation of some of the alveolar ducts may be identified. In patients who survive, the changes are modified by infiltration with a neutrophilic inflammatory reaction and often by the development of adult respiratory distress syndrome (ARDS).

Primary blast injuries to the lungs are rarely of major significance in civilian casualties from terrorist bombs. To be injured by blast, one has to be in the immediate vicinity of the explosion, say within a few meters, and at such a range, the victim is likely to die at the scene from other injuries. Also it must be borne in mind that not all lung injury is due to blast. Sometimes the lungs are bruised by direct blows on the chest by bomb fragments and debris.

Blast damage to the ear may be associated with bruising and/or rupture of the tympanic membrane and occasionally damage to the cochlea. Most victims who survive an explosion may initially complain of deafness associated with tinnitus but usually recover if the ossicles have not been damaged.

Gastrointestinal tract injury following blast is inconsistent and takes the form of hemorrhage into the peritoneum and bowel wall. Perforation of the bowel is uncommon but has been described.

Investigations of Deaths Following a Bomb Explosion

Following a terrorist bomb there may be many fatalities and the forensic pathologist dealing with such cases may have to invoke a predetermined mass-disaster plan for dealing with large numbers of bodies. The main problems are:

- identification of the victims
- confirming the number of victims
- ascertaining the causes of death
- determining the circumstances of death
- the retrieval of forensic evidence.

Identification

Surprisingly, most of the victims of terrorist bomb explosions can usually be visually identified. Mistakes can be made however when there are a number of fatalities from one bomb. Usually it is a relative of the deceased, severely traumatized by the event, who makes an incorrect identification – perhaps because of deformity of the skull or facial injuries or because the body is heavily soiled by blood and dirt (**Figure 15**). In such circumstances, if reliance is to be placed on visual identification alone, a second person, preferably not a relative, should also be requested to view the body to confirm identity. Even then, a sample of blood for DNA analysis should always be retained.

As a preliminary step in the identification process help may be obtained from distinctive clothing, although appearances can be misleading when it is burned or contaminated with plaster, oil, and blood. Jewelry may also be of assistance in making presumptive identification but would normally require confirmation by other means. Scars and tattoos, particularly if the latter are distinctive, are obviously important (**Figure 16**).

Fingerprinting bodies should never be omitted, since it may prove identity in some cases. If the victim is a known terrorist, his/her fingerprints may be held on record by the police. If an explosion victim has not been previously fingerprinted, the fingerprints taken after death may still be important if the identity of the individual is suspected. Latent prints taken from personal items which have been handled at home or at work can be compared with those taken from the body (**Figure 17**).

Dentition can also be used to establish identity provided a good dental record is available. Examination of the mouth, or if necessary of the excised upper and lower jaws, should be carried out by an appropriately experienced dental surgeon and compared with antemortem charts and X-rays.

Ideally all bodies recovered after a bomb explosion should be fully X-rayed. Old bony injuries, deformities, and prostheses may be identified as well as fragments, which may be of forensic interest. Most mortuaries are not however equipped with appropriate X-ray facilities and at a time when the hospital X-ray department may be struggling to deal with large numbers of injured casualties, it may simply not be practicable to undertake this task. Experience has shown that only rarely does postmortem radiography in such cases lead to retrieval of forensic significant material.

All bodies examined following a bomb explosion should, as a matter of routine, have material retained for DNA examination. In many cases such examination may prove unnecessary but at least it is available if required. Items such as toothbrushes and hairbrushes may provide a suitable source of antemortem DNA in individuals killed and badly mutilated in explosions. Alternatively samples may have to be obtained from the deceased's relatives.

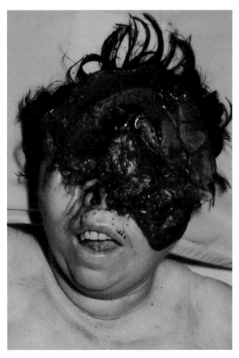

Figure 15 Severe facial injuries precluding visual identification, following a bomb explosion. Note that the absence of injury to the mouth thereby enabled a dental comparison to be carried out.

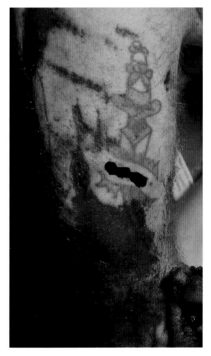

Figure 16 A distinctive tattoo, including the individual's name on the forearm. The deceased was a soldier who was killed in a bomb explosion. The extent of the injuries to the head precluded visual identification.

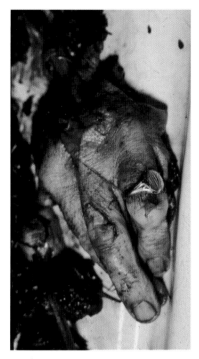

Figure 17 Amongst the mangled remains of this explosion victim was a relatively well-preserved hand from which fingerprints could be taken. Note also the engraved signet ring which was also of assistance in identifying the victim.

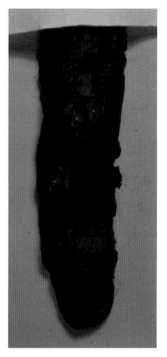

Figure 18 After an explosion in a customs shed, eight mangled bodies were recovered as well as many pieces of human tissue. Amongst the scraps of tissue was an identifiable penis. It belonged to a ninth victim, a terrorist blown up and completely disintegrated by the explosion.

Number of Bodies

When people are blown up in a civilian situation, as by a terrorist bomb, it is clearly important to ascertain the exact number of victims. Most of the dead will be sufficiently intact to be counted, but occasionally those victims near the seat of the explosion may be so disintegrated that their presence is only recognized after a careful search and examination of material collected from the scene.

In practice, it is best to start the examination with those bodies sufficiently intact to count. Any limb parts are apportioned to the appropriate bodies and portions of trunk are similarly matched. Once this has been done, attention is focused on smaller pieces of soft tissue, which are usually mangled and heavily dirt-soiled. Each piece must be thoroughly washed and carefully examined and, whilst the task might seem unrewarding, it is surprising how frequently the tissue yields important clues. On one occasion an unattached penis indicated an extra fatality, whilst on another, two prostate glands and two uterine cervices proved the existence of four further victims (**Figures 18** and **19**).

Cause of Death

When a badly injured body is retrieved after an explosion, the *prima facie* inference is that death was

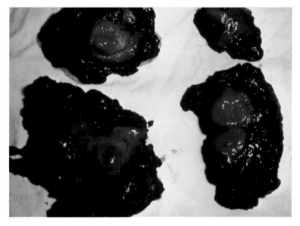

Figure 19 Two uterine cervices and two prostate glands recovered after a number of bodies were disintegrated by a large bomb – conclusive proof of at least four victims, two male and two female.

caused by the explosion and that all but a cursory external examination is required. Furthermore the examining pathologist may not be sufficiently experienced in dealing with such cases to appreciate specific types of injury and the significance of their localization on the body.

There is usually little doubt when there is severe localized explosive injury or when the triad of peppering injuries is apparent to conclude that death was due to the explosion. However, a victim who is pulled from the rubble and who bears, instead, nondestructive abrasions, lacerations, and fractures, or signs of crush asphyxia, is more likely to have been killed by falling masonry. Occasionally burns can be shown to have played a part in the fatal outcome.

The effects of blast may give rise to extensive pulmonary hemorrhage and edema which, if severe, may lead to death within hours of the explosion. Systemic air embolism may also occur as a result of air gaining the pulmonary veins after blast damage to the lungs.

Care must be taken not to miss a death from shooting. Terrorists have been known to fire indiscriminately at victims before planting a bomb, for example, in a crowded bar, and it is quite possible for a person to be fatally shot and left at the scene while others flee in panic (**Figure 20**). Likewise a householder or business owner who is resisting the planting of a bomb on his/her premises may be shot and sustain masking injuries in the subsequent explosion. Again, X-raying bodies may be of assistance in these instances by revealing the presence of bullets.

Circumstances of Death

Reconstructing the circumstances of death can be the most rewarding aspect of autopsies on explosion victims. As with other deaths involving terrorist groups, it is not unusual for an explosion to be followed

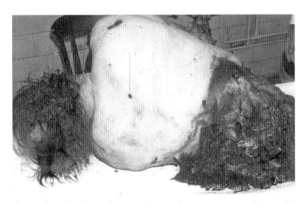

Figure 20   This man's mangled body was recovered from the scene of a bomb explosion. Note the bullet wound on the back of the chest.

by rumors and allegations, which the pathologist can often confirm or refute. When a bomb goes off prematurely – perhaps whilst being manufactured, loaded into a car, or primed – and a terrorist is killed, it may be alleged that the deceased was an innocent passer-by. When a bomb goes off whilst being transported by car, it might be said that a terrorist blown out of the vehicle was a pedestrian. When a bomb goes off inside a building, some of the dead may be terrorists planting the bomb whilst others are uninvolved innocent victims. It is thus essential, if possible, to demonstrate the relative positions of the victims and bomb.

To do this one must compare the injuries of the victims – their severity, distribution, and pattern. Interpretation rests on two factors. First, explosive force declines rapidly with distance and only those victims very near to the source are badly mutilated. Second, the force is highly directional and it is often possible to determine the position of the device in relation to the deceased – thus an explosion at ground level injures the legs of those nearby more than other parts of their bodies. Similarly, the legs especially show severe mangling injuries when an under-car booby trap device explodes (**Figure 21**).

An intelligence assessment of this kind is often invaluable in the investigation; however, unless the significance of the features is readily apparent, this kind of evidence should be used with care in court. Unusual things can happen, bizarre wounds can occur, and a particular pattern of injuries sometimes proves misleading.

Retrieval of Forensic Evidence

On occasions, fragments recovered from the bodies of explosion victims may have important forensic significance. They may help to determine the particular characteristics of the explosive device and thus implicate a specific terrorist organization. Furthermore it may be possible to link components recovered from bodies with similar items seized by the security forces in searches and raids on suspected terrorists (**Figure 22**).

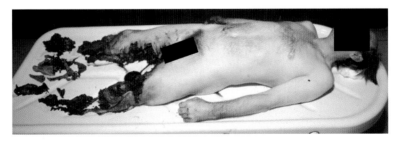

Figure 21   Mangling and traumatic amputation of the lower limbs due to an under-car booby trap device.

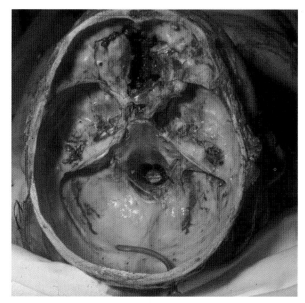

Figure 22   A nail embedded in the skull following detonation of a nail bomb. Comparison of the retrieved fragment was made against nails seized at the premises of a suspect.

As previously indicated, X-raying bodies prior to autopsy will assist in the identification and recovery of shrapnel from bodies but rarely in the experience of this author has this included specific components from the bomb itself. Recovery of fragments from soft tissue can be extremely tedious and occasionally it may be worthwhile excising the tissue and subjecting it to digestion. Trypsin or meat tenderizer can be used to facilitate this. Biological washing powder also works effectively.

Suicide Bombers

Although suicide bombers have been well recognized amongst Tamil Tigers in Sri Lanka and Palestinian extremists in the Middle East, the extent to which some organizations and their fanatical members will go was only brought home to most people as a result of the attacks in the USA on September 11, 2001.

The majority of suicide bomb attacks are of two types: either an individual, with explosives strapped to his/her body, detonates the device amongst a crowd of civilians or close to a targeted individual; or a vehicle, packed with explosives, is driven by the bomber into a specific location such as accommodation being used by civilians or military personnel.

The body of an individual strapped with explosives is invariably completely disrupted by the blast. Typically most of the trunk is blown away but remarkably the head and lower limbs remain relatively intact and are usually found some distance away from the seat of the explosion. The suicide car bomber, usually

because of the large size of the device, is completely disrupted and little of the body may be recovered. When the area is scoured the parts that are collected are usually the fairly obvious portions of the body such as a segment of spine, perhaps a foot, and pieces of scalp and skin. The internal organs are rarely recovered.

Types of Explosive Devices

Terrorist bombs come in all shapes and sizes and with varying degrees of sophistication. Experience during the "troubles" in Northern Ireland has seen the following specific types of devices used by paramilitary terrorist organizations:

- under-car booby-trap devices
- car bombs
- culvert bombs
- incendiary devices
- firebombs
- drogue bombs
- letter/package devices
- pipe bombs
- nail bombs
- mortar bombs.

Under-Car Booby-Trap Device

This small device, containing only a kilogram or so of plastic explosive, such as Semtex, is attached magnetically to the underside of a motor vehicle, usually beneath the driver's seat area (**Figure 23**). A simple timer mechanism, such as a wristwatch or parking timer, is included in the device and this in turn is activated by a mercury tilt switch that operates once the vehicle is in motion. These devices are used to eliminate specific targets, usually the driver of the vehicle, although occasionally innocent passengers are also killed or seriously injured. Mangling and

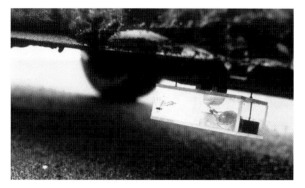

Figure 23   Under-car booby trap device. A small quantity of commercial explosive is used in these devices which are usually placed beneath the driver's seat area of the vehicle.

amputation of the lower limbs are typically seen in such cases (**Figure 21**).

Car Bombs

Vehicles of one sort or another are ideal for not only transporting and concealing a bomb but also serve as a devastating container in which to house and detonate. A car boot can be packed with a large quantity of explosive material and the vehicle driven to its intended target. A simple timer mechanism can be used to effect detonation once the bombers have safely made their escape. Destruction of the car results in multiple secondary missiles radiating from the seat of the explosion, which can cause death or serious injury. In addition, the damage to the vehicle may render useless any attempts to recover forensic evidence such as fingerprints, fibers, or low copy number DNA relating to its occupants.

Culvert Bombs

Large quantities of homemade explosive, usually made from ammonium nitrate fertilizer and sugar, were often concealed in galleys and water culverts beneath country roads in Northern Ireland by republican terrorist organizations. The security forces would then be lured to the scene, usually by an anonymous report of suspicious activity in the area. Terrorists, concealed at a vantage point some distance away, would detonate the device as the police or army patrol drove over the culvert (**Figure 24**).

Incendiary Devices

These small devices, sometimes concealed in audio cassette cases, contain a small quantity of low-order explosive, a detonator, and a simple timer (such as a wristwatch) (**Figure 25**). They are often left concealed in commercial premises and are intended to detonate when the premises have been vacated for the evening. Their purpose is primarily to cause destruction of the building and its contents by the fire, which is generated by detonation. Occasionally, nightwatchmen or security staff remaining within the premises after closing may be caught and unable to escape the ensuing conflagration.

Firebombs

These are considerably larger than incendiary devices and consist of an explosive device attached to a container of flammable liquid such as petrol (**Figure 26**). The force of the explosion causes rupture of the container and the release of inflammable vapor which then ignites. The fire associated with detonation of these devices develops rapidly and may engulf buildings within seconds, resulting in death of the occupants.

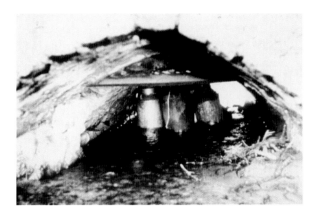

Figure 24 Typical culvert bomb beneath a road. Homemade explosive has been packed into a number of milk churns ready for detonation.

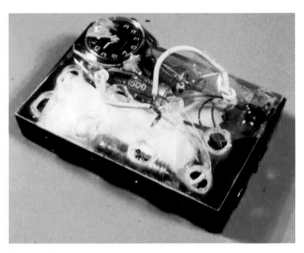

Figure 25 Incendiary device packed into an audio cassette. Note the wrist watch used as a timer.

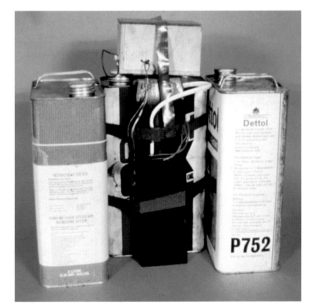

Figure 26 Firebomb. The explosive device is attached to metal containers filled with flammable liquid and designed to rupture on detonation of the device.

Drogue Bombs

These homemade devices were developed by terrorists in Northern Ireland and were intended to be dropped or thrown from the upper floors of buildings or bridges at police or military vehicles passing below. Their construction included a hollow cylindrical cooper core which melted on detonation and could penetrate the armor-plated roofs of these vehicles (**Figure 27**).

Letter/Package Devices

It is not uncommon for small explosive devices to be sent in the post to targeted individuals. The device is usually contained within a large padded envelope and detonation is usually achieved when the envelope is opened by an unsuspecting recipient. Injuries sustained in such circumstances are usually confined to the face and are often characterized by linear abrasions and lacerations radiating from a point in front of the face (**Figures 28** and **29**).

Pipe Bombs

These are fairly crude improvised devices essentially consisting of a length of metal pipe filled with low-order explosive such as that decanted from fireworks or shotgun cartridges (**Figures 30** and **31**). A simple taper fuse is attached and, once lit, the device is thrown at the intended target. Fatalities

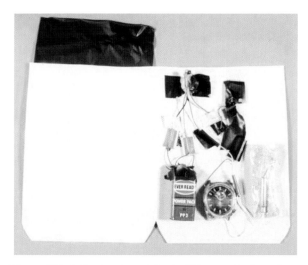

Figure 28 Letter bomb contained within a padded envelope. Note the battery and watch attached to the device.

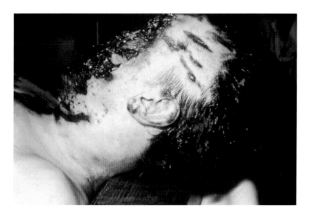

Figure 29 Facial injuries sustained when a letter bomb exploded as it was being opened.

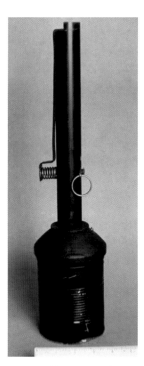

Figure 27 Drogue bomb. Homemade drogue bomb using metal food can. These devices were intended to be dropped or thrown onto passing military vehicles.

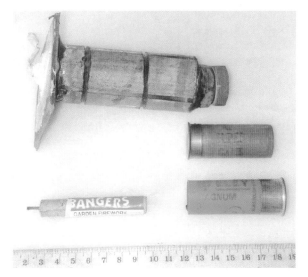

Figure 30 Pipe bomb.

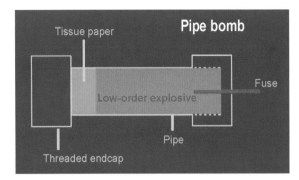

Figure 31 The pipe bomb device consists of a length of metal piping filled with low-order explosive.

have occurred in those inadvertently picking up the devices, or when the device explodes prematurely, whilst being thrown. The pattern of the injuries sustained in such cases is clearly important in determining the innocence or guilt of the casualty.

Nail Bombs

These small devices were also intended to be thrown by hand at a target, possibly a member of the security forces or a group of rioters from an opposing faction. The construction involved a small explosive charge wrapped in corrugated cardboard and containing numerous long nails. Those close to the point of detonation could sustain serious or even fatal injuries due to being struck and impaled by the contents of the device.

Mortar Bombs

These devices consist of metal cylinders packed with explosive and are designed to detonate on impact with their intended target. They are usually launched from firing tubes constructed on the back of an open lorry or a van fitted with a false roof. The advantage of this moving firing point is that it can be located relatively close to even a "protected" target and then abandoned, allowing the terrorists to make their escape before timed detonation occurs. The mortars may travel up to about 200 m but are inherently inaccurate and frequently fail to detonate on impact. It is not unusual for such devices to miss their intended target such as a police station or military camp by a long way, and instead explode in an area populated by civilians.

Conclusion

Terrorist violence, that is, violence perpetrated for political objectives, is now common throughout the world. It often has the sympathy, if not the active support, of large sections of the communities in which it occurs and such support frustrates the activities of the security forces in trying to apprehend the perpetrators and bring them to justice. It is often directed against the establishment, either the government or its law enforcement agencies. Doctors who examine the injured and pathologists who examine the dead are usually doing so in an "official" capacity and thus their impartiality may be called into question. Furthermore practitioners in some jurisdictions may feel pressurized into modifying or amending their findings to suit their authorities. To maintain credibility, it is essential that doctors undertaking this work do so in a scrupulously objective manner. All such work must be meticulously detailed and findings properly recorded for evidential purposes. The reports prepared, and the opinions offered, in such cases must be scrupulously fair and unbiased and unaffected by personal prejudice or partisan pressure of any kind. Finally, reports that are to be used in evidence for criminal proceedings must tell not only the truth but also the whole truth.

See Also

Terrorism: Medico-legal Aspects; Nuclear and Biological; Suicide Bombing, Investigation

Further Reading

Crane J (2000) Violence associated with civil disturbance. In: Mason JK, Purdue BN (eds.) *The Pathology of Trauma*, 3rd edn., pp. 75–88. London: Arnold.

Hull JB, Bowyer GW, Cooper GJ, Crane J (1994) Pattern of injury in those dying from traumatic amputation caused by bomb blast. *British Journal of Surgery* 81: 1132–1135.

Marshall TK (1976) Deaths from explosion devices. *Medicine, Science and the Law* 16: 235–239.

Maynard RL, Coppel DL, Lowry KG (1997) Blast injury of the lung. In: Cooper GJ, Dudley HAF, Gann DS, *et al.* (eds.) *Scientific Foundations of Trauma*, pp. 214–224. Oxford, UK: Butterworth.

Firearm Injuries

G M Kirk, University of KwaZulu Natal, Durban, South Africa

Introduction

Firearm wounds are a common form of trauma in many parts of the world. The accurate interpretation of these wounds is important for clinical management in the living and for medicolegal reasons in both the living and the dead. Studies in the USA and

South Africa, countries with high incidences of firearm injuries, have shown that major inaccuracies in the interpretation and documentation of firearm wounds by trauma doctors are common. An understanding of terminal ballistics and especially the nature of wounds left on the body by firearm projectiles is essential if medicolegal evidence relating to firearm injuries is to be accurate and reliable.

Classification

Firearm wounds can be classified according to the nature of the weapon, range of fire, and whether entry or exit. An examination of wounds should, in most instances, allow important information regarding their classification as well as the direction of fire to be determined (**Table 1**).

Gunshot Wounds

The most commonly encountered weapons with rifled barrels that fire individual projectiles in civilian practice are handguns (pistols and revolvers),

Table 1 Factors that may be determined by firearm wound examination

1. Confirmation that the wound is a firearm wound
2. Number of shots that struck the body
3. The nature of the weapon and ammunition
   a. Rifled weapon (handgun or rifle)
      i. Low- to medium-velocity
      ii. High-velocity
   b. Shotgun
4. The range of fire
   a. Contact
      i. Hard contact
      ii. Loose contact
   b. Near
   c. Intermediate
   d. Distant
5. Entry or exit wound
   a. Atypical features
6. The direction of fire

although hunting and assault rifles are not uncommon in many parts of the world. In terminal ballistic terms, such weapons produce gunshot wounds (as opposed to shotgun wounds, which are described later).

Entry gunshot wound The appearance of an entry gunshot wound is dependent on many factors, including the type of firearm, ammunition, distance of fire, angle of impact, passage through intermediate objects, stability of the projectile, and area of the body struck. This allows interpretations to be made from examination of the wounds (**Table 2**).

When a handgun or rifle is fired, it is not only the projectile (bullet) that is propelled from the barrel; also emerging from the end of the barrel are flame, vaporized metal, gases, smoke and soot, and burning and unburned particles of propellant powder. These all have greatly varying densities and travel different distances from the weapon. An appreciation of the effects of these components on the surface of the body of a victim of a gunshot wound is important in assessing gunshot wounds (**Table 3**).

Distant gunshot wound A distant gunshot wound is one that is fired from a range where only the bullet leaves a visible sign on the skin. In other words, there

Table 2 Differentiating typical entry and exit gunshot wounds. It is important to note that no single factor is pathognomonic or always present, and all features are seldom present together

Entry wound	Exit wound
Abrasion collar	No abrasion collar
Regular round to oval "punched-out" defect	Irregular lacerated defect
Inverted skin edges	Everted skin edges
Smaller than bullet diameter and exit wound	Larger than entry wound
Features of close-range fire	No features of close-range fire
Grease wipe on inner edge	No grease wipe
Increased carbon monoxide in tissue	No increased carbon monoxide

Table 3 Range of gunshot wounds

Range	Distance (handguns)	Distance (rifles)	Features
Contact	0 cm	0 cm	Central defect with abrasion collar Muzzle imprint Searing and blackening Stellate wound over bone
Near	<1 cm	<1 cm	Central defect with abrasion collar Searing and blackening Concentrated tattooing
Intermediate	1–65 cm	1 cm–1 m	Central defect with abrasion collar Tattooing ±Blackening
Distant	>65 cm	>1 m	Central defect with abrasion collar

is no effect from the other products of discharge, such as propellant powder or soot. The actual distance is variable and dependent on factors such as the type of weapon, length of barrel, velocity, and bullet loading. In general terms, distant wounds for handguns may be considered as those fired from greater than 40–75 cm. For rifles, the range is usually greater than 60–100 cm. No other deductions about range can be made beyond these distances.

The typical entry gunshot wound has a neat round to oval defect with a punched-out appearance and inverted skin edges (**Figure 1**). The size of the entry wound is usually slightly smaller than the diameter of the bullet and, in cases of wounds from some high-velocity rifles, it may be considerably smaller. There is usually a narrow surrounding collar of abraded skin. This is formed as the bullet strikes the skin, forcing it inward until the elasticity is exceeded and the skin tears, with the edges being abraded by the penetrating projectile. If the bullet strikes the skin perpendicularly, the abrasion collar will be concentric. If the entry is angulated, the abrasion collar will be eccentric and widest at the edge in the direction from which the bullet entered (**Figure 2**). This provides information about the direction of fire relative to the body. This factor cannot be considered reliable in areas of loose skin or pendulous parts of the body because there is no way of knowing their position when the bullet struck. Abrasion collars may be absent, especially where the skin is taut and in some high-velocity wounds. A grease wipe from the bullet may be present on the inner aspect of the wound, although this is not constant.

Intermediate-range gunshot wound Intermediate-range wounds are characterized by the effect of propellant powder grains on the skin surrounding the central hole caused by the bullet. The appearance of the central wound is the same as in distant wounds. Burning and unburned propellant powder grains impact the skin, causing superficial fine discrete punctate lesions, commonly referred to as powder tattooing or simply tattooing (**Figure 3**). In antemortem

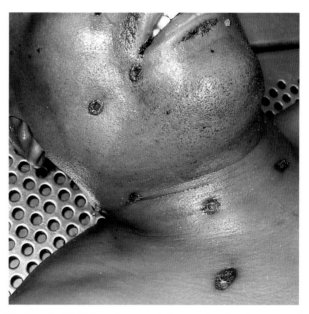

Figure 2 Multiple-entry gunshot wounds showing central defects and concentric and eccentric (bottom right) abrasion collars.

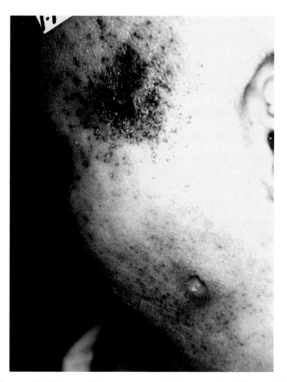

Figure 3 Intermediate-range gunshot wounds with central defects surrounded by powder tattooing. The upper wound shows more concentrated tattooing than the lower one.

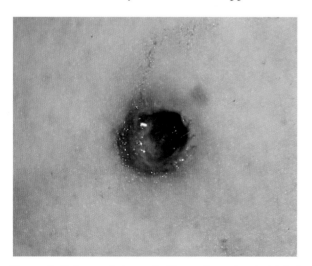

Figure 1 Entry gunshot wound with a neat round central defect and surrounding abrasion collar.

wounds, vital reaction causes tattooing to have a reddish-brown appearance. Postmortem desiccation causes the lesions to darken. The lesions cannot be wiped away. Occasionally, unburned powder grains may be present on the surface of the skin within the zone of tattooing.

The distribution of tattooing is influenced by the angle of impact of the gunshot. In perpendicular strikes, the distribution will be concentric around the central bullet wound. In angulated strikes, the distribution will be eccentric with the greater diameter furthest from the barrel. The pattern of tattooing may also be affected by intervening objects, such as clothing or jewelry, between the propellant powder and skin.

The actual range of fire in intermediate-range wounds varies depending on the type of weapon, velocity, cartridge loading, and physical nature of the propellant powder. For handguns, tattooing is usually present up to maximum distances of 40–75 cm. Where tattooing is present, a useful generalization is that the shot was fired from within an arm's length. For rifles, the maximum distance for intermediate-range wounds is 60–100 cm.

Not all gunshot wounds in the intermediate range will show tattooing. Tattooing may be absent due to intervening objects, such as clothing or dense hair. Tattooing may also be present on areas of the body that were distant from the entry wound but were adjacent when the shot was fired, such as on a hand held up to the area of wounding.

Near-contact gunshot wounds Near-contact gunshot wounds (or "near wounds") occupy a gray zone between contact and intermediate wounds. In near wounds, the flame and soot expelled along with the bullet impact on the surrounding skin. This produces a zone of soot blackening overlying seared skin surrounding the central bullet wound (**Figure 4**). The blackening, but not the searing, can be easily wiped away. Concentrated tattooing is also present but is often not apparent due to the searing effect of flame on the skin. Hair may be singed, but this is an unusual finding, probably due to hair being displaced by the expelled gas.

In angled near wounds, soot radiates out from the barrel, causing a pear-shaped area of blackening with the larger area on the side nearer the barrel (in contrast with angled loose-contact wounds) (**Figure 5**).

Contact gunshot wounds Contact gunshot wounds may be tight, where the end of the barrel is held with pressure against the skin, forming a seal even during firing, or loose, where the expelled gas forces a gap between barrel and skin, allowing the escape of some

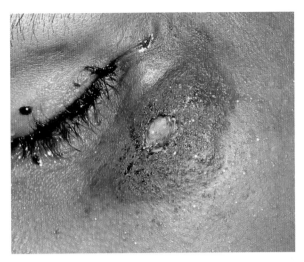

Figure 4 Near gunshot wound with a central defect, searing of the skin, soot blackening, and concentrated tattooing. Some unburned powder granules are present on the wound surface.

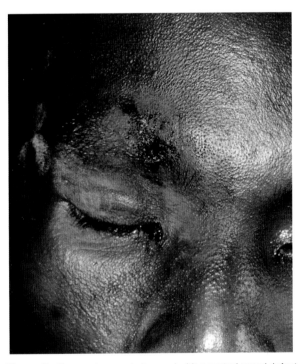

Figure 5 Near-entry gunshot wound with a central round defect and extensive surrounding blackening.

products of discharge. In both forms of contact wounds, the bullet will perforate centrally.

In tight-contact gunshot wounds, the barrel may leave an imprint abrasion (**Figure 6**). The skin within the circumference of the barrel will be seared and blackened. Except in cases where the wound is over superficial flat bone (skull, sternum, and scapulae), the bullet defect will resemble that at other ranges. Where the entry is over superficial bone, gas is forced under the skin and reflected off the bone, blowing the

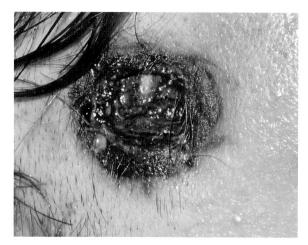

Figure 6 Tight-contact entry gunshot wound with a muzzle imprint, seared wound margins, and blackening within the wound.

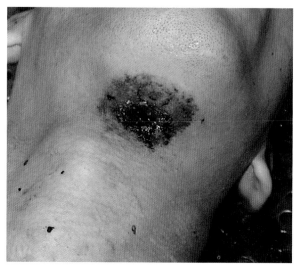

Figure 8 Loose-angled contact gunshot wound with an incomplete muzzle abrasion and eccentric blackening and searing of the skin.

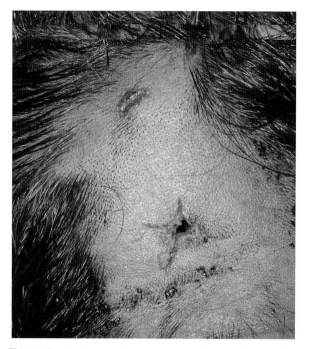

Figure 7 Contact gunshot wound over bone with a stellate laceration (lower wound). A crescentic laceration caused by the expelled cartridge case is also seen (upper wound).

skin away from the bone and causing a large irregular stellate laceration (**Figure 7**). In such cases, there is usually blackening of the underlying subcutaneous tissues, including a rim surrounding the entry fracture defect on the outer table of the bone.

Loose-contact gunshot wounds are characterized by a narrow surrounding zone of searing and blackening. A variant is the angled-contact gunshot wound, where gas and soot escape from the side of the barrel not in tight contact with the skin, causing an eccentric

area of blackening and searing (**Figure 8**). The larger diameter of this zone will be on the side opposite the angled barrel.

In some contact wounds from pistols, a 5–10-mm crescentic laceration is found within a few centimeters of the entry wound. This is caused by the expelled cartridge case striking the skin.

Atypical gunshot wounds Anything that causes the bullet to be unstable or tumble in flight may cause the entry wound to appear atypical (**Figure 9**). This most commonly occurs when the bullet has passed through an intermediary target or ricocheted off another surface before entering the body. This includes a reentry wound from a bullet that has perforated another part of the body. Such entry wounds may be irregular and unusually large, with an irregular, eccentric abrasion ring.

Another effect of a bullet perforating an intermediary target is the possible impact of fragments of that target on the skin, modifying the appearance of the entry wound. Multiple small fragments, as arise when a bullet passes though safety glass, may cause superficial lacerations around the entry wound and these are referred to as pseudotattooing (**Figure 10**). Pseudotattooing is distinguished from powder tattooing by its usually larger and more irregular appearance.

Exit gunshot wounds Exit gunshot wounds may vary greatly but are mainly differentiated from entry wounds by their more irregular, lacerated appearance (**Figure 11**). The wound edges may be everted. Exit wounds typically do not have an abrasion collar or grease wipe. Exit wounds are usually larger than

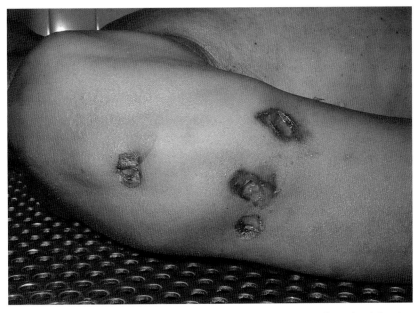

Figure 9 Atypical-entry gunshot wounds with irregular shapes. The top and middle wounds on the right mirror the profile of bullets, indicating that the bullets struck the body side-on.

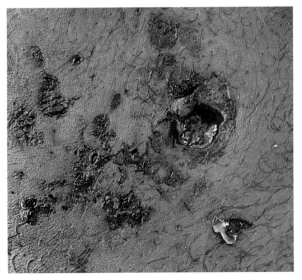

Figure 10 Atypical-entry gunshot wound with pseudotattooing. A shrapnel fragment is seen at the bottom right.

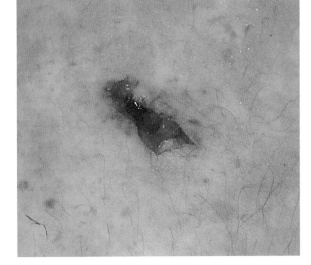

Figure 11 Exit gunshot wound with irregular shape and lacerated margins.

entry wounds, but this is highly variable and a poor discriminant on its own.

Atypical exit wounds Occasionally, an exit wound will show a broad surrounding area of abrasion. This occurs when the bullet exits through skin pressed against a firm object, such as a belt or backrest of a chair. This is referred to as a shored exit wound (**Figure 12**). Another atypical form of exit wound is the incomplete exit wound where the bullet lacerates the skin but is trapped and lodged within the skin wound. Occasionally, a single bullet may produce

more than one exit by fragmentation of either the projectile or bone, producing secondary projectiles of metallic or bony fragments.

Determining the direction of fire In single perforating gunshot wounds, the direction of fire can be readily determined by differentiating between the entry and exit wounds. If there is no exit wound, the direction may be inferred from the form of the abrasion collar surrounding the entry wound, but the wound track in the body is also an important factor to be considered. Difficulties may arise where there are

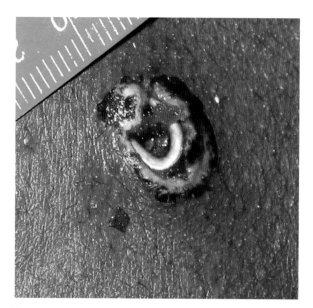

Figure 12 Atypical incomplete and shored exit gunshot wound with the bullet seen within the wound. The edges of the wound are abraded.

Table 4 Components of a shotgun discharge contributing to wounds

1. Pellets
2. Soot
3. Burning and unburned propellant powder
4. Flame
5. Hot gases, including carbon monoxide
6. Wads
7. Cartridge case fragments
8. Primer

Table 5 Range of shotgun wounds

Range	Distance	Features
Contact	0 cm	Single round hole
		Stellate wound over bone
		Muzzle imprint
		Minimal blackening and searing
		Wad in wound
Near	<15 cm	Single round hole
		Soot blackening and searing
		Wad in wound
Intermediate	15 cm–2 m	Central round or crenated wound
		Satellite pellet holes
		Tattooing
		Wad may be in wound
Distant	>2 m	Central hole (up to 6–10 m)
		Satellite pellet holes

multiple gunshot wounds, and it is not always possible to match each entry with its own exit wound. General directions of fire, however, can usually be deduced. It must be remembered that the description of gunshot directions relative to the "anatomical position" typically used in diagrams seldom reflects the position of the body in real life, which is often quite dynamic and should be correlated with evidence from the scene of the shooting.

Shotgun Wounds

A shotgun fires multiple lead pellets (shot) from a smooth-bored barrel, and these pellets emerge as a compact mass that spreads out as the distance from the barrel increases. As with gunshots, similar accompanying components are expelled along with the shot. In addition, wads and occasionally fragments of the cartridge case are also expelled (**Table 4**). A wad is a disk-shaped piece of plastic, cardboard, or felt that separates the pellets from the propellant powder. In some modern shotgun cartridges, a plastic cup replaces the wad. All these components may contribute to a shotgun wound. It must be remembered that clothing may markedly alter the appearance of wounds at closer ranges.

Entry shotgun wounds The differentiation of entry from exit shotgun wounds is usually obvious in that, in most cases, due to the relative low velocity and mass of individual pellets, the shot does not exit the body. The most important deduction to be made from the wound is the estimation of range. The differential

distances that the constituent components of a shotgun discharge travel as well as the dispersion of the pellets are used for this purpose. The choke of the shotgun influences the rate of dispersion of the pellets; thus, test firing of individual weapons is necessary for accurate range estimations, especially for distant wounds (**Table 5**).

Distant shotgun wounds Distant shotgun wounds are those in which only the pellets penetrate the body. In some cases, up to about 5 m, the wad may still strike the body, causing a laceration, abrasion, or contusion below the entry wound. Modern plastic cups usually open in flight, forming a cross shape, and on impact may leave a distinctive Maltese cross or flower petal-patterned abrasion or contusion. At distances of up to 10 m, sufficient pellets may still form a central mass to cause a larger central hole, with surrounding small satellite holes caused by dispersed individual pellets (**Figure 13**). As the range increases, the central hole will disappear and the entry wound will consist only of individual pellet holes. The diameter of dispersion of these pellet holes can be used to estimate the range by comparison with test firing the same weapon using similar ammunition. When this cannot be done, rule-of-thumb estimation can be used, but its accuracy is poor.

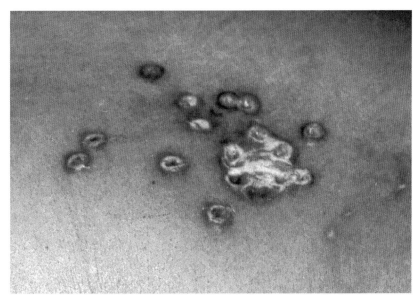

Figure 13   Distant-entry shotgun wound with individual pellet holes but still showing central clustering.

Every 2.5 cm of spread is said to be equivalent to approximately 1 m of range (or 1 inch of spread for 1 yard of range).

Intermediate-range shotgun wounds   Powder tattooing and a central wound with scalloped edges and surrounding satellite wounds characterize intermediate-range wounds. Tattooing is usually less dense than that seen in handguns due to more complete combustion of propellant powder. The maximum distance at which tattooing is seen varies with the weapon and type of powder, but tattooing is seldom present beyond 1 m.

As the central mass of pellets begins to disperse, entry wounds have a large central defect, the edges of which appear scalloped, looking somewhat "rat-nibbled" or resembling the pattern of a cookie cutter. As the range increases, some pellets make individual holes in a rim surrounding the central hole.

Blackening from soot may be present at the lower end of intermediate-range wounds, but it is usually not present beyond 30 cm. The wad is usually present within the wound track.

Near shotgun wounds   Shotgun wounds from a range of less than about 15 cm usually have a single circular hole with a smooth, or occasionally slightly scalloped, margin (**Figure 14**). Obliquely angled wounds may be oval. Concentrated powder tattooing, blackening, and singeing of the surrounding skin and hair are present. The wad is usually in the wound track.

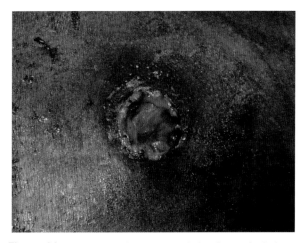

Figure 14   Near-entry shotgun wound showing a single large central defect with scalloped edges and surrounding searing and blackening of the skin.

Contact shotgun wounds   When a shotgun is fired with the barrel held against the body, a single round wound approximately the size of the bore of the weapon is produced. If the contact entry is over flat bone, as in the head, the entry wound is large and stellate due to tearing of the skin by the large amount of gas forced into the wound and reflected off the skull. Contact shotgun wounds of the head are typically very destructive.

In tight-contact wounds, a muzzle imprint may be visible and this is incontrovertible evidence of a contact wound. Soot blackening and searing are minimal unless the contact is loose, allowing some escape of flame and smoke on to the surrounding skin. Carbon monoxide in the gases of discharge may bind to myoglobin in the wound, giving the entry wound a characteristic pink coloration.

Exit shotgun wounds Exit wounds are uncommon, particularly in the trunk, due to the relatively low energy of individual pellets. Exit wounds are more common in children, in limb wounds, and in contact wounds of the head. Where they are present, the appearances are similar to those found in bullet exit wounds.

Rubber and Plastic Baton Rounds

Rubber and plastic baton rounds (bullets), which are typically used in riot-control situations, produce blunt-force injuries on impact. Rubber baton rounds cause contusions, whereas plastic baton rounds produce a characteristic wound with a discrete annular abrasion and a smaller abrasion at the center. When fired at close range, lacerations with or without penetration of the projectile and underlying fractures may occur.

Air Guns

Wounds from air guns that fire single-shaped pellets are usually small punctures resembling the individual entry of a shotgun pellet. An abrasion ring may be present. Because there is no propellant powder used in the weapon, no features of singeing, blackening, or tattooing are present, even in close-range wounds. Exit wounds are rare and when present will also resemble those of shotgun pellets.

Documentation and Forensic Interpretation of Firearm Wounds

The priorities of clinicians and forensic pathologists obviously differ when examining gunshot wounds, with the clinician's first responsibility being the treatment of the patient. However, the clinician may at a later date be expected to give testimony regarding the description and interpretation of the wounds. Hence, it is important for clinicians to recognize and accurately document wounds and their characteristics. Even if it is not possible to record all details of the wounds, a sketch of the positions, shapes, and approximate sizes of wounds can provide valuable information for later interpretation by experts. The presence or absence of features of close range should be noted. It must be remembered that one feature, soot blackening, is transient and can easily be washed away. Photography of wounds is an ideal and practical way of recording evidence that enables later examination by others.

Surgically Altered Wounds

After firearm wounds are surgically altered, such as by debridement or suturing, they may lose many or all of their characteristics, making subsequent interpretation difficult or impossible. The initial examination notes may be all that subsequent evidence can be based on.

Some deductions about entry and exit, and therefore direction of fire, may be made from internal examination when bullet fragments are present or when bone is involved in the wound track. Splinters from bone fractures may be displaced in the direction of the bullet tract. In gunshots perforating the skull, entry and exit fractures typically have different appearances. As a bullet perforates the two tables of bone that comprise the cranium, it lifts a circular rim of bone off and away from the table on the side of the direction of travel, leaving a beveled rim. Thus, entry gunshot fractures are beveled on the inner skull table, whereas exit fractures are beveled on the outer skull table.

Clothing

Clothing may significantly modify the appearance of firearm wounds on the body by trapping some components of firearm discharge. If ignored, erroneous conclusions may be made from the examination of wounds on the body. The examination of clothing should be an integral part of the examination of any firearm wound.

See Also

Ballistic Trauma, Overview and Statistics

Further Reading

Besant-Matthews PE (2000) Examination and interpretation of rifled firearm injuries. In: Mason JK, Purdue BN (eds.) *The Pathology of Trauma*, 3rd edn., pp. 47–60. London: Arnold.
Cassidy M (2000) Smooth-bore firearm injuries. In: Mason JK, Purdue BN (eds.) *The Pathology of Trauma*, 3rd edn., pp. 61–74. London: Arnold.
DiMaio JM (1999) *Gunshot Wounds,* 2nd edn., Boca Raton, FL: CRC Press.
DiMaio JM, Dana SE (1998) Gunshot wounds. In: DiMaio JM, Dana SE (eds.) *Handbook of Forensic Pathology,* pp. 107–136. Austin, TX: Landes Bioscience.
Perumal G (2001) Firearm injuries and explosions. In: Dada MA, McQuoid-Mason DJ (eds.) *Introduction to Medico-Legal Practice,* pp. 205–222. Durban, South Africa: Butterworths.
Saukko P, Knight B (2004) Gunshot and explosion deaths. In: Saukko P, Knight B (eds.) *Knight's Forensic Pathology,* 3rd edn., pp. 245–280. London: Arnold.

Sharp and Cutting-Edge Wounds

J Payne-James, Forensic Healthcare Services Ltd, London, UK
P Vanezis, The Forensic Science Service, London, UK

Introduction

Sharp-force injuries are those injuries by any weapon or implement with cutting edges or points (e.g., knives, scissors, glass). The injuries may be classified into either incised, where the cutting edge runs tangentially to the skin surface, cutting through skin and deeper anatomical structures, or stab, where the sharp edge penetrates the skin into deeper structures. An incised wound is generally longer than it is deep, whereas a stab wound is deeper than it is wide. Forces required to cause sharp injuries and the effect of such injuries are variable as a very sharp pointed object may penetrate vital structures with minimal force. The same implement may be capable of causing both stab and incised injuries, and a victim may present with a mixture of the two. Some injuries are not capable of being divided clearly into the stab or incised category, but may exhibit features of both.

Incidence

Generally injuries most frequently seen in those survivors and fatalities of sharp-force injuries are caused by implements such as knives and less commonly broken glass, although any type of agent with a sharp edge or point can cause such wounds. The type of implement varies between countries and cultures and in certain settings other implements such as axes or machetes (which may combine a sharp or sharpish edge with a heavy weight and blunt surfaces) may be used. These may produce injuries that have both sharp-force and blunt-force elements – the term "chop" wounds is sometimes applied. Sharp-force trauma, mainly resulting from the use of knives, is a common cause of nonfatal injury and is seen increasingly in emergency and trauma centers. In England and Wales the most common method of killing remains killing with a sharp instrument (2002–2003) – 27% of homicide victims were killed by this method. The sites of injury in a study of wounds from penetrating injuries in the 1990s from Glasgow showed a range of sites of wounding, with head, chest, and arms predominating (**Table 1**).

Wound Characteristics

Stab and incised wounds are generally differentiated by the fact that stab wounds are deeper rather than wider because of the mode of contact with the body, namely thrusting the knife by one means or another into the body. Incised or stab injuries are caused by the knife moving tangentially across the skin surface. This definition is of use when the dimensions of a wound can be properly assessed, for example, at autopsy. In the living victim, treatment within hospital may not properly document the size of wound prior to exploration or closure, or the depth of wound following exploration such as laparotomy or thoracotomy. Interpretation of such injury can become difficult. **Figure 1** shows a scar following a stab wound to the neck. The operation notes did not detail the depth of penetration, no major structures were damaged, and persistent bleeding was shown to originate from a small unnamed artery. The line indicates the original stab wound.

The operation scar which extended the initial stab wound obscured detail, and no documentation had been made of the preoperative wound characteristics. Such issues become very relevant in court cases where a charge of attempted murder may be argued on the perceived depth of penetration of a knife (and by inference the force used to create the wound). It is in situations such as this that proper documentation of injury, pretreatment, within the nonforensic primary care and trauma settings, can be extremely helpful.

It should also be appreciated that a knife, glass, or other object or fragment with a sharp edge is capable of producing a cleanly cut wound resulting in a stab or an incision. Perhaps the most common error that nonforensic personnel make is using the term laceration (skin splitting or tearing after blunt-force injury) for an incised or stab wound when describing a "cut" which they have treated. "Cuts" may

Table 1 Distribution of wounds by body region

Body region	Percentage of all wounds
Head (face and scalp)	22.3
Neck	6.5
Shoulders	2.7
Chest	22.3
Abdomen	12.4
Groin	1
Thighs	7.9
Buttocks	4.9
Arms	19.9

Modified from Bleetman A, Watson CH, Horsfall I, Champion SM (2003) Wounding patterns and human performance in knife attacks: optimising the protection provided by knife resistant body armour. *Journal of Clinical Forensic Medicine* 10: 243–248.

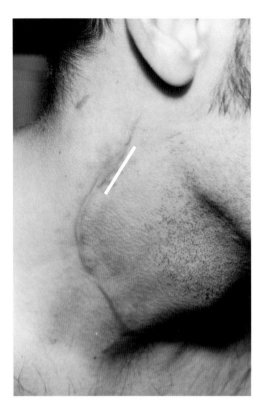

Figure 1 Scar following a stab wound to the neck (line indicates site of wound, remainder of scar is due to surgical intervention).

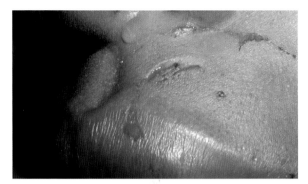

Figure 2 Small laceration with associated swelling after punch to face.

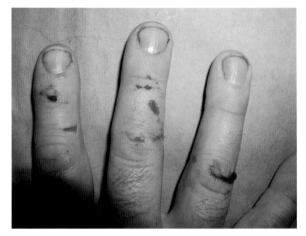

Figure 3 Fingers of a male after having broken a window with a punch with his hand.

be divided into those caused by blunt-impact injury – lacerations – and those caused by sharp implements or edges – "incisions" or incised-type and stabs. The distinction between incised wounds, stabs, and lacerations is of the greatest importance medicolegally as causation (blunt impact or sharp implement) is often the key to the outcome of a case. Although in clinical treatment terms this is a minor issue, it can be extremely relevant in the medicolegal and forensic setting. Lack of understanding of the difference and its significance between lacerations and sharp-force wounds is probably the most common mistake made by nonforensic doctors at all levels when providing statement or reports for courts.

Heavy implements with a sharp surface such as an axe or machete result in a combination of cutting injuries associated with crushing of underlying tissue and frequently fractures if there is underlying bone. Sometimes, however, a lacerated wound is the predominant component rather than a clean-cut wound.

Lacerations versus Sharp-Force Cuts

Lacerations are caused by blunt-force impacts compressing and splitting the skin, or occasionally by shearing force. Lacerations most commonly occur where underlying bone is prominent – classically at

the orbital margin. After treatment, that is, suture or gluing, it is often impossible to distinguish between a laceration and an incised wound, which is why adequate documentation before treatment is essential. The most significant difference that can distinguish between lacerations and incised wounds is that incised wounds have clean distinct edges. Lacerations may have macroscopically clean and distinct edges, but not under magnification. Generally lacerations have irregular or macerated edges – residual skin bridging (particularly at the ends) – and may have other features of blunt-impact injury associated, e.g., swelling, reddening, and bruising. **Figure 2** shows a small laceration with associated swelling and irregularity of the wound edge after a punch to the face.

Incised Wounds

Incised-type wounds may be caused by anything with a sharp edge, including knives and broken glass. If glass breaks at the time of impact, multiple cuts from sharp glass shards may be seen. **Figure 3** shows the fingers of a male arrested for breaking into a house, having broken a window with his hand. The illustration shows multiple small incised wounds.

Incised wounds crossing irregular surfaces may be irregular in depth, but their linearity will assist in confirming causation. **Figure 4** shows the dorsum of a hand across which a sharp knife had been drawn.

Assaults with broken glasses or bottles are commonly seen in emergency medicine, maxillofacial, and plastic surgery clinics. The characteristics of such injury are multiple irregular incised-type wounds of variable depth and severity. **Figure 5** shows a male who had a broken bottle thrust in his face. The wound edges are all clean with no skin bridging, confirming that sharp edges caused these injuries.

Figure 6 shows another typical "glassing" injury after treatment and suture: the wounds were much more superficial and irregular. This particular injury was caused when an intact glass was thrust to the side of the face, breaking on impact.

Figure 7 is another example of the type of injury seen when an intact glass object is impacted on the face, breaking on impact. The periorbital hematoma and the cut indicated by the arrow which is more likely to represent a laceration is caused by the (blunt) impact of glass striking, and the multiple incised-type wounds are caused by the pieces of broken glass after breakage.

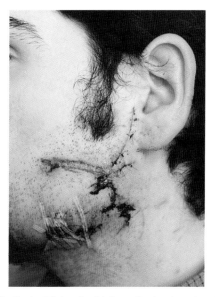

Figure 6 Typical "glassing" injury after treatment and suture.

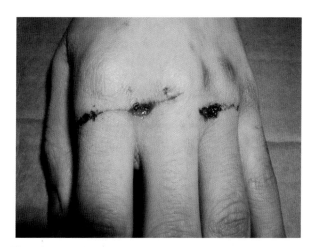

Figure 4 Dorsum of a hand and fingers across which a sharp knife had been drawn.

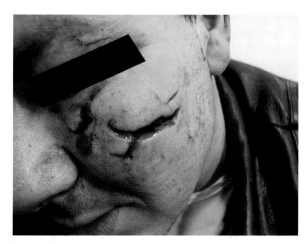

Figure 5 Male who had a broken bottle thrust in his face.

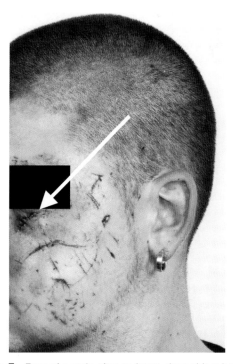

Figure 7 Face of a male after an intact glass object broke on impact on the face.

With glassing injuries it is extremely important to try and identify from witness accounts and examination of the scene whether the glass or bottle was broken prior to impact, or on impact. Issues such as these become extremely important in court cases where intent (to maximize injury) may be determined on the interpretation of the injury patterns.

Sharp blades may have features of their own which give rise to a patterned appearance. **Figure 8** illustrates the sutured incised wound of a male who alleged he had been assaulted with a serrated bread knife. This was confirmed by review of the injury where a repeated regular pattern could be observed along the length of the scar, which matched exactly with the serration pattern on the bread knife used in the attack.

Heavy weapons with sharp blades (e.g., meat cleavers, machetes, swords) are capable of causing major injury with damage to soft tissues and bone.

A mixture of blunt and sharp injury may be present and lacerations and incised wounds may be evident. Slash wounds ("slicing" or "striping") may be caused by the above implements with the intention of killing or simply disfiguring. Often the face is the target. Stanley knives, razor blades, and other very sharp instruments may be used, creating clean cuts that can be repaired surgically but leave clean scars. **Figure 9A** shows a scar that was repaired surgically from a wound in which a sharp blade was used. The continuity across irregular surfaces indicates that pressure must have been applied throughout the length of the injury.

Figures 9B and **9C** show the initial appearance of a wound caused by a single blade slash cut across the face and the subsequent appearance after suture. Clearly there is a difference in emotive value between the two injuries and it is for the forensic examiner to make clear to the court the seriousness or otherwise of injuries that are sustained during assaults.

Figure 10 shows scarring following a serious assault with a machete about 1 year previously. The victim did not attend hospital and simply dressed the wounds until healed.

Death and loss of body parts may be the result of chop wounds. Compound fractures have been described – the term "bony laceration" has been used, although "bony incision" may be a better term.

Certain incised wounds have particular medicolegal relevance. These are incised wounds to the neck, wrist, and specific wounds to other parts of the body.

Incised Wounds in Specific Sites

Neck

Incised wounds to the neck are generally either homicidal or suicidal and only occasionally accidental. Accidental wounds are seen particularly in traffic accidents where such injuries are caused by fragments of glass.

The distinction between homicidal and suicidal wounds can be difficult and sometimes unascertainable at autopsy alone. It is essential before an

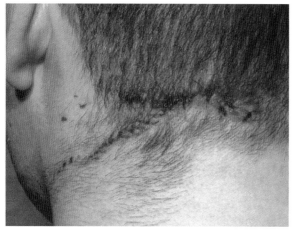

Figure 8 Sutured incised wound after assault with a serrated bread knife.

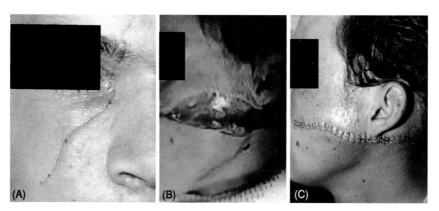

Figure 9 (A) Scar caused by a sharp blade that was surgically repaired. (B) The initial appearance of a wound caused by a single blade slash cut across the face and (C) the subsequent appearance after suture.

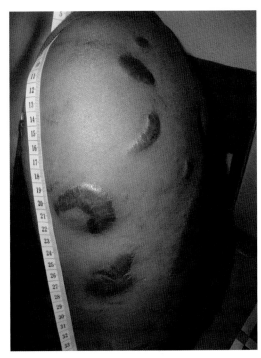

Figure 10 Scarring following an assault with a machete about 1 year previously.

opinion is given that account is taken of the circumstances surrounding the deceased's movements shortly before death, his/her personal history, and a thorough examination of the scene of discovery of the body.

There are a number of characteristic features in terms of appearance and distribution of incised neck wounds that may be of assistance to the pathologist in making the distinction between self-infliction or attack by an assailant. When made by right-handed individuals, self-inflicted injuries normally begin high on the left side of the neck and pass downward across the front to end on the right side. They are deeper at their origin and then tail off on the right. Such wounds may also be horizontal, lying across the front of the neck. They are usually linear and clean-cut, since the skin is likely to be put under tension. Separate shallow wounds, "tentative" or "hesitation" wounds, are strongly indicative of self-infliction. There may be associated incised wounds to the wrist or occasionally elsewhere. There may be evidence of healed self-harm scars indicating previous attempts at self-harm. Some self-inflicted incised wounds may be extremely deep, extending as far as a and leaving score marks on the cervical vertebrae.

As a rule, homicidal wounds do not have the more organized "planned" appearance of self-inflicted wounds and are unaccompanied by tentative injuries, but may be frequently accompanied by incised wounds

that are difficult to interpret without accompanying obvious self-inflicted injuries. Generally, homicidal wounds are more haphazardly placed on the neck and, in some cases, have more irregular edges. In addition such wounds tend to be deeper, although this is by no means invariably so. Accompanying stab wounds may also be present on the neck and other parts of the body, as well as defense cuts to the backs of the arms and hands. There may also be non-cutting injuries to the body which may have contributed to the cause of death.

Accidental incised wounds may be caused by glass in road traffic accidents. Such wounds are frequently accompanied by numerous small abrasions from glass fragments and particles of glass may be found in wounds if carefully searched for.

Wrists

Multiple and commonly parallel incised wounds to the ventral aspect of the wrist and lower forearm are typical of self-inflicted injury as a means of deliberate self-harm. They frequently accompany other self-inflicted cutting wounds to other parts of the body and often old healed wounds may be evident. Although the victim may be aiming to sever a major artery in the wrist, usually the resulting wounds are more superficial. Incised wounds to the dorsal surface of the wrists are occasionally seen in cases of self-inflicted injury but, depending on their number and distribution, they may well be defensive injuries.

Other Sites

Planned incised wounds to various parts of the body, including the face and trunk, may well form part of torture, or of cultural rituals. It is important to distinguish these in those still living by inquiring of the individual, and in fatalities asking friends, family, or cultural experts to determine whether they are relevant to the death.

Stab Wounds

Forensic pathologists and physicians are frequently asked to determine the degree of force used in homicidal and nonfatal stabbing. It is almost impossible to quantify in a precise way and therefore a more qualitative approach may be used. Generally, an impact with greater force is more likely to produce severe injury than an impact of lesser force.

There are a large number of factors or conditions that need to be taken into account when assessing injury severity. These factors range from and influence the movement of the knife up to the point of impact with the skin and from the skin to the point of termination and withdrawal from the body. These phases must be considered in conjunction with: (1) the properties of the knife; (2) the way the assailant delivers the blow, in terms of speed and direction; and (3) the movement or reaction of the victim to the assault. It is important to convey to the nonforensic investigator that this is a dynamic process that changes moment by moment. **Table 2** summarizes the main factors to consider when assessing force required.

It was previously believed that, once the skin had been pierced, unless the knife impacted against bone, virtually no resistance was offered by the internal soft tissues, including the major organs. More recent work has suggested that the scenario is more complex than previously appreciated. It appears that once the skin has been pierced, significant resistance may be offered by the internal organs and other soft tissues. Once the knife has impacted on the skin and even after piercing it, there still needs to be a firm hand on the knife to push the weapon further into the body, because it has been slowed down by the resistance offered by the skin. In an accidental stabbing or where a knife has been thrown, less penetration into the body is to be expected. In the case of accidental stabbing, it is much more likely that, once resistance is offered by the skin, then there would not be a follow-through thrust, as in a deliberate movement. To produce such a further

deliberate movement, the weapon would need to be anchored or held firmly. To produce impalement on to a knife there would need to be enough momentum by the victim moving toward the knife and it would need to be fixed firmly in some way. When a knife is thrown at a person, the main resistance will be by the skin, causing significant loss of its kinetic energy. Because there would be no follow-through, penetration into the body may not be deep because of the further resistance of the internal tissue.

Generally the best approach to assist those investigating such wounds is to advise that the force required is in the following range – weak, weak/moderate, moderate, moderate/severe, or severe.

Wound Assessment

In a case involving sharp-force trauma, assessment of the injuries should take into account the following:

- the number of wounds
- their location and relationship to each other
- their character.

Characteristics of Surface Wounds

Assessment of stab wound characteristics will frequently assist the forensic examiner in identifying the type of implement involved, its shape, size, and any possible individual features such as a broken or bent blade tip or anomalous serrations on the blade. Additionally review of possible implements will allow a determination of whether an implement was capable of causing the injury described. **Figure 11A** shows a piece of glass alleged to have created the wound seen on the thigh in **Figure 11B**. The depth of the wound was measured at operation and, even allowing for compression, the piece of glass was too wide at all relevant points to have been responsible for creating the wound seen in **Figure 11B**. The crime-scene officers were asked to look for and were able to identify the weapon that had caused the injury.

Stab wounds on the surface of the body may show a wide variety of morphological characteristics, depending on the type of implement used, cutting surface, sharpness, width, and shape of the blade. Most stab wounds seen in the UK result from knives with a single sharp-edged blade. Occasionally, broken glass, screwdrivers, and other pointed objects are used. Most stab wounds caused by knives tend to have clean-cut edges with one or both ends appearing pointed. If the blade is single-edged the nonpointed end may be either squared off or split (fishtail) in appearance. **Figure 12** shows an example of a "fishtail" caused by a single-sided blade, although there is evidence to suggest that a double-edged blade moving

Table 2 Main factors influencing outcome of stabbing

Factor	Additional comment
Intrinsic properties of knife	
Shape of knife	Including length, extent of blade, single blade/double blade/serrated blade, sharp tip, round tip, hilt?
Sharpness of knife	Razorsharp? Degree of sharpness?
Weight of knife	
Delivery of blow by assailant	
Velocity of thrust	Is force kept up throughout thrust?
Type/direction of thrust	Overarm, underarm?
Movement of knife up to point of impact over which victim has influence	
Clothing	Amount of clothing, body protector?
Movement of victim	Towards, away from, deflecting?
Movement of knife through skin into body	
Skin resistance	
Underlying organs	Fat, muscle, body cavity, bone, solid organs, e.g., liver?
Movement of organs	On respiration?

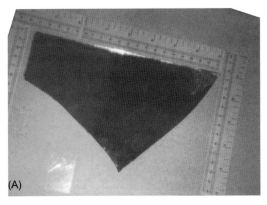
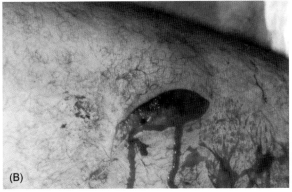

Figure 11   (A) A piece of glass alleged to have created the wound (B) seen on the thigh.

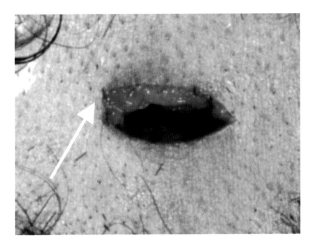

Figure 12   A "fishtail" caused by a single-sided blade.

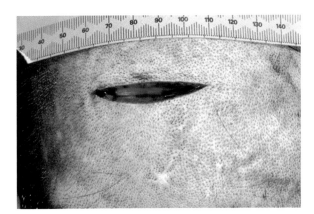

Figure 13   A tangential stab wound to the crown of the head with underlying scoring of the cranium.

with rotational force in the wound may have created a similar appearance.

Figure 12 shows a stab wound caused by a knife with a single cutting edge. The right side of the wound is caused by the cutting side of the blade and the more ragged square/fishtail end, indicated by the arrow, is from the noncutting side.

A wound overlying bone, especially over the skull, requires care in its interpretation. It is not unusual to find a laceration of the skin resulting from a blunt impact having clean edges and a very similar superficial appearance to an incised or stab injury. The reason for this is that the skin, being close to a bony surface, becomes easily stretched during impact, thus tending to split cleanly. A thorough exploration of the wound to detect bridging tissue as one would observe within a laceration is essential. With sharp-force trauma one may see scoring by the weapon on the outer table of the skull. **Figure 13** shows a tangential stab wound to the crown of the head with underlying scoring of the cranium. This can be confirmed at autopsy but may not be able to be

confirmed in a living victim, and the differentiation between a laceration and an incised wound depends on accurate assessment of the cut itself and absence of associated blunt injury. However, with a "chop" wound it may be almost impossible to determine in the living.

Bruising may also surround the wound as a result of impaction by the hilt of the knife. Sometimes the wound may show abraded edges or a clear hilt pattern.

Often wounds show a notch or change of direction along the margin on the skin. This is caused by relative movement of the knife and the body during the stabbing action, thus causing the exit track of the wound to be slightly modified. **Figure 14** shows a stab wound showing a slight central notch on its upper margin. The lower margin shows "shelving," with underlying tissue visible. Such wounds give the investigator an indication of the direction of the track of the wound.

Figure 15 shows a stab wound with a central notch giving the appearance of a V-shape, again caused by the dynamic movement of assailant, victim, and knife.

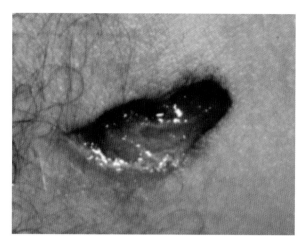

Figure 14   A stab wound showing a slight central notch on its upper margin.

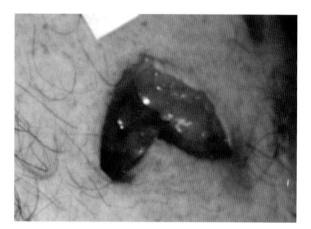

Figure 15   A stab wound with a central notch.

Other Information

There are a number of factors to assess in determining the mechanism of injury. Assessment of clothes has been referred to in relation to injuries caused by deliberate self-harm. In assault cases, careful examination of the defects of the items of clothing by a sharp weapon such as a knife and matching these up with the wounds on the victim can help in assessing the number of times the victim has been stabbed and the direction of the stab (**Figure 12**). Where possible – this is generally easier in the deceased victim than the living where clothes may have been cut off or discarded during first aid or resuscitation – the forensic examiner should take the opportunity to examine the clothing and the various tears produced by a knife, in conjunction with the wounds found on the body and the implement supposedly used. The number of cuts in clothes may not correspond to the number of wounds on the body. This may be for a

number of reasons, including that the weapon may impact on an outer garment but not reach the skin, clothing may be folded, the knife may cause more than one cut from the same thrust, and clothing at the point of impact may not be present, for example, it may have been pulled away from its normal position for various reasons.

Assessment of Wound Tracks

As with assessment of many injuries, detailed and accurate assessment is done better in the deceased victim than the living victim because treatment and repair may obscure information, and nonforensic personnel have different agendas when documenting the type of injury. Although the characteristics of a stab wound on the surface of the body give a great deal of information, as discussed above, it is desirable to examine the track of a particular wound, which can be done at autopsy, or to attempt to describe it anatomically in the living survivor.

Ideally the following factors should be determined or commented upon:

1. the direction of impact on to the body
2. the depth of an injury resulting from stabbing
3. the force used to inflict the injury, taking into account the various structures injured
4. injured structures and their bearing on morbidity and mortality
5. in cases of multiple stabbing, to assess which surface wounds are responsible for which internal injuries.

The depth, or more accurately, the length of the track of the wound may give some guidance as to the depth to which the blade of the knife has penetrated. Nevertheless, it should be appreciated that a number of factors affect the estimation of the length of the track, which first, is only an approximation and second, depending on the site, may be valueless in correlating with the length of blade that has penetrated the body. This is particularly the case with abdominal and neck wounds. In chest wounds one must allow for the elasticity of the ribs, especially in younger subjects.

Figure 16A shows external injuries following multiple stab wounds on the left side of the chest. The probe indicates the initial entry through the arm then to the chest wall. **Figure 16B** shows the track of the wound continued into the upper lobe of the left lung.

Outcome of Injury

The forensic examiner needs to be able to interpret first, the injuries seen and second, the potential for

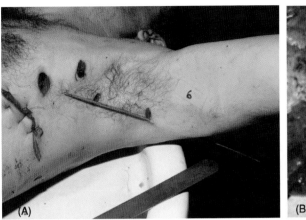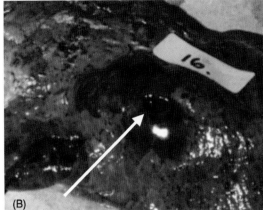

Figure 16 (A) External injuries following multiple stab wounds on the left side of the chest; (B) the track of the wound continued into the upper lobe of the left lung.

injury that could have or might have been the outcome in both living and deceased. **Table 3** identifies the potential outcome of even single sharp-force or stab traumas required to take into account the various possible effects of sharp-force trauma, including the impact of medical intervention on the overall outcome and possible contribution to morbidity and mortality. The list below is not intended to be comprehensive but includes the more recognized effects of sharp-force trauma – acute, subacute, and chronic.

Subacute and chronic complications include:

- infection
- loss of or diminished function
- aneurysm
- dissection
- ischemia
- fistula
- diaphragmatic hernia
- adhesions
- chronic inflammation.

Defense Wounds

Certain types of injuries may be described as "defense" injuries. These are injuries that are typically seen when an individual has tried to defend him/herself against an attack, and are the results of instinctive reactions to assault. When attacked with blunt objects most individuals will attempt to protect their eyes, head, and neck by raising their arms, flexing their elbows, and covering the head and neck. As a result the exposed surfaces of the arms become the impact point for blows. Thus the extensor surface of the forearms (the ulnar side) may receive blows, as may the lateral/posterior aspects of the upper arm, and the dorsum of the hands. Similarly the outer and

Table 3 Potential effects of sharp force trauma

Acute effects include:
- Hypovolemic shock from blood loss
- Tamponade
- Direct effect of injury to organ function, e.g. heart, spinal cord
- Air embolism
- Asphyxia from airway obstruction from hematoma
- Aspiration of blood
- Pneumothorax
- Hemothorax

Subacute and chronic complications include:
- Infection
- Loss of or diminished function
- Aneurysm
- Dissection
- Ischemia
- Fistula
- Diaphragmatic hernia
- Adhesions
- Chronic inflammation

posterior aspects of lower limbs and back may be injured as an individual curls into a ball, with flexion of spine, knees, and hips to protect the anterior part of the body.

In addition to the above, in sharp-force attacks another natural reaction is to try and disarm the attacker, often by grabbing the knife blade. This results in cuts to the palm and ulnar aspect of the hand. On some occasions the hands or arms may be raised to protect the body against the stabbing motion, resulting in stab wounds to the defense areas, which in some cases may be through and through because of the sharpness of the blade. **Figure 17** shows the palmar and dorsal surface of a hand and the sutured through and through cut where the victim had put his hand palmar surface out to ward off a knife attack. Note that the alignment is the same, confirming that this was from a single stab.

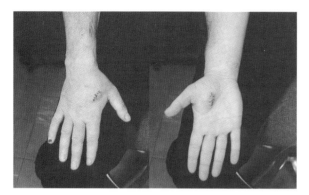

Figure 17   The palmar and dorsal surface of a hand after a knife attack.

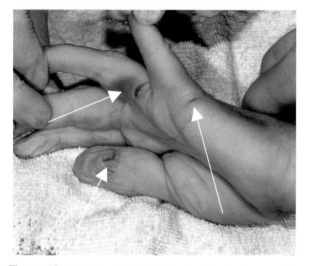

Figure 18   Injuries to the palms and ventral surfaces of the fingers.

Figure 18 shows injuries to the palms and ventral surfaces of the fingers. Such wounds indicate that the victim tried to grab hold of the weapon between all the fingers with the thumb in apposition, or predominantly between the forefinger and the thumb.

In the latter situation care should be taken to differentiate between injuries caused by the knife slipping through the hand of the assailant holding a knife thus injuring his/her own hand, or from a genuine defense injury suffered by the victim.

The number of defense wounds tends to increase as the number of stab wounds to the victim increases and defense wounds in stab wound cases may be present in about 40% of victims.

Homicidal versus Suicidal Stabbing

The assessment of any stabbing case requires great attention to detail, particularly where there is a possibility that the injuries may be self-inflicted. In the living victim it is easier to determine a relevant history but in fatalities there may be times when the two categories are difficult to distinguish on pathological grounds. The circumstances, appearance of the scene, and any background information play an important role in resolving the problem and the autopsy findings should all be examined, taking into consideration all these factors. **Table 4** summarizes some of the factors that may differentiate between the two categories.

Summary

Sharp-force trauma may present in many different ways, with both living and deceased victims. Living

Table 4   Factors to assist in the differentiation between homicidal and suicidal stabbing

Factor	Homicide	Suicide
Scene		
Signs of disturbance	Likely	Very unlikely
Knife near body	Unlikely	Almost always
Body		
Clothing pulled above wound	Unusual	Very common
Stab through clothing	Very common	Unusual
Single or very few deep wounds seen	Can be any number from one upwards	Common
Multiple deep wounds	Common	Uncommon
Body laid out neatly	Uncommon (unless restrained)	Common
Irregularly placed multiple wounds	Very common	Uncommon, tend to be in single region
Tentative wounds	Not seen (unless torture involved)	Common
Defense wounds	Common (almost half of cases)	No
Additional fresh marks of self-harm	No	Sometimes
Old marks of self-harm	Sometimes	Common
Location of injury in site accessible to reach	Possible	Commonly, chest, abdomen, neck, and wrist
Other types of injury (e.g., blunt impact)	Possible, particularly if there was a struggle	Unusual unless unrelated

victims are able to provide accounts of what happened, but the characteristics of the injury may be poorly documented. For deceased victims the characteristics of the injury can be documented clearly, although the account of what happened may be lacking. In each case of sharp-force trauma, from the most minor to the most serious, accurate documentation, detailed review of available history, and interpretation of the findings with an understanding of the mechanism of injury will enable the investigators and courts to come to the most appropriate determination of outcome.

See Also

Deaths: Trauma, Head and Spine; Trauma, Thorax; Trauma, Abdominal Cavity; Trauma, Musculo-skeletal System; **Deliberate Self-Harm, Patterns**; **Injury, Fatal and Nonfatal:** Blunt Injury; **Suicide:** Etiology, Methods and Statistics

Further Reading

Bhattacharjee N, Arefin SM, Mazumder SM, Khan MK (1997) Cut throat injury: a retrospective study of 26 cases. *Bangladesh Medical Research Council Bulletin* 23: 87–89.

Bleetman A, Watson CH, Horsfall I, Champion SM (2003) Wounding patterns and human performance in knife attacks: optimising the protection provided by knife resistant body armour. *Journal of Clinical Forensic Medicine* 10: 243–248.

Chadwick EKJ, Nicol AC, Lane JV, Gray TGF (1999) Biomechanics of knife stab attacks. *Forensic Science International* 105: 35–44.

Horsfall I, Prosser PD, Watson CH, Champion SM (1999) An assessment of human performance in stabbing. *Forensic Science International* 102: 79–89.

Hunt AC, Cowling RJ (1991) Murder by stabbing. *Forensic Science International* 52: 107–112.

Karlsson T (1998) Homicidal and suicidal sharp force fatalities in Stockholm, Sweden. Orientation of entrance wounds in stabs gives information in the classification. *Forensic Science International* 93: 21–32.

Katkici Ü, Özkök MS, Örsal M (1994) An autopsy evaluation of defence wounds in 195 homicidal deaths due to stabbing. *Journal of the Forensic Science Society* 34: 237–240.

Milroy CM, Rutty GN (1997) If a wound is "neatly incised" it is not a laceration (letter). *British Medical Journal* 315: 1312.

Missliwetz J, Denk W (1994) Assault and homicide by chop blow: a series of 11 cases. *Journal of Clinical Forensic Medicine* 1: 133–138.

Murray LA, Green MA (1987) Hilts and knives: a survey of 10 years of fatal stabbings. *Medicine, Science and the Law* 27: 182–184.

National Statistics (2004) *Crime in England and Wales: 2002/2003.* Supplementary volume 1. *Homicide and Gun Crime.* London.

O'Callaghan PT, Jones MD, James DS, *et al.* (1999) Dynamics of stab wounds: force required for penetration of various cadaveric human tissues. 104: 173–178.

Ong BB (1999) The pattern of homicidal slash/chop injuries: a 10 year retrospective study in University Hospital, Kuala Lumpur. *Journal of Clinical and Forensic Medicine* 24–29.

Ormstad K, Karlsson T, Enkler L, Law B, Rajs J (1986) Patterns in sharp force fatalities – a comprehensive forensic medical study. *Journal of Forensic Sciences* 31: 529–542.

Payne-James JJ (2002) Assault and injury in the living. In: Payne-James JJ, Busuttil A, Smock W (eds.) *Forensic Medicine: Clinical and Pathological Aspects.* London: Greenwich Medical Media.

Rogde S, Hougen HP, Poulsen K (2000) Homicide by sharp force in two Scandinavian capitals. *Forensic Science International* 109: 135–145.

Rouse DA (1994) Patterns of stab wounds: a six year study. *Medicine, Science and the Law* 34: 67–71.

Start RD, Milroy CM, Green MA (1992) Suicide by self-stabbing. *Forensic Science International* 56: 89–94.

Vanezis P, West IE (1983) Tentative injuries in self-stabbing. *Forensic Science International* 21: 65–70.

INJURY, RECREATIONAL

Contents

Water Sports

P Lunetta, University of Helsinki, Helsinki, Finland

Introduction

Boating and activities on water are among the oldest human activities and have been an important component of the earliest cultures' life and transport. The development of watercraft, starting from the earliest primitive forms (floating devices, rafts made of wood or reed bundles and buoyed by inflated animal skins, bark canoes, dugouts), up to the nineteenth century, when steam propulsion ousted sail craft, has embraced a wide set of human activities, from locomotion, fishing, and transportation to exploration, colonization, trading, and the military.

During the twentieth century, recreational sailing and motor boating developed greatly, especially in high-income countries. In the USA, more than 60 million people engage in recreational boating activities, with over 13 million registered boats across the country, including 1 million personal watercraft. In Europe, France, which is the world's second largest leisure boating market, counts almost 1 million pleasure boats, and smaller countries such as Finland or the Netherlands each have up to 400 000–600 000 registered boats.

The present article focuses on water-related traffic accidents during leisure activities; this is an increasingly recognized setting in developed countries for high injury-related mortality and morbidity. It does not cover water-transport accidents unrelated to recreational activities, although in developing countries these represent a major public health problem connected to migration, transportation, occupation, and sustenance fishing.

Epidemiology

The US Department of Homeland Security (formerly Department of Transportation) maintains a unique boating accident report database system, which provides annual nationwide information on fatal and nonfatal recreational boating accidents. No comparable reporting systems exist in the European Union or in other developed countries. World Health Organization standard data are available for many countries worldwide but provide no information on water-transport-related mortality or boating-related drowning. In addition to the USA, the most comprehensive data on recreational boating-related morbidity and mortality come from in-depth studies performed in high-income countries, especially Canada, Australia, and New Zealand, and in Europe, Finland. In some countries, national statistics offices tabulate and report mortality data according to the *International Classification of Disease* and provide specific data for water-traffic accidents, resulting in either drowning or another cause of death. Comparative studies on drowning rates between countries are, however, hampered by registration systems at different levels and, at least in part, by differences in coding practices.

In the USA (population 291.9 million), during the period 1997 to 2002, there were 43 903 accidents involving recreational boating, which injured 26 173 and claimed 4502 victims (**Table 1**). This corresponds to an annual average of 7317 accidents, with 4362 injured and 750 fatalities. Boating fatalities concern mostly middle-aged males, with most victims being 30–39-year-olds, and the highest number injured among 20–29-year-olds. Boating is a rare cause of death among children: fewer than 3% of victims are under 12. Marked differences are, however, observed concerning age and sex distribution between countries and even among different regions of the same country.

Overall, recreational boating accidents occur more often during the warmest season at weekends when exposure is higher; however, some studies report higher fatality rates for accidents occurring during the fall and winter months, likely due to reduced survival possibilities in cold water and under adverse weather conditions.

In Nordic countries, although no reporting system for boating accidents exists, boating-related mortality data are rather extensive due to the high medicolegal autopsy rate and separate tabulation by national statistics offices of water traffic-related fatalities,

Table 1 Boating-related accidents[a] in the USA, 1997–2002

Year	Total no. of accidents	Killed	Drowned	Killed in alcohol-related accidents	Injured	Registered boats	Killed per 100 000 registered boats
1997	8047	821	588	223	4555	12 312 982	6.7
1998	8061	815	574	217	4612	12 565 930	6.5
1999	7931	734	517	191	4315	12 738 271	5.8
2000	7740	701	519	215	4355	12 782 143	5.5
2001	6419	681	498	232	4274	12 876 346	5.3
2002	5705	750	524	284	4062	13 040 726	5.8

[a]Accidents involving property damages less than US$2000 and with only slight injury that require no medical treatment beyond first aid are not included.
Adapted from US Department of Homeland Security (2003) *Boating Statistics 2002*. Commandat Publication P16754. 16, US Coast Guard, Washington.

land-traffic fatalities, and drowning. In Finland (population 5.3 million), where more than 98% of boating fatalities undergo a full medicolegal autopsy, water traffic accounted for 110 victims annually during 1970 and 2000, almost one-third of all drownings. Boating is therefore the most frequent single activity related to drowning in Finland; boating-related drownings peak in an older age group (50–54-year-olds) than in the USA, and the male-to-female ratio is much higher (21:1) than in nonboating drowning (9:1). The typical Finnish victim can be described as a middle-aged male who, under the influence of alcohol, operates a small motorboat on a lake during the warm season. In Finland, ad hoc investigation teams composed of police officers, boat engineers, and forensic pathologists have extensively analyzed circumstances (hours, day of the week, month, body of water, weather conditions, and water temperature) related to leisure-boating fatal accidents, vessels (type, condition, overcrowding), and human factors (operator experience, swimming ability, disease, alcohol).

In most countries, drowning represents the overwhelming cause (more than 90%) of boating-related fatalities, and in many of them boating is the leading activity causing drowning. Accordingly, boating-related drowning in Canada or Finland represents 30–40% of all drownings, in New Zealand and Denmark 20–30%, in the USA and Australia 10–20%, but in the UK, Germany, and Italy less than 10%.

Vessel and Accident Types

The entire range of recreational vessels (open or cabin motorboat, sailing boat, rowboat, pontoon boat, houseboat, personal watercraft, jet boat, airboat, inflatable, canoe/kayak, even cruise ships) can be involved in boating accidents. The involvement of a given vessel in a boating accident depends on the total number of similar vessels circulating and exposure

time for boaters. These variables vary markedly from one country to another and even between regions of the same country, depending on geographical, climate, and economic factors.

In the USA, for instance, 60–65% of vessels involved in fatalities are open or cabin motorboats, and almost 10% are personal watercraft, with rowboats representing less than 5% of the vessels involved. When considering nonfatal boating accidents, personal watercraft account for up to 30–35% of the cases. In Canada powerboats represent 60% of the vessels involved in fatalities, canoes are involved in 10–15% of cases, rowboats in 3%, and personal watercraft in only 2%. In Finland, the use of personal watercraft is rather limited and related accidents are still very rare, whereas rowboats are involved in up to 30% of fatal accidents, which most frequently occur on lakes during the summer cottage season.

The most frequent types of boating accident include capsizing, falling overboard, collision, and sinking. Collisions may involve a fixed or floating object or another vessel. Other causes of boating accidents involve being struck by a boat, motor, or propeller, falling into boat, fire or explosion, water-skier mishap, or carbon monoxide poisoning. The accident type, and its consequences, greatly depends on the type of vessel. Capsizing, for instance, involves preferentially open motorboats, rowboats, or canoes or kayaks, not cabin motorboats or personal watercraft; falling overboard is more frequent in open motorboats, rowboats, or personal watercraft; collision or being struck by a boat involves personal watercrafts; being struck by a propeller involves cabin or open motorboats; and fire or explosion occurs in cabin motorboats. Water-skiing-related injuries are caused by falls into water, by boat propeller blades, collisions with a boat or fixed obstacle, or by towropes.

The probability for each type of accident to be fatal varies widely, also in relation to circumstantial and

Table 2 Common types of boating accident and percentage of fatalities

Types of boating accidents	Fatalities (%)
Capsizing	49.8
Falling overboard	34.9
Sinking	12.5
Collisions	6.3
Explosion/fire	2.5

Adapted from US Department of Homeland Security (2003) *Boating Statistics 2002*. Commandat Publication P16754. 16, US Coast Guard, Washington.

Table 3 Main contributing factors of boating-related accidents and fatalities in the USA in 2002

Contributing factors	Accidents (n)	Fatalities n	Fatalities %
Operator-controllable	3758	414	11.0
Operator inattention	718	41	5.7
Careless/reckless operation	636	53	8.3
Operator inexperience	533	46	8.6
Excessive speed	455	29	6.4
Passenger/skier behavior	341	32	9.4
No proper lookout	331	22	6.6
Alcohol use	267	95	35.6
Other	477	96	20.1
Environmental	714	170	23.8
Hazard waterway	418	99	23.7
Weather	228	66	28.9
Congested waterway	61	1	1.6
Dam/lock	7	4	57.1
Vessel machinery/equipment	435	35	8.0
Other/unknown	676	131	19.4
Total	5705	750	13.1

Adapted from US Department of Homeland Security (2003) *Boating Statistics 2002*. Commandat Publication P16754. 16, US Coast Guard, Washington.

individual factors. In the USA, for instance, a collision with another vessel is, overall, the most frequent type of boating accident, but capsizing or a fall overboard claims the highest number of lives and accounts for over half of all fatalities (**Table 2**).

Risk Factors

Boating-related accidents result from the complex relationship between personal, environmental, and equipment factors (**Table 3**). The risk factors associated with the different types of boating accident, in addition to those related to vessel machinery and equipment, include environmental, and operator- and passenger-dependent factors. Environmental factors comprise weather conditions, hazardous water, and congested waterways. Boater-dependent factors include operator and passenger negligence,

inexperience, and risk-taking attitudes. According to several studies, the two most important individual risk factors for boating-related fatal accidents are not wearing a personal flotation device (PFD) and alcohol consumption on board. In most series, over 80–90% of victims of boating-related drowning are not wearing a PFD, and a large proportion (up to 90%) could have been saved if a PFD was worn. The role of alcohol will be considered in detail in the following paragraphs.

Boating and Alcohol

The relation between boat accidents and alcohol has been documented in different countries and various settings, with most studies reporting alcohol involvement in 25–50% of boating drownings, a percentage higher than for most other unintentional injury deaths. As for the frequency of alcohol-related boating deaths, in the USA, during 2000 and 2001 alcohol was involved in approximately one-third of all 1382 recreational boating fatalities. In Maryland and North Carolina, of 221 recreational boating fatalities from 1990 to 1998, 36% had a blood alcohol concentration (BAC) $> 50 \, \text{mg} \, \text{dl}^{-1}$. In Canada in 1999, 32% of the 122 victims of boating-related drowning had a BAC $> 80 \, \text{mg} \, \text{dl}^{-1}$. In Finland, despite the introduction of a legal BAC limit for boat operators ($150 \, \text{mg} \, \text{dl}^{-1}$ in 1976, further reduced to $100 \, \text{mg} \, \text{dl}^{-1}$ in 1994), alcohol is based on a 92% postmortem testing rate, still a major contributor to boat fatalities, with up to 78% of victims 15–64 years old being alcohol-positive. During the period 1998–2000, of 704 Finnish drowning victims of all ages, 405 (57.5%) had a BAC $\geq 50 \, \text{mg} \, \text{dl}^{-1}$, 386 (54.8%) $\geq 100 \, \text{mg} \, \text{dl}^{-1}$, and 133 (18.9%) $\geq 250 \, \text{mg} \, \text{dl}^{-1}$ (**Table 4**).

Direct Biological and Other Indirect Effects

Alcohol is usually involved in boating-related accidents because of its impairment of human performance during watercraft operation in tasks involving cognitive and psychomotor skills. Importantly, in contrast to land traffic, alcohol impairs the performances not only of boat operators, but also of passengers, by increasing their risk of falling overboard and, once in the water, by reducing their capacity to swim and thus survival possibilities, especially in cold weather. Moreover, the inebriated boater also poses a risk to those nearby, who may be other drinkers or sober persons, including those not on board. Although the effects of alcohol show a dose–response effect, it must be stressed there is no BAC threshold below which no performance impairment occurs. Moreover, because for the same alcohol consumption,

Table 4 Boating-related fatal accidents in Finland and their association with alcohol, 1997–2002

Boating-related drowning				Other boating-related fatalities		
Years	n	n/100 000	% associated with alcohol	n	n/100 000	% associated with alcohol
1995	81	1.6	52	9	0.2	1
1996	50	1.0	35	3	0.1	1
1997	64	1.2	37	1	<0.1	0
1998	74	1.4	NA	7	0.1	NA
1999	57	1.1	38	8	0.2	5
2000	68	1.3	39	5	0.1	3
2001	64	1.2	36	3	0.1	0
2002	65	1.2	40	4	0.1	0

NA, not available.
Adapted from Statistics Finland (1996–2003) *Cause of Death, 1995 to 2002.* SUT Health, Helsink.

resultant BAC levels and tolerance vary from person to person, BAC *per se*, although important in legal definition, is not a good parameter of performance impairment.

Alcohol use has other effects unrelated to its direct effects on physiological performance. It increases one's sense of confidence, reduces perception and response to hazards, and may hamper decision-making regarding safety. Those under the influence of alcohol may be more prone to risk-taking behaviors, and thus operate a boat in dangerous situations or fail to use appropriate safety devices. The injury risk may even be increased during the "hangover" period when BAC is very low or negative. Alcohol may also influence injury severity and outcome, and reduce the likelihood of survival. For instance, those under the influence may have less effective reflexes to avoid head injury during falls and in a cold climate, impaired protective mechanisms against hypothermia. For chronic alcohol abusers, after a near-drowning episode, malnutrition, and a reduced immune response may promote infections.

Study Design and Methodological Issues

The quality of data on the association between alcohol and boating varies considerably, most studies being more descriptive than analytical. Criteria used to define alcohol-positive boating drowning, population selected, and age range, and proportion of victims tested represent important issues for comparability of data. Legislation on investigation of cause of death and the rate of medicolegal autopsy and of postmortem toxicology are all critical for reliable data and international comparisons. While countries such as Finland have a high (up to 95–99%) autopsy rate for injury deaths, and for most of these deaths, determine BAC, other countries have considerable legislative and practical limitations on postmortem BAC determination. In the UK, for instance, extensive postmortem alcohol testing is not

allowed under the Human Tissue Act; in the USA, testing rates vary widely on a state-by-state basis; and in southern Europe, autopsies and toxicological analysis are ordered, case-by-case, by the prosecutor in charge.

The association between alcohol and fatal boating accidents can be explored with a wide variety of study designs. Most studies are simply descriptive and illustrate the proportion of deaths or injuries at various levels of BAC. Moreover, when a low BAC limit (e.g., $50 \, \text{mg} \, \text{dl}^{-1}$) defines a case as alcohol-positive, the study will provide a conservative estimate, since impairment may even occur at a lower BAC level. Many studies only consider the alcohol involvement of the victim, although BAC-negative victims, as previously mentioned, can die from the action of an inebriated boater.

The association between alcohol and boating injuries does not always imply a direct role of alcohol in such injuries. Because several potential confounding factors may coexist, the multivariate statistical analysis should identify independent effects of alcohol. To measure excess risk of injury and death associated with various BAC levels, case-control studies are necessary, although practical difficulties exist concerning extensive measurement of BAC in controls. Control groups can comprise fatalities from other causes (relative effect of alcohol), nonfatal injuries (effect of alcohol on the probability that injury will be fatal), or noninjured persons (effect of alcohol on the probability of sustaining an injury).

Specific methodological issues that must be briefly addressed are the treatment of missing values and postmortem alcohol production. Since in most studies only a certain percentage of victims are tested for BAC, the values will be overestimated if calculated on the basis of the cases tested, and be underestimated if based on all the study material. If the untested group differs from the tested group, this approach will bias the effects of alcohol involvement, because missing

BAC values can either be randomly distributed or not. Imputations for missing values are statistical methods used to estimate the true nature of missing cases but their results must be interpreted prudently.

The validity of postmortem BAC data, that is, how well the measured BAC reflects the BAC at the time of injury or death, is an important medicolegal and epidemiological issue. The first problem is represented by postmortem endogenous alcohol production. After death, bacteria from the gut may penetrate the systemic vessels, where glucose and lactose act as substrates for bacterial fermentation which may be enhanced by high environmental temperature, hyperglycemia, septicemia, or severe disruption of body parts. Postmortem alcohol production rarely exceeds $40-50\,mg\,dl^{-1}$. Selection criteria proposed for avoiding false-positives include blood sampling within 24 h postmortem or sampling within 48 h postmortem with BAC results $>100\,mg\,dl^{-1}$. More recently, adjustment procedures to compensate for postmortem alcohol production have been proposed for bodies submerged in water for up to 1 week. Evaluation of false-positive cases can be achieved by comparing BAC with alcohol values in urine and vitreous humor, since normally urine does not contain any substrate for fermentation, and vitreous humor is resistant to postmortem bacterial invasion. In high-profile medicolegal cases, blood culture coupled with a fermentation test can help to confirm postmortem ethanol production. Two other potential factors interfere with the validity of postmortem BAC values: (1) postmortem redistribution of alcohol from the stomach and small bowel to the heart and great blood vessels, requiring alcohol samples always to be obtained from peripheral vessels; and (2) delayed blood testing after the injury, with the result that the alcohol has been partially metabolized: the victim may have drunk during the interval between injury and death, or intravenous fluids may have been admisered before blood testing.

Cause of Death and Medicolegal Investigation

The majority of boating-related fatal accidents are due to drowning, with the remaining fatalities generally resulting from blunt and incised wound, hypothermia, or carbon monoxide intoxication. In most studies, drowning represents more than 90% of all fatalities in boating accidents; and hypothermia, especially during the cold season and without a PFD, can be an important contributing factor. These fatalities are generally associated with capsizing, sinking, or falling overboard. In other boating accidents, propeller-related injuries, blunt injury, neck and spinal

trauma, or burns can cause severe morbidity or be fatal. Propeller injuries cause major amputations in 15–20% of cases, with a similar percentage of fatalities, and can involve boaters overboard as well as water skiers, divers, and swimmers. Bacterial marine flora contamination of the amputation wound may critically influence the outcome. Carbon monoxide poisoning mostly occurs aboard old cabin watercraft powered by a gasoline engine and with no carbon monoxide detector; however, carbon monoxide poisoning can also occur in a semienclosed environment or in the open air due to engine exhaust gases. These injuries, although not at the time fatal, may, due to loss of consciousness or impairment in swimming capability, lead to death by drowning or hypothermia (**Table 5**).

Together with water-skiing, PWD (personal watercraft device), which, has become increasingly popular during the past decade, especially in the USA, is the only type of recreational boating activity for which the leading cause of death and injury is not drowning but blunt trauma, including head and other internal injury, and fractures and lacerations, most often in the lower extremities.

When a victim of a putative boating accident is found in water, police and medicolegal investigations must identify the body, evaluate the postmortem submersion time, and determine the cause of death. Addressing these issues requires the localization of the site of death, which may be close to the place where the body was found, a more remote aquatic setting, or, in the case of a cadaver's disposal, far away on a boat or dry land. Diagnosis of cause of death relies upon accurate assessment of postmortem autopsy findings, individual characteristics of the victims, environmental aspects, and circumstances surrounding death.

Table 5 Boating-related fatal accidents and life-jacket wear in the USA, 1997–2002

| Cause of death | Wearing a PFD (n) | Not wearing PFD | | Total (n) |
		n	%	
Drowning	82	442	84.3	524
Trauma	63	101	61.6	164
Hypothermia	9	10	52.6	19
Carbon monoxide	0	8	100.0	8
Other	5	24	82.8	29
Unknown	0	6	100.0	6

PFD, personal flotation device.
Adapted from US Department of Homeland Security (2003) *Boating Statistics 2002*. Commandat Publication P16754. 16, US Coast Guard, Washington.

During the investigation of a boating-related fatality, a wide range of events has to be adequately considered, to reconstruct the events that led the victim into the water. Traumatic lesions and pathological processes sustained on board, during a fall from a watercraft, or while already in the water, must be thoroughly considered, since any of these may have triggered or may contribute to the fatal outcome. Differentiation between antemortem and postmortem lesions may be difficult due to the washout effect of water on soft-tissue hemorrhages in vital lesions. Even when the cause of death is ascertained, its manner may remain difficult to assess. For instance, a boater, perhaps under the influence of alcohol, may not only fall accidentally overboard, but may voluntarily jump into the water or be pushed overboard. In many of these cases, the forensic pathologist will have to exclude these possibilities and accurately determine the manner of death.

Prevention

Surveillance in boating-related accidents consists in the systematic collection, analysis, and interpretation of data relevant to identify populations exposed, and risk and protective factors. It aims to design, evaluate, and implement prevention programs. Countermeasures focus on previously analyzed risk factors and include education and legal interventions aiming; (1) to increase vessel safety (maintenance, equipment); (2) to promote safety behavior on board (use of PFD, sobriety) and in water settings in general; (3) to improve swimming proficiency; and (4) to increase skill in resuscitation in both lifeguards and the general community. Since improved swimming proficiency may result in a greater exposure to risk, it must necessarily be linked to the promotion of safe behavior in water settings.

Broad-based countermeasures to reduce alcohol use are also needed as part of any strategy to reduce morbidity and mortality in water settings. Legal control of access to alcohol is a common strategy to reduce alcohol-related injuries, and, in turn, may be enforced and implemented by local policy and community interventions. These include total prohibition, monopolies, taxation of alcoholic beverages, legal drinking-age limits, regulation of alcohol outlets and advertising, limitations of days and hours of sale, and BAC legal limits for boat operators. However, laws prohibiting boat operators from drinking while boating fail to recognize the increased risk for inebriated passengers, for example in falling overboard. Countermeasures reducing drinking by all boat occupants would therefore be more likely to reduce boating fatalities.

Establishment of national surveillance multidisciplinary systems for boating accidents is essential for effective preventive countermeasures. Medical examiners, within the limits of the existing laws, can play a significant role in surveillance and prevention by providing accurate reports of victims' injuries and supporting wide BAC testing. In addition to improved surveillance systems, a strong need exists for high-quality study designs to disentangle the cause and effect of any likely risk factors and to monitor the effects of preventive countermeasures, since any favorable trend may also be related to decreased exposure to risk and improved trauma care.

See Also

Autopsy, Findings: Drowning; **Crime-scene Investigation and Examination:** Underwater Crime Scene; **Injury, Fatal and Nonfatal:** Blunt Injury

Airborne Sports

K Yonemitsu and S Tsunenari, Kumamoto University, Kumamoto, Japan

Introduction

Airbone sports include many kinds of recreational aviation sports, which allow people to fly with or without a power supply. Such sports include hot-air balloon, glider (glider, hangglider, and paraglider), ultralight plane, gyroplane (gyrocopter), and skydiving. Investigation of commercial air crashes involving numerous victims is one of the most important fields in forensic pathology and medicine, and such literature is sometimes available, emphasizing the process of personal identification. However, recreational skysports accidents and injuries are rarely described in detail in forensic textbooks, although the number of such accidents is not small. This article provides general information on airborne sports and the forensic aspects of related injuries.

Various Types of Airbone Sport

Hot-Air Balloon

The idea of riding aloft on air was born when Archimedes discovered the law of buoyancy in the third century BC. In 1783, balloon flying became a widely known pursuit and the first public demonstration of a hot-air balloon was given by the Montgolfier brothers. The first recorded fatality in a balloon accident occurred in 1785 during an attempt to reach England from France. Hydrogen or helium balloons have long been used for scientific and war purposes. In the 1960s hot-air ballooning was revived as a recreational sky sport. The development of a small, lightweight, propane burner allowed the heat source to be carried on board (**Figure 1A**).

Gliders

A standard glider is a light plane without an engine that can only fly after it is pulled into the air by another plane or propelled by another mechanical system such as a winch. Recently, hanggliders and paragliders have become popular.

In 1891, Otto Lilienthal in Germany succeeded in reproducible gliding flights. His methodical strategy "from jump to flight" was adopted by the Wright brothers, who made the world's first powered and controlled flights. After World War II, Professor Francis Rogallo invented a flexible hangglider parachute, which was the forerunner of present hanggliding.

From the 1970s, the hangglider (**Figure 1B**) became a fashionable leisure sport in many countries. In the late 1980s, the paraglider also became popular, because it is lighter, more portable, quicker to rig, and capable of slower flight than the hangglider. The paraglider consists of a double-layered cloth with partitions. It has several lines (risers) to control the flight. Pulling one line results in a change of direction and pulling both lines acts as a brake (**Figure 1C**).

Ultralight Plane and Gyroplane

Developments in engineering have led to the invention of the ultralight plane. There are three types: (1) airplane type; (2) hangglider type; and (3) paraglider type (**Figure 2A–C**). These are classified as ultralight planes and flights are regulated by the authorities. However, powered hanggliders and paragliders are not classified as ultralight planes, because they have no wheels for taking off and landing.

The gyroplane (gyrocopter) is in the same category of rotor craft as a helicopter. Unlike a helicopter, the rotors are not actually powered – all they need to keep moving is a flow of air over their surfaces. Also unlike a helicopter, a gyroplane has a propeller which is powered by an engine to generate thrust which moves the machine forward (**Figure 2D**).

Legal regulations of airborne sports activities differ from country to country. Generally, hot-air balloons, ultralight airplanes, gyroplanes, and gliders are classified as aircraft, and they need to be registered and certified airworthy by authorities such as the Federal Aviation Administration (FAA) in the USA. Hanggliders and paragliders do not have to be registered by the aviation authorities, but the pilot has to undergo proper training programs to fly, as well as submitting a health certificate.

Accident Statistics

Databases for national and international commercial aircraft accidents are available, but there are no systematic worldwide databases for airborne-sports accidents. The US National Transportation Safety

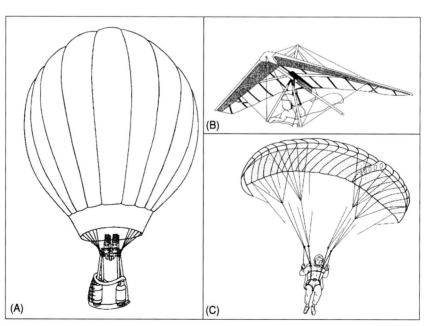

Figure 1   (A) Hot-air balloon, (B) hangglider, (C) paraglider.

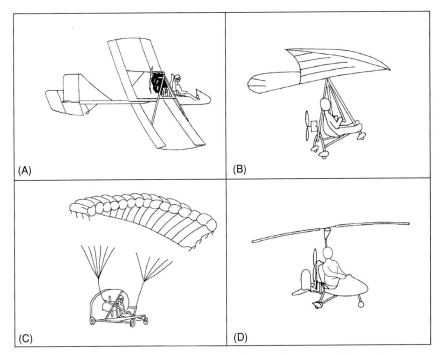

Figure 2 Ultralight planes: (A) airplane type, (B) hangglider type, (C) paraglider type, and (D) gyroplane.

Table 1 Mean number of airborne-sports accidents and fatalities in the USA per year in each decade. Data from the US National Transportation Safety Board

	Balloon	Glider	Ultralight plane	Gyroplane
1960s	0.8 (0.3)	25.4 (2.7)	0 (0)	9.9 (3.1)
1970s	9.7 (1.7)	63.2 (6.8)	0 (0)	18.1 (5.1)
1980s	27.9 (1.6)	53.2 (8.5)	19.9 (9.5)	13.3 (5.7)
1990s	19.3 (1.8)	35.7 (4.7)	3.9 (1.4)	9.0 (4.2)

Figures in parentheses represent fatalities.

Board provides aviation accident statistics for the USA. **Table 1** shows average numbers of accidents and fatalities in the USA caused by balloons, gliders, ultralight planes, and gyroplanes per year in each decade. Accidents by glider and gyroplane reached a peak in the 1970s while those for ultralight planes and balloons peaked in the 1980s. The average numbers of accidents for the four sky sports decreased in the 1990s. In 2002, the number of accidents in the USA were balloon: nine cases with one fatality; glider: 31 with six fatalities; ultralight plane: one with no fatality; and gyroplane: 14 with six fatalities. In contrast, in Canada in 2002, there were 36 ultralight plane accidents with 12 fatalities and accidents by glider, balloons, and gyrocopters were 10 cases with three fatalities.

There are no official databases for hangglider or paraglider accidents. However, several reports are available. For example, 409 accidents involving paragliders were reported in Germany between 1997 and 1999. Over the study period, there were substantial decreases in the accident numbers – 166 cases in 1997, 127 in 1998, and 116 in 1999 – while the number of licenced pilots has remained steady since 1993.

Causes of Accidents

Contributing factors for hot-air balloon accidents are: (1) pilot errors; (2) electrical power lines; (3) problems with propane fuel tanks; and (4) weather conditions. The most common pilot errors are inappropriate in-flight planning, misjudgment of weather, selection of unsuitable landing sites, and incorrect positioning of the pilot or passengers inside the balloon basket. Hitting electrical power lines contributes to a large portion of hot-air ballooning deaths. Contact with power lines causes the basket to overturn, and the pilots and passengers fall to their deaths. When confronted with the possibility of power line contact, pilots are instructed to deflate immediately, because it is safer to be on, or close to, the ground when power line contact is made. Falling from high in the air would cause serious injuries.

The causes of paraglider accidents include poor training and lack of experience, especially in weather-induced danger, as well as carelessness and overconfidence. Paraglider pilots often sustain serious injuries from a high-speed impact caused by the gravitational forces attained as a result of the glider spinning out of control after the canopy collapses. About one-third of accidents are caused by incorrect use of the brake lines, resulting in stalling. Accidents during takeoff are also common. Taking off with a partially opened glider may result in a crash. Mountainous areas and terrain with stones, holes, and bushes are particularly stressful for the pilot, who has to look where to place their feet while simultaneously checking if the paraglider has opened properly.

There are two general categories of ultralight aircraft accident: aircraft-related and operator-related. Operator-related factors are more difficult to control by legislation. Some users of ultralight aircraft want a thrilling flight with the minimum training, whereas in fact they need the maturity to become capable of being a professional or military pilot.

Injuries and Cause of Death

High-velocity airborne-sports accidents cause severe multiple trauma and injuries which often include neurologically significant spinal trauma. Fractures of more than one bone or one region are very common. In cases involving several isolated injuries, each injury could be fatal on its own. It is often difficult to determine which injury actually caused death. Multiple injuries are frequently listed as the immediate cause of death, followed by head injury, and internal injury of the thorax, abdomen, or pelvis. Burns and drowning can also be a cause of death.

Most fatalities involving hot-air balloon contact with electric power lines result from blunt-force injuries when the balloon occupants fall or jump to the ground. Electrocution seldom occurs because the pilot rarely comes into direct contact with the electrical wires and only a portion of the balloon conducts electricity.

According to the 10th International Statistical Classification of Diseases and Related Health Problems (ICD-10), the underlying cause of death for those who died in aviation crashes related to airborne sports is coded as one of the following: V95.1 (ultralight plane or powered glider), V96.0 (balloon), V96.1 (hangglider), and V96.2 (glider).

Forensic Autopsy

Autopsy is the only way to reveal all the factors contributing to an accident. Any relevant preexisting disease or consumption of alcohol, drugs, or medication will result in impairment of the pilot's ability to fly. These factors, which can only be discovered by autopsy, are essential to reconstruct an accident. In most cases, the main purpose of the medical investigation of the deceased would be to ascertain whether disease or toxicological findings could have precipitated the crash. Medical factors do play a significant role in accident causation because most sky sports are single-pilot-operated, and incapacitation of the pilot can lead to a crash. Investigation of natural diseases in pilots as a cause of accident and the mechanisms causing fatal injuries will help to assess preventive measures against airborne-sports accidents. Cardiovascular disease has been well studied in relation to aircraft accidents and flight safety, particularly coronary atherosclerosis, which has the potential to cause sudden incapacitation or death.

Sometimes observation of certain injuries can lead to improved structural and safety features which

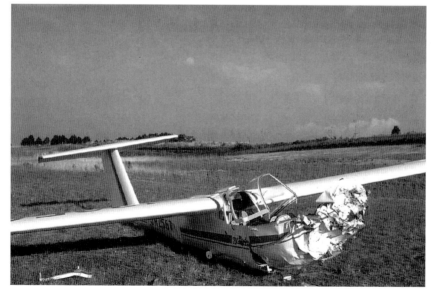

Figure 3   Case 1: the crashed glider.

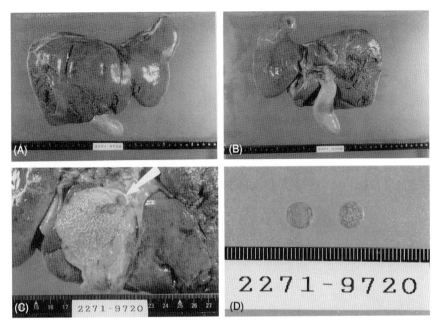

Figure 4 Case 1: autopsy findings of the pilot. (A) Lacerations of the liver (anterior view), (B) swelling and edema of the gallbladder (posterior view), (C) two gallstones in the gallbladder and the common bile duct (arrow), and (D) the two gallstones (scale = 1 mm).

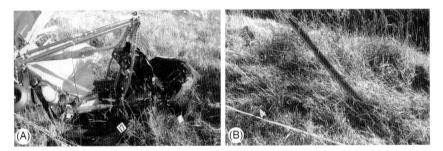

Figure 5 Case 2: the accident scene. (A) Crashed ultralight plane; (B) wire fences on the ground.

could prevent deaths. Also, knowledge of the trauma sustained in an aircraft impact can focus the clinical management of injured survivors. The interpretation of the significance of a postmortem finding in accident causation should be integrated with other pertinent information gathered during the investigation. Communication between the various investigators is essential. Forensic pathologists would benefit from sharing information with forensic aircraft engineers in addition to an autopsy of the victim. Knowledge of the environmental conditions and a review of the statements of witnesses and survivors can be evaluated and correlated with autopsy findings.

Alcohol and Drugs

Flying under the influence of alcohol and other drugs is strictly regulated in all countries. For example, the US FAA allows for a maximum blood alcohol level of 0.04% by weight to operate a balloon, and no alcoholic beverage may be consumed within 8 h of flying (FAA regulation 91.17). In Germany, the limit of alcohol in the blood for paraglider pilots is lower than that for drivers on the road. A blood alcohol level of 0.05% in a pilot will result in conviction. Any impairment caused by alcohol, drugs, or medication can have fatal consequences. This was confirmed by Stevens, who found that pilot errors were responsible for 36 of 55 air crashes in England. The presence of intoxicating substances can only be demonstrated by toxicological analysis.

Case Studies

Case 1

A glider (L23 Super Blaniks, USA) crashed to the ground from an altitude of 60–80 m just after

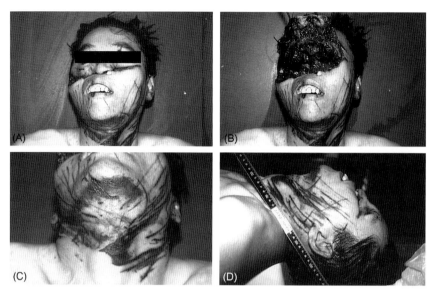

Figure 6 Case 2: the pilot's injuries. (A, B) A laceration on the face caused by the wire fence stanchion and (C, D) linear abrasions on the neck caused by the wire fences.

being pulled up to the sky by a winch (**Figure 3**). A 78-year-old man died: he was the copilot of the airplane and he was receiving a flight tuition from a 73-year-old teaching pilot. The deceased had nitroglycerine tablets in his pocket. Forensic autopsy revealed that the cause of death was a complete dislocation of the first cervical vertebra. There was no abnormal histopathology in the cardiovascular system except for slight focal myocardial fibrosis. The gallbladder was very swollen and edematous and had 75 ml of bile and two small gallstones in it. One of the stones was impacted in the gall duct (**Figure 4**). The cause of accident was not clear from the autopsy, but acute abdominal pain due to gallstones may have been the main trigger of the accident. This man was not healthy enough to fly.

Case 2

An ultralight plane (Drifter XP-503, USA) crashed on to a grass field (**Figure 5**). A 38-year-old pilot in the front seat died, and a passenger in the back seat was injured. There was a deep laceration on the face of the deceased, caused by a wire fence stanchion on the grass field (**Figure 6**). Multiple linear abrasions on both sides of the face were made by barbed wire between the stanchions. The cause of death was severe contusions to the frontal lobe of cerebrum with skull fractures. No histopathological changes were observed in other organs. The cause of accident was attributed to unskillful control of the plane by the deceased. He had just qualified as a pilot 15 days before the accident, and his total flight time was only 25 h 15 min.

See Also

Aviation Accidents, Role of Pathologist; Aviation Medicine, Illness and Limitations For Flying

Further Reading

Aguilar J (1980) Forensic science investigation of a balloon accident. *Journal of Forensic Science* 25: 522–527.

Copeland AR (1987) Ultralight aircraft fatalities: report of five cases. *American Journal of Forensic Medicine and Pathology* 8: 296–298.

Cowl CT, Jones MP, Lynch CF, et al. (1998) Factors associated with fatalities and injuries from hot-air balloon crashes. *Journal of the American Medical Association* 279: 1011–1014.

Faschig G, Schippinger G, Pretscher R (1997) Paragliding accidents in remote areas. *Wilderness and Environmental Medicine* 8: 129–133.

Frankenfield DL, Baker SP (1994) Epidemiology of hot-air balloon crashes in the US, 1984–1988. *Aviation, Space, and Environmental Medicine* 65(1): 3–6.

Guohua Li, Baker SP (1997) Injury patterns in aviation-related fatalities. *American Journal of Forensic Medicine and Pathology* 18: 265–270.

Hamada K, Kibayashi K, Ng'walali PM, Honjyo K, Tsunenari S (2000) Aircraft crashes in sky sports. Report of two autopsy cases and review of the accidents during 1981 to 1997 in Japan. *Japanese Journal of Legal Medicine* 54: 241–246.

McConnell TS, Smialek JE, Capron RG III (1985) Investigation of hot-air balloon fatalities. *Journal of Forensic Science* 30: 350–363.

Schulze W, Richter J, Schulze B, Esenwein SA, Buttner-Janz K (2002) Injury prophylaxis in paragliding. *British Journal of Sports Medicine* 36: 365–369.

INJURY, TRANSPORTATION

Contents
Motor Vehicle
Air Disasters

Motor Vehicle

I Nordrum, Norwegian University of Science and
Technology, Trondheim, Norway

Introduction

Accidents involving motor vehicles may cause any
number and degree of injuries. Some injuries result in
immediate death, others lead to disablement, and
many are trivial. The injury can vary from a simple
small abrasion to a complex combination of blunt injuries, sharp and cutting-edge wounds, or even burn
injuries, affecting one or several regions of the body.

According to the World Health Organization
(WHO), 1.26 million people died as a result of
road traffic injuries worldwide in the year 2000. In
the same year road traffic accidents ranked as the
ninth leading cause of mortality and morbidity.
WHO estimates that by the year 2020 these accidents
will rank at third place, even though many high-
income countries have reduced the burden of injuries
from traffic accidents. Most road traffic deaths occur
in Southeast Asia, but Africa has the highest death
rate – 28 deaths per 100 000 population. Comparing
these deaths by level of motorization reveals that, for
example, Sweden has 1.3 deaths per 10 000 vehicles
while some African countries have more than 100
deaths per 10 000 vehicles.

Proximity to trauma care facilities and their quality
affect the outcome following accidents. Morbidity
after road traffic accidents differs significantly between
high- and low-income countries.

Among the factors influencing the risk of being
involved in a motor vehicle accident and its outcome
are road design, speed limit, road environment,
weather conditions, such as rain, fog, and snow, and
vehicle safety and maintenance.

Types of Accident

Transportation injuries by motor vehicle involve cars,
trucks, and motorized two-wheel vehicles such as
motorcycles and scooters. A wide range of accidents
can occur. The accident may be a single motor vehicle
accident involving only those in or on the vehicle, or it
can be a more complex situation involving other
motorized vehicles, bicycles, or pedestrians.

Typical situations are driving off the road, collision
with another motor vehicle, or with pedestrians.
Collision with another motor vehicle may involve
a front-to-front crash situation, a side-impact or a
rear-impact crash, or various combinations of the
above.

Human Factors Contributing to Accidents and Injuries

Driver failure is the most important cause of motor
vehicle accidents. High speed or driving while under
the influence of alcohol, drugs, or medication is the
most common reason for driver failure, and this is an
increasingly important public health issue.

Suicide by use of motor vehicle is well known.
Driving into an oncoming vehicle, usually at high
speed, can result in a severely mutilated body.
Driving off the road, or throwing oneself in front
of a vehicle, are other ways of committing suicide
involving motor vehicles. Homicidal traffic accidents
are seldom encountered.

Various diseases may affect the ability and awareness of a driver, cyclist, or pedestrian. Ischemic heart
disease is the most important disease in this context. However, other diseases such as stroke, epilepsy,
bronchial asthma, and diabetes mellitus can contribute to the occurrence of an accident. Sequelae after
illness and old injuries can affect the competence of
the driver, and may thus be relevant to the cause of
an accident.

Inappropriate use, or lack of use, of safety devices
such as seatbelts, child restraints, and helmets affects
the outcome of an accident. Likewise, clothing and
factors such as age, weight, and height partly determine the type of injuries that occur as consequences
of an accident.

Forces Involved in Accidents

Forces involved in motor vehicle accidents are a function of velocity and stopping distance. The impact
and extent of injuries to the body are proportional

to the velocity, and inversely proportional to the stopping distance. The injuring effect of the so-called G-forces upon the body is a complex issue depending on many variables.

G-forces exerted upon a body can be estimated if the change in velocity is linear. A simple formula with a constant velocity and stopping distance can be used to calculate the G-forces. The force of gravity upon the body is 1 g, which is equivalent to the body weight. The magnitude of forces involved in motor vehicle accidents even at low velocities is considerable, with possible serious consequences. For instance, the force inflicted upon a body after a dead stop from 50 km h^{-1} is about 40 g.

The forces exerted upon a body involved in a motor vehicle accident are often complex, involving varying combinations of deceleration, rotation, and acceleration forces. The effect of a given G-force upon the body depends on the area, shape, and surface of the object(s), where and at which angle the object(s) hit the body, and subsequently which part of the body is being moved in relation to another.

General Injuries

Injuries after an accident involving motor vehicles are a consequence of speed, surroundings, characteristics of vehicles involved, safety devices, protection gear, and the characteristics of the body itself.

Blunt and sharp injuries of any size, number, and combinations, ranging from minimal injuries not requiring treatment, to mutilating and fatal injuries, are encountered. External and internal injuries may not always correspond. Sometimes there may be extensive findings on the body surface, but clinically or at autopsy there are limited findings of internal injuries. On the other hand, deadly wounds such as lacerations and ruptures of internal organs can occur without any marks on the surface of the body.

The anatomical consequences of blunt force are abrasions, bruises, contusions, avulsions, lacerations, ruptures, and fractures.

Blunt force can also affect the function of organs without leaving anatomical marks. Important examples are fatal cardiac arrhythmia after an impact to the chest, and concussion of the brain after an impact to the head. Concussion of the brain can result in unconsciousness and secondary life-threatening consequences such as hypothermia or continuing bleeding from wounds.

Compression of the chest from being pressed against or between structures can leave few anatomic changes on the body. The changes may be limited to some marks on the skin, a few fractures to the ribs, and some hemorrhages in the lungs.

Internal laceration injuries appear when soft tissue, or organs, moves in relation to other soft tissue or organs, given sufficient kinetic energy caused by a rapid change in speed. Different degrees of fixation of internal organs to surrounding structures contribute to determining the pattern and severity of injuries. Artificial soft-tissue cavities may be the result of blunt injuries to the thigh and buttock. Bleeding into such cavities may be so copious as to cause death. Deceleration forces of a certain magnitude can cause such injuries.

Two classical and fatal injuries to the chest and head are worth mentioning: first, traumatic rupture of the aorta, which is caused by forceful deceleration. This transverse sharp-edged rupture, or laceration, affects a part of or all of the circumference and is typically located distal to the left subclavian artery, leading to hemorrhage into the mediastinum or pleural cavity. The other is the "hinge" fracture of the skull that typically runs through both petrous bones and the sella turcica of the base of the skull. These fractures are often caused by sideways violent impact. The impact causing these fractures may not injure the soft tissue outside the skull or the brain itself.

Extensive abrasions to the skin are typically seen when a person decelerates on a rough road surface. There are often multiple parallel superficial abrasions or cuts, also called "brush abrasions," classically running more or less along the body axis. Friction burns may accompany such abrasions. Motorcyclists, persons ejected from cars, pedestrians, or cyclists thrown or shoved forward after the primary impact from a motor vehicle, may suffer such injuries. Dicing abrasions to the head can be seen after impacting on gravel-covered surfaces or on a car windshield.

Sharp forces can result in amputation of limbs and a variety of sharp-edged and penetrating wounds to various part of the body.

Injuries to Pedestrians

Pedestrians hit by a car are usually in an upright position when the primary impact occurs. The pedestrian typically acquires injuries to the legs as skin wounds and fractures, but also injuries to the knees and thighs, from the primary impact caused by the front part of a car. Injuries to the head from a secondary impact to the hood or windscreen are frequently seen. If the motorist brakes forcefully, the pedestrian may slide to the ground in front of the car, and subsequently be run over, or dragged along the ground by the car.

The sequence and number of secondary impacts vary. They depend on the speed, and the height and shape of the front of the vehicle, which can vary considerably. It should be noted that the term secondary impact is sometimes used to describe contact with the ground rather than the second contact between the body and the car.

Sometimes the pedestrian may be in a prone position before being run over, due for instance to drunkenness or an incapacitating acute disease.

Injuries to the skin may sometimes have a distinct pattern corresponding to a specific structure on the vehicle. In a hit-and-run accident, possible vehicle-identifying injuries and marks such as tire marks are of importance. Remnants of car enamel may be found on the clothes or on the body.

Injuries to Cyclists

Accidents involving motorcyclists are typically high-energy accidents with corresponding forceful deceleration and severity of injuries. If the deceleration forces run along the body axis, this may lead to a ring fracture around the foramen magnum. Such fractures are also seen in other accidents with so-called vertical deceleration. External wounds are often limited if the motorcyclist is wearing protective clothing such as gloves, jacket, trousers, and helmet. If the body is not appropriately protected, classical brush abrasions may occur. Injuries to pedal cyclists depend on the energy involved, protection gear such as helmet, other vehicles, and the surroundings.

Injuries to Occupants of Motor Vehicles

Injuries to occupants of motor vehicles are, in general, similar to those described earlier. Here, some emphasis is placed mainly on safety devices. Devices such as seatbelts and airbags affect the extent and consequences of injuries to those in the vehicle.

Seatbelts, especially three-point belts, are the single most important safety device in a car. Three-point belts in both front and back seats are common in many countries today. The use of seatbelts has reduced the number of fatal injuries. Two-point hip or diagonal belts are less effective than three-point belts.

Airbags provide additional safety. They reduce serious facial and head injuries, and injuries to other regions of the body, from the interior of the car. The most important effect of airbags, however, seems to be a limitation of nonfatal injuries when used together with appropriate seatbelts. Even though airbags prevent injuries, it should be remembered that they can also cause injuries, and even death. Airbags do not reduce the amount of deceleration forces but rather distribute these forces over a larger area. It is therefore important to be aware of the possibility of serious internal injuries after high-energy deceleration forces with minimal external injuries to the body.

Children represent a special problem with regard to airbags. It is important to avoid placing a rearward-facing safety car seat for children in a car seat protected with an airbag, because the child can die of injuries from the airbag if it inflates.

Head restraints prevent hyperextension of the neck to a certain degree. Such hyperextension, or whiplash, most commonly happens when a car is run into from behind. The movement can result in the whiplash syndrome, especially when the car does not have head restraints. The syndrome is characterized by a number of symptoms but few signs or findings.

Characteristics of the accident, together with safety devices and the interior of the vehicle, are vitally important as regards the injuries the occupants acquire. Fatality secondary to the accident itself, such as drowning due to submersion, burns following the vehicle catching fire, or asphyxiation after being trapped strapped upside-down, can occur.

Marks from the shoulder strap of a seatbelts can indicate whether the person was sitting in a left- or right-hand seat, but are not always found when belts have been used. Comparing the pattern of injuries with the interior of the car can help to determine whether the injured person was the driver.

Internal Findings

The internal organs should be inspected *in situ*, eviscerated, and dissected systematically.

Before opening the chest and pleural cavities, the possibility of a pneumothorax should be remembered, and appropriate investigation methods applied. Bear in mind also the possible presence of crepitations and small bubbles in the soft tissue, signifying subcutaneous emphysema, whether due to the accident or to an attempted resuscitation.

In the majority of cases the internal findings will readily explain the cause of death, which may be due to injuries to the head, chest, abdomen, and limbs.

In some deaths important internal changes may be overlooked or not emphasized enough by the dissecting procedure. This may involve changes in the anatomy, explaining why the individual died from trauma, or may be the result of a disease process that has possible implications for the accidental events. A few examples can be mentioned here. Traumatic dissection of the coronary arteries and carotid arteries can occur. The coronary arteries should be examined properly with crosscutting, perhaps especially among the elderly. The arteries should be decalcified if necessary. A fresh thrombus could explain why the accident happened.

Cardiopulmonary resuscitation can cause a variety of injuries, such as fractures to the ribs, and laceration and hemorrhage of both hollow and solid organs. The heart may have superficial petechial hemorrhages and ruptures, even to the left ventricular wall. Microscopic examination may reveal contraction bands in the myocytes near the epicardial surface after resuscitation.

Interpretation of Injuries in Relation to the Accident

Before beginning to examine an injured body, and then interpreting the findings, as much relevant information about the circumstances around the accident and the accident itself, including photo documentation, should be acquired.

Interpretation of injuries and diseases is important to both relatives and investigative authorities, and may have important criminal and insurance implications.

Were the injuries the cause of death, or was the person already dead or incapacitated by acute illness? Was the person influenced by alcohol or drugs? Was the ruptured aortic aneurysm the cause of the accident, or did it rupture due to a moderate blunt trauma to the chest in the accident? What could have been the sequence of the injuries, and what objects could be responsible for a particular wound? Was it possible to decide from the injuries whether the person was the driver or a passenger? Were the pattern and localization of wounds consistent with being hit from behind? Was the person incapacitated or killed on the spot, or could he/she have moved a certain distance? Remember, though, that both the survival time and acting capability (capacity to move) can be longer and more extensive than we sometimes imagine. Was the immediate cause of death hypo- or hyperthermia because the person was immobilized under the vehicle? Could the person's life have been saved if the rescue unit had arrived earlier?

These questions are but a few examples of what one will regularly have to consider. Alternative explanations as to the causes and consequences of injuries, and the sequence in which they might have occurred, should be discussed. The demand for reconstruction of accidents varies from country to country. Similarly, the expectations of unequivocal conclusions and their consequences also vary. Experience reaffirms that the complexity of the issues discussed in this article often precludes an unequivocal conclusion.

Further Perspectives

Insurance policy and compensatory damage claims will perhaps have a greater influence on the investigation of the circumstances of the accident, the extent of examination of the injured, and the number of accident reconstructions in the future.

Since driving under the influence or alcohol, drugs, or medication is an increasing problem, it is important to emphasize adequate collection, analysis, and interpretation of samples of blood, urine, and preferably also vitreous humor.

Whole-body computed tomographic scan is an interesting area that should be explored further. Such imaging has the potential to reveal detailed and important information about the skeleton and soft tissue in a number of cases.

See Also

Road Traffic Accidents, Airbag-Related Injuries and Deaths

Further Reading

DiMaio VJ, DiMaio D (2001) *Forensic Pathology.* Boca Raton, FL: CRC Press.

Eck JC, Hodges SD, Humphreys SC (2001) Review: whiplash: a review of a commonly misunderstood injury. *American Journal of Medicine* 110: 651–656.

Finbeiner WE, Ursell PC, Davis RL (2004) *Autopsy Pathology. A Manual and Atlas.* Philadelphia, PA: Churchill Livingstone.

Payne-James J, Busuttil A, Smock W (2003) *Forensic Medicine: Clinical and Pathological Aspects.* London: GMM.

Sato Y, Ohshima T, Kondo T (2002) Review: air bag injuries – a literature review in consideration of demands in forensic autopsies. *Forensic Science International* 128: 162–167.

Saukko P, Knight B (2004) *Knight's Forensic Pathology,* 3rd edn. London: Arnold.

Tomczak PD, Buikstra JE (1999) Analysis of blunt trauma injuries: vertical deceleration versus horizontal deceleration injuries. *Journal of Forensic Science* 44: 253–262.

World Health Organization (2001) *A 5-year WHO Strategy for Road Traffic Injury Prevention.* Geneva, Switzerland: WHO.

Air Disasters

M Gregersen, Institute of Forensic Medicine, University of Århus, Århus, Denmark

Introduction

Aircraft accidents attract intense public interest. The steady increase in size of passenger aircrafts has made it imperative that any aircraft disaster be investigated thoroughly.

The first fatal aircraft accident was in 1908 when Orville Wright's airplane crashed and the passenger Thomas Selfridge was killed. In Tenerife in 1977 two jumbo jets crashed on the runway and 583 people lost their lives.

In the September 11, 2001 disaster, crew and passengers on four planes died but at the same time several thousands lost their lives on the ground.

Stevens has stated: "It is impossible to prevent accidents without analyses of their cause, their potential for causing death, and injuries cannot be reduced if it is not known precisely how injuries are sustained and how they are produced. It is rational, therefore, that accidents should be the subject of routine and comprehensive scientific investigations."

The investigations of aircraft disasters are performed by national investigation teams, and forensic scientists play an important part in this connection.

The role of the forensic pathologist is to look for natural disease or abnormality in the operating crew which may have caused impaired function and provide a possible or probable medical or nonmedical cause for the event. In addition the pathologist aims to make a judgment of what happened in the aircraft before the event, at impact, and after the event.

Identification is an essential part in cases of disaster and will often be performed by identification teams in line with Interpol's regulations and advice.

Detailed autopsies of all bodies are the main source of medical evidence. The postmortem findings must be correlated with the medical histories of the aircrew, the laboratory results, the victims' clothing, and the scene of the disaster. Furthermore, and most importantly, the medical and pathological evidence must be correlated with and interpreted in the light of what was found by nonmedical investigators.

The technical investigations will often continue for months or years and include investigations of partly destroyed items from the airplane. The forensic pathologist often finishes work within days or weeks and the conclusion made by the forensic pathologist can be of help to the technicians.

It is recommended that technicians consult with the forensic pathologist until the case is closed.

Types of Disaster

Aircraft disasters can be divided into three main groups in which the injuries, to some degree, are different.

Disasters on the Ground

Disasters on the ground can occur while the airplane is standing or moving on platforms or runways, but may also involve collision with other airplanes, vehicles, or buildings, or there may be technical causes on the airplane. Fire is often seen in such accidents.

These accidents often result in few fatalities and many people survive as possibilities for rescue are good within the airport area.

Death may be due to mechanical trauma; deceleration traumas are rare. Fire is another important factor and many deaths are due to carbon monoxide poisoning or burns.

Disasters with Primary Impact Toward the Ground

Disasters with primary impact toward the ground are the most common and often occur in connection with take-off or landing in the airport area or its neighborhood and quite often out of range of rescue facilities. Although the airplane is not at full cruising speed and is at lower altitude, the speed at impact is extremely high and the force of gravity will be great.

These accidents are characterized by the fact that the airplane and its remains are often located within a small area. Fire frequently complicates the situation and is a destroying factor. The accidents may result in many fatalities but, depending on the circumstances, there can be survivors, who are often severely hurt by the accident or the following fire.

The causes of this type of accident are often human error or technical problems, for instance, lower flying altitude than prescribed or bad weather.

The damage depends on the circumstances. Some accidents may be caused by a collision with hills or buildings, while others involve landing at too high a speed in a field or a forest.

An aircraft accident may also cause fatalities on the ground.

A Gulfstream with a crew of four, and five passengers on board, was out of control before landing, possibly because of heavy turbulence, and the plane hit the ground and was destroyed (**Figure 1**). Nine bodies were disintegrated and more than 1000 pieces of human origin were found, but no person could be identified. The remains of organs did not give any clue as to the cause of the accident.

Disasters in Mid-Air

Collisions between two airplanes, an aircraft hit by a missile, explosions on board a plane, technical causes, as well as suicides and hijacking, are all brought to mind in this connection. Many of these events happen without any warning signal from the pilot – suddenly the airplane just disappears.

If the event happens at great altitude the plane will often be more or less disintegrated in the air and bodies and parts of the airplane will be spread over a huge area, often many square kilometers. No one survives. If the plane has disintegrated, many of the bodies have had a free fall through the air. There may also be victims on the ground.

Airplane Types

Accidents and their consequences also depend on the type of airplane:

1. Commercial planes carry up to several hundreds of passengers and their crew.
2. Light airplanes are used for transportation and sport and are often privately owned. They fly at low altitude and low speed, with only a few on board. Accidents are quite frequent (**Figure 2**).

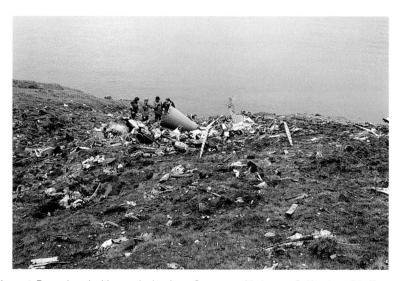

Figure 1   The site of impact. Reproduced with permission from Gregersen M, Jensen S, Knudsen PJ. *The crash of the Partnair Convair 340/580 in the Skagerrak: identification of the deceased.* Aviat Space Environ Med. 66. 1995.

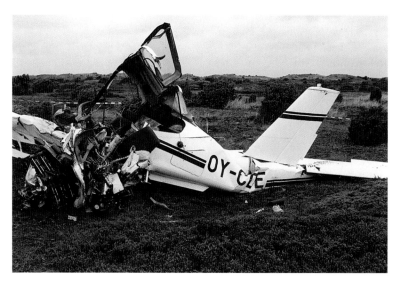

Figure 2   On landing a small airplane went out of control and crashed. The pilot and two passengers died from multiple injuries, one passenger survived with severe cranial lesions.

3. Helicopters are used by civilians for transportation and occupational work. They operate at low speed and low altitude and are vulnerable because of their rotors. If a helicopter loses power it may drop straight down. There are often survivors of such accidents.

4. Gliders fly on thermal energy and are used for sports; accidents are quite frequent. A glider becomes airborne with the help of a wire or an engine-aircraft; some gliders have small engines for take-off or for moving around. There are usually 1–2 persons on board, and a glider operates at very low speed and low altitude. Most accidents happen in connection with take-off.

5. Paragliders, parachutes, and hot-air balloons are not real airplanes; they generally cause the same kind of injuries as are seen in a fall from a building.

Identification

The identification of bodies is essential and often very difficult in mass disasters.

It is important that the forensic expert is at the scene of the disaster and takes part in the collection and identification of the bodies.

Manner of Death

Most flying incidents are accidental. It is very difficult to prove suicide during a forensic investigation and such a decision must be based on background information such as earlier attempts and psychiatric disorder. Homicide may be due to terrorism or sabotage.

Types of Injury

Injuries in aircraft accidents are usually very severe with a fatal outcome, but there may be survivors and the types of injury are the same.

The degree of physical traumas experienced in aircraft accidents is often enormous and may result in blunt injury; sharp injury, explosions, these are important factors in identifying the cause of the disaster. Burns are often seen as complicating injuries, and may be from chemical and/or toxic substances. Gunshot injuries may be identified.

Crew and passenger injuries often reveal the cause of the accident (e.g. cuts from propellers).

Frequently there are multiple injuries to the body, which may be fragmented. In other cases bodies are found intact but with severe defects and deformations, many with extensive internal injuries and multiple fractures of the bones, and destruction of the cranium, organ rupture. It is often difficult to draw definate conclusions.

The technical investigation team is especially interested in the direction of the impact. The pathologist can help by identifying injuries from contact with instruments and compression fractures or other injuries which may indicate the direction.

Explosions, Gunshots, or Other Injuries Inflicted by Others

Explosions can cause different types of lesion, such as burns and blast injuries in the airways, which may be difficult to differentiate from other lesions caused by the disaster. It is important to review the surface of the body, and to X-ray the body to look for metals or other foreign materials.

Disintegration of the airplane may also generate numerous particles and foreign bodies that may be difficult to differentiate from materials from an explosion.

X-rays will also show possible firearm projectiles. It may be impossible to differentiate stab or incision wounds from accident lesions.

Pre- and Postmortem Lesions

It is important to know whether the lesions occurred pre- or postmortem and if the pilots were alive during the accident. It is important to look for vital signs like hemorrhage and contusions, indicating that people survived the accident for at least some time.

Bone-marrow embolus in pulmonary vessels and fat embolism may indicate vital injuries to bones, while soot in the distal airways and carbon monoxide in the blood may indicate that the person was alive when the fire started.

Pilots and Crew

The crew should be identified as soon as possible and a detailed autopsy performed with microscopy, toxicological analyses, and X-ray imaging.

Lesions seen on pilots may be from the console instruments and may provide information about the direction of the impact. In small-aircraft accidents, fractures of the legs and arms and compression fractures of the spinal column may provide information on the impact.

Who was the active pilot? This is often known from the position in the plane, but wounds and fractures of the hands may indicate who had his/her hands on the control column.

Safety belts often cause marks on the bodies; passengers use lapbelts, while the crew use H-belts.

Case study   On descent a cargo-aircraft with a crew of three crashed in the hills. The plane had a long horizontal impact, as if it had an unforeseen landing in the hills. The captain was found about 50 m from the wreck, which was almost burnt out. In the remains of the cockpit two bodies with severe burns were found.

The captain had injuries to his face from contact with an instrument, indicating that he had been thrown against the console at impact (**Figure 3**). He had no marks from an H-belt. The technicians also suspected that he had not used his H-belt.

Injuries in Mid-Air Disasters

If an airplane gets into trouble at high altitude it may result in impact with the ground in a similar manner as accidents during take-off and landing. The disaster may also result in complete or partial disintegration of the airplane in mid-air: decompression will occur in the cabin, and the temperature will drop rapidly. There are risks of injury during descent, as well as free falls of individuals from a high altitude.

It is likely that people sustain injuries during the break-up, which may be seen as vital lesions. In a free fall characteristically the clothes can be torn off the person by air resistance, while ties, as well as rings and watch straps, are left on the body. When people hit the ground the injuries sustained depend on the terrain: impact with water usually protects against larger injuries to the surface of the body, but can cause particular extensive skin lesions.

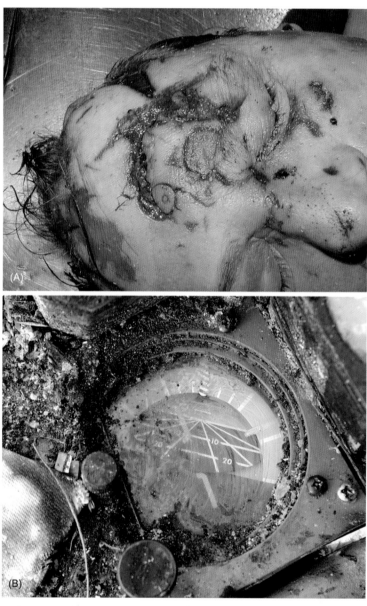

Figure 3   (A, B) The commander's face with rounded injuries, possibly from the horizon on the console. Reproduced with permission from Gregersen M, Jensen S, Knudsen PJ. *The crash of the Partnair Convair 340/580 in the Skagerrak: identification of the deceased.* Aviat Space Environ Med. 66. 1995.

Burns

In many accidents the crew and passengers are often totally burnt. The location of the burns may indicate the nature of the fire on the airplane and can be combined with the passenger's position in the cabin.

Burns make it difficult to detect other lesions, as well as other findings, which may be useful for identification. Burns can be the cause of death, especially in aircraft accidents on the ground.

Case study   A Cessna air plane with a pilot and three passengers surprisingly tried to land down the wind and hit the runway too close to the end, took off again, and shortly after hit some trees; the airplane fell on its back and caught fire. At autopsy all victims had severe burns. The pilot had minor fractures of his cranium and some ribs, small subarachnoid hemorrhages and hemothorax; he had 8% carbon monoxide hemoglobin. The cause of death was determined to be burns in connection with minor injuries. There were no signs of disease or intoxication that could explain his line of action.

One passenger had extensive fractures of his ribs, laceration of aorta, heart, lung, liver, and spleen and 2000 ml blood in his thorax. The cause of death was deemed to be multiple injuries.

Another passenger had a fractured rib, slight contusion of a lung, and soot particles in his airways. The cause of death was burns.

The last passenger, a 7-year-old boy, had no injuries and died from severe burns.

Drowning

Drowning has been the cause of death in a few cases where there have been a landing or impact on the sea as illustrated in the two case studies below.

Case study 1   A small airplane (Cherokee Warrior 151) with four people on board disappeared in heavy fog. Three days later one of the passengers was found in the sea. Five months later the airplane was found with the pilot and one passenger in the cabin. The autopsies showed no injuries: the cause of death was considered to be drowning.

Case study 2   In an ultralight airplane the small engine stopped, probably because of a loose wire to a spark plug. Because of trees in the area the pilot made a forced landing in a small lake; the pilot saved his own life, but his passenger was found dead in his seat inside the plane that was found lying on its back on the bottom of the lake. An autopsy showed signs of drowning, but no injuries.

The plane had not been cleared for use; the pilot had some training in flying but did not yet have a license, which could be a cause of the accident and the fatal outcome.

Hypothermia and frostbite   Hypothermia and frostbite are seen in airplane crashes on the sea, in the mountains, and in Arctic areas. In mid-air disasters, especially combined with free falls, unprotected individuals will also be at risk of frostbite.

Intoxication

Samples should be taken for toxicology analysis even if it is difficult in bodies with multiple lesions. Alcohol intoxication has played a role in several aircraft accidents, especially with small airplanes.

Toxic substances from the airplane may interfere, for instance jet fuel and hydraulic oil can cause corrosive burns.

Drugs   There are regulations as to which drugs are permitted for pilots. This will vary according to jurisdiction.

Fumes   In small airplanes where the engine is in front, carbon monoxide intoxication is possible; in modern and larger planes carbon monoxide and cyanide may be generated in a fire. In such cases it is essential to discover whether the pilot survived for some time or whether he/she died immediately after crashing.

Suffocation is of minor importance in civilian accidents.

Case study   An airplane with two pilots and six passengers disappeared after it had reached cruising level. Later it was found in a desert area. Autopsies and analyses did not explain the accident. At the last point of radio contact the pilot's voice had sounded strange, indicating that he might be in an anoxic condition. No technical explanation was found: a leak in the pressurized cabin is one possibility.

Diseases

Full autopsy of the crew should look for possible signs of disease that could influence the accident. Some pilots have atherosclerotic lesions of the coronary artery, but this is not conclusive; an acute disease such as coronary thrombus or ruptured aneurysm is more informative. In addition, signs of acute infection can be important. It is mandatory to carry out microscopic examination of all organs of the pilot, for instance to look for myocarditis.

Generally, it is difficult to extrapolate from disease signs to function, and findings should be correlated to the results of the investigation on the site and to clinical information from the pilot's physician.

Case study   A 66-year-old man with a license to fly small airplanes was grounded because of slight diabetes. He was not known to have any heart disease. Nevertheless, he invited three friends for a flight in his airplane. Just after take-off the plane hit some trees and crashed. All were killed and had multiple injuries.

The pilot's autopsy revealed an enlarged heart (550 g) with extensive fibrosis in the myocardium, but no acute infarction. The coronary arteries revealed atherosclerosis with severe stenosis. The liver was large and fatty, suggesting alcohol abuse. The blood alcohol concentration was 106 mg 100 mL^{-1} and the concentration in the urine was 157 mg 100 mL^{-1}.

It was concluded that heart disease and alcohol intoxication were important factors in the accident.

The Final Forensic Pathology Report

The report must contain: (1) a detailed description of the autopsy findings; (2) the results of other forensic analyses; (3) a description of the work with the technical investigation team, including their questions to the pathologist; (4) a conclusion on the cause and manner of death; (5) possible or probable medical and nonmedical causes for the accident; and (6) a correlation between the injuries and the results of the technical findings and investigations.

Two examples illustrate the value of forensic examinations in connection with the investigation of aircraft accidents.

A Mid-Air Accident

A Convair 340/580 turbo-prop aircraft, with a crew of five and carrying 50 passengers, was at its cruising altitude of 6700 m and speed (500 km h^{-1}) when communication with the plane ceased without warning and it disappeared from the radar. Shortly after, ships found debris and 31 bodies floating in the water within quite a small area (**Figure 4**). These constitute group 1.

Later a vessel collected wreckage and bodies from the sea bed at a depth of 70–90 m.

Over the next 4 weeks 16 complete bodies were picked up and one was washed up on the shore (group 2); later two bodies were found by fishermen (not included in the two groups).

All bodies were identified by disaster victim identification teams.

Medicolegal autopsies were performed on all bodies, concentrating on finding clues as to the cause of the accident.

In both groups the bodies were externally intact, although some external injuries were seen.

In group 1 fewer than half wore clothes or remnants of clothes; the remaining bodies were almost or completely naked. The male casualties often retained by a tie as the only piece of clothing. Shoes and wrist watches were almost all missing (**Figure 5**).

Group 1 showed the most conspicuous external changes. In 24 (77%) there were moist, grayish areas of the skin that later turned parchment-like, with underlying severe lesions of the subcutaneous tissue; these lesions were found on only one side of the body (**Figure 6**).

Only one was severely deformed by impact injuries, while several had bruises and hemorrhages on their hands.

In group 2, a large percentage had intact or almost intact clothes. Only one had the same extensive damage to the skin as in group 1 (**Figure 7**).

The injuries in the two groups are listed in **Tables 1** and **2**.

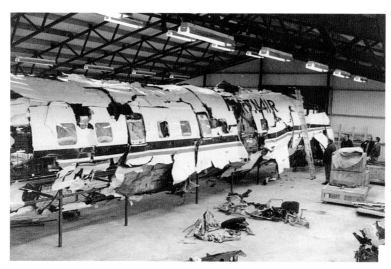

Figure 4   The fuselage of the aircraft after reconstruction.

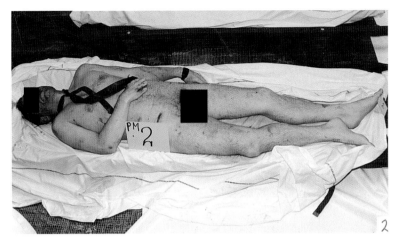

Figure 5 Group 1: the body is externally intact, but naked apart from the tightly knotted tie. Reproduced with permission from Gregersen M, Jensen S, Knudsen PJ. *The crash of the Partnair Convair 340/580 in the Skagerrak: identification of the deceased.* Aviat Space Environ Med. 66. 1995.

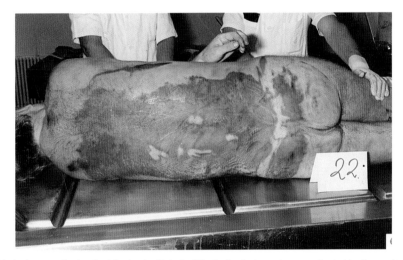

Figure 6 Group 1: skin lesions on the back of the body. Note that the buttocks have been protected by the underwear. Reproduced with permission from Gregersen M, Jensen S, Knudsen PJ. *The crash of the Partnair Convair 340/580 in the Skagerrak: identification of the deceased.* Aviat Space Environ Med. 66. 1995.

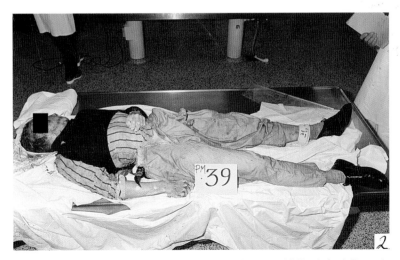

Figure 7 Group 2: the body is somewhat decomposed by sea water, but intact and fully clothed. Reproduced with permission from Gregersen M, Jensen S, Knudsen PJ. *The crash of the Partnair Convair 340/580 in the Skagerrak: identification of the deceased.* Aviat Space Environ Med. 66. 1995.

Table 1   Fractures: number of victims with one or more fractures of bones

Fracture	Group 1 (n = 31)	Percentage	Group 2 (n = 17)	Percentage	Total (n = 48)	Percentage
Skull	30	97	16	94	46	96
Face	25	81	15	88	40	83
Hyoid bone	16	52	12	71	28	58
Thyroid cartilage	9	29	6	35	15	31
Sternum	23	74	11	65	34	71
Clavicle	13	42	6	35	19	40
Ribs	31	100	17	100	48	100
Spine	26	84	14	82	40	83
Pelvis	30	97	12	71	42	88
Upper arm	19	61	8	47	27	56
Forearm	14	45	7	41	21	44
Hand	5	16	4	24	9	19
Thigh	17	55	11	65	28	58
Lower leg	22	71	8	47	30	63
Foot	3	10	5	29	8	17

Table 2   Lesions: number of victims with one or more lesions of the organs listed

Lesion	Group 1 (n = 31)	Percentage	Group 2 (n = 17)	Percentage	Total (n = 48)	Percentage
Brain	21	68	13	76	34	71
Heart	29	94	13	76	42	88
Aorta	27	87	13	76	40	83
Lungs	31	100	16	94	47	98
Upper airway	17	55	9	53	26	54
Liver	29	94	17	100	46	96
Spleen	26	84	16	94	42	88
Kidney	11	35	6	35	17	35
Gastrointestinal tract	14	45	10	59	24	50
Bladder	9	29	6	35	15	31
Diaphragm	11	35	10	59	21	44
Perineum	5	16	1	6	6	13
Other	6	19	4	14	10	21

Seatbelt lesions were found in 22, including the pilot.

In two passengers superficial lesions and small fragments looked like explosion damage; later it was proved that the fragments came from the airplane. Otherwise the findings could not support the idea that the plane had been hit by an explosion: there were no lesions that could have been caused by propellers working loose and cutting the fuselage (**Figure 8**).

It could be concluded that group 2 had mainly been located in the front part of the plane. The nonexplosive disintegration that happened over water yielded a number of reasonably intact victims, but it appeared that group 1 entered the water after an unprotected fall, while group 2 were protected by parts of the wreckage. This supports the opinion on the skin marks in group 1 and is in fact a result of impact with the surface of the sea; the loss of clothes is partly an effect of falling through the air and partly an effect of contact with the water. Alternative suggestions for the skin lesions involved the tearing of the clothes,

chemical burns from fuel or similar materials, or the effects of cold – all of which would probably not be limited to one side of the body.

Wounds and fractures to the pilot's hands support the theory that he was in his seat, holding the controls at the time of impact.

The autopsy findings strongly suggest that there were three stages in the accident: (1) a sudden and violent event – presumably disintegration of the aircraft in mid-air – where the casualties received superficial lesions and some fractures; (2) a descent phase where some people had a free fall in the air, losing their clothes (group 1), and some were protected by large fragments of the aircraft (group 2); (3) the bodies hitting the sea, causing most of the injuries and immediate fatal outcome. No medical reason for the accident was found, neither was there any evidence of an explosion, fire, or the propellers breaking off and penetrating the cabin.

The findings must be evaluated in the light of the technical investigations and it is believed that

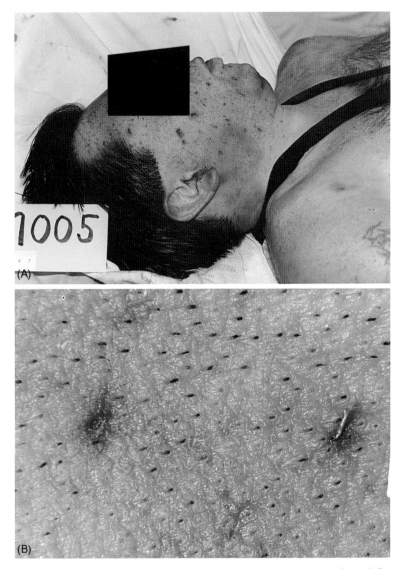

Figure 8 (A, B) A passenger with multiple small injuries on the face, one containing a piece of metal. Reproduced with permission from Gregersen M, Jensen S, Knudsen PJ. *The crash of the Partnair Convair 340/580 in the Skagerrak: identification of the deceased.* Aviat Space Environ Med. 66. 1995.

the evidence from the autopsies would supplement this.

Some of our theories about the crash later on – 3.5 years after the crash – were confirmed by the technicians when the accident report was published. A technical error in the tail of the airplane was the cause of the accident.

A Glider Accident

A pupil in the front seat and an instructor in the rear seat in a twin-seated glider were practicing abnormal flight positions (**Figure 9**). At an altitude of 250 m the glider was brought into a right turn with a severe bank that continued in a spin. A few seconds later the glider hit the ground. Both pilots were found dead in the plane. The glider was partly disintegrated and

the front control column was broken while the rear one was intact (**Figures 10** and **11**).

The instructor, a 52-year-old man, had suffered from hypertension, which had been treated, and his pilot's certificate had been restored to him.

The pupil, a 45-year-old man, had an abnormal rotation test a few days before at a medical examination, and further examinations were planned.

Autopsy of the instructor showed fractures of the cranium, facial bones, ribs, and sternum; compression fractures of the lumbar vertebrae; fracture of the pelvis; severe cerebral lacerations; and contusions of the lungs. There were no injuries to his hands. Only slight atherosclerosis was found.

It could be concluded that at impact he was thrown forward and his head hit the instrument

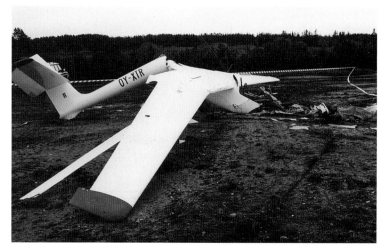

Figure 9 The crashed glider.

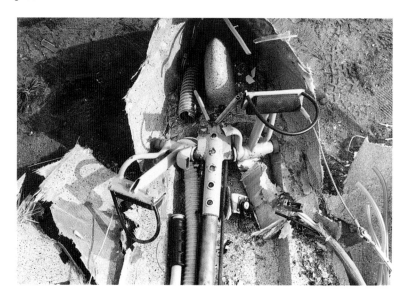

Figure 10 Front seat area: the control column is broken and the cabin is destroyed.

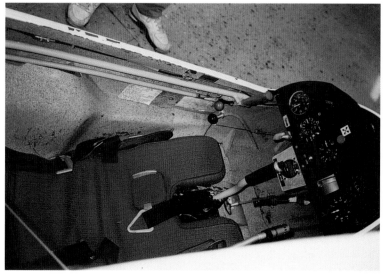

Figure 11 The rear seat with intact console and control column.

console; the compression fractures could also indicate vertical compression of the body. There were no signs that he had been handling the control column with his hands.

Autopsy of the pupil also showed severe injuries of the thorax with multiple fractures of the ribs, rupture of the aorta, and injuries to the heart; he had fractures of the pelvis, legs, right forearm and upper arm, cranium, and facial bones. He had contusions on his right hand, which might be caused by the control column in his hands. He had atherosclerosis with some stenosis of his coronary arteries but no occlusions.

The coronary artery disease cannot be excluded as an important factor in the accident.

Blood alcohol concentration was zero for both pilots.

The autopsies and the technical examinations indicated that the pupil had his feet on the front pedals, which may have prevented the instructor taking over.

The asymmetry demonstrated in the rotation test cannot be excluded as an important factor in the accident.

See Also

Aviation Accidents, Role of Pathologist; **Aviation Medicine, Illness and Limitations For Flying**; **Crime-scene Investigation and Examination:** Major

Incident Scene Management; Recovery of Human Remains; **Injury, Fatal and Nonfatal:** Blunt Injury; **Mass Disasters:** Role of Forensic Pathologists; **Terrorism:** Medico-legal Aspects

Further Reading

Brogdon BG (1998) *Forensic Radiology.* Boca Raton, FL: CRC Press.

DiMaio VJ, DiMaio D (2001) *Forensic Pathology,* 2nd edn. Boca Raton, FL: CRC Press.

Interpol (2003) *Disaster Victim Identification Guide.* Lyons, France: Interpol.

Job M, Tesch M (1999) *Air Disaster.* vol. 3. Sydney, Australia: Australian Aviation.

Krause SS (1996) *Aircraft Safety. Accident Investigations, Analyses and Applications.* New York: McGraw-Hill Professional.

Mason JK (1962) *Aviation Accident Pathology. A Study of Fatalities.* London: Butterworths.

Reals WJ (1977) Air diasaster trauma. In: Tedeschi CG, Eckert WG, Tedechi LG (eds.) *Forensic Medicine – A Study in Trauma and Environmental Hazards.* Philadelphia, PA: WB Saunders.

Stevens PJ (1970) *Fatal Civil Aircraft Accidents. Their Medical and Pathological Investigation.* Bristol, UK: John Wright.

Walthers JM, Robert L, Sumvalt III, Walters J (2000) *Aircraft Accident Analysis. Final Reports.* New York: McGraw-Hill Professional.

INJURIES AND DEATHS DURING POLICE OPERATIONS

Contents

Shootings During Police Stops and Arrests

T S Corey, University of Louisville School of Medicine and Office of the Kentucky Medical Examiner, Louisville, KY, USA

Introduction

As an enforcer of the law, with a legal mandate and specific training in the use of deadly force, the police officer occupies a unique position in society. Depending on the times, the economic environment, and the particular social setting, the relationship of the police with civilian groups within a given community may vary from openly hostile and distrustful to cooperative and mutually appreciative. One of the most important elements of any sound, objective forensic investigative procedure is transparency – any and all investigative procedures should be adequately documented to permit future evaluation by other experts or investigators at a later time. This is of paramount importance in incidents involving use of deadly force by police.

The death of a civilian during an encounter with police may be a flash point in a given community if there is preexisting tension between the police and the community. Further, such an event usually results in intense investigative coverage by the media, with ensuing community-wide, national, or even international coverage. Establishing a multiagency investigative protocol prior to such incidents will help ensure rapid, thorough investigation when they occur. Organized, competent investigation will thus reassure the public that police officers are held to high standards, and must obey the law as well as enforce it. Honest and complete reporting of the results of such investigations helps reassure a given community that the mission of the police is to serve and protect.

Establishing a written protocol for the investigation of police-involved shootings ensures standardization of procedures, and thorough collection of all pertinent evidence. While each incident will have unique factors that must be considered on a case-by-case basis, there are many factors common to all such incidents that should be covered in any protocol developed.

All death investigations should be undertaken as a team effort with interagency cooperation of multiple agencies and disciplines. If information is not shared, then errors may result in conclusions generated from incomplete investigation and/or information. Nowhere is this team approach more important than in police-involved deaths. Previous preparation for such events helps ensure a rapid, smooth, organized investigative response that may assist in allaying the concerns of the community. In the United States and some other countries, due to varying statutes, regulations, and death investigation systems, there is no national investigative protocol for these events. In contrast, the systems in place in England and Wales ensure that every police death is investigated through: (1) the Independent Police Complaints Commission; and (2) the coronial system before a jury.

Forensic investigation of police-involved shootings involves much more than just a postmortem examination. Other important elements include:

- assessment of the scene
- gathering of historical information
- collection of trace evidence.

Further, not all persons shot by police die, and cases involving surviving but seriously injured persons should undergo the same organized, thorough investigation. This article covers police-involved shootings. However, the reader is encouraged to remember that other types of deaths in custody or during arrest require the same basic, thorough approach.

Assessment of the Scene

As discussed elsewhere in this text, the importance of the scene information as a vital, integrative portion of the information considered in the formulation of opinions cannot be overemphasized. First and foremost in any developed protocol, the scene integrity should be preserved as soon as the situation is under control, and all persons (civilians and law enforcement officers) are no longer at risk. This scene preservation involves the cordoning-off of a scene perimeter and controlled access to the area. Some investigators advocate a two-layered perimeter, with a wide external perimeter limited to investigating officials, and a smaller internal perimeter with access thereto limited to the lead detective, and those invited by him/her. In such a scenario, those invited into the inner perimeter could include, at various times, a videographer, evidence technicians, the firearms examiner, and the coroner/medical examiner. But even in the best of circumstances, with rapid cordoning-off of a scene perimeter, and controlled and limited subsequent access, it may not be possible to preserve the scene as it appeared when the incident occurred. Such subsequent scene alterations may occur for a variety of reasons not under the control of the investigating agency. Such factors include:

- weather-related changes such as rain or wind in outdoor scenes
- alterations caused by the necessary actions of emergency medical personnel attending to the wounded and/or dying
- involvement of well-intentioned bystanders moving in to the scene in an attempt to assist the injured persons.

Ideally, the forensic pathologist will have the opportunity to visit the shooting scene, and will be able to walk through the scene with the lead detective. If on-site examination is not possible because of geography, staffing levels, or local protocol, then the forensic pathologist should be provided with complete and proper photographic documentation, with accompanying video footage (with appropriate narration) of the scene.

Today, in many urban areas and along major expressways, there may be surveillance cameras monitoring street corners, intersections, or major roadways. Further, many businesses and public transportation vehicles are equipped with video monitoring devices. Many law enforcement agencies now equip patrol cars with in-car cameras to record events during traffic stops. All of these may be potential sources of video documentation of the actual shooting event.

Based on the information available from multiple sources, it may be possible to reconstruct the scene and sequence of events. Information useful for this undertaking may include witness accounts, shell-casing locations, blood stain pattern locations and characteristics, trace evidence on clothing, and ranges and paths of gunshot wounds. Obviously, the components necessary for an adequate scene reconstruction are not immediately available. Therefore, scene reconstruction is usually best conducted days to weeks to even months after the shooting incident, to ensure availability of all necessary information. At the time of reconstruction, it may be helpful to utilize laser sites to establish lines of fire and paths of projectiles. Further, with the advancement of computer graphics, it may be possible to recreate the scene and events using three-dimensional models.

Historical Information

Historical information regarding the sequence of events of the shooting and the events preceding it should be gathered from all potential sources. These sources may include:

- radio transmissions before, during, and after the shooting
- statements from the officers present at the shooting (taped statements if they are available to the criminal/forensic investigator)
- tape-recorded witness statements
- cell phone records/transmissions
- tapes or transmissions of any undercover recording devices
- media interviews.

Radio transmissions represent a good source of information regarding precise timing of events, and may further provide details forgotten by officers later during investigative interviews. Depending on the nature and timing of the firing of guns, the actual sequence of the shots fired may be available on the radio transmission.

In many agencies, the officers involved in a shooting may be required to give a taped statement as part of the administrative probe, but this may not be made available to the criminal/forensic investigator. If taped or written statements are available, they should be reviewed by the lead detective. Depending on the specifics of the case and the nature and location of the wounds, the pathologist may wish to review the statements, to correlate the wound patterns observed on the body.

All witnesses present at the time of the shooting (including the victim if he/she survives) should be interviewed. It is highly desirable to obtain such witness statements on tape as soon as possible, as memories may fade, and details may become less clear than in the period immediately following the shooting. Tape-recording such interviews protects both the investigator and the witness, as it provides concrete evidence of the events as perceived by the witness before the passage of time. Another potential source of information includes the treating emergency medical personnel. Information sources in this area include first-responder emergency medical technicians, and hospital nurses and physicians. The victim may have spoken to medical personnel about the event, or the medical personnel may have observed injuries or evidence, such as soot surrounding a gunshot entrance wound.

In today's world, mobile telephones are in constant use by a significant percentage of the population. As such, telephones possessed by the police, the decedent (or living victim), and other persons present at the scene may provide an additional source of information. Another potential source of recorded information would include any undercover recording device being used by the officer(s) at the time of the shooting.

Witnesses at the scene may give interviews to the media, which may be quite extensive. It is useful for the lead detective to be aware of all such media interviews, with assistance from the Public Information Office of the agency. The detective may review those television/newspaper/radio interviews, to look for concordance with the information supplied to the police, and also to check for additional information that the interviewee may have failed to tell investigators. If the information in the interview seems particularly germane, the investigator may wish to pursue retrieval and review of any "outtake" segments of the broadcast interview.

Trace Evidence

In many officer-involved shootings, scenarios that seem relatively straightforward to investigators at the time of the incident may become muddled with the passage of time and the influence of outside sources in these (at times) highly politically charged cases. Adequate and thorough documentation and collection of appropriate trace evidence allow the record to "speak for itself," and allow independent review by outside sources at a later time.

Often, blood stain evidence may help reconstruct the sequence of events. In officer-involved shootings, blood stain evidence may assist in determining a number of factors, including:

- location of victim at time of shooting
- position of victim at time of shooting, and following shooting

- movement of victim following shooting
- movement or action of others following shooting.

In any officer-involved shooting scene with blood stain patterns, all patterns should be documented multiple times. Distant orientation photographs will allow placement of the pattern within the scene. Closer photographs will allow characterization of the overall pattern, and its relation to surrounding or adjacent objects. Finally, close-up, detailed photographs allow documentation of the individual blood spatters by both shape and size. It should be noted that photographic documentation should be made with the lens perpendicular to the blood stain pattern. This is especially important in the detailed, close-up photograph. Further, a scale should be included in each documentation view. Again, it is especially important that a scale be included in the close-up photographs – this will allow knowledge of the actual size of individual spatters. In outdoor scenes in hostile weather conditions such as rain or snow, patterns will not survive and thus should be documented as soon as possible. In cases in which the pattern exists on a removable portion of the scene, it is strongly encouraged that such material be collected and thus preserved. Thus it is recommended that thorough scene processing include consideration of removal of sections of drywall or carpet if these items demonstrate significant patterns that will be crucial to the investigation of the case.

As previously discussed, the shooting scene should be restricted and isolated as soon as possible. Access to the physical scene should be restricted as much as possible pending review by the lead detective and (if possible) the firearms examiner. The location(s) of shell casings and projectiles, along with other evidence, may be crucially important in the reconstruction of events. Shell casings are light and relatively small – they are easily kicked from their original position by well-meaning parties walking in the crime scene proper. Further, projectiles may be easily kicked and subsequently lost without adequate protection of the integrity of the scene. Even with prompt and proper scene isolation, such items may have been displaced during the event itself, or during the ensuing medical response.

The involved officer must be considered as a source of trace evidence as well. In jurisdictions in which gunshot residue tests are routinely performed, appropriate samples should be collected from both the officer and the shooting victim as soon as possible. If the incident involved a physical altercation prior to gunfire, any and all injuries or evidence of clothing defects (ripped shirts, lost buttons, etc.) should be documented well and expeditiously. At times, the absence of injury may be of significance. Therefore, it is recommended that all involved parties be examined by a forensic physician, and that not only injuries but absence thereof be documented.

Even in cases in which the officer does not report physical contact with the suspect, complete photographic documentation of the officer's clothing and shoes should automatically occur. It is strongly recommended that all of the officer's exterior clothing and shoes be collected and maintained as evidence, as information may subsequently develop that will require examination of such items.

In most instances, it is recommended that all guns be collected from all officers present at the time of the shooting – even if the case appears relatively straightforward and there appears to be a clearly identified individual shooter. Until such time as the firearms examiner determines that the projectiles were indeed fired from the individual weapon, all guns present at the time of the shooting may be considered as potential weapons. Depending on the circumstances, this may not be practical – for example, if a shooting occurs at a public event with many officers in attendance and a relatively clear-cut event, it would be burdensome and unnecessary to collect all weapons. However, in a shooting occurring in an isolated environment with only two or three officers present, it may be practical and advisable to collect all firearms.

Adequate front, side, and back-view "stand-up" photographs are obtained of all officers involved in a shooting. Additionally it is recommended that close-up views of the officer's shoes be taken from multiple angles. Any areas with blood stains or other trace evidence should be documented as previously described for the scene itself, with multiple photographs from multiple vantage points, all containing a measurement scale.

If the officers at the scene at the time of the shooting have been injured in the course of events, they should be evaluated not only for treatment of their injury but also for adequate forensic documentation of the injury. Even small injuries that do not require medical treatment may be of crucial forensic importance in evaluating the credibility of the information provided by those present at the time of the shooting (**Figure 1**).

The Living Victim

Depending on the country or region involved, various legal maneuvers may be required to obtain the necessary information for forensic medical evaluation of the living victim. Because some of the information sought may be time-sensitive, it is preferable to have a

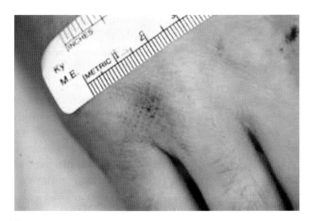

Figure 1 Fabric weave pattern on the dorsal surface of a hand sustained by ''punching'' the clothing covered torso of another person with the fist. This type of small injury does not need treatment, but is very important in verifying witness accounts.

protocol developed, cleared by legal advisors, and in place prior to the occurrence of such an event within a community. The various records and/or tests sought in a living person involved in a police shooting are basically the same as those involving fatalities. Such records and procedures may include:

- review of complete medical records (including emergency response and transport records, radiographs, and pathology reports)
- physical examination of the patient, with photographic and diagrammatic documentation
- procurement of a sample for possible DNA testing – this sample may vary (blood or buccal swabs) depending on the capabilities and procedures at the local crime lab
- collection of swabs for gunshot residue analysis.

As with autopsy examinations, the examination and findings are documented in several forms. These multiple forms may include verbal account of the examination and findings (narrative or checklist depending on local customary procedures), photographs, and diagrams. Radiographs taken as in the course of medical treatment serve as yet another source of documentation, as does the medical record. If possible, the gunshot wounds should be documented as soon as possible, in the Emergency Department, before the treating surgeons debride the wounds. If the wounds are debrided, the tissue removed should be sent to pathology – microscopic examination may help in the determination of entrance versus exit, and range of fire. Any bullets or projectile fragments removed at surgery should be collected from the Pathology Department, with appropriate chain-of-custody documentation. In addition to the gunshot wounds, any and all other wounds should be documented as well. These may include abrasions and contusions that do

not require medical intervention, and thus are unlikely to be documented elsewhere. It may be those medically insignificant wounds that have the greatest forensic significance in providing physical evidence that supports or refutes the historical information provided.

The clothing worn by the patient at the time of the shooting must be collected. This should include the shoes. The clothing may be examined by the firearms examiner to elucidate the distance between the muzzle and person – the range of fire exhibited by the gunshot wound trace evidence. The clothing may demonstrate salient blood stain patterns, and may be of use in determining paths of projectiles in cases of multiple wounds. Further, the clothing provides corroborative evidence of the anatomic location and nature of the wounds on the body. In perforating gunshot wounds, the projectile may even be located within the clothing. All personal items in or with the clothing should be examined and assessed for relevance to the case. Personal items with particular importance may include drugs or weapons.

Blood and urine from admission to hospital should be collected by investigators as soon as possible, with documentation of chain of custody of such specimens. During hospitalization and treatment, the living patient will continue to metabolize ethanol or other drugs.

The forensic physician will be able to assess the paths of the projectiles through review of all available records (including operative reports and radiographs), and physical examination. Any other injuries may be assessed in the same manner. If feasible, it is advisable to reevaluate the patient after 24–48 h to see if pattern injuries have emerged.

Examination of the Decedent

If the person is dead at the scene, alteration of the appearance of the body should be avoided as much as possible. The hands of the decedent are bagged in plain small paper bags for transportation. The bags are removed at autopsy, and trace evidence, including collection of swabs for gunshot residue testing, may be performed. At the scene, all clothing and associated objects should be left in place and transported with the body. This may include handcuffs if present, so that the pathologist has the opportunity to view the body in a condition that is as close as possible to the condition at the time of the shooting. It is advisable to wrap the body in a clean, new, white sheet prior to placement in the body bag, to preserve any trace evidence that may be present. The pathologist will examine and process the body for trace evidence collection prior to placement on the autopsy table.

The lead investigator should attend the autopsy examination. This is especially important if the pathologist has not had the opportunity to attend and examine the scene of the shooting. At autopsy, the investigator should be prepared to provide the pathologist with information, including:

- the current understanding/knowledge of the sequence of events of the shooting
- information regarding the sequence of events following the shooting (e.g., was the body exposed to high environmental temperatures and/or sunshine for hours as the scene was processed?)
- any known activity of the decedent following the shooting.

The body is photographed in the condition in which it was received. Photographic documentation then continues throughout the process, with documentation of the anterior and posterior body surfaces, and all wounds or other salient findings. Some agencies even videotape the autopsy procedure. Prior to removal of the clothing and dissection, the body undergoes radiographic examination to identify the location and number of retained projectiles. All clothing is then removed and collected, and correlated with the wounds on the body. During clothing removal, care is taken to ensure preservation of defects pertaining to wounds on the body.

At external examination of the body, gunshot wounds may be arbitrarily numerically designated for record-keeping purposes, without reference to order of fire. A wound diagram is a tremendous asset in cases of multiple wounds, as the locations and reference numbers are recorded on the diagram. During the internal examination, the paths of the projectiles are determined with the organs *in situ* in the body cavities. The projectile paths are then verified through stepwise dissection of organs. All projectiles retained in the body should be recovered at autopsy – these should be properly documented and then turned over to the law enforcement officials, with maintenance of chain of custody.

At autopsy, the pathologist further documents and interprets all other injuries and natural disease processes. Blood (preferably peripheral) and urine are collected and submitted for toxicologic analysis. If the decedent underwent resuscitation procedures, with receipt of large volumes of intravenous fluids, it may be necessary to obtain and submit the admission blood specimen at the hospital and postmortem vitreous fluid for analysis of ethanol concentration. Additional blood is collected for preservation on a standard card for possible serology or DNA testing. If the decedent was transfused prior to death, it may be necessary to collect a less traditional specimen. It is advisable to discuss the potential of this scenario with the crime laboratory, and seek advice on other specimens suitable for analysis at that particular laboratory.

Depending on the historical information available and the physical findings, the pathologist may need to perform additional dissections to document the presence or absence of injury. Such additional dissections may include the posterior soft tissue (as performed in infant autopsies as well for illustrations of the dissection), and shaving of the scalp hair. Other dissections may involve additional incisions over the head or extremities to document projectile paths and injuries, or recover bullets or fragments.

Summary

In summary, thorough investigation of officer-involved shootings requires an extensive collaborative effort by many members of different agencies. Proactive development of a multiagency response protocol may help the investigation and aftermath of police-involved shootings to proceed more smoothly. Some suggestions for items to be included in a protocol are found in **Table 1**. Complete and thorough investigation can only occur in an atmosphere of interagency collaboration and cooperation. All available information must be assessed and correlated into logical and defensible opinions regarding the sequence of events and interpretation of findings.

All involved agencies should have an established protocol for dealing with requests for information from the media and others. If press releases need to be issued it is imperative that the family be notified of the findings before this information is released to the general public through the media.

When such cases are finally adjudicated, the forensic physician is cautioned to remain neutral regarding the outcome of any criminal investigation; this is especially important to remember in countries with an adversarial method of operation in criminal court proceedings. Further, unless also a sworn law enforcement officer, the forensic physician is cautioned not to render opinions regarding the appropriateness or inappropriateness of the use of deadly force in a given scenario. The medicolegal definition of homicide as "death of one occurring as a result of the intentional act(s) of another" should be emphasized to the media and family members so that the lay public does not equate the pathologist's term "homicide" with "murder." Finally, forensic physicians must always be open to new findings, and be willing to reevaluate opinions if credible new evidence emerges. A prepared, organized competent investigation of

Table 1 Template for investigative protocol for officer-involved shootings

1. Establish safe environment
2. Establish scene perimeter(s) and control access
3. Investigative law enforcement: notify appropriate agencies from prepared call list:
   (a) District attorney or equivalent
   (b) Coroner/medical examiner
   (c) Pathologist (if not addressed in (b))
   (d) Crime laboratory personnel:
       i. Evidence technicians
       ii. Firearms examiner
4. Document scene in multiple forms:
   (a) Photographs
   (b) Video
   (c) Notes for narrative reports
5. Collect trace evidence at scene
6. Collect historical information from all available sources
7. Examine clothing and wounds of officers
8. Collect officer's clothing and shoes
9. Collect firearms of all officers present at time of shooting
10. Obtain proper legal authorization for examination of shooting victim (living person or decedent) according to local laws and protocols
11. Collect trace evidence (including clothing) from decedent or patient
12. Examine decedent or patient – document any and all injuries, along with range of fire and path(s) of projectiles
13. Procure necessary standard samples such as DNA standard cards from appropriate parties
14. Discuss what, when, and by whom with regard to information released to the media (ensure that families are informed first)
15. Meet to discuss facts of case with multiple agencies present
16. Consider scene reenactment, with pathologist and firearms examiner in attendance

police-involved shootings may help alleviate community concerns, and foster cooperative symbiotic relationships between the forensic investigators, police, and the community.

See Also

Autopsy: Medico-legal Considerations; Adult; **Crime-scene Investigation and Examination:** Death-scene Investigation, United States of America; **Custody:** Death in, United Kingdom and Continental Europe; **Histopathology**; **Injury, Fatal and Nonfatal:** Blunt Injury; **Serology:** Bloodstain Pattern Analysis; **Toxicology:** Methods of Analysis, Antemortem

Further Reading

DiMaio VJM (1999) *Gunshot Wounds: Practical Aspects of Firearms, Ballistics, and Forensic Techniques.* New York: CRC Press.

DiMaio VJ, DiMaio D (2001) *Forensic Pathology,* 2nd edn. New York: CRC Press.

Geberth V (1996) *Practical Homicide Investigation: Tactics, Procedures, and Forensic Techniques,* 3rd edn. New York: CRC Press.

Henry TE Blunt force injuries. In: Froede R (ed.) *Handbook of Forensic Pathology,* 2nd edn., pp. 139–146. Northfield, IL: College of American Pathologists.

Klinger D (2004) *Into the Kill Zone.* San Francisco, CA: Jossey-Bass.

Luke JL, Reay DT (1992) The perils of investigating and certifying deaths in police custody. *The American Journal of Forensic Medicine and Pathology* 13(2): 98–100.

Pilant L (1993) Less-than-lethal weapons: new solutions for law enforcement. International Association of Chiefs of Police.

Police Complaints Authority (2003) *Review of Shootings by Police in England and Wales from 1998 to 2001.* Norwich, UK: Stationery Office.

Reay DT (2003) Deaths in custody. In: Froede R (ed.) *Handbook of Forensic Pathology,* 2nd edn., pp. 195–202. Northfield, IL: College of American Pathologists.

Stone IC, Holt J, Gillett M (1991) Coordination of resources in office-involved shootings. *Journal of Forensic Sciences* 36(1): 40–46.

Van Kirk DJ (2001) *Vehicular Accident Investigation and Reconstruction.* New York: CRC Press.

Wawro PAS, Hardy WR (2002) Penetration of the chest by less-than-lethal "beanbag" shotgun rounds. *Journal of Trauma* 52: 767–768.

Special Weapons and Training Teams

T S Corey, University of Louisville School of Medicine and Office of the Kentucky Medical Examiner, Louisville, KY, USA

D F Burbrink II, Louisville Metropolitan Police Department, Louisville, KY, USA

Introduction

Most experts would agree that the police unit known as a SWAT (special weapons and tactics) team was developed in response to an incident in the USA at the University of Texas on August 1, 1966, known to many as the "Texas tower incident." On this date, a civilian named Charles Whitman armed himself with several high-powered weapons and climbed into a bell tower on the campus of the University of Texas. In the ensuing 96 minutes of terror, Mr. Whitman killed 16 people and wounded 30 more. The event finally ended when he was killed by resourceful police officers who gained access to the tower. This ordeal galvanized police around the nation to consider new strategies and tactics to respond to this type of threat in a community. Those involved in the forensic investigation of police-involved shootings need a basic knowledge of SWAT teams – an understanding of the organization and commonly used weaponry improves the investigation of SWAT-related incidents.

Early SWAT teams were composed of police with additional knowledge in the use of high-velocity rifles or machine guns – these officers were often deer hunters, combat veterans from the Vietnam war, or long-gun match shooters. In the early stages of SWAT team formation, the emphasis was on weapons, rather than tactics.

The Los Angeles Police Department (LAPD) in the USA is considered by most to be the founder of the modern SWAT team. LAPD was the first to develop extensive tactics and protocols to enter and secure residences, clear rooms, and deal with barricaded subjects and hostage situations. Some of the most publicized incidents involving SWAT teams occurred in Los Angeles, including: (1) an extensive shooting event known as the Black Panthers shootout in December 1969; (2) a gun battle involving an organization known as the Symbionese Liberation Army in May 1974; and (3) an event following a bank robbery known as the North Hollywood Bank shootout in February 1997. Today, many people throughout the world are familiar with the term "SWAT team" and such organizational teams are found worldwide. In fact, SWAT teams have become so common and such an integral part of police strategy that there is an entire industry of support products manufactured specifically for them. Globally, as the threat of terrorism increases, the roles and responsibilities of SWAT teams will increase accordingly.

A SWAT team is usually a special organizational unit within a police department. Officers assigned to SWAT usually receive specialized training, are equipped with special weapons in addition to those carried by patrol officers, and are subjected to more rigorous physical fitness requirements than most officers.

In the USA, most teams along the east coast have a separate hostage negotiation team, while west-coast teams have negotiators for hostage situations actually assigned to the SWAT team.

SWAT teams respond to a variety of events and situations; there are several broad categories of events that necessitate activation and response of the SWAT team, known as a "SWAT call-out." Situations generally considered of sufficient gravity and danger to activate a SWAT team include:

- hostage-taking events
- situations involving barricaded subjects who may be wanted by the police

- barricaded individuals who are expressing suicidal ideations
- service of arrest warrants/search warrants that are considered high-risk
- assistance to federal or international agencies in dignitary protection activities
- any call that may be of potentially high risk, or which may require an unusual response.

Organizational Structures

SWAT teams are organized in a variety of ways, depending upon the needs and resources of the community served. Organizational structures include:

- Full-time teams, with officers performing duties solely pertaining to SWAT
- Parttime teams, in which the officers' primary duties are assigned variously throughout the department, and the officers only act together as a unit for training and call-outs
- Multijurisdictional teams in which several small departments (each too small individually to organize its own parttime team) pool resources and staff to form a parttime team that will respond to any event within the jurisdictional areas of all participating agencies.

Full-time teams may be found in large police departments serving large metropolitan areas. Full-time SWAT officers are exclusively assigned to respond to incidents requiring SWAT team intervention – these officers do not have other assigned duties. Full-time SWAT officers train daily, have high standards of physical fitness, and are the prototype of the public perception of SWAT team officers.

Some full-time teams have other responsibilities along with the traditional SWAT calls. New York Police Department's Special Services Unit handles all calls traditionally assigned to SWAT, and further responds to other situations requiring specialized training, including bridge-related rescues, building collapse rescues, extractions from motor vehicles, and water rescues. In other large departments, SWAT teams are aligned with bomb squads, dignitary protection units, street crime units, or warrant service units. These organizational units may be referred to as hybrid teams.

Parttime teams are in place in many mid-sized metropolitan areas. These teams meet and organize for SWAT calls and dedicated SWAT training sessions, but the officers have other daily responsibilities. In such parttime teams, officers are assigned to various patrol and investigative functions throughout the department. During a SWAT call, the officers leave their usual assignments and gather to execute a SWAT response.

Multijurisdictional teams are associated with small departments that do not have the staff, resources, or response volume to create a parttime team. These small agencies elect to pool their staff and resources to form a team that serves the geographic regions of jurisdiction of all participating agencies, and thus responds to traditional SWAT calls. This allows for a SWAT response to critical incidents but does not deplete the agency in the typical daily handling of calls for service. The officers have primary responsibilities within the geographic area of jurisdiction of their assigned department, but gather as a regional response team for critical incidents. Each agency provides personnel and equipment to form the team. Multijurisdictional teams have signed written agreements delineating duties, responsibilities, and liabilities in multijurisdictional responses.

Situations Calling for SWAT Team Response

In hostage situations, one person (usually armed with a gun or other weapon) is holding another person or persons against their will. Movies and television dramatize these situations as a sophisticated career criminal holding someone else for a ransom or for a trade of goods. In reality, these events usually arise in situations involving either domestic violence or work-related violence. Domestic violence-related SWAT incidents are extremely dangerous, as these situations are highly volatile due to the emotional basis of the crime. Further, it is not unusual for the perpetrator to be intoxicated to some degree, rendering that person more emotionally labile. These may be considered among the most stressful of SWAT calls, as the fate of the innocent people held hostage depends on the actions of the SWAT team, and the perpetrator's response to those actions. As stated above, the perpetrator may be intoxicated, and thus less predictable. These calls may last for hours on end, and then suddenly depend upon a quick response at a moment's notice. The SWAT officers must be alert and ready to respond for extended periods of time; this causes extreme fatigue, both mentally and physically. More rarely, a subject committing a crime (such as a bank robbery) is unable to accomplish the planned escape and takes a hostage as a negotiating tool – a bargaining chip. Generally, these situations are more predictable than the domestic violence-related events, as the perpetrator's goal is more "business" than personal – there is generally no emotional connection between the perpetrator and the hostage, and the motive of the hostage-taking

action is to enable eventual escape, rather than being the end-process of a volatile emotional relationship.

A barricaded subject situation often involves a person wanted for a crime, who has been located and confined, but who is attempting to control a few last hours of freedom. The subject may realize that, with the SWAT team in attendance, the end result will be incarceration – the perpetrator's goal is not necessarily escape, but rather, delay in being arrested and placed in custody. Depending on the initial crime for which the individual is wanted, and the personality and motives of the perpetrator, these situations may be resolved quickly or may continue for a protracted length of time. In general, the violence of the initial offense serves as an indicator of the difficulty and course of the situation necessitating SWAT team response.

In another type of scenario, a barricaded subject call may involve a person who is suicidal or delusional. Due to drug use, mental illness, or a combination thereof, these subjects may be extremely unpredictable, making negotiations difficult, and the potential for self-harm and/or harm to others a real possibility.

High-risk warrants are search warrants that have some factor or circumstance causing an increased risk to safety of the police and community. Examples include:

- Barricaded entrances requiring special breaching equipment
- Attack dogs known to be on site
- Heavily armed subjects, or subjects with known access to automatic weapons.

The policy and procedure of the individual department will dictate what is considered a high-risk warrant. Some departments utilize a matrix to assist in the determination of high-risk status requiring SWAT team response.

Dignitary protection assistance usually involves visits to communities by high-ranking government officials. In the USA, the Secret Service has the primary responsibility for protection, but may seek assistance from local agencies. In such events, a SWAT team member is assigned to work with a Secret Service agent to provide general background and layout information, and to assist in logistics. Members of the local SWAT team are kept on-call nearby, as a potential response team, should anything untoward occur. If an incident occurs, the Secret Service is responsible for the safety of the protectee and thus concentrates on the safe departure of the protectee. In such a situation, the local agency will be called to assist in resolution of the ensuing situation, while the Secret Service focuses on the safe departure of the protectee.

Additional situations sometimes involving SWAT teams include "undercover buys" of illegal goods, and arrests. SWAT teams may be assigned to security duties in high-profile trials. They may be used in high-crime areas to assist with patrol. SWAT teams are often called out to assist in police response and protection in public demonstrations or protests. Anything that falls out of the norm of the usual police activities may be assigned to the SWAT team.

SWAT Team Organization

SWAT teams will vary in size depending on the needs and resources of the community. Most SWAT teams will have a similar organizational structure, with certain team members assigned to certain functions. These various assignments include:

- SWAT commander
- second commander
- entry personnel
- snipers
- perimeter officers.

Although cross-trained in many areas, all team members usually have a role to which they are regularly assigned, and in which they have trained extensively as part of the team.

SWAT Team Firearms

As mentioned earlier, most SWAT teams have an array of weapons not in use in standard police patrol work. All SWAT team members are armed with a handgun, with which they must demonstrate shooting proficiency on a regularly scheduled basis. In firearms proficiency testing, the usual passing grade for a patrol officer qualification ranges around 75–80%. In contrast, SWAT team members must qualify at 90% or higher. Further, SWAT teams use training scenarios in which the weapons malfunction; in these scenarios, the SWAT officer must "clear" the weapon (correct the malfunction), and then fire a predetermined number of shots with accuracy and precision within a given timeframe.

SWAT teams traditionally carry handguns of .40 caliber or larger; in some jurisdictions, these weapons may differ from that carried by patrol officers. Larger-caliber weapons are used in an effort to enhance "stopping power." Many departments supply the larger-caliber handguns to all sworn personnel for this reason. However, the most important determining factor in threat elimination in cases requiring use of firearms is anatomic location of the gunshot wound(s). For this reason, many SWAT teams spend up to 50% of training time on shooting scenarios.

Accuracy and precision of aim are tantamount in SWAT response.

SWAT teams usually possess several types of shotguns. In most departments, the weapon of choice is a Remington 870 shotgun. This weapon can hold five rounds of 00 buckshot, deer slugs, "ferret rounds" of gas, or a combination of all of these rounds. Many SWAT teams also use a Benelli automatic shotgun – this dynamic weapon recharges itself after each shot, so the user simply pulls the trigger to continue firing. However, this type of weapon will usually not accommodate less traditional ammunition such as "ferret rounds" or sock rounds.

As mentioned above, a common organizational position on a SWAT team is that of a sniper. Most snipers are equipped with long rifles of .308 caliber or larger. Large-caliber weapons are employed because many of the instances when snipers will have to fire their weapon will involve long muzzle-to-target distance, and often through glass. Good SWAT sniper teams will practice shooting targets set up behind all different types of glass. A type of glass notoriously difficult to penetrate with accuracy is automobile windshield glass. As a safety feature, windshield glass is laminated – consisting of both glass and plastic to prevent flying glass shards in motor vehicle collisions. This configuration of glass and plastic may lead to deflection of projectiles of smaller caliber or lower velocity. SWAT snipers generally do not use weapons with higher caliber than .308 because these higher-caliber weapons may overpenetrate – SWAT incidents often occur in relatively populated areas. The goal in civilian law enforcement is, of course, to eliminate hostile threats without hurting surrounding persons or property. The goal of ammunition in law enforcement in civilian settings is to penetrate the target, and then remain in that target, rather than exiting to strike another surface.

SWAT snipers train for all types of weather and temperature. Most SWAT snipers receive additional training specifically related to sniper activities, in addition to regular training with the entire SWAT team. SWAT sniper targets are usually very small. Snipers must maintain accuracy in shot placement at distances over 100 m. In training, a goal is to place five shots into a target such that all defects are covered by a single 50-cent piece from 100 m.

Qualities for perimeter weapons include shot placement accuracy with penetration at distance ranging around 25–50 m. A common weapon of choice for the perimeter is the M-16 military rifle. This is a very reliable, accurate weapon with good penetration through glass, without overpenetration through the intended target. It is easy to operate, and can be fired numerous times without cleaning while maintaining accuracy. The M-16 is important as a perimeter weapon as it maintains accuracy and reliability, and yet is durable enough to perform in many weather conditions.

SWAT team members assigned to making entry into a building often carry submachine guns. Commonly used weapons include the Heckler & Koch MP-5 and the Colt submachine gun. These weapons fire 9-mm or 40 caliber rounds. They are fully automatic weapons – as long as the trigger is depressed, the weapon will continue to fire until it is empty. These weapons generally have a selector switch that allows the weapon to be in a single-shot mode, or in the case of the MP-5, a three-shot mode. These weapons are usually equipped with 30-round magazines, and the rate of fire is such that the 30-round magazine is emptied in less than 8 s when the weapon is operated in the fully automatic mode. Submachine guns are smaller and more compact than the M-16 rifle, and have collapsible stocks. This means that the weapon can be made even smaller if need be. They are good in close quarters because they are small and not extremely heavy. They are used as entry weapons because they are extremely accurate at less than 25 m and easy to load and unload. Lighting packages may be added to them very easily without compromising the weight or the sight picture.

Special Equipment – Less Lethal Weapons

One of the biggest recent advances in the police industry and especially in SWAT is the development and utilization of less lethal rounds and weapons. These weapons and rounds are used as an alternative to gunfire, in an attempt to subdue subjects without causing serious traumatic injury. However, whenever an officer is using a less lethal round, there should be a cover person with the capability of using lethal force. There have been a number of less lethal options on the market for years and development is still continuing in this field. Some of the types of less lethal weapon currently in use by police agencies in the USA include:

- nightstick
- PR-24
- ASP (a type of collapsible metal baton)
- oleoresin capsicum (OC) spray
- OC canisters that are hand-launched
- beanbag rounds
- sock rounds
- soft baton rounds
- hard baton rounds
- pepper ball launchers
- tasers
- stinger balls.

The above types of less lethal ammunition are commonly used on noncompliant, aggressive individuals, and generally are effective through pain compliance.

In some countries, rubber bullets and/or water cannons are used as crowd dispersal agents, and are not covered in this article.

The nightstick is generally a cylindrical object made of wood or hard plastic that is used as an impact weapon against a combative individual; officers are trained to strike a subject in designated body regions. Most SWAT teams do not use this weapon in the normal course of SWAT tactics but it is used in routine police work.

The PR-24 is a hard plastic nightstick with a small handle perpendicular to the long axis of the instrument. This instrument is used in jails and prisons, but is seldom used in routine police work due to its bulky shape.

The ASP, a collapsible metal baton, is the third type of impact weapon. It has replaced the nightstick and the PR-24 in most departments. It collapses in telescope fashion to less than 30 cm (12 in.) in length, and thus may be carried on the officer's utility belt. It is perhaps the most common impact weapon in use by police departments in the USA today, but it is not used commonly in SWAT team operations.

OC spray canisters are carried by most law enforcement personnel throughout the USA. OC spray applied to the eye area incapacitates individuals by causing local irritation and profuse tearing. The canister may be sprayed with sufficient accuracy from a distance of up to 2.5–3 m (8–10 ft). The product disperses as a stream, but may be affected by wind in outdoor settings. SWAT teams often utilize OC spray to gain control of noncompliant individuals inside dwellings and to gain control of persons during difficult takedowns. This method of control works very well on most people, and effectively stops aggressive action. However, one of the authors has had several anecdotal experiences in which OC spray has been applied liberally with little or no effect. OC spray also works very well on aggressive dogs encountered at scenes. The drawback of OC spray is the lingering effect in the immediate vicinity – after it is released into the air, there is a smaller but noticeable effect on all persons in close proximity. This may be especially problematic in small rooms.

Hand-launched OC canisters may be used effectively on barricaded subjects. These canisters are thrown in close proximity to the subject; upon impact, they immediately release a large amount of OC powder which covers the subject. The effects of the powder are similar to the spray, causing discomfort to the nose and eyes, and tearing. The powder settles on to the floor and surrounding objects; it becomes airborne again when someone moves through the area. This may be advantageous, as movement by the individual will result in additional exposure to OC. However, this same quality may be a disadvantage to the apprehending officer, who will have some exposure to the OC powder as well.

Aptly named, beanbag rounds are small 5×5 cm (2×2 in.) square cloth containing BB shot; they are launched from a shotgun. Because of its shape, the beanbag is not aerodynamic. These less lethal projectiles are relatively accurate for 4.5–7.5 m (15–25 ft) or less, but tend to twist off-target at greater distances. Further, if the beanbag impacts the person's skin surface on edge, rather than flat, lacerations may occur. Because of these two issues, beanbags have been largely replaced by the second generation, sock rounds, which are also fired from a shotgun. If striking the skin surface on edge, beanbag rounds often create relatively linear superficial lacerations. When the beanbag round impacts the skin surface on the flat broad surface, a square-pattern contusion is often produced.

Currently, sock rounds are used by most SWAT teams. They are accurate at distances of up to 20 m. Sock rounds consist of BB shot encased in a loose nylon "sock" secured below "tails" present to facilitate increased accuracy. The sock round may be used in situations involving physically aggressive noncompliant subjects. Both beanbag rounds and sock rounds are effective in convincing people to comply because of the pain they cause, without causing serious physical injury. However, some people, due to drug intoxication, mental illness, or a combination thereof, may not be affected by these weapons. Sock rounds produce pattern contusions that mirror the shape and size of the impacting object.

Soft baton rounds are composed of hard foam rubber, and may be fired from a shotgun or a launcher (40 mm launcher or multilauncher). Launchers are not carried as entry weapons and are not very precise. They are primarily used to introduce chemical agents through large windows, rather than as impact weapons. Their main application is in crowd control rather than SWAT events.

Hard baton rounds are composed of hard rubber or wood. As with soft baton rounds, these are used with the above-described launchers, and are more applicable to crowd control or dispersal than SWAT events.

Pepper ball launchers are similar to paintball guns; they are loaded with small OC pepper balls that sting and disperse OC gas upon impact. The pepper balls are similar in size to traditional paintball rounds. They may be quite effective, but as with sock rounds and beanbag rounds, they may be relatively ineffective on individuals not exhibiting normal pain responses. Pepper balls produce blunt-force pattern injuries that most often display a circular ring of abrasion, with a diameter similar to that of the pepper ball itself.

Tasers have been in use by law enforcement for many years, and have evolved. The latest generation of tasers is more accurate and more powerful than their predecessors. They now have memory devices to prevent unreported discharges, and thus lessen the potential for abuse. Today's taser fires two barbs that superficially embed in the target surface. After the barbs embed, an electrical shock is dispersed through the two barbs into the person. Tasers may be accurate to distances of around 6 m (21 feet). Unlike other forms of less lethal weaponry, the electrical shock from the taser effectively stops voluntary movement for a very brief period of time. The duration of the initial electrical discharge is around 5–7 s; if the subject returns to a state of aggressive noncompliance, additional electrical impulses may be delivered, each around 3–5 s in duration. The effects are immediate and brief – no follow-up medical treatment is required. Heavy clothing does not diminish the effectiveness, as long as both barbs are embedded in the material. Many law enforcement agencies are turning to tasers as first-line response weapons, to lessen the potential for police shootings, especially those with fatal outcomes. Tasers represent yet another less lethal weapon for SWAT members to consider when dealing with aggressive, combative subjects.

Stinger balls are large plastic or rubber balls that are used to assist in entry into a building. They are thrown by hand into a building. Stinger balls have small explosive charges that disperse both gas and small hard plastic beads that sting the person's lower legs. Stinger balls may be quite hazardous to anyone who is on the ground or at a low level. They are generally used in crowd control situations where most of the people are upright and the goal is crowd dispersal. Some SWAT teams use them for entries into locations, but they may affect the footing of the entering SWAT team members, due to the multiple loose hard plastic pieces scattered about the floor.

Additional Equipment and Devices

SWAT teams use distraction devices upon entry into buildings. These hard metal objects make a large noise or bang, and emit a bright flash of light that temporarily disorients and distracts those caught unaware. They are quite effective, and have the additional advantage of frightening away even the most aggressive dogs. One of the disadvantages of these devices is the very real risk of subsequent fire, if the distraction device deploys on or near a flammable surface such as upholstered furniture. In recent years, manufacturers have enacted many modifications to diminish the risk of fire, but these devices will emit heat and a large flash. Most SWAT teams include fire extinguishers in their entry equipment when distraction devices are used.

A variety of types of tear gas are available for use by SWAT teams. Most of the gases produced today are nonflammable and do not increase the risk of fire. Once such agents have been introduced into a scene, the SWAT team must operate in gas masks. Gas masks cause several potential problems, including reductions in visibility and communication. Most SWAT teams practice precision shooting while wearing their gas masks in training to overcome these problems.

On occasion, SWAT teams have used fire hoses to cause a person to lose balance and footing, or to knock a weapon from an assailant's hand. SWAT teams should train with these hoses because, as firefighters will confirm, these instruments can be very difficult to manage, and have the potential to inflict serious injury to the subject.

SWAT teams utilize ballistic bunkers or shields on entries or searches. Large shields may measure 1.5 m (5 ft) in height and 1 m (3 ft) in width, while smaller shields measure approximately 1 × 0.75 m (3 × 2.5 ft). They are of sufficient strength to deflect a projectile fired from a handgun, but will be penetrated by bullets fired from high-powered rifles. Bunkers have been used to immobilize subjects armed with blunt-force instruments. However, caution must be exercised, as this maneuver may cause blunt-force injury to the subject.

When a SWAT team is forced to intercede in an event, the possibility of injury exists, simply because of the overwhelming nature of the force necessarily used by SWAT teams. When firearms are used by SWAT members, the end result is often the death of the individual, since, because of their extensive firearms training, SWAT members are very accurate. Pattern injuries associated with less lethal weaponry have been discussed previously. Other injuries associated with SWAT incidents are often referred to as "takedown injuries" sustained when an uncooperative person must be subdued by physical force. Many times, these takedowns are enacted with the use of a bunker, as it provides protection for the officer. Most of the injuries associated with takedowns are minor blunt-force injuries in the form of contusions and abrasions associated with impact with the ground. The force utilized in these events may be equated with that of a hard tackle in football, albeit without the pads. Many times the impacting surface is concrete or asphalt – these unforgiving surfaces add to the superficial blunt-force injuries incurred by the person. The vast majority of injuries sustained in this way are minor and superficial.

Summary

SWAT teams represent a specialty force within a police department. The structure and function of the SWAT team differ from that of the general patrol force. SWAT team officers are equipped with different types of weaponry, and are trained to organize and react in ways that are different from the organizational structure of the general department. An understanding of the organizational structure, training, and weaponry of SWAT teams assists the forensic investigator in evaluating injuries or fatalities occurring during events involving SWAT team response.

See Also

Chemical Crowd Control Agents; **Excited Delirium**; **Injuries and Deaths During Police Operations:** Shootings During Police Stops and Arrests; **Occupational Health: Police**; **Restraint Techniques, Injuries and Death**

Further Readings

Burbrink DF (1999) Matrix system to classify warrants. *The Tactical Edge* Fall: pp. 31–32.

DiMaio VJM (2004) *Gunshot Wounds: Practical Aspects of Firearms, Ballistics, and Forensic Techniques.* New York: CRC Press.

DiMaio VJ, DiMaio D (2001) *Forensic Pathology,* 2nd edn. New York: CRC Press.

Gabor T (1993) Rethinking SWAT. *FBI Law Enforcement Bulletin.* April.

Geberth V (1996) *Practical Homicide Investigation: Tactics, Procedures, and Forensic Techniques,* 3rd edn. New York: CRC Press.

Henry TE. Blunt force injuries. In: Froede R (ed). *Handbook of Forensic Pathology,* 2nd edn., pp. 139–146. Northfield, IL: College of American Pathologists.

Luke JL, Reay DT (1992) The perils of investigating and certifying deaths in police custody. *The American Journal of Forensic Medicine and Pathology* 13(2): 98–100.

McCarthy R (1990) Reducing the risk in high risk warrant service. *The Police Chief* July.

Pilant L (1993) Less-than-lethal weapons: new solutions for law enforcement. International Association of Chiefs of Police. December.

Reay DT (2003) Deaths in custody. In: Froede R (ed.) *Handbook of Forensic Pathology,* 2nd edn., pp. 195–202. Northfield, IL: College of American Pathologists.

Stone IC, Holt J, Gillett M (1991) Coordination of resources in office-involved shootings. *Journal of Forensic Sciences* 36(1): 40–46.

Wawro PAS, Hardy WR (2002) Penetration of the chest by less-than-lethal "beanbag" shotgun rounds. *Journal of Trauma* 52: 767–768.

INTERNET

Contents
Forensic Medicine
Toxicology

Forensic Medicine

G N Rutty, Forensic Pathology Unit, Leicester, UK

Introduction

The internet as we know it today in the twenty-first century is far removed from its original conceptual idea. Historically the internet originated in the late 1960s and early 1970s when it was developed by the USA during the Cold War. Its original purpose was as a means of communication between key institutions within the USA following a nuclear attack. Considering the computer software and hardware available at the time of its original development, it was a pure text-based system. It was not, in fact, until the early 1990s when the graphical interface of the worldwide web (www) was developed that the internet as we know it today was born. The development of the graphical interface led to interest from the general public and the expansion of use of the internet. Prior to this it had not been readily available to most of the population. The increase in demand for use of the internet also coincided with a new generation of computers and appropriate software; the personal computer moved into our lives both within the work and home environment and more recently on to our handheld palmtops and mobile phones. Thus, following 1992, its role within the provision of medical services became apparent and since then the system as a provider of information and communication between health professionals, amongst the general population, and in the commercial sector has expanded exponentially.

Terminology

For the purposes of this article there are three types of system, which may be available to the forensic practitioner either singly or in combination. They are defined within the internet hyperdictionary as follows:

1. The internet/www: this term refers to a computer network consisting of a worldwide network of computer networks that use the TCP/IP (Transmission Control Protocol/Internet Protocol) network protocols to facilitate data transmission and exchange.

2. An intranet: this is a restricted computer network or private network created using worldwide software. It is any network within an organization that provides access to that of the internet but is not necessarily connected to the internet. The commonest examples of this are organizations such as the UK National Health Service (NHS) that provides one or more www servers on a TCP/IP network for distribution of information within the NHS.

3. An extranet: this is the extension of a company's intranet out on to the internet, for example, to allow selected customers, suppliers, and mobile workers to access the company's private data and applications via the www. This is in contrast to, and usually in addition to, the company's public website, which is accessible to everyone. The difference can be somewhat blurred but generally an extranet implies real-time access through a firewall of some kind. Such facilities require careful attention to security but are becoming an increasingly important means of delivering services and communicating efficiently.

Thus, by gaining access to one or more of these networks the forensic practitioner can start to make use of the full potential of the computer-based communications.

The Internet and Forensic Practitioners

Nowadays it would be unusual for a forensic practitioner not to have access to the internet, an intranet, or an extranet. This could be via a personal computer either at the workplace or at home, on a palmtop, laptop, or notebook computer, or via a mobile phone. The question is, however, why would a forensic practitioner consider or wish to access the internet for work rather than purely for leisure purposes? The remainder of this article will discuss possible uses of the internet in forensic practice.

Communication

The mainstay system of communication for the internet is e-mail. The ability to send text and images anywhere in the world via the internet has undoubtedly been one of the most significant modern human developments. With the development of secure password-protected encrypted systems, confidential documents can now be sent and delivered within a matter of minutes to colleges across the world. This could include statements for court or cases for urgent opinions. However, e-mail is not without problems, and to date has not replaced more traditional forms of document carriage. The recipient does not know that the author of the e-mail is who it says. Although the IP address of the computer from which it was sent can be checked and traced, the person who actually typed it can be challenged. This is a particular problem within the world of internet pedophilia where the pedophile "grooms" the victim by making the child think he or she is talking to another child. The ability to send multiple copies of the same letter all at the same time to multiple recipients is open to abuse, for example within an office environment and may lead to individuals reading other people's correspondence. The mail may not bear a true signature and the size of the images or text may be restricted by firewalls or the recipient's server. As these are electronic communications they can contain viruses that can be rapidly disseminated throughout the world, which in turn may have catastrophic results on computer systems of individuals, companies, or institutions.

Other forms of communication also exist within the internet. Webcams and video conferencing allow the transmission of still and real-time images with or without voice between the host and recipient. This could be within an office or home environment or at a scene of crime or modern forensic mortuary. The presence of the senior investigating police officer at the scene of crime or mortuary may become a thing of the past as he or she can be updated or watch procedures occurring at distant sites from the comfort of the incident room.

Journals

At the time of writing we are at a crossroads in the history of medical and scientific journals. Medical journals are the traditional accepted way of disseminating new knowledge within forensic practice. This could be in the form of editorials, peer-reviewed articles, case reports, letters, or rapid communications. Journals are dedicated to specific areas of forensic practice and may or may not be associated with national or international associations. Traditionally access to them is either through personal subscription or via a library. The internet, however, has changed access to journals as we know them forever.

The use of the internet allows the forensic practitioner three different means of accessing information via journals:

1. Journal subscription. Journals can still be received in their entire hard-copy format that, depending on the journal, may contain color or black-and-white images and text. However, these days most journals can also be received via the internet. Those holding personal or institutional subscriptions will, via passwords, be able to access their journals online, although some journals choose to have free access to all. As they are in an electronic format there is no longer restriction on the length of the article or the use of color photographs as the cost of printing, production, and circulation is removed. Access to archived back issues of journals removes the necessity to visit library facilities or to store hard copies of journals within offices in forensic institutions. Many journals now publish articles on the internet prior to hard-copy publication, leading to more rapid dissemination of peer-reviewed information.
2. Abstracts. Most journals publish abstracts of their articles on the internet and they are free to be accessed by anyone. This allows wider dissemination of information amongst the scientific community, although access to the full journal article may be restricted by the journal owner and access only granted on a "fee-for-paper" basis unless you subscribe to the journal. The abstracts and citations are also held by a number of global electronic indexing facilities such as PubMed or Medline, allowing rapid searching for articles by use of keywords, journals, or authors' details: this allows rapid accumulations of information related to cases through an electronic medium. Thus practitioners can rapidly research cases that they have not encountered before or review the known knowledge in a case where the defense may be putting forward an alternative scenario/causation.
3. ETOCs. ETOC stands for "electronic table of contents." A significant number of journals are now available to be accessed through the internet using the ETOC system. This system is free of charge and allows users to specify by a keyword their area of expertise or interest. The system then identifies all available journals that are accessible through the internet in the chosen field and then, whenever one of the identified journals is published, forwards to the user via e-mail the table of contents of the journal. Each article within the contents table may then be hyperlinked to the abstract, journal, or paper. In this way users can gain access to the content tables and articles of

large numbers of journals without subscribing to them or visiting the library. These are often in areas which may be peripheral to their main field of expertise and yet may contain articles that are relevant to them from time to time. Thus the forensic practitioner has a wider access to information throughout the world on a day-to-day basis.

Education

Sitting in a classroom and being spoon-fed information and facts is a thing of the past thanks to the internet. Many institutions throughout the world now offer postgraduate education via distance learning. The use of systems such as Blackboard allows students to undertake learning distant from the institution where they are registered to study. By logging into the password-protected area of the tutor's web-page students are given coursework such as essays, reading lists, lectures, or tutorials at set times through the course just as if they were attending the institution. Thus the forensic practitioner can undertake under- or postgraduate courses at universities anywhere in the world.

Many universities and institutions now have their libraries and collections accessible through the internet. It is this global access to information or the ability to contact and discuss case material with peers throughout the world that brings the entire world's knowledge of a subject to the fingertips of the forensic practitioner.

Peer Review

Many areas of forensic practice require reports or material to be peer-reviewed before statements are released for use in court. Example areas include forensic science and forensic pathology within the UK, where it is becoming the norm that statements to be used in the prosecution of individuals are not released to the courts without all work being checked by a peer. Traditionally this requires the second person to go through all hard-copy paperwork, slides, laboratory work, or images of the original practitioner. If this takes place within a host institution where both individuals work, then access to this material may be easy, although if the peer review is to occur by a person working distant from the original practitioner then the transportation of large quantities of sensitive material may be impractical or preclude this process. The question as to whether peer review should be undertaken by colleagues within the same work environment or by independent individuals has not been satisfactorily answered to date. As more and more work, of all types, is stored in electronic format, including paper documents, laboratory reports, photographs, video streaming, and histological slides, then the use of the internet means that all of this information can be accessed and peer-reviewed via computer by a peer working at a distant site. The report can be checked online, electronically signed, and sent to the courts having been independently reviewed by the peer without the need to use traditional means of document carriage. However, some bodies (e.g. legal firms) may not accept documents transmitted via e-mail.

Quality Assurance Schemes

Internal and external quality assurance (EQA) schemes can be developed by use of the internet. For example, in the case of forensic pathology, these tend to be distant learning packages (DLPs) rather than EQA, as the subject remains, to date, opinion-based rather than evidence-based. Things will change. One has to be very careful how one sets up an internet-based EQA as any image or text-based system must allow users to be able to demonstrate their knowledge rather than using multiple-choice-type answers which could lead users to fail if insufficient information is available to them to interpret the question or several possible answers are available. This is why DLP is currently preferred.

Where the internet does come into its own is that a practitioner can opt to participate in multiple EQAs or DLPs in different parts of the world by online access: this may be required for continuous professional development (CPD) and revalidation to practice. Electronic submission of answers, certificates, or questionnaires to a professional body to acquire CPD credits is extremely easy using the internet.

Commercial

The commercial element of the internet can be seen as a benefit or a drawback depending on which side of the fence you are on. If you enter a keyword into an internet search engine you will usually be overloaded with "hits," most of which will be individuals or companies offering commercial services in that field. This may be what you are looking for, for example if you need to source someone to represent you in a case or seek the services of an "expert" within a given forensic field. Trying to find someone specialized in a highly selective field of expertise has undoubtedly been simplified by the internet. It has become as simple as using a telephone directory and, unlike a paper-based telephone directory, it will even have a map of where to drop off the material for the opinion. However, if you are seeking general information on a subject but then have to wade through hundreds or thousands of commercial adverts, it is at times a time-consuming task.

Societies, Associations, and Professional Bodies

To practice a forensic practitioner must be in a position to keep up-to-date with current and new knowledge within his/her field of chosen expertise. One way of doing this is to be a member of one or more of the range of national and international societies and associations related to forensic, science, or medical practice. It would be unusual for these groups not to have a web-based facility these days. These are used to inform potential members of the benefits of membership and help give an insight into the given field. They will have contact details of members, notice boards, and chat rooms for dissemination of information, journal reviews, similar site links and, in some cases, draft policy documents or national guidelines will be circulated for consideration, opinion, and views via member-only areas of the sites. They will advertise the contents of their forthcoming meetings with links provided to allow online abstract submission, hotel and venue details and booking forms, as well as flight and accommodation information. Thus they have become mini travel agents for the society/association. They may also carry job advertisements, recruitment drives, or best-practice advice for practitioners.

Many professional bodies are now making use of extranets, for example, the police, security services, forensic pathologists, scientists, and the courts. In the case of forensic pathology original notes, images, histology, and video can be downloaded to secure national storage centers for the purpose of security, data collection, research, and peer review. Court documents can be generated, reviewed and dispatched from anywhere in the world as long as there is a telephone connection into which to plug your laptop. Rapid, confidential secure communication with all entries being logged for disclosure and tracking purposes ensures consistency between practitioners within any field of forensics.

Meetings

Scientific meetings may be advertised on stand-alone sites or, more commonly, in association with the above group sites. In the old days if you couldn't make the meeting, especially if it was in a foreign country, then you may have missed out considerably on the activities within your profession. However, these days many more organized or large associations/societies will include facilities for distant online discussion at the meetings as well as video conferencing to allow absent colleagues to view or participate in the meeting. Those at the meeting can keep in contact with their place of work by cybercafé-type computer facilities within the conference venue.

Summary

As the internet continues to expand, diversify, and develop, the forensic practitioner will be able to gain access to a world of knowledge and communication that could only have been dreamed about by those who came before us. This is a brief summary of some of these opportunities.

See Also

Computer Crime and Digital Evidence

Toxicology

A Aggrawal, Maulana Azad Medical College, New Delhi, India

Introduction

The internet has become a colossal online library, where required information can be obtained by the touch of a button. The emergence of search engines, such as Google, AltaVista, Yahoo, etc., has added immensely to its utility. Information on every conceivable subject is available on the internet today. Toxicology is no exception. Professionals and laymen alike can use the internet to retrieve much valuable information regarding toxicology.

Using the Search Tools on the Net

Search Engines

There are special search engines meant specifically for toxicologists, e.g., ChemFinder (http://chemfinder.camsoft.com/). By entering a CAS registry number in the search box, ChemFinder will provide information by searching hundreds of chemical-related sites. This free search engine is provided by CambridgeSoft, a commercial firm which sells software and chemical information resources.

Web Directories

Another useful way to search for meaningful toxicology websites is to use web directories. These are collections of web pages of a similar theme arranged in a hierarchical system and, in some cases, even annotated.

Yahoo! (http://www.yahoo.com/) maintains a large directory of toxicology sites, in a hierarchical order. A search by the author in late 2003 showed 42 toxicology sites maintained in six categories, such as, environmental toxicology, forensics, institutes, journals, organizations, and schools, departments, and programs. Other useful directories are Open Directory Project (ODP) (http://www.dmoz.org/), Galaxy (http://galaxy.einet.net/), LookSmart (http://www.looksmart.com/), Snap (http://www.snap.com/), About.com (http://home.about.com/index.htm), Lycos (http://www.lycos.com/), eBlast (http://www.britannica.com/), Magellan Internet Guide (http://www.mckinley.com/magellan/), The Argus Clearing House (http://www.clearinghouse.net/), Buble Link (http://bubl.ac.uk/link/), Infomine (http://infomine.ucr.edu/Main.html), Librarians' Index to the Internet (http://lii.org/), and 192 Directory (http://www.192directory.co.uk/).

Toxicology Data Network (Toxnet®)

One of the biggest needs of toxicologists today is a broad database on toxicology, which can be searched easily to retrieve relevant and appropriate information. Toxnet® (http://toxnet.nlm.nih.gov) is such a database. Started in 1985, it is an integrated system of several different databases organized into four groups. It is maintained by the Toxicology and Environmental Health Information Program (TEHIP) in the Division of Specialized Information Services (SIS) of the National Library of Medicine (NLM). The four groups of databases within Toxnet® are: (1) databases providing toxicological data, such as GENE-TOX, (2) bibliographic information, such as Toxline®, (3) chemical releases to the environment, such as Toxics Release Inventory (TRI), and (4) nomenclature information on chemicals, such as NCI-3D. The Toxnet "Multiple databases" option allows for simultaneous searching of HSDB, IRIS, CCRIS, and GENE-TOX. Toxnet® databases are accessible free of charge. More information is available at http://tehip@teh.nlm.nih.gov or (http://sis.nlm.nih.gov/). Factsheets on these databases are available online as well as by request to http://publicinfo@nlm.nih.gov. **Table 1** summarizes the various Toxnet® databases classified according to groups. The Toxnet® training manual can be downloaded free of cost from http://www.sis.nlm.nih.gov/Tox/ToxLecture.html. Both pdf (portable document format; 9.9 MB) and ppt (PowerPoint presentation; 4.2 MB) files are available.

Other Online Databases

Toxnet® is undoubtedly one of the largest databases on the internet related to toxicology. However, there are other databases on the net that can be used profitably.

Elsevier Science runs ScienceDirect® at www.sciencedirect.com, which offers users browse and

Table 1 Toxnet® databases

No	Database	Type	Short description
1	HSDB®	Data	Hazardous substances databank. Human and animal toxicology data on over 5000 potentially hazardous chemicals
2	IRIS	Data	Integrated risk information system. Toxicological data on more than 500 chemicals that are primarily chemicals in commerce that are of regulatory interest
3	CCRIS	Data	Chemical carcinogenesis research information system
4	GENE-TOX	Data	Genetic toxicology database from the US Environmental Protection Agency
5	Tox Town	Data	An interactive guide to commonly encountered toxic substances, people's health, and the environment
6	Haz-Map	Data	An occupational toxicology database designed primarily for health and safety professionals
7	EMIC	Data	Environmental mutagen information center
8	TOXLINE®	Literature	Literature on biochemical, pharmacological, physiological, and toxicological effects of drugs and other chemicals
9	DART/ETIC	Literature	Developmental and reproductive toxicology and environmental teratology information center
10	TRI	Chemical release	Toxic release inventories from EPA for various years
11	CHEMIDPLUS	Chemical information	Chemical names, synonyms, structures, regulatory list information, and links to other databases
12	HSD structures	Chemical information	Two-dimensional chemical structures of chemicals in HSDB
13	NCI-3D	Chemical information	Two- and three-dimensional chemical structures from National Cancer Institute

Modified from Young RR (2002) Genetic toxicology: web resources. *Toxicology* 173: 103–121.

search functionality based on Lexis®-Nexis technology®. ScienceDirect® provides seamless access to abstracts from more than 10 000 journals, including the Elsevier Science family of products, BIOSIS Previews®, Ei Compendex®, Beilstein, INSPEC®, and EMBASE. Access to abstracts is free but payment is required for access to full text.

Elsevier Science also runs a comprehensive scientific search engine, Scirus (http://www.scirus.com). Scirus covers more than 60 million scientific pages from free and fee-for-access-controlled scientific information sources. It searches both web and membership sources, concentrating on those with scientific content. Sources include Neuroscion, BioMed Central, MEDLINE, BioMedNet, Beilstein on ChemWeb, Patients, and ScienceDirect®. The EMBASE service is available at http://embase.com. It provides access to the Excerpta Medica database.

Environmental Toxicology

Environmental toxicology is the study of the ecological effects of anthropogenic substances (e.g., pesticides) released into the environment. A number of websites are devoted to this topic. One of the largest sites devoted to this is ECOTOX (http://www.epa.gov/ecotox). It is a large database comprising more than 320 000 individual effect records abstracted from 17 195 peer-reviewed publications representing over 7800 chemicals and 5300 aquatic and terrestrial species. The database is updated quarterly. ECOTOX database is available in its entirety at http://www.epa.gov/ecotox/data_download/data_download.htm.

Environmental Defense Scorecard (http://www.scorecard.org/) collects data from more than 300 state and federal databases to profile environmental pollution problems and the health effects of toxic chemicals. It provides information on 6800 chemicals released by manufacturing companies.

ECOSAR, a Windows-based application, developed by the US Environmental Protection Agency (EPA), Office of Pesticide Pollution and Toxics (OPPTS), Office of Pollution Prevention and Toxics (OPPT), can be used in estimating the toxicity of single chemicals to primarily aquatic organisms. The program uses quantitative structure–activity relationships (QSARs). It can be downloaded from the web free of cost as part of the EPI Suite™ (v3.11) (http://www.epa.gov/oppt/exposure/docs/episuitedl.htm).

ERED (Environmental residue-effects database) at http://www.wes.army.mil/el/ered/ is a database of test results, where both tissue contaminant concentration and observed toxic responses are reported. The database includes ecotoxicology literature published from 1964 to 1998. Currently, it has over 3400 records abstracted from over 700 publications, covering more than 200 compounds and 180 aquatic species.

The Agency for Toxic Substances and Disease Registry (ATSDR) produces "toxicological profiles" for hazardous substances found at National Priorities List (NPL) sites. These hazardous substances are ranked based on frequency of occurrence at NPL sites, toxicity, and potential for human exposure. Toxicological profiles are developed from a priority list of 275 substances. ATSDR also prepares toxicological profiles for the Department of Defense (DOD) and the Department of Energy (DOE) on substances related to federal sites. At the time of writing, more than 250 toxicological profiles of various chemicals had been published. More information (including complete toxicological profiles) can be obtained at the ATSDR site at http://www.atsdr.cdc.gov/.

Three self-guided tutorials on toxicology, mainly covering environmental toxicology are available for all at http://www.sis.nlm.nih.gov/Tox/ToxTutor.html.

Food Toxicology

Food toxicity deals with adverse reactions developed by the consumption of food. The toxicity observed may be due to food additives, pesticide residues, environmental contaminants, food allergens, or natural toxins. Since most of these are being dealt with in separate articles, only internet resources related to food additives and toxicity resulting from them are described here.

All humans are consumers of food, and it is their natural instinct to know what chemicals are added to it to enhance its flavor, color, or shelf life. Some food additives are considered to be "generally recognized as safe" (GRAS) while others are more strictly regulated. All countries have their own regulatory agencies that exercise control over food additives. In the USA, the FDA has primary responsibility for the regulation and approval of food additives.

The FDA's Center for Food Safety and Applied Nutrition has a comprehensive website at http://www.cfsan.fda.gov/~lrd/foodadd.html. It provides consumer information at (http://www.cfsan.fda.gov/~dms/opa-bckg.html) and includes information on such food additives as monosodium glutamate. Members of the food industry can also get useful information from the FDA site. A list of technical documents is available at http://www.cfsan.fda.gov/~dms/opa-tech.html. It contains information on a wide variety of subjects, such as guidelines for submitting food additive petitions, petition status, inspection results, notification programs, and threshold of regulation exemptions. The site also contains a valuable database at http://www.cfsan.fda.gov/~dms/opa-indt.html. This database gives information about a number of "indirect" additives used in food contact substances such as adhesives and components of coatings, paper and paperboard components, polymers, and adjuvants and production aids. These are generally substances that come into contact with food as part of packaging or processing equipment, but are not intended to be added directly to food.

However, the data that may be of more immediate concern to toxicologists are available from the Everything Added to Food in the United States (EAFUS) food additive database. This database comprises of chemical and toxicological information on over 2000 substances directly added to food, including substances regulated by the FDA as direct, "secondary" direct, and color additives, and GRAS and prior-sanctioned substances.

There are a number of other organizations providing information on food toxicology. These are the UK Institute of Food Science and Technology (http://www.ifst.org/ifstfaq3.htm) and the International Food Information Council Foundation (http://ific.org/mediaguide/). These two sites contain a vast variety of consumer-friendly educational materials on food additives.

Genetic Toxicology

The biggest online database on genetic toxicology is undoubtedly GENETOX, a part of Toxnet® discussed already. An important area in genetic toxicology concerns the regulatory guidelines that apply to hazard assessment of new drugs. Harmonized guidelines have been developed for preclinical genotoxicity testing of drugs before they are used in humans. Almost all drugs in development must be tested by a battery of genetic toxicology tests that include a bacterial reverse mutation assay, an *in vivo* rodent bone marrow micronucleus assay, and either an *in vitro* mammalian cell gene mutation assay or an *in vitro* mammalian cell chromosome aberration assay. The complete guidelines are available at http://www.ifpma.org/ich5s.html. Good laboratory practice (GLP) are available at http://www.fda.gov/ora/compliance–ref/bimo/default.htm.

Various websites related to professional genetic toxicology societies and journals related to genetic toxicology are discussed in sections dealing with toxicology societies, and online toxicology journals.

Drug Toxicity

Information on drug toxicity is used primarily by three categories of consumers: (1) patients who want to be aware of possible side-effects of drugs they are taking, (2) physicians, who need to be aware of various drug interactions and their toxicities, which could help in better treatment and provide more viable alternatives for treatment, and (3) R&D scientists who are in the process of developing newer drugs. They need to know the toxic potentials of various new molecules in the development process. Various softwares are now available online, which can do this job easily.

There are information resources on the web today catering to everyone. Consumers can access a very useful resource R_x list (http://www.rxlist.com/) for information on side-effects and drug interactions for more than 1300 products. The site provides an A–Z listing of these drugs and their toxicities at http://www.rxlist.com/cgi/generic/brand.htm. Recent additions to R_x List monographs are given in a separate table. A neat search box is provided through which the consumer can search for toxicity of any drug. Another good site for the consumers is provided by The Institute for Safe Medication Practice (http://www.ismp.org). It is a non-profit organization involved in reporting medication errors and adverse events associated with drugs. The aim is to prevent future similar occurrences.

For physicians, key information on drug–drug interactions can be accessed through a number of sites such as www.drkoop.com and the drug-checker system, http://www.pharmacytimes.com. The former is a very user-friendly site and can profitably be used by nontechnical persons as well. A search box is provided over the top-left, where one can enter the name of the drug to read about its toxicity.

Perhaps the biggest beneficiaries of the internet in the field of drug toxicity are the R&D scientists, who can use a number of online applications to predict toxicity of newer molecules. These are sometimes referred to as "new chemical entities" or NCEs and "new molecular entities" or NMEs. One of the key steps in the development of a new drug molecule is the evaluation of its so-called "ADME/tox" profile (absorption, distribution, metabolism, excretion, toxicity). Previously done by actual experimentation entailing high costs, this can now be done easily and much more economically by simulation software, most of which is available online. These softwares generally make use of the structure–activity relationship (SAR). SAR is a computer-based technique that allows chemical testing based solely on a chemical's molecular structure. It is one component of the more comprehensive QSAR, which is capable of quantifying the type of relationship identified. Although quite complicated in their working, essentially most of these software compare the chemical structures of

NCEs and NMEs with those whose toxicity is already known. A prediction on toxicity of the new molecules is based on the similarity between the two structures. A number of QSAR-based software programs are available online. One is Accelrys' TOPKAT (available at http://www.accelrys.com/products/topkat/). *dsNavigator*, a suite of internet-based applications for adverse event compilation and reporting is available at http://www.biopharm.com/prod5dsNav.html and http://www.drugsafety.com. Other similar software are Hazard Expert available from Compudrug at http://www.compudrug.com, M-CASE and Casetox available from Multicase Inc. at http://www.multicase.com, *C2.ADME* from Accelrys at http://www.accelrys.com/cerius2/c2adme.html and *MetabolExpert* available from CompuDrug at http://www.compudrug.com.

ToxScope is a new virtual decision-making software that provides access to 150 000 chemical structures and expert statistical analysis of complex data to speed the process and cut the high costs of drug discovery. The ToxScope databases encompass acute toxicity, hepatotoxicity, mutagenicity, and carcinogenicity. It is made available by LeadScope Inc, in collaboration with ddplatform LLC. More information about this software is available at http://www.hpcwire.com/dsstar/01/0612/103161.html.

"Registry of toxic effects of chemical substances" (RTECS) at http://www.ccohs.ca/products/databases/rtecs.html is a database that provides toxicological information with citations on over 150 000 chemical substances. Among other data, the detailed profiles also include toxicological data and reviews. Six types of toxicity data are included in the file: (1) primary irritation, (2) mutagenic effects, (3) reproductive effects, (4) tumorigenic effects, (5) acute toxicity, and (6) other multiple dose toxicity. It was first published on 28 June 1971. Known as "toxic substances list" at that time, it included toxicological data for ~5000 chemicals.

Pesticide Toxicology

Pesticides released into the environment are a major concern today. There are a number of websites specifically devoted to pesticide toxicology. A useful site about pesticides in a nontechnical language is the EXTOXNET (http://ace.orst.edu/info/extoxnet/). EXTOXNET is a cooperative effort of University of California–Davis, Oregon State University, Michigan State University, Cornell University, and the University of Idaho. Primary files are maintained and archived at Oregon State University. The EXTOXNET database is divided into several parts. Specific information on pesticides is provided in what they

call PIPs (pesticide information profiles). It is available at http://ace.orst.edu/info/extoxnet/pips.html. Toxicology information briefs (TIBs) contain a discussion of certain concepts in toxicology and environmental chemistry. TIBs are available at http://ace.orst.edu/info/extoxnet/tibs/tibs.html. Other topic areas include toxicology issues of concern (TICs), fact sheets, news about toxicology issues, newsletters, resources for toxicology information, and technical information. The PIPs page also has an alphabetical listing of all the cataloged active ingredients.

Other useful resources are EPA biopesticides (http://www.epa.gov/pesticides/biopesticides/), EPA office of pesticide programs (http://www.epa.gov/pesticides), EPA OP insecticide tolerance reassessment (http://www.epa.gov/pesticide/op), and EPA pesticide reregistration status (http://www.epa.gov/pesticides/reregistration/status.htm).

Developmental and Reproductive Toxicity

Developmental and reproductive toxicity studies deal with risks faced by the fetus, when the pregnant mother is exposed to poisons and toxic agents. Several websites are now devoted to developmental toxicity. The Center for the Evaluation of Risks to Human Reproduction (CERHR) has its website at http://cerhr.niehs.nih.gov. It was established by the NTP/NIEHS (National Toxicology Program/National Institute of Environmental Health Sciences) in 1998 to provide scientific assessments of the potential for environmental agents to cause adverse effects on human reproduction and development. It reviews the developmental toxicity of several chemicals. The reports are available at its website.

A web-based resource on developmental toxicology (http://www.devtox.org/index.htm) has been developed by German agencies and the WHO Collaborating Center for Developmental Toxicology under the auspices of the Harmonization Project. This online resource contains harmonized terminology (nomenclature) for developmental toxicology along with images of anomalies to aid classification, and associated background documents.

Reprotox® (http://reprotox.org/) is a computerized database that was developed by A. R. Scialli (an obstetrician with expertise in clinical teratology) and associates at the Reproductive Toraicology Center in Bethesda, MA, for use by scientists, healthcare professionals, and governmental agencies. It is a component of the Reprorisk System® of Micromedex, Inc. (http://www.micromedex.com) and is available via the internet by subscription only. This database provides up-to-date information on reproductive toxicity data related to a number of chemicals and environmental agents, including medications and recreational drugs.

FETAX (Frog Embryo Teratogenic Assay – *Xenopus*) is a developmental toxicity test conducted on the South African clawed frog *Xenopus laevis*. Information about this and other similar tests is available at http://usacehr.detrick.army.mil/aeam/Methods/Dev_Frog/default.asp.

Veterinary Toxicology

The first animal poison control center in the world was the ASPCA Animal Poison Control Center (http://www.napcc.aspca.org/).

The American Board of Veterinary Toxicology (ABVT) is at http://abvt.org. The ABVT consists of a group of trained veterinarians whose aim is to educate the public, professional veterinarians, and veterinary medical students about toxicologic hazards to pets, livestock, and wildlife. The American Association of Veterinary Laboratory Diagnosticians is at www.aavld.org. If offers links to veterinary diagnostic laboratories in the US that offer extensive veterinary toxicologic testing.

The food animal residue avoidance database (FARAD) at http://www.farad.org/ is a computer-based decision support system. It has been designed to provide livestock producers, extension specialists, and veterinarians with practical information on how to avoid drug, pesticide, and environmental contaminant residue problems. Information can be obtained from this site by both producers and veterinarians.

Details about the Veterinary Toxicology Residency Program are available at www.cvm.uiuc.edu/vb/toxres/. This program is run by the University of Illinois College of Veterinary Medicine. The College maintains an outdoor garden specifically for toxic plants (http://www.library.uiuc.edu/vex/vetdocs/toxic.htm). This gives residents, veterinary students, and practitioners opportunities to identify plants poisonous to livestock, companion animals, and human beings at all stages of growth and maturation over the growing season. "Plants causing sudden death" (http://www.ivis.org/special_books/Knight/chap1/chapter_frm.asp?LA=1) is a full-text document describing plant species that can cause sudden death in animals.

Nitrate and nitrite poisoning in livestock (http://www.agric.nsw.gov.au/reader/an-health/a0967.htm) is a resource provided by the New South Wales Department of Agriculture, Australia, in July 2003 as part of its "Agfact" series. Written by Dr Sarah Robson (a veterinary officer), this site provides information on nitrate and nitrite poisoning in livestock.

Zootoxins deal with toxins produced by animals. One useful website on this subject is sponsored by the Department of Environmental Health and Safety at Oklahoma State University at http://www.pp.okstate.edu/ehs/links/poison.htm.

There is a discussion group on veterinary toxicology. It is called VetTox. For details, one can contact the moderator Dr. Merl Raisbeck at http://raisbeck@uwyo.edu.

Toxicology Associations and Societies

Many toxicological societies now have their own websites. These websites give information about their aims and objectives, constitution, memorandum of association, memberships, annual meetings, professional and academic activities, subscription fees, etc. It would not be possible to give the names and URLs of all professional toxicological societies, because there are several. **Table 2** lists a few representative societies. Many of these societies have their own links pages, through which the visitor will be able to visit further societies and associations.

Online Toxicology Journals

A number of toxicology journals are now available online. Full-text access requires membership in many cases, while a few are available free online. The *Journal of Analytical Toxicology* (http://www.jatox.com) provides abstracts free of cost, but full text is available for a fee.

The European Journal of Genetic Toxicology (http://www.swan.ac.uk/cget/ejgt1.htm) is an online journal published by the European Environmental Mutagen Society (EEMS). It is an international multidisciplinary journal aimed at bringing together research and overviews of research and regulatory activities into the mechanisms of action and consequences of exposure of living organisms to genotoxic chemicals and radiations.

The International Journal of Toxicology (http://landaus.com/toxicology/journal.htm) publishes refereed papers covering the entire field of toxicology, including research in risk assessment, general toxicology, carcinogenicity, safety evaluation, reproductive and genetic toxicology, epidemiology and clinical toxicology, mechanisms of toxicity, new approaches to toxicological testing, and alternatives to animal testing. Reviews and major symposia in the field are included.

Inhalation Toxicology (http://www.tandf.co.uk/journals/titles/08958378.html) is a peer-reviewed monthly publication providing a key forum for

Table 2 Some representative professional toxicology associations and societies with their URLs

No.	Society	URL
1	American Academy of Clinical Toxicology	http://www.clintox.org/
2	American Association of Poison Control Centers	http://www.aapcc.org/
3	American Board of Forensic Toxicology	http://www.abft.org/
4	American Board of Toxicology	http://www.abtox.org
5	American Board of Veterinary Toxicology	http://www.abvt.org/
6	American College of Medical Toxicology	http://www.acmt.net/
7	American College of Toxicology	http://www.actox.org/
8	Argentine Toxicologial Association (Asociación Toxicológica Argentina) (in Spanish)	http://www.ataonline.org.ar
9	ASIATOX (Asian Society of Toxicology)	http://yes.snu.ac.kr/asiatox/
10	Association for Development, Study and Advice in Toxicology (Association pour le Développement, l'Etude et le Conseil en Toxicologie)	http://www.lptc.u-bordeaux.fr/pages-perso/adectox/Adec_Homepage_en.htm
11	Association for Research in Toxicology (Association pour la Recherche en Toxicologie) (in French)	http://www.aret.asso.fr/
12	Association of Government Toxicologist	http://www.agovtox.org/
13	Australasian Society of Clinical and Experimental Pharmacologists and Toxicologists	http://www.ascept.org/
14	Behavioral Toxicology Society	http://www.behavioraltoxicology.org/
15	British Toxicology Society	http://www.thebts.org/
16	California Association of Toxicologists	http://www.cal-tox.org/
17	Canadian Society of Toxicology	http://meds.queensu.ca/stcweb/
18	Estonian Society of Toxicology (Eesti Toksikoloogia Selts) (in Estonian, with some English)	http://www.estsoctox.ee/
19	European Association of Poison Centres and Clinical Toxicologists	http://www.eapcct.org/
20	EUROTOX-Association of European Toxicologists and European Societies of Toxicology	http://www.eurotox.com/
21	Finnish Society of Toxicology	http://www.uta.fi/fst/
22	French Society of Genetic Toxicology (Société Française de Toxicologie Génétique) (in French and English)	http://www.sftg.org/
23	French Society of Toxicology	http://www.ccr.jussieu.fr/sft/index.htm
24	Genetic and Environmental Toxicology Association of Northern California	http://www.ems-us.org/geta/index.html
25	German Society for Experimental and Clinical Pharmacology and Toxicology (Deutsche Gesellschaft für experimentelle und klinische Pharmakologie und Toxikologie) (in German)	http://www.dgpt-online.de/
26	International Association of Forensic Toxicologists	http://www.tiaft.org/
27	International Society of Regulatory Toxicology and Pharmacology	http://www.isrtp.org/
28	International Union of Toxicology (IUTOX)	http://www.iutox.org/
29	Irish Society of Toxicology	http://www.toxicologyireland.com/
30	Italian Society of Toxicology	http://users.unimi.it/~spharm/sit/SIThome.html
31	London Toxicology Group (LTG)	http://ramindy.sghms.ac.uk/~ltg/links.htm
32	Netherlands Society of Toxicology (Nederlandse Vereniging voor Toxicologie) (in Dutch)	http://www.toxicologie.nl/
33	Norwegian Society of Pharmacology and Toxicology	http://www.farmakoterapi.uio.no/nsft/
34	Society of Clinical Toxicology (Société de Toxicologie Clinique) (in French)	http://www.toxicologie-clinique.org/
35	Society of Environmental Toxicology and Chemistry	http://www.setac.org/
36	Society of Forensic Toxicologists	http://www.soft-tox.org/
37	Society of Toxicologic Pathologists	http://www.toxpath.org/
38	Society of Toxicology	http://www.toxicology.org/
39	Swedish Society of Toxicology	http://www.imm.ki.se/sft/
40	The Genetic Toxicology Association	http://www.ems-us.org/gta/index.html
41	Turkish Society of Toxicology	http://www.turktox.org.tr
42	Ukrainian Toxicology Society	http://www.medved.kiev.ua/utox/info_en.htm

Modified and updated from Kehrer JP and Mirsalis J (2001) Professional toxicology societies: web based resources. *Toxicology* 157: 67–76.

the latest accomplishments and advancements in concepts, approaches, and procedures presently being used to evaluate the health risk associated with airborne chemicals.

Archives of Environmental Contamination and Toxicology (http://link.springer.de/link/service/journals/00244/) is published by Springer-Verlag and contains peer-reviewed papers on environmental toxicology. More information about this journal is available at http://link.springer.de/link/service/journals/00244/about.html.

The *International Journal of Drug Testing* (http://www. criminology.fsu.edu/journal) is an online peer-reviewed journal edited by Mieczkowski. Another journal is *Anil Aggrawal's Internet Journal of Forensic Medicine and Toxicology* at http://www.geradts.com/~anil/index.html. This biannual journal was started on February 25, 2000, and has an international board of editors. There are currently 25 professionals on the editorial board, including at least one forensic professional from each of the six continents. The journal publishes original papers, theses, book reviews and dissertations in full and also has a regular undergraduate and postgraduate section.

Some representative toxicology journals available online are given in **Table 3**. In addition to these, http://www.freemedicaljournals.com/ provides a list of about seven free online toxicology journals, including three in French and more information can be obtained by browsing.

Toxicology Books and Atlases on the Internet

A number of free toxicology books are available on the internet for download and more information can be obtained by browsing http://freebooks4doctors. com/. More information on free e-books can be obtained by browsing http://www.bizzydays.com/freeebooks.htm. However, this site has books on other subjects as well, including nonmedical subjects; browsing for a while is needed to get the required book.

A number of sites allow one to download books on payment basis. One such site is OVID (gateway.ovid. com), which has a number of toxicology books in its database (including books like, *The 5-Minute Toxicology Consult* and *The 5-Minute Emergency Medicine Consult*). These books can be downloaded for a small fee. PROQUEST (http://www.umi.com/proquest) is another online database, which also allows downloading of a number of books. Both OVID and PROQUEST also allow downloading of journal articles, from several forensic and toxicology journals, such as *American Journal of Forensic Medicine and Pathology*.

A number of poisonous plants atlases are available on the internet free of cost. Most useful among them are *Poisonous Plants of North Carolina* by Dr. Alice B. Russell and colleagues of the Department of Horticultural Science (http://www.ces. ncsu.edu/depts/hort/consumer/poison/images/), high-resolution engravings of poisonous plants by the Southwest School of Botanical Medicine (http://www.kmxq.com/hrbmoore/Illustrations/Illust.html), pictures provided by University of Pennsylvania School of Veterinary Medicine (http://cal.vet.upenn. edu/poison/), *Poisonous Plants of Pennsylvania* (http://caltest.nbc.upenn.edu/poison/Brett/AgBook/AgHome.htm) and "Poisonous plants" home page of Cornell University (http://www.ansci.cornell.edu/plants/). There is also an interesting poisonous animals atlas dealing mainly with poisonous frogs at http://www.colonet.com/frogs/. Best Toxicology Books at http://www.geradts.com/~anil/btb/index. html reviews only toxicology books.

Online Toxicology News

There was a methyl isocyanate (MIC) gas leak in Bhopal, India on 2 December, 1984 in which 2000 people died. Papers in India were agog with news regarding this disaster. It was a significant news related to toxicology, but not many people around the world got to know about it. In the rest of the world, the event got a very small coverage in the national papers or a few seconds on TV and radio, if at all. If anyone missed the news, the information was lost. Certainly it was very difficult for anyone to get this news in detail, after, say, one month. There was no internet at that time. In such a scenario, researchers (in other countries) doing research in MIC could very easily be deprived of this significant event.

With the development of the internet, the situation has completely changed. There are an estimated 10 000 daily newspapers, and several more general-interest magazines around the world. Now search for, e.g., MIC disaster, can be done easily not only for the current but also for the previous years by *electronic library systems*. One of the best electronic libraries is the eLibrary tracker (http://ask.elibrary.com/). Sponsored by Electric Library. It searches each day for any topic needed and emails the latest headlines automatically. 1stHeadlines (http://www.1stHeadlines.com) indexes 415 newspapers, broadcast and online sources, and Moreover. com (http://w.moreover.com/) (please note there is just one "w" in the address, not "www") indexes articles from about 1500 sources. Proquest mentioned above also allows readers to access a number

Table 3   Some representative toxicology journals available on the internet

No.	Journal	URL (at the time of writing)
1	Adverse Drug Reactions and Toxicological Reviews	http://www.adis.com/page.asp?ObjectID=154
2	Anil Aggrawal's Internet Journal of Forensic Medicine and Toxicology	http://www.geradts.com/~anil/index.html
3	Annual Review of Pharmacology and Toxicology	http://pharmtox.annualreviews.org/
4	Archives of Environmental Contamination and Toxicology	http://link.springer-ny.com/link/service/journals/00244/
5	Archives of Toxicology	http://link.springer.de/link/service/journals/00204/
6	Best Toxicology Books	http://www.geradts.com/~anil/btb/index.html
7	Bulletin of Environmental Contamination and Toxicology	http://link.springer.de/link/service/journals/00128/
8	Cell Biology and Toxicology	http://kapis.www.wkap.nl/journalhome.htm/0742-2091
9	Chemical Research in Toxicology	http://pubs.acs.org/journals/crtoec/index.html
10	Comments on Toxicology	http://www.tandf.co.uk/journals/titles/08865140.html
11	Critical Reviews in Toxicology	http://www.crcjournals.com/ejournals/issues/issue_archive.asp?section=1053
12	Current Advances in Toxicology	http://www.elsevier.com/inca/publications/store/7/3/9/
13	Drug and Chemical Toxicology	http://www.dekker.com/servlet/product/productid/DCT
14	Ecotoxicology	http://www.kluweronline.com/issn/0963-9292
15	Ecotoxicology and Environmental Safety	http://www.elsevier.com/locate/issn/0147-6513
16	Environmental Toxicology and Pharmacology	http://www.elsevier.com/inca/publications/store/5/2/3/0/2/4/
17	European Journal of Genetic Toxicology	http://www.swan.ac.uk/cget/ejgt1.htm
18	Experimental and Toxicologic Pathology	http://www.urbanfischer.de/journals/exptoxpath/et_patho.htm
19	Food Additives and Contaminants	http://www.tandf.co.uk/journals/titles/0265203x.html
20	Human and Experimental Toxicology	http://www.arnoldpublishers.com/journals/pages/exp_tox/aut.htr
21	Immunopharmacology and Immunotoxicology	http://www.dekker.com/servlet/product/productid/IPH
22	In Vitro and Molecular Toxicology	http://www.liebertpub.com/ivt/default1.asp
23	Inhalation Toxicology	http://www.tandf.co.uk/journals/titles/08958378.html
24	International Journal of Drug Testing	http://www.criminology.fsu.edu/journal
25	International Journal of Toxicology	http://landaus.com/toxicology/journal.htm
26	Journal of Analytical Toxicology	http://www.jatox.com/
27	Journal of Applied Toxicology	http://www.interscience.wiley.com/jpages/0260-437X/
28	Journal of Biochemical and Molecular Toxicology	http://www.interscience.wiley.com/jpages/1095-6670/
29	Journal of Environmental Pathology, Toxicology and Oncology	http://www.begellhouse.com/journals/0ff459a57a4c08d0.html
30	Journal of Toxicology – Cutaneous and Ocular Toxicology	http://www.dekker.com/servlet/product/productid/CUS
31	Journal of Toxicology and Environmental Health Part A	http://www.tandf.co.uk/journals/titles/15287394.html
32	Pharmacology and Toxicology	http://www.munksgaard.dk/tidsskrifter.nsf/a3b40ef0ca9b8d86c1256a160050049f/c6c5ae8d31463c59c1256a1c004870e9?OpenDocument
33	Regulatory Toxicology and Pharmacology	http://www.elsevier.com/locate/issn/0273-2300
34	Reviews in Toxicology	http://www.iospress.nl/site/html/13826980.html
35	Toxicologic Pathology	http://www.tandf.co.uk/journals/titles/01926233.html
36	Toxicological and Environmental Chemistry	http://www.tandf.co.uk/journals/titles/02772248.html
37	Toxicological Sciences	http://toxsci.oupjournals.org/
38	Toxicology	http://www.elsevier.com/inca/publications/store/5/0/5/5/1/8/
39	Toxicology and Applied Pharmacology	http://www.tandf.co.uk/journals/titles/10937404.html
40	Toxicology and Industrial Health	http://www.arnoldpublishers.com/journals/pages/tox_ind/07482337.htm
41	Toxicology in Vitro	http://www.elsevier.com/inca/publications/store/8/0/0
42	Toxicology Letters	http://www.elsevier.com/inca/publications/store/5/0/5/5/1/9/
43	Toxicology Mechanisms and Methods	http://www.tandf.co.uk/journals/titles/15376516.html
44	Toxicon	http://www.elsevier.com/inca/publications/store/2/5/9/
45	Xenobiotica	http://www.tandf.co.uk/journals/tf/00498254.html

of newspapers for toxicology news. The Newspaper Association of America (http://www.naa.org) lists 1150 US papers and 200 non-US papers. Editor and Publisher magazine (http://www.editorandpublisher.com/ editorandpublisher/index.jsp) has 4600 newspapers worldwide, which can be searched online.

Online Theses and Dissertations

An interesting recent development is the availability of a number of theses and dissertations submitted to various universities online. They are known as electronic theses and dissertations (ETDs). To know more about ETDs, it is useful to browse a site entitled *About Electronic Theses and Dissertations* (http://etext.lib.virginia.edu/ETD/about/). Ranging on all subjects, many ETDs deal with toxicology.

Toxicology Sites for the Layman

Although a majority of sites mentioned above are meant primarily for professional toxicologists, there are a number of other sites meant specifically for the layman. One of the most popular is *Anil Aggrawal's Forensic Toxicology page* (http://www.geradts.com/~anil/index.html). This site is in the form of a discussion between an expert forensic pathologist and a very curious 15-year-old youngster Tarun. Most of the time the pathologist is in the postmortem room just about to begin the postmortem examination on the dead body of a person, who is suspected of having died from poisoning. Tarun sees the body and starts asking questions of the pathologist. As the pathologist keeps dissecting the body, he keeps answering Tarun's questions, discussing with him the signs, symptoms, pathological findings, etc., of poisons. By the time the postmortem is complete the poison which killed the person is determined. One poison is dealt with in one discussion. The site is a collection of 50 such discussions. A total of 49 poisons are discussed, the first discussion being on the history of poisons. Poisons discussed range from such commonly known as arsenic and Spanish fly to such exotic ones as cicutoxin and gold. Although basically meant for lay people, these discussions would interest a professional toxicologist as well, for the various interesting historical sidelights given in each discussion.

Crime and Clues (http://crimeandclues.com) is a very popular and useful site which includes a number of articles related to toxicology. Other useful sites primarily for the layman are "Poisonous plants and animals" (http://library.thinkquest.org/C007974), "Dictionary of Botanical Epithets" (http://www.winternet.com/~chuckg/), Botanical.com – A Modern Herbal by Mrs. M. Grieve (http://www.botanical.com/botanical/mgmh), "Minnesota Poison Control System" (http://www.mnpoison.org/index.htm) and "Edible and Poisonous Mushrooms" (http://www.conservation.state.mo.us/nathis/mushrooms/mushroom/).

Toxicology Quiz Sites

Quiz is one of the most interesting ways not only to test one's knowledge but also to gain additional information. A number of toxicology quizzes are being run on various sites both for lay persons and professional toxicologists alike. One of the best is Dalefield's toxicology quiz at http://www.dalefield.com/toxicology/.

Other useful sites are "Tox trivia" at http://www.Pharmacy.Arizona.EDU/centers/poisoncenter/trivia/questions/, "Hazardous Substances Review Toxicology Quiz" at http://macpost.odr.georgetown.edu/ehands/News698.html, and "School of Veterinary Medicine, Tuskegee University Toxicology quiz" at http://192.203.127.60/quiz/physiology/Toxicology.html. Anil Aggrawal's "Forensic Toxicology" page, and "Minnesota Poison Control System" mentioned above also have a number of tox trivia and toxicology quizzes, including picture quizzes.

Toxicology Newsgroups and Fora

There are a number of toxicology newsgroups, including: http://www.bio.net/charters/toxicol, http://www.bio.net/hypermail/toxicol/current, and http://groups.yahoo.com/group/cr_po.

NLM's division of SIS runs a small announcement list called NLM-Tox-Enviro-Health-L. The purpose of the announcement list is to broadcast updates on SIS's resources, services, and outreach in toxicology and environmental health. The NLM-Tox-Enviro-Health-L archives allow users to search list postings, and to modify subscription options. More information is available at http://www.sis.nlm.nih.gov/Tox/ToxListServ.html.

Conclusion

The internet is a very strong medium for dissemination of information and toxicologists have made good use of it. Today there are a number of websites, newsgroups, online journals, searchable databases, and other web-based services solely devoted to toxicology and its various subspecialties. The relevant information is no longer limited to libraries; it is not difficult to search for information either, as compared to past. All information that is needed is available at the touch of a button. However where and how to look for information on the internet is key. Indeed, the internet has completely changed the way that toxicology is viewed today.

See Also

Internet: Forensic Medicine

Further Reading

Aggrawal A. Anil Aggrawal's Forensic Toxicology Page (http://www.geradts.com/~anil/index.html).

Aggrawal A. Best Toxicology Books (http://www.geradts.com/~anil/btb/index.html).

Aggrawal A (moderator). Criminal Poisoning Discussion Forum. (http://groups.yahoo.com/group/cr po).

Nelson LS (2001) A guide to clinical toxicology resources available on the internet: forensics. *Journal of Toxicology – Clinical Toxicology* 39(7): 745–746.

Wexler P (2000) *Information Resources in Toxicology*. San Diego, CA: Academic Press.

Wexler P (ed.) (2001) Special issue: digital information and tools, Part I .*Toxicology* 157(1–2): 1–164.

Wexler P (ed.) (2002) Special issue: digital information and tools, Part II – Web resources in special toxicology topics. *Toxicology* 173(1–2): 1–192.

Wexler P (ed.) (2003) Special issue: digital information and tools, Part III – global web resources. *Toxicology* 190(1–2): 1–142.

Wexler P (2003) A forum to highlight internet resources of note for toxicologists. *Toxicology* 184: 241–242.

J

JUDICIAL PUNISHMENT

H A N El-Fawal, Mercy College, Dobbs Ferry, NY, USA

Introduction

In the context of this encyclopedia, judicial punishment refers to physical punishment, including corporal punishment and/or capital punishment. Judicial punishment has long been, and will likely continue to be, a topic of heated debates. The intention here is to give a historical perspective on judicial punishment as it applies to capital punishment, rather than expound one view or another. As part of this historical perspective, this article is an overview of the stance taken by the three Abrahamic faiths: Judaism, Christianity, and Islam. The underlying justification for this approach is that even societies that proclaim themselves secular, or even atheistic, are informed in their conduct and views by their heritage and that of their forebears. An American may not of necessity be a churchgoer to be influenced by Judeo-Christian tradition. Furthermore, in recent years religion has become a major part of the debate, as witnessed by several national and international conferences such as the series A Call for Reckoning: Religion and the Death Penalty, sponsored by the Pew Forum on Religion and Public Life.

Judicial Punishment in the Torah and in Contemporary Judaism

The Tanach or Tanakh is the Hebrew acronym for the Jewish Bible. This name is derived from the initial letters of its three main sections: the Torah, Neviim, and Ketuvim. The Protestant Old Testament consists only of the Tanach, although the arrangement is not identical and there are some differences in text. For example, the Old Testament includes some books that have extra paragraphs that do not exist in the Jewish version. The Catholic and Orthodox Old Testaments are more extensive than the Tanach, by six books.

Rabbinical Judaism holds that the books of the Tanach, the written law, were transmitted in parallel with an oral tradition. This came to be known as the "oral law." They point to the text of the Torah, Pentateuch, or first five books of the Old Testament, where many words are left undefined, and to procedures that are not elaborated on with detailed instructions. The assumption is that the reader should refer to oral sources. Initially, it was forbidden to write this oral law. This restriction was lifted when it became apparent that it was the only way to ensure that the law could be preserved. Rabbi Judah HaNasi reduced oral tradition to written form around 200 CE in what become known as the Mishnah (Repetition). Interestingly, the Mishnah shows a lack of citation of a scriptural basis for its laws. However, the link between Tanach and Mishnah is drawn from the commentaries of rabbis, over the next four centuries, on the Mishnah that were edited together into the compilations known as the Talmud (550 CE). Halakha (Jewish law and custom) is therefore not based on a literal reading of the Tanach, or Revelation, but on the combined oral and written tradition of the rabbis. Jewish law, therefore, developed in its written form 130–480 years after the fall of the Jerusalem Temple at the hands of Rome.

The Torah required the death penalty for at least 37 different transgressions, some religious, and others civil. The first of these is murder: "Whoso sheddeth man's blood, by man shall his blood be shed: for in the image of God made he man (Genesis 9:6)." However, the Talmud argues that the burden of proof was so stringent, including two eyewitnesses, that it was rarely carried out. *Ratsach* (in Hebrew) and *phoneuo* (in Greek) refer to premeditated murder, with the penalty being death (Leviticus 24:17; 24:21; Numbers 35:16; Deuteronomy 17:6).

The Biblical texts of Exodus, Leviticus, Numbers, and Deuteronomy promulgate another 613 laws, and expand the range of crimes punishable by death other than murder.

Religious Grounds

Religious grounds applied to Israelites and non-Israelites and included apostasy (Exodus 22:20; Numbers 25:1–15), a stranger entering the temple (Numbers 1:51; 3:10; 18:7; and 17:13), non-Israelite missionaries (Deuteronomy 13:1–10), communication with the dead through mediums (Leviticus 20:27), and for black magic (Exodus 22:18).

Sexual Grounds

Sexual grounds included adultery, and applied to the two parties (Leviticus 20:10; Deuteronomy 22:22), incest (Leviticus 20:11–17), temple prostitution, possibly pagan homosexual behavior (Leviticus 20:13; Deuteronomy 22:24), bestiality – the sentence applied to both human and beast (Leviticus 20:15; Exodus 22:19), premarital sex, applied only to the woman (Deuteronomy 22:13–21), *ménage à trois* with another woman and one's mother (Deuteronomy 20:14), infidelity to a woman's fiancé (Deuteronomy 22: 23–24), rape of an engaged woman, where the male is punished (Deuteronomy 22:25) (if the victim was single, he is required to marry her and pay a dowry), and for prostitution by a priest's daughter (Leviticus 21:9).

Other Crimes

For killing a male or female slave, no specific punishment is given. However, for kidnapping with the intention of selling someone into slavery, death is the penalty (Exodus 21:16; Deuteronomy 24:7). Sacrificing one's children to a pagan god (Leviticus 20:2–5), cursing or shaming one's parents (Exodus 21:17; Leviticus 20:9), abusing one's parents (Exodus 21:15), deaths caused by one's livestock (Exodus 21:29), where the offending animal is also put to death, blasphemy in the Lord's name (Leviticus 24:16), working on the sabbath (Exodus 35:2), ignoring the judgment of a priest or judge (Deuteronomy 17:12), perjury (Deuteronomy 19:15–21), death of a pregnant woman during an altercation (Exodus 21:22–23), an uncircumcised male (Genesis 17:14), ritual animal sacrifice other than at the temple (Leviticus 17:1–9), gluttony and excessive drinking (Deuteronomy 21:20), and going to temple in an unclean state (Numbers 19:13) could all earn one the death penalty.

Capital punishment according to the Torah could be carried out by burning (Genesis 38:24; Leviticus 20:14; 21:9), stoning (Leviticus 20:2, 27; 24:14; Numbers 14:10; 15: 33–36; Deuteronomy 13:10; 17:5; 22:21, 24), hanging (Genesis 40:22; Deuteronomy 21:22–23), and sword or spear (Exodus 19:13). The convicted could be executed by witnesses (Deuteronomy 13:9; 17:7) or by the congregation (Numbers 15:35–36; Deuteronomy 13:9), and it was done speedily (Leviticus 10:1–2).

In contrast to the Torah, Rabbinical Judaism relies heavily on Talmudic teaching and has abrogated for itself the right to determine when and how the law of punishment should be implemented. The underlying reason often given for this is the absence of a functioning temple and a standing priesthood to administer the Mosaic law since the fall of the Temple in 68–70 CE at Roman hands. In practice this refers to the absence of Jewish governance and authority since the diaspora, although historical records indicate enclaves of Judaism that applied some form of Mosaic law in the Near East up to the eighth century and in Spain as late as the fourteenth century.

Rabbinical Judaism, not scripture, indicates that the death penalty was only to be used in extremely rare cases. Two witnesses were required to the crime. Furthermore, the witnesses must establish that they verbally warned the person that he/she would be liable for the death penalty, and that the perpetrator had to acknowledge that he/she was warned, but went ahead and committed the sin regardless. However, the individual was not allowed to testify against him/herself. Therefore, the death penalty was effectively legislated out of existence, since meeting the conditions of guilt and conviction were rendered impractical and untenable. This Talmudic opinion is expressed in the Sanhedrin tractate.

Nevertheless, *Halakha* as voiced by orthodox rabbis recognizes the possible need for the death penalty. In the same Sanhedrin tractate, the murderer was to be imprisoned, even if all the rules of evidence were not satisfied, and their death should be hastened through malnutrition. The great Spanish Jewish Rabbi Maimonodes further codified this view in the Law of Murderers. Discussing the responsibilities and obligations of the court, Maimonides says: "It is forbidden for the court to take pity on the murderer, for they should not say. 'One has already been killed, what purpose is there in killing this one?' and they will become derelict in their duty to execute him." This suggests that showing compassion to a murderer is in itself cruelty to society for failing to eliminate a potential danger or providing a deterrent.

The Rashba (Rabbi Shlomo Ben Adret, the Rabbi of Spain in the fourteenth century) permitted the handing-over of Jews to non-Jewish authorities, which was generally forbidden, to face the justice of the land if it was to protect the lives of others. The Talmud (Makkot tractate) states that a criminal guilty of a capital crime is put to death, even if he/she repents, since repentance is between the criminal and God, and not between the criminal and society. This is what distinguishes divine justice (paying the debt to God) from human justice, which is based on past actions where repentance cannot undo what has been done. True repentance of the perpetrator can only be achieved when forgiven by the victim, and the victim cannot forgive in this lifetime.

In contrast, conservative Judaism, as exemplified by the Rabbinical Assembly, argues against the death penalty is based on the fallibility of humanity and replaces the punishment with imprisonment without parole. Those among conservative and reformed Judaism quote the Mishnah, where it says: "A Sanhedrin that executes once in seven years is called murderous." Rabbi Eleazer ben Azaryah pronounces harsher judgment by saying: "once in seventy years," and Rabbis Tarfon and Akibah are even harsher: "Were we in the Sanhedrin, no one would have ever been executed." Rabbi Simon ben Gamliel's retort to this in the same Mishnah, "they too increase shedders of blood in Israel," is ignored.

At a recent conference on religion and the death penalty, D Novak, J Richard, and D Shiff Chair of Jewish Studies at the University of Toronto, summed it up as follows:

> Rashba wrote in a response, 'it seems to me that this is for the preservation of society (mequyyam ha'olam), because it bases everything on the laws collected in the Torah, and only does what the Torah prescribes as punishment in these and similar offenses, then society will be destroyed, for we require witnesses and hatra'ah. It is as the rabbis said that Jerusalem was destroyed only because they based their judgment on the law of the Torah'.

This radical interpretation of Rashba is based on two rabbinic precedents. The first is that the Mishnah expresses the principle of the "maintenance of society (tiqqun ha'olam)" as a ground for changing earlier laws, which if allowed to remain unchanged would lead to social breakdown in one way or another. The second precedent is an aggadic passage indicating that at times the needs of society require one to go "beyond the boundaries of the Law (lifnim me-shurat ha-din)." "Now this concept is usually interpreted to mean that a more lenient ruling is called for in place of the strict letter of the law. Rashba, on the other hand, takes the destruction of Jerusalem as a paradigm of the breakdown of society in general, and he attributes this to the fact that the authorities, by sticking to the letter of the law of capital punishment, contributed to the breakdown of law and order. They should have seen the danger to society in such permissiveness and been harsher, which he sees as the spirit of the law. Apparently, laxity in applying the law removed its deterrent intention.

In the USA, Judaism, regardless of its sectarian differences, is fairly united in supporting a moratorium on the death penalty since it does disproportionately target the poor and racial minorities, and in many instances unjustly, through skewed jury selection.

Judicial Punishment in Christianity

Christianity, as reflected in the four canonical gospels, does not bring new laws to the capital punishment debate. Many contemporary Christian denominations claim that Jesus abrogated the support or need for a death penalty when he is reported to have said: "Ye have heard that it hath been said, An eye for an eye, and a tooth for a tooth: But I say unto you that ye resist not evil: but whosoever shall smite thee on thy right cheek, turn to him the other cheek also" (Matthew 5:38–39). This is apparently an invitation for forgiveness and not an invitation to murder. However, it is also reported that Jesus said: "Think not that I am come to destroy the law, or the prophets: I am not come to destroy, but to fulfil. For verily I say unto you, Til heaven and earth pass, one jot or one tittle shall in no wise pass from the law, till all be fulfilled. Whosoever therefore shall break one of these least commandments, and shall teach men so, he shall be called the least in the kingdom of heaven: but whosoever shall do and teach them, the same shall be called great in the kingdom of heaven" (Matthew 17–19).

Arguably, in Pauline Christology, it is the death penalty that provides the opportunity for vicarious atonement per Deuteronomy 21:23: "for he that is hanged is accursed of God" as Jesus was convicted by the Sanhedrin for blasphemy. Paul extols this in Galatians 3:13: "Christ has redeemed us from the curse of the law, being made a curse for us: for it is written, Cursed is everyone that hangeth on a tree." Yet it is Paul who in Romans 13:1–7 preaches to his followers that they need to obey the secular rulers since all power comes from God, and since these rulers are in power, therefore, they must be sanctioned by God.

The Church has defended the right of the state to impose capital punishment for certain crimes. In the late second and third centuries, Tertullian and Lactantius, respectively, affirmed that, in the case of murder, divine law consistently required a life for a life. The Council of Ephesus (431 CE) in settling the Nestorian controversy enacted a legal code specifying capital crimes. While Augustine, among others, acknowledged the role of the state in mediating capital sanctions, various councils from the seventh (Eleventh Council of Toledo) to the thirteenth century (Fourth Lateran Council) followed the lead of Leo the Great (fifth century) in seeking to forbid clerics from engagement in matters of capital justice, but to leave it to the temporal authorities. In general, the Church recognized capital punishment. This is bolstered by the opinion of theologians such as Thomas Aquinas who wrote: "The common good is better than the good of the individual … The life of certain pestilent fellows is a hindrance to the common good, that is, to the concord of human society. Such persons therefore are to be withdrawn by death from the society of men." In point of fact, when the Church was the secular state, for all intents and purposes, making or unmaking kings, it often labeled dissenters as heretics or apostates and used its power in the temporal world to exterminate groups such as the Cathars and even its once-beloved Knights Templar. It also extended to the literal "witch hunts" which were mirrored in Protestant Puritan New England of the American colonies.

The Protestant Reformation also endorsed the death penalty. The Schleitheim Confession (1527) and Lutheran Formula of Concord (1580) are but two examples. Protestantism is where much of contemporary opposition to capital punishment originates. Penal excesses did result in opposition during the age of Enlightenment. This included figures such as Benjamin Franklin, Thomas Paine, Voltaire, and Jean Jacques Rousseau. However, this was secular humanist opposition, and not religious. Even in the American Constitution, it is argued that when the Eighth Amendment was enacted in 1791, the death penalty in America was already in place, and so could not be considered "unusual." Therefore, this Amendment on "cruel and unusual punishment" is not intended to apply to capital punishment *per se*.

In addressing Italian Catholic jurists in 1952, Pope Pius XII reaffirmed the Church's historic recognition of retribution and therapeutic penology, noting that: "the state does not dispose of the individual's right to live. Rather, it is reserved to the public authority to deprive the criminal of the benefit of life, when already, by his crime, he has deprived himself of the right to live." Referring to Romans 13:4, the Pontiff also noted "in conformity with what sources of revelation and traditional doctrine teach regarding the coercive power of legitimate human authority."

Recently, the current Pontiff, John Paul II, while not excluding the death penalty in *Evangelium Vitae* (1995), restricted it to unusual extreme cases, and advised that bloodless means were always to be preferred if they could sufficiently protect society against the criminal. In accordance with these statements, the Catholic Catechism was revised. Many Catholics, including prominent bishops, face the dilemma of reconciling this new stand with their adherence to the traditions of the early Church fathers. The argument is made that this declaration is in response to the use of the death penalty that is often disproportionate in the populations that are targeted or to the crime that is being punished.

Judicial Punishment in Sharii'ah and Islam

Islam draws its laws from the Quran, for the Muslim the verbatim Word of God, and the *Sunnah*, the authenticated sayings (*Hadith*) or actions of the Messenger Mohammed. The authority of these sources is dealt with in Sharii'ah Law in this encyclopedia. Because these sources of Sharii'ah are also the vehicle of worship in Islam, all Muslims are aware of the consequences of their actions. Ignorance cannot be claimed. The purpose of Sharii'ah is to preserve life, family, society, belief, and intellect. Those crimes subject to judicial punishment are, therefore, those that tear at the fabric of the sanctity of life, family, society, belief, and intellect.

Islam sees itself as a continuation of the revelations received by Moses, the Israelite prophets, and Jesus. As such, in matters of judicial punishment it combines the strictness of the Torah with the compassion of the Gospel. The Quran, the Muslim scripture, states: "And We ordained therein [in the Torah] for them: 'Life for life, eye for eye, nose for nose, tooth for tooth, and wounds for equal wounds.' But if anyone remits the retaliation by way of charity, it shall be for him an expiation. And whoever does not judge by that which God has revealed, such are the wrong doers" (Quran 5:45).

Judicial punishment in Islam falls under a category known as Haddud (plural of Hadd), meaning limits. The author of these limits and the punishments for transgression are the realm of God alone. Haddud crimes are not exclusively crimes that involve capital punishment, but may include instances of corporal punishment or exile. Those crimes carrying a penalty of death include murder, adultery (by married individuals), and open rebellion against the Muslim community (a meaning not communicated by the word apostasy). This latter case refers to open incitement against the Islamic community. It is equated with treason, since Islam does not recognize a dichotomy of sacred and secular in a nation where Muslims are in the majority. Other Haddud crimes, not carrying the death penalty, are slandering women, theft, robbery, and public intoxication. Here we deal with the death penalty in the case of murder and punishment in the case of theft, since these are often what grab the headlines in the international media. It is important to make a distinction that what will be outlined here is what Islamic doctrine, as per its sources, teaches, and not what states defined internationally as Islamic do. Much of the laws found in these countries are derived from Napoleonic law and not Sharii'ah.

The standard of proof in Hadd crimes is quite stringent (known in Arabic as Taghleedh). The Islamic judge cannot enforce the prescribed Hadd punishment unless the person gives an uncoerced confession, or if there are sufficient witnesses to the crime. Often the witnesses are the subject of great scrutiny to determine impartiality and soundness of reputation. In point of fact, a person who slanders a woman as to her moral conduct, without providing four other witnesses to that conduct, is himself punished, and his testimony is never accepted again (Quran 24:4). In an Islamic court there is no such concept as plea-bargaining or immunity for testimony. For most Hadd crimes two witnesses are required, and in the case of adultery, four (this is an example of Taghleedh, suggesting that repentance is better than confession and punishment). Furthermore, it is incumbent on the judge to seek higher proof of the crime as to motive, particularly in capital offenses.

Premeditated or Intentional Murder

Murder is the ultimate crime since it is a denial of life, which is the sole property of God: "And do not kill the soul which God has forbidden, except in justice. If one is killed wrongfully [premeditated], We have given their heir authority, but he is not to seek excess. He will surely find a champion [in the Law]" (Quran 17:33). The meaning of "We have given their heir authority" is elaborated on in what is known as Qesas (law of equity in punishment): "O you who believe! Al-Qesas has been ordained for you in the case of murder: the free for the free; the servant for the servant, the female for the female [this heralds back to the Mosaic code]. But if the killer is forgiven by the brother [family of the victim] and requests reparation (diya) in fairness let it be given in fairness. This is an alleviation [of the burden of taking a life] and a mercy from your Lord. Whoever transgresses after this [member of victim's family] he shall have a painful torment [in the hereafter]. There is [the saving of] life for you in Qesas O people of understanding. Perhaps you will be heedful" (Quran 2:178–179). Therefore, there is punishment and closure if that is the desire of the victim's family. However, unlike other systems of justice, commuting the sentence does not rely on exhausting appeals to higher courts until the twelfth hour and after 30 years of incarceration. Commuting the sentence relies on the victim's family, which may request reparations

(diya). This diya is often translated as blood money, which is erroneous. It is restitution for harm done to the victim's family, which may include young children – and is in lieu of the perpetrator's life, not in addition – and for depriving the family of their loved one. This is why the verse says: "There is [the saving of] life for you in Qesas O people of understanding." It is ironic that in the notorious OJ Simpson case of the 1990s, Simpson was acquitted in the criminal court for murder, but held liable for the deaths of both his wife and R Goldman in the civil court and responsible for compensation (diya) of 8.5 million dollars to R Goldman's family. No one considered this blood money.

The position of Sharii'ah on punishment for murder is also exemplified in a Hadith of the Messenger Mohammed. A man came to the Messenger Mohammed dragging another man by a strap, and announcing: "This man killed my brother!" The Messenger Mohammed asked, "Did you kill him?" Whereupon the accused said, "Yes. He and I were cutting down the leaves of the trees, he abused me and enraged me, and so I hit him with my axe." The Messenger Mohammed asked, "Do you have anything to pay in compensation?" On receiving a negative, he then asked, "What of your family or tribe?" The man answered: "I am more insignificant to my tribe than this axe." So the Messenger Mohammed gave the strap back to the victim's brother and said, "He is yours [i.e., yours to punish]." After the man left, Mohammed turned to his companions and said "If he kills him, he is no better than he is." Whereupon one of the companions rushed after the man and informed him of this. The victim's brother returned to the Messenger and said, "I heard that you said that if I killed him, I am no better than him." The Messenger Mohammed asked, "Would it not be better for you that he carry your sin and that of your brother?" And he set the man free.

Islam also provides compensation for injury or harm, as exemplified by the Hadith: "If a relative is killed or suffers injury, you may choose retaliation, forgiveness, or compensation. If anyone desires more, then suppress him/her. Anyone who exceeds these limits will have a grave penalty."

These references are an invitation to clemency where clemency is warranted, since it is not likely that such a perpetrator would commit this crime again. This, however, may not always be the case. Crimes such as serial murder, rape, and pedophilia do not leave room for forgiveness.

In the USA we often hear criticism of the death penalty being applied to juveniles, the mentally retarded, or insane (not referring to those who trot out expert witnesses for a single documentation of insanity). In 2004 the Juvenile Justice Center of the American Bar Association (ABA), reported that there are 73 persons on death row who were juveniles (aged 16–17) at the time of their crime. Twenty-two have been executed since reinstatement of the death penalty in 1976. The state of Texas holds the record for 13 executions of juvenile offenders and was the only jurisdiction to carry it out in 2002. However, 22 states have provisions for juvenile executions in their laws. According to the ABA only the USA and Iran formally recognize the practice. It is refreshing to see that this concern has been anticipated in Islam. The Messenger Mohammed said: "There are three whose actions are not recorded [not held responsible for]: a sleeper till they awake, the mentally deranged till they are restored to reason, and the child until they attain puberty." The Muslim jurist Malik comments: "It is generally agreed that in our way there is no retaliation against children. Their intention is accidental. The Haddud are not obliged for them if they have not reached puberty." What may pose a challenge for some Islamic jurists is choosing the definition of puberty as mental rather than biological maturity.

Punishment for Theft

Contrary to the popular image many have of Islam, it is no cavalier affair to pass judgment for the intentional severing of a person's hand. In fact those most eligible, according to Sharii'ah, are more likely to be those dealing in depreciated mutual funds, or intentional fraud, rather than the homeless and hungry. Seven conditions must be met in order for an Islamic jurist to pass such a judgment. These include: (1) two reputable witnesses, with no contradiction or error in their testimonies; (2) the value of stolen goods must exceed the equivalent buying value (in today's society) of a quarter dinar (4.25 g of gold); (3) it must be stolen from a secure place (i.e., this shows intention and effort on the part of the thief, as in breaking and entering); (4) it cannot be food; (5) it cannot be from one's family; (6) there should be no doubt as to the provenance of the goods (i.e., whether or not it may be the thief's property or disputed property between the thief and another); and (7) it must not be something that is prohibited under Islamic law (i.e., not drugs or intoxicants, which changes the nature of the crime). The Quranic injunction is: "As for the male thief and female thief, cut their hand as recompense for their deed, an example from God [deterrent], and God is All-Powerful, All-Wise. But whosoever repents after his crime and does right, then God accepts his/her repentance. God is Oft-Forgiving, Most Merciful" (Quran 5:38–39).

Capital Judicial Punishment in Contemporary Society

Hanging was practiced in many countries until the beginning of the 1960s. The last hanging in Scotland was in 1963, and in England in 1964. The death penalty was abolished in England in 1965 and this abolition was confirmed in 1969. However, it was reserved for the crimes of treason, piracy with violence, and arson until 1998, when these ceased to be capital crimes. Hanging continues to be used in several countries, including Egypt, Iran, Japan, Jordan, Kuwait, Malaysia, Nigeria, Pakistan, Singapore, and Zimbabwe.

Beheading, by guillotining, was also popular in several countries, in addition to France. It was exported to Algeria, Belgium, Germany, Greece, Switzerland, Sweden, and Vietnam. What became West Germany abolished the death penalty in 1951 and had its last guillotining in 1949. In France, the death penalty was finally abolished in 1981. Beheading by sword is currently only practiced in Saudi Arabia, although the Congo and Arab Emirates do have it in their criminal law.

Execution by shooting is carried out in China, Kazakhstan, occupied Palestine, Thailand, Uganda, Vietnam, and Yemen. Execution by shooting is prevalent in 70 countries.

The USA is the only major country that uses lethal injection and the electric chair. Lapidation (stoning), although legal in six countries, was not used in 2002.

A summary of executions, based on data primarily from Amnesty International, is presented in **Table 1**. On record, only seven countries practice the death penalty for those committing crimes as juveniles (i.e., under the age of 18), although only applied in the USA and Iran. These countries include Congo, Iran, Nigeria, Pakistan, Saudi Arabia, the USA, and Yemen. In 2003, China, Pakistan and Yemen raised

Table 1 Numbers executed worldwide from 1998 to 2003 (data summarized from Amnesty International Reports)

Year	1998	1999	2000	2001	2002	2003
Number of executions	2258	1813	1457	3048[a]	1526[b]	1146[c]
Number of countries	37	31	28	31	31	28

[a]2468 in China; 139 in Iran; 79 in Saudi Arabia; 66 in the USA.
[b]1060 in China; 113 in Iran; 71 in the USA (33 in Texas alone, the remainder in 12 states, although 38 states have the death penalty), 47 in Saudi Arabia.
[c]726 in China; 108 in Iran; 65 in the USA (the 900th execution since 1977 was in March 2004); 64 in Vietnam.

the minimum age to 18, in their legal code, and Iran is in the process of doing so. Nearly all executions of individuals who were juveniles at the time of their crime take place in the USA. All countries, except the USA and Somalia, subscribe to the United Nations Convention on the Rights of the Child, forbidding capital punishment for juveniles. In 2002, two perpetrators convicted as juveniles were executed by lethal injection in the state of Texas. The US Supreme Court recently refused to ban the execution of juveniles.

In the 1990s, in the USA there was a vigorous drive for a moratorium on the death penalty by both secular and religious leaders. This drive stemmed from the belief that three factors influence the sentencing for capital punishment: (1) geography; (2) race; and (3) income. The geographical argument is that the death penalty in the USA is a product of southern culture. For example, 62 of the 71 executions in 2002 occurred south of the Mason–Dixie line. Outside the south only California and Ohio executed anyone. Since 1976, when the death penalty was resumed, two out of three executions took place in only five states: Florida, Missouri, Oklahoma, Texas, and Virginia. In late 2003, Amnesty International was campaigning to stay the execution of Kevin Zimmerman on December 10 in Texas; Charles Singleton on January 6, 2004 in Arkansas (he was believed to suffer from mental illness); and Hung Thanh Le, a Vietnamese, on January 6, 2004 in Oklahoma. All three executions took place in 2004, although the last was postponed until March.

Another reason for the call for a moratorium is spurred by Governor George Ryan of Illinois, traditionally a death-penalty supporter, who declared a moratorium in his state. This was in response to the exoneration of 13 convicted murderers since 1985, based on new evidence and/or DNA testing, and fear of executing an innocent person. Further impetus for the moratorium was provided by a Columbia University (New York) study reporting a 68% error in sentencing based on a survey of capital cases. PG Cassell, a University of Utah law professor, points out that what the Columbia University study neglects to mention is that they failed to find a single case where an innocent person was executed. Therefore, the rate of mistaken execution was zero. Supporters of the death penalty argue that exoneration of some on death row proves that the system works. An interesting caveat to all of this is the question raised by some as to what makes an average incarceration of 25 years followed by execution or life imprisonment more humane than the death penalty?

Opponents of the death penalty point out that racial minorities, particularly blacks, are disproportionately represented in the prison system, probably as a result of racial profiling. According to statistics from the US Census Bureau, Bureau of Justice and Statistics, and the Federal Bureau of Investigation, 42% of those on death row nationwide are black, compared to 56% white, and 2% of other ethnic groups. Blacks comprise only 13% of the US population.

The third argument offered for a moratorium is the disparity in representation for low-income defendants. These lack the resources to engage an experienced defense attorney, and therefore must rely on the overworked, understaffed, and underpaid public defenders office.

Worldwide, 76 countries have abolished the death penalty. This includes almost all European countries, since this is a condition of being a member of the European Union. The Council of Europe has also made this a condition, although it does accept a moratorium as a temporary measure. Russia is one such country that has declared a moratorium, although it has the death penalty on the books. Belarus is not a Council member and retains the death penalty. Australia, Canada, and most South American countries have also abolished the death penalty. Taiwan has abolished the death penalty for kidnapping, gang robbery, and other violent crimes short of murder. There are 15 countries that maintain it for exceptional circumstances, and 21 countries that have lapsed in its application. The death penalty is maintained in both law and practice by 83 countries.

It is important to insert a word of caution here. These statistics are based on reports available to international organizations, such as Amnesty International. They do not include data on political and religious persecution. They do not include data for state-sanctioned killing, justified by security, or capital murder in the form of genocide. They also do not include data on wrongful death that may result from abuse of power by the authorities. These are often forms of extrajudicial punishment.

Conclusion

Judicial punishment, in the form of capital punishment, remains, and will likely remain, a controversial sphere. Although Judeo-Christian scripture sanctions capital punishment for over 30 different transgressions, adherents of the represented faiths have denominational and sectarian differences. Judaism, with its emphasis on Talmudic tradition, the absence of a temple or temple priesthood, is of two minds: those who uphold the sanctity of the law, and those who believe it no longer applies under current conditions. As for Christianity, while preaching forgiveness, the Church, particularly Catholicism (although not exclusively), recognizes secular authority, as it also recognizes that authority's excesses. Islam, despite its detractors, limits the scope of the death penalty to three transgressions; paramount among these is murder. Islam provides a system of clemency to the perpetrator and reparation for the victim's family. Common secular law finds itself in a quandary, torn between its perception of justice and the fallibility of human conduct, and possible excesses, in practice. Common law, as much as it claims to be divorced from the religious, is informed by individuals' religious background. Regardless of religious or secular law, we often preach what we do not practice, much to the loss of the individual, society, and humanity as a whole.

See Also

Court Systems: Sharii'ah Law; Law, China; Law, Japan; Law, United Kingdom; Law, United States of America

Further Reading

Abou E, l-Fadl K (1998) Political crimes in Islamic and western jurisprudence. *University of California at Davis Journal of International Law and Policy* 4: 1.

Al-Qaradawi Y (1989) *The Lawful and Prohibited in Islam.* Indianapolis, IN: American Trust Publications.

Bailey LR (1987) *Capital Punishment: What the Bible Says.* Nashville, TN: Abingdon Press.

Banner S (2002) *The Death Penalty: An American History.* Cambridge, MA: Harvard University Press.

Dow DR, Dow M (2002) *Machinery of Death. The Reality of America's Death Penalty Regime.* New York: Routledge.

Hassanain MM (1990) *The Criminal Law Policy in Islamic Legislation.* Riyadh, Saudi Arabia: Institute of Islamic and Arabic Sciences in America.

Holy Bible (1985) *King James Version.* Oxford, UK: Oxford University Press.

Holy Quran (1999) *Abd Allah Yusuf Ali (translator).* Indianapolis, IN: American Trust Publications.

Kamali MH (1999) Law and society, the interpretation of revelation and reason in the shariah. In: Esposito JL (ed.) *The Oxford History of Islam*, pp. 107–153. Oxford, UK: Oxford University Press.

Megivern JJ (1997) *The Death Penalty: An Historical and Theological Survey.* New York: Paulist Press.

Michigan State University and Death Penalty Information Center (2000) *Arguments for and Against the Death Penalty.* New York: Michigan State University and Death Penalty Information Center.

Novak D (1983) *The Image of the Non-Jew in Judaism: An Historical and Constructive Study of the Noahide Laws.* Lewiston: Edwin Mellen Press.

O'Donovan O (1997) The death penalty in Evangelium Vitae. In: Hutter R, Dieter T (eds.) *Ecumenical Ventures in Ethics: Protestants Engage Pope John Paul II's Moral Encyclicals*, pp. 216–236. Grand Rapids, CA: Eerdmans.

Sahih Bukhari (1994) *Muhsin Khan M (translator).* Riyadh, Saudi Arabia: Darrussalam.

Scherman N (ed.) (1996) Tanach. In: *The Stone Edition*, Brooklyn, NY: Mesorah Publications, Ltd.

Skotnicki A (2000) *Religion and the Development of the American Penal System.* Lanham: University Press of America.

L

LEGAL DEFINITIONS OF DEATH

R Gaebler and R Dworkin, Indiana University School of Law, Bloomington, IN, USA

Introduction

Until the 1960s, jurists were not particularly concerned with the task of legally defining death. Up to that time it was self-evident that death occurs when cardiopulmonary functions permanently cease, and there was relatively little need to determine the precise moment of death. In common-law jurisdictions a murder conviction could only be obtained if the victim died within a year and a day of the offending blow, and for estate distribution purposes it was sometimes necessary to know which of two or more persons died first when both or all were victims of a common disaster. However, for the most part, the timing of death was unimportant, and the common-sense notion of cessation of cardiopulmonary function sufficed. After all, the lungs and heart comprise the means by which oxygenated blood is delivered to the rest of the human body, without which all human tissue soon dies.

The movement for a precise legal definition of death arose for three distinct reasons. First, the invention of mechanical devices, such as the ventilator, made it possible to induce respiration and blood circulation in patients who were no longer able to perform these functions autonomously due to irreversible destruction of the brain. Second, the advent of organ transplantation as a practical therapy led to the use of cadaver organs for that purpose. Third, the development of the electroencephalogram and agreed-upon medical criteria made it possible to determine that a person who still retained naturally or artificially supported heart and lung function could no longer return to a cognitive, sapient life.

In light of these developments, jurists have been pressed over the past 30 years to develop legal criteria of death that would permit the removal of nontwin organs and the removal of life support from brain-dead patients. As a result, the undoubted trend has been toward accepting whole-brain death, i.e., permanent cessation of functions by the cerebrum, cerebellum, and brainstem, as the legal definition of death. Many countries now have statutes or regulations that incorporate this standard, establishing the procedures for declaring patients legally dead and the circumstances under which some or all of their organs may be removed for transplantation.

Despite the overall trend outlined above, death definition statutes differ in several interesting respects. They differ in the extent to which they focus on transplantation and in the type and specificity of the definition of death they incorporate. In addition, transplantation statutes differ with respect to whether or not they adopt a unitary definition of death. A unitary definition is usually thought of as one that defines death solely in terms of a single criterion or set of criteria (e.g., whole-brain death, higher brain death, permanent cessation of respiration). However, statutes also differ with respect to whether they require a unitary result, given that a particular criterion or set of criteria has been met. In other words, will a statute embodying a brain-death standard always lead to the conclusion that the patient is dead after it has been determined in any given case that he/she has met the criteria of whole-brain death? Perhaps surprisingly, not all statutes insist upon this type of unity.

In addition to the factors that distinguish from one another the legal definitions of death embodied in statutes, there is also the interesting question of how these statutes in general compare to norms embodied in traditional, religious systems of law. The claim has been made that modern transplantation statutes bypass the sanctity of life ethic common to the world's great religions. However, religious legal systems have themselves responded in different ways, adopting for the most part whole-brain death definitions of death. Within their respective religious traditions, these definitions are authoritatively regarded as wholly compatible with the sanctity of life ethic, rather than as a new, incompatible ethic.

Definition of Death in Religious Legal Systems

There is no provision in the 1983 Code of Canon Law concerning the definition of death. Therefore, one cannot say that there is any explicit, binding norm within the Catholic tradition. However, in an address to the Eighteenth International Congress of the Transplantation Society (2000), Pope John Paul II defined death as the literal disintegration of the unitary person, resulting from the separation of the soul from the corporeal body. The Pope expressed indifference as to the criteria a professional health worker might employ to determine that a patient has arrived at the state of death, as long as certain proof is provided, albeit through inference only, of the disintegration of the person into his/her spiritual and corporeal parts. Speaking in particular of the neurological criterion for inferring the fact of death, Pope John Paul II stated that it "consists in establishing, according to the clearly determined parameters commonly held by the international scientific community, the complete and irreversible cessation of all brain activity in the cerebrum, cerebellum, and brain stem." Thus, it would seem that the Catholic Church accepts both the traditional cardiopulmonary and the modern whole-brain death criteria, on the ground that both, when properly applied, provide a sound evidentiary basis for the conclusion that death, i.e., the separation of the soul from the body, has occurred.

It should be noted that this position has received criticism within the Catholic community. Criticism tends to focus on three factors: (1) that there are no clearly determined parameters within the scientific community, nor any that are commonly held; (2) that no set of criteria can be rigorously applied without incorporating the traditional definition of death, since complete and irreversible cessation of all brain activity presupposes the destruction of the circulatory and respiratory functions as well; and (3) that the myriad sets of criteria proposed have become increasingly permissive.

The first of these criticisms is true up to a point. There is less certainty within the scientific community than was the case just ten years ago. However, recent concerns about the whole-brain death criterion are a natural reaction to its success in gaining widespread currency, and only serve to highlight that success. The second criticism is related to the first, since it reflects scientific skepticism about the whole-brain death standard. It is based on the fact that determination of death via electroencephalogram cannot detect the activities of cells deep within the brain. Therefore some cells may still be living. This supposition is consistent with outward physical evidence manifested by brainstem-dead patients, suggesting the presence of some neuron activity, even in dead brainstems. The third criticism ignores the fact that, while professing indifference toward the technical decisions involved in establishing criteria, the Pope's statement did carefully limit neurological criteria to those that confirm the existence of whole-brain death.

The situation in Islamic law closely resembles that in contemporary Catholic thought. There is no revealed or otherwise authoritative definition of death. The traditional definition of death in Islam, as in Catholicism, is separation of the soul from the body. The traditional criteria for determining that death has occurred are cessation of heartbeat and pulse. However, recent Islamic jurisprudence has concluded that the whole-brain death criterion is not in conflict with the definition of death. In fact, there is some indication in Islamic jurisprudence that the soul is especially associated with the functions of thought and volition, and that whole-brain death is therefore a better criterion of death than the cessation of cardiopulmonary functions.

In 1986, the Academy of Islamic Jurisprudence, a specialized body within the pan-Islamic Organization of Islamic Conferences, adopted a resolution, according to which a person is considered legally dead either when complete and irreversible cessation of the heart or respiration occurs, or when complete and irreversible cessation of all functions of the brain occurs, and the brain is in a state of degeneration. Brain death is defined as including death of the brainstem. The Academy has no powers of enforcement to carry out its resolutions, nor are they binding. However, its pronouncements are influential, and clearly have found their way into national legislation within the Islamic world. In Saudi Arabia, the Senior Ulama Commission's Decision no. 99 (1982) permits removal of organs if transplantation seems likely to succeed and organ removal poses no risk to the donor. Though obviously intended originally to regulate donations from live donors, this decision has been interpreted to permit removal of organs from patients considered legally dead from the time of determination of whole-brain death. The Council of Islamic Jurisprudence in Iran, in its Rulings Concerning Organ Transplantation, held that the criterion of death is cessation of the "normal" pulse and heartbeat, and that revival of the pulse through electronic intervention does not constitute life. Organs may therefore be removed from a whole-brain-dead patient, if he/she has so provided in a will. A number of other Islamic nations, including at least Kuwait, Tunisia, and Turkey have transplantation statutes and related regulations permitting removal of organs from whole-brain-dead patients. Some of these statutes refer to current scientific knowledge for the criteria of death. In its 1985 statement on The End of Life, the Islamic Organization of Medical Sciences adopted a whole-brain death standard for determining when the patient has died. It reconfirmed this standard in 1996. Therefore, statutes referring to current medical knowledge incorporate the whole-brain standard of death indirectly.

Jewish law contains a more explicit, scriptural definition of death than either the Roman Catholic or Islamic religions. Both the Talmud and later authoritative codifications of the Talmud by Maimonides and Joseph Caro confirm that the criterion of death is the permanent cessation of respiration. Moreover, the weight of religious authority imposes upon the doctor a duty to heal and on the patient a corresponding duty to permit him/herself to be healed, since God owns the body and soul. Protection of the integrity of the body and soul applies equally to healthy and sick because both are equally created in the image of God. This sanctity of life principle is embedded in Israeli law both in the Basic Law on Human Dignity and Liberty (1992, amended 1994) and in the Penal Code. The former explicitly recognizes the "sanctity of life," and states that "there shall be no violation of the life, body, or dignity of any person as such." The Penal Code states that any act or criminally negligent omission in the performance of a duty will be regarded as having caused death if it hastens the death of one suffering from injury or illness, and imposes upon doctors an unqualified duty to care for their patients.

In addition, the permissibility of euthanasia is deeply embedded in Jewish legal tradition, despite the sanctity of life principle. According to a well-known gloss on the Shulchan Aruch of Joseph Caro, it is permitted to remove an impediment that is preventing a soul from departing. Thus, according to one recent analysis, the relevant distinction in discharging one's duty to the sick is not between act and omission, but between acts that hasten death and those that remove some factor holding back the soul's departure. There is some disagreement on the scope of this principle, concerning whether it only applies to patients who are in the final stages of dying, whether it permits the cessation of usual treatments (e.g., provision of food and oxygen) as well as unusual treatments, and whether it is only permissible if the patient is suffering great pain. However, it seems that most contemporary commentators believe this principle permits the disconnection of a terminally ill patient from a respirator. This is confirmed by *Shefer* v. *Israel* (1993), the only Israeli Supreme Court decision to address the issue (**Table 1**).

Thus, in practical terms Jewish law arrives at the same conclusion as Islamic and Roman Catholic law, that it is permissible to remove organs from patients

Table 1 Court decisions determining criteria of death

UK	*R.* v. *Potter*, Times, 26 July 1963
	R. v. *Malcherek*, *R.* v. *Steel*, [1981] 2 All ER 422, [1981] WLR 690 (CA)
	Re A [1992] 3 Med LR 303 (Fam D)
Israel	*Shefer* v. *State of Israel* [1994] IsrSC 48(1) 87, [1992–1994] Isr LR 170
USA	In re T.A.C.P., 609 So. 2d 588 (Fla. 1992)

who have suffered permanent whole-brain death. However, it is not entirely clear whether such patients are regarded as dead in Jewish law. In a 1987 directive concerning Brain Death and Heart Transplants, the Rabbinical Council of Israel found that complete and irreversible cessation of respiration can be inferred from confirmation that the entire brain has been destroyed, including the brainstem. From this it follows that a whole-brain-dead patient is legally dead according to the traditional criterion for determining death. Alternatively, the principle that it is permissible to remove an impediment to the soul's departure implies that the patient is still alive until the respirator is turned off.

Because Jewish law, at least to some degree, views removal of artificial respiration from a brain-dead patient as an acceptable form of euthanasia, Israeli courts have been preoccupied with the question of whether this exception might be widened. In a recent case, the District Court of Tel Aviv granted the requests of two patients suffering from amyotrophic lateral sclerosis that they not be given any life-sustaining treatment when they slipped into a persistent vegetative state. The sanctity of life principle would forbid this in Roman Catholic and Islamic law on the grounds that a patient suffering persistent vegetative state is not yet dead.

Taxonomy of Definitions

It is typical of transplantation statutes and regulations to include definitions of the criteria according to which responsible healthcare professionals are to determine that a patient has died. Such statutes and regulations tend to fall into one of two categories. In the first category are many that provide definitions of whole-brain death only. For example, the statutes or regulations of Argentina, Colombia, Hungary, Norway, Peru, Russia, Spain, and Sri Lanka fall into this category, as does the Canadian model act. The Norwegian regulation is the clearest in this regard, explicitly defining whole-brain death as the exclusive definition of death, and indicating that verification of the traditional criterion (i.e., cardiopulmonary failure) constitutes proof of whole-brain death as well. Other statutes and regulations in this category are less clear, often implying that whole-brain death is an alternative to the traditional criterion. For example, the Canadian model statute states that death "includes brain death." In the second category are statutes and regulations that expressly define death as either the permanent cessation of cardiopulmonary functions or whole-brain death. The statutes and applicable regulations of Australia, France, Germany, Greece, Italy, Mexico, Panama, and the Philippines, among others, fall into this category. The Bulgarian statute employs a single definition that can be interpreted as either whole-brain or cardiopulmonary death, referring to "clearly established irreversible biological death." In contrast, the Ecuadorean statute seemingly requires attending doctors to determine both whole-brain and cardiopulmonary death.

As of 1994, the number of countries with statutes or regulations incorporating brain death either as the sole or alternative legal definition of the criterion of death stood at 28, according to one source, and that number has surely risen since (**Table 2**). It should be noted that, in some countries, such as Australia, Canada, and the USA, competence to legislate in this area falls within the jurisdiction of states and provinces, rather than the federal government; therefore there are many statutes in these countries, rather than a single statute. Finally, it should also be noted that only a few of the statutes defining the criteria of death also state that those criteria are mandatory. For example, the Hungarian statute states that the fact of death "must be considered as established" in the event that the attending doctor determines that the patient has suffered destruction of the entire brain. Where statutes do not make the enumerated criteria mandatory, it is entirely a question of interpretation whether the attending doctor must follow them.

Another group of statutes and regulations establish a standard indirectly, by referring to scientific consensus for the definition of death. For example, the Turkish statute requires that death be determined "in accordance with contemporary medical knowledge and procedures." The Belgian, Bolivian, and Tunisian statutes, among others, also fall into this category. Statutes of this type may be regarded as incorporating the whole-brain death standard by reference, since virtually all national, medical standard-setting bodies have adopted it. In addition, the World Medical Association adopted the whole-brain death standard in its 1968 Declaration on Death.

At the other extreme are statutes and regulations that provide no definition of death. For example, the UK Human Tissues Act (1961) states only that organs may be removed by a doctor after he has "satisfied himself by personal examination of the body that life is extinct." In lieu of providing a definition, some

Table 2 Statutes and regulations determining criteria of death

Argentina	Law no. 21541, s.21 (1977)
Belgium	Law on the removal and transplantation of organs, s.11 (1986)
Bolivia	Regulations on the use of organs and tissues, s.7 (1982)
Bulgaria	Ordinance no. 15, Ministry of Public Health, s.4 (1976)
Canada	Uniform Human Tissue Donation Act (1990)
Colombia	Decree no. 1172, s.9 (1989)
Ecuador	Law no. 64, s.2 (1987)
France	Decree no. 96-1041 (1996), codified in Code of Public Health, ss.671-7-1 to 671-7-4
Germany	Law on Transplantation, ss.3,5 (1997)
Greece	Law no. 1383 (1983)
Hungary	Ordinance no. 18, annex 2 (1972)
Israel	Basic Law: Human Dignity and Liberty (1992–4); Penal Code, ss.299,309,322 (1977)
Italy	Law no. 644, s.4 (1975)
Japan	Law no. 104 (1997)
Kuwait	Ministerial order no. 253 (1989)
Mexico	General Law on Health, s.317 (1983)
Norway	Regulation on the definition of death in connection with the law on transplantation, s.1 (1977)
Panama	Law no. 10, ss.7,8 (1983)
Peru	Law no. 23415, s.5 (1982); Civil Code, article 61
Philippines	Organ Donation Act, s.J (1991)
Russian Federation	Law on the transplantation of human organs and/or tissues, s.9 (1992)
Saudi Arabia	Senior Ulama Commission Decision no. 99 (1982)
Singapore	Act no. 22, Interpretation Act s.2A (1998)
Spain	Law no. 30, s.5(1) (1979)
Sri Lanka	Transplantation of Human Tissues Act, no. 48, s.15 (1987)
Sweden	Law no. 269, concerning criterion for determination of human death (1987); National Social Welfare Board Regulations concerning Medical Care, no. 269 (1987)
Tunisia	Law no. 91-22, s.15 (1991)
Turkey	Law no. 2238, s.11 (1979)
UK	Human Tissue Act, ss.4,4A (1961)
USA	Uniform Determination of Death Act, 12A Uniform Laws Annotated 593 (1996 and 2003 Supp.)

statutes specify fairly elaborate procedures that must be followed in determining death. Oftentimes the determination must be made by a commission of three doctors, occasionally required to include a neurologist or other particular specialist.

In the UK and other similar nations, the definition of the criteria to be used in determining death for the purpose of authorizing organ donation must be derived from some other source. English common law has supplied the definition of death from cases, though not from cases interpreting the Human Tissues Act. In an initial false step, a doctor charged with manslaughter was convicted of simple assault for turning off a respirator after removing a kidney from a whole-brain-dead patient. In two later, consolidated cases not involving transplantation, the Appeals Court upheld lower court rulings that there was no evidence to suggest that patients were still alive when their respirators were removed, since the record showed that doctors had followed "normal and conventional" procedures to establish whole-brain death. The Appeals Court side-stepped the lower courts' conclusion as to the time of death. However, the Appeals Court did overrule Potter by holding that shutting off the respirator did not break the chain of causation leading from original assaults to ultimate death (*R.* v. *Malcherek, R.* v. *Steel*, 1981). Finally, in Re A (1992) (**Table 1**) the court unambiguously held that death of the brainstem constitutes legal death, and in *Airedale NHS Trust* v. *Bland* (1993) decreed that "a person is not clinically dead so long as the brainstem retains its function."

Consideration of the various approaches taken by transplantation statutes to the definition of death raises several important questions. First, in deferring to current medical knowledge for the definition of death, how far should statutes go in codifying that knowledge? The definition of death itself, which underlies any acceptable definitions of the criteria for determining when death has occurred, is a philosophical and religious, rather than medical matter. Therefore, statutes do well to state explicitly which standard applies, whether it be whole-brain death, cardiopulmonary death, or both, without reference to medical opinion. Alternatively, statutes and accompanying regulations that go further, setting out in detail precisely which clinical tests are to be carried out, and in what manner, in order to determine that death has occurred, perhaps stray too far into clinical detail and risk freezing the law at one point in technological and scientific development. Better to incorporate the best current medical practice by reference, leaving it to the appropriate medical bodies to define precisely what those practices are. This is particularly so since what constitutes best practice is subject to continuous development.

Another significant question involves the applicability of the definition contained in transplantation or general definition statutes to the many contexts in which the definition of death is of legal consequence. Such contexts include matters related to contracts, ownership of property, testamentary bequests, inheritance, debts, trusteeships, maintenance, and termination of marriage, among others. In order to establish a uniform standard, some nations have incorporated the brain-death standard in general all-purpose statutes. Among these nations are Peru, Singapore, and Sweden. However, it is quite

likely that different definitions of the criteria of death will appeal to reason in different contexts. Definitions of the criteria of death contained in transplantation statutes ought to be strictly construed to apply only to cases arising under those statutes. In common-law systems, flexible and adaptive case law ought to be encouraged to develop a variety of context-specific definitions of the criteria of death as needed. In legal systems that do contain a single, statutory definition of the criteria of death, it may be necessary to develop evidentiary presumptions applicable to specific situations, for example, a presumption of death in the case of a spouse who has been missing for a specified period of years.

Different to the question of whether legal systems ought to have a unitary definition across the entire spectrum of possible contexts is whether transplantation statutes ought themselves to have a unitary definition of death. The Japanese Law Concerning Organ Transplantation (1997) is interesting because it requires the donor to express previous consent both to the legal diagnosis of death by reason of whole-brain death and to removal of specified organs. In the absence of express prior consent, death will only be diagnosed according to the traditional, cardiopulmonary criteria. The statute thus permits the donor to choose which of two legal definitions of death he/she wishes to apply to him/herself. Within the limits imposed by the statute, this approach provides a very sensible form of religious accommodation.

The Definition of Death in the USA

At present, the American approach comes fairly close to adopting context-specific definitions of death. Many states have adopted general definitions that purport to apply in all contexts. The Commissioners on Uniform State Laws have adopted a model death definition statute that has been adopted by 32 states, the District of Columbia, and the Virgin Islands. It defines an individual as dead when that person has sustained irreversible cessation of either circulatory and respiratory functions or "all functions of the entire brain, including the brainstem."

However, the American situation is less monolithic than this general approach seems to suggest. First, the Uniform Act itself provides different criteria for determining whether a person is dead without specifying the circumstances in which one or the other criterion is to be used. Thus, for example, one is left to wonder whether a person who has sustained irreversible cessation of "unassisted" circulatory and respiratory function is dead. More importantly, many issues that seem to revolve around the question of whether a person is dead are not resolved by the statutes. Thus, for example, if a person has been missing for a long time, presumptive death statutes treat the person as dead for purposes of distributing his/her estate or allowing a spouse to remarry, without regard to the missing person's circulatory, respiratory, or brain function. Also, in Florida the State Supreme Court held that an anencephalic infant was not dead for the purposes of permitting her organs to be removed for transplantation (**Table 1**). This leaves open the question of whether such an infant might be treated as dead for other purposes. For example, would an anencephalic infant be viewed as dead if the question were whether she had to be treated at an emergency room or resuscitated? Such questions cannot be resolved by definition.

Whole-Brain Death versus Persistent Vegetative State

Virtually all legal definitions of brain death distinguish between whole-brain death, involving destruction of the brainstem as well as the cerebellum and cerebrum, and higher brain death only. Patients who suffer the latter, or persistent vegetative state, are not regarded as dead. On what basis is this distinction made? If a patient were unable to breathe without a respirator, but nevertheless retained consciousness, no definition would regard that person as dead. Thus, it is the concept of death as the permanent annihilation of all human consciousness, rather than the fact that the patient is no longer able to breathe without assistance, that underlies brain death as the criterion of legal death. Yet the patient who suffers from persistent vegetative state suffers such annihilation as well. The rationale underlying the distinction in the world's legal systems must be that continued respiration and circulation, unaided by mechanical means, forecloses the conclusion that loss of all consciousness is irreversible and therefore permanent. The distinction is also supported by a dualist conception of life, according to which autonomous respiration involves too much physical activity, and too much integration between physical and mental activity, to constitute the state of death.

See Also

Coma, Definitions and Differential Diagnoses: Pediatric; Adult; **Organ and Tissue Transplantation, Ethical and Practical Issues; Religious Attitudes to Death**

Further Reading

Ad Hoc Committee of the Harvard Medical School to Examine the Definition of Brain Death (1968) A definition of irreversible coma, 205 *Journal of the American Medical Association* 337–340.

Alexander MC, Leon RC (1972) A statutory definition of the standards for determining human death: an appraisal and a proposal. *University of Pennsylvania Law Review* 121: 87–118.

Breman SL, Delgado R (1981) Death: multiple definitions or a single standard? *Southern California Law Review* 54: 1323–1355.

Dworkin RB (1973) Death in context. *Indiana Law Journal* 48: 623–639.

Moosa E (1999) Languages of change in Islamic law: redefining death in modernity. *Islamic Studies* 38: 305–342.

Neeman Y, Sacks E *Euthanasia: The Approach of the Courts in Israel and the Application of Jewish Law Principles.* Jewish Virtual Library, American-Israeli Cooperative Enterprise.

Pallis C, Harley DH (1996) *ABC of Brain Stem Death.* London: BMJ Publishing.

Potts M, Byrne PA, Nilges RG (2000) *Beyond Brain Death, The Case Against Brain Based Criteria for Human Death.* Dordrecht: Kluwer.

President's Commission for the Study of Ethical Problems in Medicine and Biomedical and Behavioral Research (1981) *Defining Death: Medical, Legal, and Ethical Issues in the Determination of Death.* Washington, DC: The Commission.

Singer P (1994) *Rethinking Life and Death.* New York: St. Martins Press.

Shewmon DA (1998) Brain stem death, brain death, and death: a critical re-evaluation of the purported evidence, 14. *Issues in Law and Medicine* 14: 125–145.

World Health Organization (1994) *Legislative Responses to Organ Transplantation.* Dordrecht: Nijhoff.

MASS DISASTERS

Contents
Role of Forensic Pathologists
Organization
Principles of Identification

Role of Forensic Pathologists

M I Jumbelic, Upstate Medical University, Syracuse, NY, USA

Introduction

It is very difficult to conceptualize the forensic processing of a mass disaster. Unfortunately, this must be done more and more in this modern era. In the 1990s and more recently, there have been major mass fatality incidents (MFIs) including the TWA airline Flight 800 crash off Long Island, New York, in 1996, the unspeakable destruction of the World Trade Center twin towers in New York City, in 2001, and the 10 simultaneous bombings of commuter trains in Madrid, in 2004. Each event, with its unique multitude of casualties, creates its own set of hardships and circumstances. However, forensic scientists must see the common thread and apply professional protocols even in the face of extreme adversity.

Forensic pathologists, in particular, are called upon to perform perhaps the most gruesome of duties – detailing the physical aspects of the human carnage and helping to identify those who have perished. Families deserve that much – the return of their loved one and the knowledge of how he or she died. This article will document the involvement of forensic pathologists in the mass disaster scenario and how they can proceed with calm, and efficiency, applying forensic techniques in a sea (often quite literally) of fatalities (**Figure 1**).

Definition

Forensic pathology is the study of postmortem processes and focuses on investigations and autopsies to determine how people die. This discipline is involved with the medicolegal world and the certification of deaths. It is a special branch of the broader discipline of anatomic pathology, emphasizing the gross and microscopic analysis of human tissue taken at the time of surgical or autopsy procedures.

There are two main authorities overseeing death investigation in the USA, the medical examiner and the coroner. Forensic pathologists can serve as medical examiners working for municipal and state governments as the sole authority in explaining and certifying all sudden, unexpected, or unnatural deaths. Forensic pathologists can also serve as consultants to elected coroners providing pathologic expertise to the death investigation while the coroner remains the certifying authority. The goal of each system is the same, namely the determination of the cause and manner of death for an individual dying in sudden, suspicious, or traumatic circumstances. Unfortunately, the difference in the jurisdictional structure leads to a lack of uniformity in attaining this goal.

Forensic pathologists are physicians and as such take the Hippocratic oath to "do no harm." This applies to all patients, the dead as well as the living. Forensic pathologists are the deceased's advocate, speaking for them when they can no longer speak for themselves. Therefore, even though the magnitude of decedents at an MFI can be overwhelming, forensic pathologists must still apply this credo.

Mass Fatality Incidents (MFIs)

An MFI is considered technically to be any incident resulting in the death of more than one person. However, the practical definition of an MFI is the actual number of deceased determined to be an MFI on a

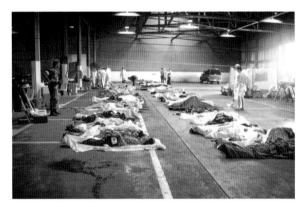

Figure 1   Temporary morgue. Recovered bodies from the Korean Airlines crash in Guam, August 1997, line the floor of the temporary morgue facility at the US Naval base.

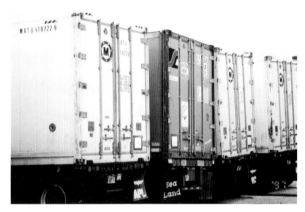

Figure 2   Refrigerated trucks. These vehicles are used for the temporary storage of human remains when the local morgue body cooler capacity is exceeded.

local level and should be defined by the death investigation team prior to the occurrence of an incident. For example, for Onondaga County and three surrounding Central New York Counties of approximately 1 million population, an MFI is considered to be any incident that results in the death of 10 or more people.

A mass disaster, another term sometimes used synonymously with MFI, is really any incident that exceeds available local resources. Thus, in a small rural jurisdiction, a two-vehicle crash with six fatalities might be classified as both an MFI and a disaster. While in a large urban center with a 3 million population, 15 deaths from an industrial accident might not be considered an MFI, though there are mass fatalities, and would be handled through routine processes (**Figure 2**).

The forensic pathologist brings a necessary expertise to an MFI. Two distinct priorities of every death investigation must also be addressed during an MFI – "identification" and "investigation." For all decedents, the same questions apply – the cause of the death and the identity of the person. The core training and daily experience of the forensic pathologist makes him or her well suited to answer these questions.

Philosophically, it may be asked what is the value of investigating the cause of death in certain obvious tragedies. For example, because the Twin Towers collapsed thousands of people died. Although the massive destruction is the cause of death, the forensic imperative goes well beyond the obvious. It is through the process of methodical death investigation that the forensic pathologist might uncover the sequencing of events preceding the death, as well as unsafe occupational, environmental, or transportation issues. Documenting the injuries and the mechanism of death provides answers to inevitable questions related to a

decedent's pain and suffering and leads to changes in design of aircraft, buildings, rescue equipment, and consumer products. Careful scientific analysis also ensures accurate identification of individuals. This forensic approach, to look for answers in the face of human tragedy, provides information to grieving families and on a larger scale, to their communities. Hidden benefits might emerge from a thorough investigation with detailed examinations and autopsies.

It is up to the forensic pathologist to ensure that professional protocols and procedures are followed, decedents properly identified, and the accurate cause and manner of death assigned. It is important to know whether someone died of blunt trauma injuries, or asphyxia due to mechanical compression, or carbon monoxide poisoning from a fire. Though it is not always possible to separate out these individual causes, it is the job of the forensic pathologist to try, even in the face of extreme adversity.

A special approach is needed for the forensic pathologist to properly address the challenging situation of an MFI. It is not easy to draw up an unwavering blueprint of what to do. The following represents a guideline that the forensic pathologist will use and the recommended roles to follow throughout a mass disaster. It should be remembered throughout that flexibility and adaptation are key to a successful operation. Investigating an MFI is literally an attempt to create order out of chaos, which makes each MFI unique.

Notification

The forensic pathologist's work begins at the time of notification of the MFI. The usual method of death notification will be expanded to include information critical for the emergency response. A standard death notification form includes caller's identity, date, time, and call-back number, specific data about the type of incident, and the agency handling the scene. In an MFI, information about the approximate number of fatalities, exact location of the incident, access routes to use, noteworthy conditions requiring special equipment or specially trained responders, exact location of the command post and staging areas, and the notification tree for appropriate personnel has to be collected.

Every office should have an emergency telephone tree so that each employee knows whom he or she is responsible to notify. Telephone numbers of personnel should be updated as needed on a regular basis and distributed to all staff members. The forensic pathologist needs to be familiar with this process as well as to have telephone numbers of governmental officials, medical personnel, and law enforcement agencies for contact at any time. This allows communication to take place in a timely and efficient fashion.

Advance Team

The first issue confronting the advance team is to ascertain the safety of the scene before actually entering it. The team should be prepared to follow specific biological, chemical, and radiation hazardous materials guidelines for any specialized treatment required in the handling and recovery of decedents. Details provided by the initial emergency responders and law enforcement investigative agencies guide the approaches the team will follow. For example, if there is a possible secondary explosive device, then the recovery of the dead is delayed until the immediate threat to life is handled by properly trained specialists.

The advance team includes the forensic pathologist and makes a preliminary assessment about the MFI. This assessment will consider the condition of the remains with the amount of fragmentation, commingling of the bodies, the state of decomposition, and alteration by the environment. Other items of importance that the team will assess are the incident locale, investigative questions, need for retention of evidence, community concerns, and available resources.

The forensic pathologist provides important expertise to the advance team since he/she is familiar with the normal postmortem processes, the effect of environment and trauma on the human body, proper evidence recovery, and the type of equipment and personnel needed for various tasks.

The advance team makes recommendations to establish a decision tree based on the specific circumstances of the mass disaster. This decision tree will address the constitution and differentiation of common tissue, nonidentifiable remains, and potentially identifiable decedents. Minimal examination will be done with the common tissue. These categories should be clearly defined in advance so that confusion does not result during triage. Every professional must follow the decision tree to avoid inconsistent actions at the autopsy table. When clearly delineated at the onset, it will be easier for everyone to follow a professional protocol.

Recovery of Bodies

An MFI usually begins as a rescue operation. One of the essential qualities of being human is our ability to hope. It is one of the hardest emotional aspects of the operation as efforts turn from rescue to recovery; when casualties become fatalities (**Figure 3**). However, once this occurs, the necessary structure must be put in place to accurately identify where bodies are recovered.

The forensic pathologist can help to establish a scene grid quickly to identify where remains are uncovered. This grid may use geographical positioning system (GPS) coordinates, geographic points (NE, SW, etc.), or other specific, physical descriptors. It must be a reproducible, permanent, and relevant framework used consistently by all throughout the entire recovery and investigation. Grid coordinates ensure that the pathologist's documentation of injury

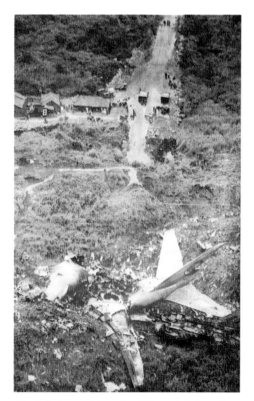

Figure 3 Aviation accident site. This aerial shot of a crashed jetliner reveals severe destruction of the aircraft and wide dispersal of bodies. The road in the upper portion of the photo was created by the military in order to reach the crash site.

will have greater meaning during later analysis. For example, if in one particular segment of the grid, all bodies are intact with minimal trauma, engineers and accident reconstructionists would investigate the physical reasons why this has occurred. Likewise an absence of a pattern may also be informative.

Generally, the human remains will be transported to a temporary morgue for examination. They should be respectfully placed in appropriately sized evidence or body bags and clearly labeled with the grid coordinates. The paper trail has begun and now each decedent can be placed historically back to the scene of the incident. Scientific relevance starts with the scene grid, so that the data collected by the forensic pathologist at the time of autopsy can be correlated to the incident milieu.

Disaster Manual

When an MFI occurs, it is the local jurisdiction that has responsibility for the retrieval, identification, determination of cause and manner of death, and death certification of each decedent. Every jurisdiction must be equipped with a disaster manual in advance with a consideration of available resources, types of disasters that might occur, and the community plan in the event of such an occurrence. A convenient list of available resources with contact numbers should be included in the manual to aid in swift communication. A recommended outline of topics covered in the manual is listed in **Table 1**.

Any forensic pathologist suddenly faced with an MFI in their jurisdiction will have a monumental set of demands and responsibilities. Those forensic pathologists familiar with emergency jurisdictional procedures can more easily establish contact with the local disaster management team and authorities in the command center. It is useful to work with emergency rescue and hospital personnel, and government and public health officials in a simulated exercise, utilizing the incident command system, and testing the lines of communication prior to a tragedy striking the community.

Triage

Triage involves the prioritizing of services and resources. A primary morgue station should be assembled to include experts from forensic pathology and anthropology, evidence collection, photography, and DNA (forensic biology/serology). This is where the preliminary physical examination of the remains is performed with photographic and X-ray documentation. The remains will be classified as human and potentially identifiable using classic forensic or DNA techniques, or as common tissue with no further

Table 1   Disaster manual: table of contents

I	Definition
II	Authority
III	Security
IV	Philosophy
V	Notification
VI	Advance team
VII	Establishment of morgue
VIII	Family Assistance Center
IX	Personnel
X	Consultants and volunteers
XI	Scene processing
XII	Transportation
XIII	Body processing
XIV	Identification
XV	Release of bodies and personal property
XVI	Records management
XVII	Media
XVIII	Communication
XIX	Critical Incident Stress Debriefing (CISD)
XX	Communication flowchart
XXI	Resource list including websites
XXII	State emergency management agencies
XXIII	Biologic, chemical, and radiologic agents

Table 2   List of nonhuman remains[a] recovered from the World Trade Center and brought to temporary morgue at Ground Zero, New York City, September 2001

Banana
Fig
Tomato
Beef ribs
Lamb chops
Insulation
Wig hair
Jelly
Turkey lunch meat
Kidney
Heart
Thoracic aorta
Small intestine with mesentery
Colon

[a]Initially thought to be human by recovery workers, but careful examination revealed the nonhuman nature of the material.

identification. No further examination will be done with remains labeled as common tissue.

Not all remains recovered at the time of a disaster will be human. An example of this is provided by the list of nonhuman material recovered at the World Trade Center (**Table 2**). In particular, nonhuman bones can confuse workers during recovery and may be initially mistaken as human. Rescue workers may recover discarded food (for example, squid or fish).

Specialists at the triage station can make the scientific decision to authorize disposal of the nonhuman remains, creating a more efficient workflow. If there is any question about the origin of the remains, then further examination should be performed including X-ray, histology, or DNA analysis.

Potentially identifiable human remains are the priority. Each specialist at the triage station provides unique expertise. The forensic pathologist provides soft tissue analysis, while the forensic anthropologist performs skeletal, jaw, and teeth evaluation. Evidence technicians can identify important trace materials while DNA biologists can select the best sites for viable tissue for testing. Photographers document the remains, evidence, and associated property as they are received. X-ray technicians assist with providing quality radiographic films.

At the preliminary examination, a presumptive identification might be made from associated property with the remains, such as clothing, an airline boarding pass, or jewelry. A distinction must be made between clothing and jewelry that are actually on the body part (e.g., a ring on a finger, a helmet on a head) and those items that are near or adherent (e.g., a wallet melded to nearby burned soft tissue, a badge next to an arm). Property physically on the body part is much more useful in a preliminary identification. It can point investigators in the right direction and limit the number of possible victims that this decedent may be. However, the physical property is only a clue to identification. It is not a scientific method for forensic identification of the remains. Consideration of property only (without corroborative scientific evaluation) may lead to false identification. For instance, a deceased first responder may have grabbed a coworker's helmet when responding to the initial emergency.

Computer Assistance

Computer databases are essential to help catalog, organize, and search the mass of information that is gathered at the disaster site. This has been enhanced by the increasing power of laptops, digital cameras, wireless networks, and the internet. For example, the case number and grid data can be immediately entered into a computer as soon as the remains are brought to the morgue. Preliminary examinations can then be entered into a laptop computer at the triage station including the important physical characteristics of the recovered decedent. Identification/case management programs are available and can be obtained prior to an MFI (e.g., WINID®, VIP®).

Concurrently, there is another aspect of the data recovery operation under way – the family assistance center. It is there that the victims' families are interviewed and provide extensive antemortem information about their deceased loved ones. This information includes past medical and surgical histories, physical characteristics, and clothing and jewelry descriptions that are then entered into a computer database. If this database is networked and shared between the family assistance center and the morgue, then a timely comparison of antemortem and postmortem data can be performed. This ultimately leads to proper scientific identifications.

Identification

The identification process utilizes classic forensic techniques to compare antemortem records and postmortem examination data (dental, radiographic, medical, and fingerprint analyses). In addition, DNA testing may be used to compare living relatives or the decedent's own cells left behind in a hairbrush, or toothbrush with DNA of tissue recovered from the human remains. Visual identification or the use of personal property found on the decedent does not meet the standard of a positive forensic identification.

A positive identification is that conclusion of the person's identity that reaches 95% certainty. In legal parlance, this is defined as "within a reasonable degree of scientific certainty."

A presumptive identification is a preliminary determination that narrows down the possible identities of the deceased. For example, following an autopsy, the deceased is known to be an elderly female with prior gallbladder, and appendix surgeries, permanently tattooed eyebrows, and an old amputation of the right big toe. In addition, within the pants pocket, still on the deceased's body, is a boarding pass with the name of Jane Doe. This information provides a likely but still preliminary identity. Further formal scientific examination (fingerprint, dental, and radiographic analyses) is needed to elevate this to the level of a positive identification.

Presumptive identifications are more likely to occur in instances where the decedents' bodies are fairly intact. However, there may be fragmentation and amputations with multiple body parts of a single individual recovered separately. Attention is then directed to remains that provide unique identifiers including hands for fingerprints, teeth for dental records, bones and soft tissue with surgical/metal appliances or prostheses, portions of skulls with teeth or sinuses, vertebrae and ribs, and old fracture sites. These body parts are considered potentially identifiable based on unique physical characteristics of the type and location of tissue. When the classic techniques of forensic identification are vigorously applied, the need for DNA analysis is lessened and the time required for individual identification shortened.

Some human remains recovered may exhibit no individually identifiable characteristics. Small fragments of bone or soft tissue may bear no recognizable feature. It is unfeasible and untenable to perform DNA testing on all recovered human materials. This is especially true with severe fragmentation resulting from high-velocity impacts. In addition, some remains may be sufficiently incinerated to consist only of powdery gray cremated material. These are scientifically unidentifiable as they are without viable cellular material for DNA testing. Some body parts and tissue fragments will be labeled as common tissue and never traced back to a specific individual. This is an unfortunate but important realization that must be made.

The local jurisdiction must ultimately make the difficult decision how far to continue with the identification process, once all forensic scientific efforts have been utilized. Local resources and the availability of DNA testing will also have an impact on this decision. One scenario might be that fragments of tissue unidentifiable by classic forensic identification modalities (dental, fingerprint, radiology), and measure less than $15 \times 15 \times 15$ cm, will be considered common tissue and no further testing will be done.

Nevertheless, every body part and fragment of tissue should be recorded even if not extensively examined. This documentation is helpful in understanding events and in assessing how many individuals perished.

A daily identification meeting should be held among the scientific specialists and the local authority responsible for certifying the death. This team should approve each individual identification and document the primary forensic method utilized. This ensures that all specialties (pathology, anthropology, fingerprint, dental, etc.) agree on the age, gender, ancestry, and identity of the person. This minimizes the possibility of a misidentification, and provides clear documentation of how each person has been identified.

Release of Bodies

Once the formal identification, examination, evidence collection, and investigative tasks concerning the individual decedent have been accomplished, the death certificate may be signed in accordance with local law. Notification of the next of kin of the decedent should be made in person through the family assistance center when possible. Details of the condition of the body and the remains recovered should be sensitively explained to the family. It is unwise to let them learn of this during their formal time of grieving at the funeral home.

Families will be asked to sign a release authorization that contains the name of their chosen funeral home. This release should also include information on whether or not the family wishes to be notified if any additional remains of their loved one are recovered. It is much easier to ask the family at this time, than several months later. If they do not wish to be notified, then any other remains recovered from that decedent will be considered as common tissue. Local law and custom will address how the common tissue should be handled.

Once the death certificate is signed along with the release authorization, the funeral home may claim the remains. Funeral directors should show identification and acknowledge possession of the decedent and any personal property that is turned over to them.

Personal Property and Evidence

Personal property intimately associated with the decedent that is not deemed evidence is turned over to the next of kin or the funeral director at the time of release of the body. Inventory of unassociated property is taken and cataloged with the hope of reassociating it with the proper family. This is a long-term effort and may require the support of a private agency with the resources to accomplish this task.

Evidence collection begins at the scene of the incident and continues to the triage station of the morgue. Law enforcement personnel responsible for the criminal investigation take custody of any material having evidentiary value. This is done in conjunction with other scientific specialists so that minimal manipulation of the body occurs.

Delegation of Duties

An MFI requires special assignments of responsibility in addition to normal duties. The forensic pathologist may assume leadership and administrative duties as well as performing autopsies. Thus the forensic pathologist must have scientific knowledge, management skills, and the requisite authority. Three vital leadership roles that require the expertise of the forensic pathologist include the commander responsible for overall management of the disaster, commander of daily operations, and morgue team leader who also serves as safety officer.

The commander of the MFI establishes required protocols for autopsies and examinations, approves all final identifications, signs all death certificates, releases information to the media, and coordinates with other command leaders to allocate resources and personnel. The commander of daily operations is responsible for ensuring that normal day-to-day functions of death investigation continue, and implements requests for outside assistance as needed. The morgue team leader is responsible for overall management of the morgue, creating a safe environment for the performance of autopsies, and assigns and supervises appropriate personnel, consultants, and volunteers for the morgue.

Other team leadership duties involve finance and logistics, search and recovery, records, identification, and family assistance, and these may be handled by other forensic specialists including death investigators. The chain of command should be enforced with personnel reporting to their designated supervisor with any problems, requests, or recommendations.

Communication

Effective interpersonal communication can enhance efficiency, reduce mistakes, and improve productivity. The forensic pathologist as medical examiner is often best equipped to coordinate daily group briefings to update staff on recovery statistics (number of body bags, number of identifications), changes in procedure, and any logistical issues. Such regular updates help workers maintain focus on their mission, boost morale, and limit rumors and fears.

A more extensive meeting can be held at the beginning of the operation and provide details about expectations and procedures along with a thorough review of the established facts of the investigation, and the purpose of the mission. Having workers sign confidentiality statements at this time is helpful in reinforcing an ethical standard of conduct.

Concluding informational sessions provide closure and a sense of accomplishment to people who have worked hard, often separated from their families and isolated from their normal routine.

Intersectional daily briefings by team leaders will ensure that each section (pathology, anthropology, dental, fingerprints, radiology, DNA) is aware of the issues of the other specialties and are updated with current concerns or changes in procedure. Brief intrasectional meetings at the change of shift will enhance efficiency, and encourage cooperation. Both provide opportunities for input and change in the challenging and stressful environment of a disaster.

Families of the victims must also be updated on a regular basis and receive accurate and timely information from the appropriately knowledgeable source. Often this is the forensic pathologist, who is prepared to address the medical issues and can

provide accurate numbers concerning decedents recovered and subsequently identified.

Community interest and media attention is heightened during an MFI. News briefings are essential but should be held after the family meetings and restricted to information that does not infringe on the rights of the victims or the work of the criminal justice system. It is wise to designate a Public Information Officer who will be the sole person authorized to communicate with the media.

International incidents, or those disasters that occur in one country but may involve the citizens of many nations, require special consideration. The legal jurisdiction will be the responsibility of the country where the incident occurred. However, many countries may have a strong interest in the investigative and forensic process. It is important to have representatives from those countries kept informed of the process. This may be done through the incident country's established agency to deal with foreign governments. It is also important to have interpreters available to facilitate communication, both for families, and foreign government representatives.

Pathology Protocol

The main pathologic procedures that will be performed on decedents include external examination, autopsy, and specialized autopsy. Decisions on which victims will be autopsied are based on prevailing laws and customs. Consideration should be given to the autopsy of all unidentified bodies, those without obvious cause of death, and a set percentage of remaining victims to provide meaningful statistical information. All bodies should receive as thorough an autopsy as is possible.

An external examination is a detailed viewing of the outside of the deceased's body, front to back and head to toe. Blunt and sharp force trauma, burns, patterned markings due to restraint, and explosive injury may all be seen on the skin of the decedent.

The autopsy incorporates the careful external examination with surgical incisions of the head and body to expose and evaluate internal organs. The internal organs are dissected, weighed, and examined individually. This internal examination may further delineate the extent of those injuries noted externally as well as preexistent natural disease.

Both types of examinations provide information as to the decedent's identity by revealing tattoos, unique physical characteristics, and old trauma and prior surgical scars. Additional testing such as X-ray and toxicologic studies may provide further important information, such as demonstrating occult fractures and quantifying alcohol or drug levels.

Basic anatomic findings in victims of a mass fatality often involve damage from blunt force, fire, and smoke inhalation. These injurious changes are carefully documented, with attention to their pattern, location, and areas of sparing. Interestingly, external burning of the body may not have caused death; rather the black, sooty material in the airway would indicate the person was alive in the fire and inspired toxic gases. Blood can be tested for the predominant toxic gas, carbon monoxide. Similarly, a decedent may appear relatively intact on the outside, with only a few scrapes and bruises, yet have fatal internal hemorrhaging from the aorta or liver.

In transportation disasters, special consideration must be given to those responsible for controlling the vehicle in question. The autopsy should attempt to answer questions on human performance and document visual problems, preexisting medical conditions with consideration of incapacitation and cause of death, a detailed description of stomach contents, injuries of the hands and feet due to possible contact and/or control of the throttle, yoke, or rudders, evidence of restraints, seatbelts, and the presence of any medications (**Figures 4** and **5**).

In an event the MFI involves a biologic, chemical, or radiologic agent, then special procedures may be required in the morgue. Examinations of the deceased should be limited and focused on obtaining fluids and tissues for evidentiary purposes.

Certain communicable or infectious diseases may necessitate the use of a more advanced biosafety level facility and specialized equipment such as high efficiency particulate air (HEPA) filter self-contained respiratory units (**Figure 6**). The Centers for Disease Control in Atlanta, Georgia, USA, can advise pathologists on appropriate autopsy techniques for individual biologic agents. State and local public health departments are also sources of information concerning prophylactic or postexposure antibiotic and/ or immunization treatments.

Chemical agents may require specific decontamination procedures either in the field or in the morgue. Certain toxins require that the stomach is opened under a fume hood, while others require holding the body 24 hours prior to performing the

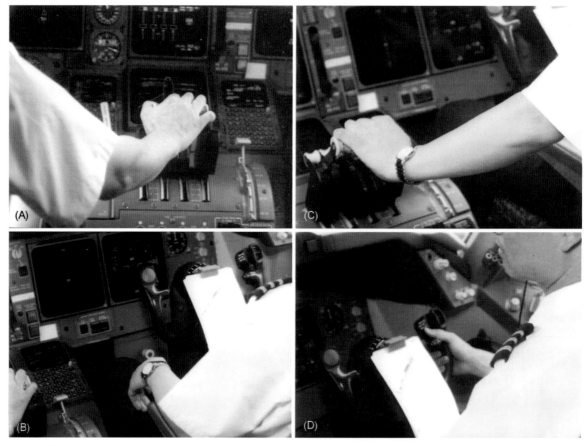

Figure 4 Flight deck of jet plane. (A) Captain demonstrates hand position when he is in control of the aircraft during take off and landing. (B) First Officer demonstrates hand position when at rest while the captain is in control to the aircraft. (C and D) First Officer demonstrates hand positions when he, and not the captain, is in control of the aircraft during take off and landing.

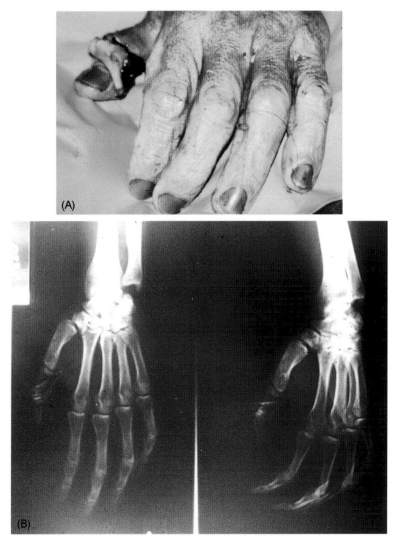

Figure 5 Hand of first officer from aviation accident. (A) The hand reveals avulsion of the left thumb. (B) X-rays of the same hand reveals underlying fractures of the middle and distal phalanges of the left thumb. Injuries on the hands of the flight deck crew must be carefully evaluated as they may indicate contact with the controls and who was in control of the aircraft at the time of the crash.

autopsy. Local hazardous materials teams are best suited to determine the necessary procedures. Radiologic agents may require decontamination and radiation monitoring with personal dosimeters for morgue workers. Environmental health agencies are knowledgeable about the monitoring for chemical or radiologic exposures that may occur in the morgue.

The documentation of the pathologic findings should be written and may be noted on an international DVI form or a local adaptation, such as the Pathology Examination Form of the Disaster Mortuary Operational Response Team in the USA.

Security

High-level security must be quickly established at the recovery scene, morgue, and family assistance centers. Personnel must wear specific identification badges with access privileges marked on each badge. Forensic pathologists may require access to all sites depending on their duties.

Law enforcement agencies should cordon crime scene perimeters at the disaster site. Curious observers must be prohibited from viewing the area. Families must be provided privacy at the family assistance center, away from media scrutiny. At all times the decedents must be treated with respect and confidentiality.

Critical Incident Stress Debriefing (CISD)

All MFI recoveries take their emotional toll on rescue and recovery workers. Sorting through endless carnage puts the pathology workers at particular risk.

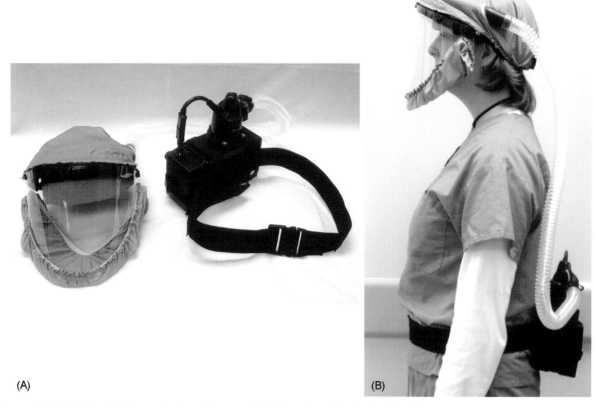

(A)   (B)

Figure 6 HEPA-filtered self-contained respiratory unit. (A) Overview showing the black battery-operated filter unit and attached plastic air hose and mask. (B) Side view showing medical personnel donning the respiratory unit that brings the filtered air past the wearer's face beneath the face shield. This unit is worn by morgue personnel to control exposure to infectious airborne pathogens.

Therefore, it is imperative to realize susceptibilities to the psychological stress of the work. Mental health professionals can assist workers in coping with their emotions and recognize possible trouble signs of grief overload and exhaustion.

See Also

Autopsy: Procedures and Standards; Pediatric; Adult; **Aviation Accidents, Role of Pathologist**; **Crime-scene Investigation and Examination:** Major Incident Scene Management; **Death Investigation Systems:** United States of America; **DNA:** Basic Principles; **Identification:** Prints, Finger and Palm; Prints, Ear; Facial; **Injury, Transportation:** Air Disasters; **Mass Disasters:** Organization; Principles of Identification; **Odontology:** Overview; **Terrorism:** Medico-legal Aspects; Suicide Bombing, Investigation

Further Reading

Bass WM (1995) *Human Osteology: A Laboratory and Field Manual*, 4th edn. Columbia, MI: Missouri Archeological Society.

Brogdon BG (1998) *Forensic Radiology.* Boca Raton, FL: CRC Press.

Eliopulos LN (1993) *Death Investigator's Handbook: A Field Guide to Crime Scene Processing, Forensic Evaluations, and Investigative Techniques.* Boulder, CO: Paladin Press.

Ellison DH (2000) *Handbook of Chemical and Biological Warfare Agents.* Boca Raton, FL: CRC Press.

Fierro MF (ed.) (1986) *CAP Handbook for Postmortem Examination of Unidentified Remains: Developing Identification of Well-Preserved, Decomposed, Burned, and Skeletonized Remains.* Skokie, IL: College of American Pathologists.

Hutchins GM (ed.) (1994) *An Introduction to Autopsy Technique.* Northfield, IL: College of American Pathologists.

Jensen RA (2000) *Mass Fatality and Casualty Incidents: A Field Guide.* Boca Raton, FL: CRC Press.

Mason JK (1993) *The Pathology of Trauma*, 2nd edn. London: Edward Arnold.

National Disaster Medical System (1998) *Disaster Mortuary Operational Response Team: Team Member Handbook.* Washington, DC: US Public Health Service.

National Transportation Safety Board (1999) *Federal Family Assistance Plan for Aviation Disasters.* Washington, DC: National Transportation Safety Board.

National Transportation Safety Board, in coordination with National Disaster Medical System (1999) *Morgue Protocols for Transportation Disasters*. Washington, DC: National Transportation Safety Board.

Spitz WU, Fisher RS (eds.) (1980) *Medicolegal Investigation of Death: Guidelines for the Application of Pathology to Crime Investigation*, 2nd edn. Springfield, IL: Thomas Books.

Stimson PG, Mertz CA (eds.) (1997) *Forensic Dentistry*. Boca Raton, FL: CRC Press.

Ubelaker DH (1999) *Human Skeletal Remains: Excavation, Analysis, Interpretation*, 3rd edn. Washington, DC: Taxaxacum.

Westveer AE (1997) *US Department of Justice, Federal Bureau of Investigation: Managing Death Investigation*. Washington, DC: US Department of Justice.

Organization

J Levinson, John Jay College of Criminal Justice, New York, NY, USA

Introduction

Definition of Mass Casualty

There are numerous definitions of a mass-casualty incident. The definition used here is an incident that requires a response beyond standard deployment. Thus, an incident in a small jurisdiction can be termed a mass casualty, whereas the same incident in a larger jurisdiction may be handled by the routine work force.

Organization

This article deals with the general organization of a mass-casualty incident response. As the above definition suggests, the deployment requirements for such a response are different from those needed for a regular crime scene. Medical aspects are part of that response and cannot be treated separately. They must be understood in the context of the general incident response.

Response Goal

The essential goal of a response is to restore life to normalcy. In a typical incident, this includes removing any dangers (hazmat (hazardous material), fire, etc.) and evacuating casualties and fatalities. Often in incidents occurring in a remote and unpopulated area, there is little or no disruption of daily routine.

Treatment of the injured, fatalities and identification of fatalities, however, are still prerequisites to reestablishing normal living patterns.

In a terrorist incident, the primary objective of the perpetrator(s) is the disruption of normal life. Thus, in such an incident there is often political pressure on response authorities to restore the area to normalcy and defeat the terrorist perpetrator, even at the expense of meticulous evidence collection.

Command

A basic rule of mass casualty management is that one single organization, best determined as part of pre-incident planning, has ultimate responsibility at the scene(s). Although this article refers to the "scene" as a matter of convenience, it should be noted that one incident can have multiple scenes. This is true, for example, in an air crash in which parts of the plane(s) fall at a significant distance from each other. This happened, for example, on December 16, 1960, when United Airlines and TWA flights collided over New York: one plane fell in Brooklyn and the other in Staten Island. In such a case, each scene can have its own commander, who reports to an overall incident commander.

A currently popular management system is the incident command system (ICS), a flexible framework originally developed for use by fire departments and now with versions adapted to other incident responders. A benefit of ICS is its ability to expand or contract forces as incident needs change.

Relations with the Media

Relations with the media start before an incident. Local reporters should be given a basic understanding of mass-casualty emergency planning, so that they understand the basics of disaster response. It is difficult to give such background during a response. Many disaster plans include sample press releases prepared in advance. These releases have a basic text with blanks to be filled in.

During an incident the commander's spokesperson acts as the coordinator of various agencies' representatives. This includes hospitals, ambulance services, and forensic medical institutes. When organized properly, each spokesperson will provide the same approved information, but from his/her agency's work perspective, thus giving the media various sources to quote.

A basic guideline is that incident command should be as forthcoming with information as possible. If incident command cannot supply information, reporters will find material for their stories elsewhere. By its nature, the information provided by representatives is slower than information received from private sources. The primary reason is that a spokesperson can never release news until it has been properly verified.

Information regarding criminal investigations should be withheld from the public, and the names of victims should not be released until families are officially notified. This can be time-consuming, particularly when next-of-kin are abroad or on vacation.

Press conferences should be scheduled regularly, particularly in an incident that continues for a long period of time. They should not be cancelled, even if there is no significant "news."

Photography, in the form of both video and stills, is part of news. Pictures can be provided to the press, but it is usually better to provide photo opportunities, provided they do not hamper the rescue and response effort.

It is a reality that media coverage (primarily the written press) determines the historical legacy of an incident and not what, in fact, really transpired.

Organizational Responsibility

Various organizations work under the authority of the incident commander, almost as autonomous units. If, for example, the incident commander is a senior police officer, fire and medical responders will work autonomously in their professional spheres. It is the function of the commander to coordinate the framework for working: this involves access/exit traffic patterns, unit staging areas, intergroup communications, and work priorities.

As a practical matter, there tend to be fewer problems of coordination between local police, fire, and the ambulance services, since they are accustomed to working together on a daily basis. More problems are encountered when external backup units are brought in, or with other groups who do not attend routine incidents.

On-Site: Nonmedical

First on Scene

The function of the first responder on site is to survey the situation and to report the situation to appropriate authorities. This is particularly difficult for a medical responder, who is sometimes tempted to begin treating the injured. Accurate reporting is the best way to insure the arrival of the appropriate number and type of responders.

It is common for there to be a certain amount of confusion in the initial postincident period of response, as forces arrive, and a command structure is established.

Police Functions

One of the first tasks of police at a mass-casualty incident is to establish traffic patterns, so that other emergency vehicles can have relatively unhindered access to the area, then rapid exit to destinations such as hospitals. This includes designating parking areas, so that the vehicles of responders do not hinder traffic. An extension of this function is the rerouting of general traffic away from the incident area, with appropriate notice to the public, usually by radio and mobile phone announcements.

Another police task is to cordon off the incident area, limiting access to authorized personnel only. The objectives are to allow efficient work and to provide basic security of information and evidence. Closing off the immediate area also prevents unscrupulous media representatives from conducting interviews with those victims needing or receiving medical attention. This task is extremely difficult, since it also involves tactfully removing volunteers who were essential immediately after the incident took place and witnesses who need to be interrogated. There is also not an absolute list of responders who are authorized to be present; the list varies according to the progress of the response. For example, after victims have been removed from the site, only a small medical contingent is necessary – and then for first aid.

Additional functions in which police often play a role are incident reconstruction (in the case of specialized incidents such as aviation, often delegated to agencies established for the purpose) and locating out-of-area relatives through law enforcement liaison channels.

Fire Functions

The obvious duty of the fire department is to extinguish all fires. This includes notification to responders that particular areas are safe for entry and monitoring the scene to ascertain that no additional fires break out (e.g., in cases where there is a fuel spill).

In some jurisdictions the fire department is assigned a role in first aid and extrication, since they normally perform these functions.

Staging Areas

An efficient organizational plan is to divide the mass-casualty area into two or three zones. The inner zone is that area of direct response. Only active responders are allowed into this zone to minimize confusion and allow the least interference with work. In many cases the number of workers allowed in this zone is pragmatically restricted by space. Depending on the size of the incident, one or two outer holding zones are established; it is there that responders wait with their equipment before they are told to move forward.

Some disaster work is sequential and not simultaneous. Fire fighting, for example, often precedes the introduction of medical responders into the affected area. Dealing with the injured precedes handling the dead.

Evidence

A mass-casualty site is a potential crime scene. One approach is that it should be considered a crime scene until proven otherwise. How can an earthquake, for example, be considered a crime scene? There have been numerous examples of the collapse of a building due to the use of substandard construction materials.

Suicide terrorist attacks should also be treated as a crime scene, even though the bomber has been killed. In the vast majority of such incidents, there is a group of people who manufactured the explosive device, planned the incident, and transported the bomber. Proper evidence collection will assist in their arrest and prosecution.

Although medical necessity certainly justifies moving evidence, photographic recording of the scene as early into the incident as possible can be a major help in incident reconstruction.

Other Functions

A variety of nonemergency functionaries have roles at a mass-casualty incident. These range from insurance adjustors to structural engineers. Each function has to be evaluated independently in terms of entry to the scene. The structural engineer might be needed immediately to decide if a building is safe to enter; the insurance adjustor can be admitted much later.

Disaster Myths

There are many myths and misconceptions about behavior after a mass-casualty incident. Taking these myths into consideration during planning results in a more realistic response.

Rarely, for example, is there panic. Victims can be selfish in their desire to save themselves, even to the extent of pushing others aside, but it is only when there is no clear escape route that they sometimes make irrational (i.e., "panic") decisions.

Contrary to popular conception, victims who are not seriously injured are not helpless. Many save both themselves and others before professional rescuers arrive. This is also true for passers-by, who often play a critical role in rescue before trained personnel come to the scene. Part of planning is

the orderly replacement of volunteers by professional staff.

Another myth is that of looting, the open and wanton stealing of property. This is an extremely rare phenomenon. Much more common is quiet and surreptitious theft, often within the definition of souvenir hunting.

On-Site: Medical

Ambulance Deployment

There are two approaches to routine ambulance deployment. One is to station ambulances at a dispatch center from which they are sent to various incidents. Another is to park ambulances in neighborhoods, often at the house of the driver, who is dispatched through a communications network. The latter system has the advantage of quick response due to dispersal throughout a city; in addition, the simultaneous arrival of numerous ambulances is often counterproductive, since they cannot all receive patients at the same time.

Another idea now being tested is the use of motorcycles carrying limited supplies to a mass casualty site. These motorcycles generally arrive before regular ambulances. Negative considerations in this approach are the minimal amount of time saved and lack of equipment. Another point of concern is that ambulances arrive and quickly depart from the scene; motorcycles are parked, thus complicating scene management.

Victim Treatment

In a mass-casualty situation the basic goal is "to do the most good for the largest number of people." This differs from standard medicine, where the goal is to save lives. In practical terms, when the injured outnumber the medical staff available, doctors sometimes have to forgo the intensive treatment of a patient who might otherwise be saved, so that more patients can be treated. This change in medical emphasis is often a root cause of postincident psychological trauma for medical responders.

A second goal is the identification of the dead (disaster victim identification (DVI)), which requires cooperation between police and legal–medicine personnel. From an organizational perspective, the police are often tasked with collecting background information about the disaster and antemortem information. Forensic medical personnel are tasked with collecting most postmortem information and comparing it for identification purposes. Needless to say, there must be coordination between the two functions, so that there is an emphasis on the collection of antemortem information corresponding to medical needs.

In popular language, there is sometimes confusion between mass casualty (injury) and mass fatality (death). It is very common that a large incident will include both casualties and fatalities.

Triage

A triage or examination area is established for the rapid examination of victims extricated from a disaster site. Such an area is located close to, but at a safe distance from, the mass casualty incident. In triage a priority evacuation system can be established when victims outnumber ambulances, allowing for the most seriously injured to be evacuated first. A common technique in triage is to fasten commercially available preprinted labels to victims, indicating the priority of their evacuation.

When the number of ambulances available equals or exceeds the number of victims, the "scoop-and-run" system is often used for evacuation. In such cases, victims are removed from triage in the order they arrive. Prioritization of treatment becomes a hospital function.

It is common for medical staff to attempt rudimentary stabilization of patients in the triage area, before they are transported to hospital.

Medical Precautions

Mass-casualty sites often include numerous medical hazards, ranging from sharp metal edges to bodily fluids. Potential responders should maintain up-to-date inoculations such as tetanus and hepatitis. In addition, they should be supplied with protective clothing, often of the disposable type.

There is no one kind of protective clothing that is appropriate for all hazardous situations; thus, supply must be both adequate and flexible. A general guideline for quantity of all response equipment is a sufficient supply until additional materials can be obtained. In most cases this will include 24/7 emergency arrangements with commercial sources. When sharp edges (e.g., bent and torn metal) are present, thick-soled shoes and heavy gloves are recommended. In hazmat incidents, sometimes an entire closed-system breathing apparatus is required.

Record-Keeping

A record is kept of victim dispatch to hospital. This will necessarily be incomplete due to those who are less seriously injured being evacuated independently, but it will be of major assistance in bringing order to the evacuation procedure. These records should be compared and verified with hospital reception records.

In many cases hospitals record the reception of patients by their type of injury and the treatment needed. Records should always include the incident involved, so that victims of the mass-casualty incident can be separated for record-keeping purposes from other hospital patients.

Decontamination

There are numerous types of hazmat mass-casualty possibilities, ranging from commercial industrial accidents to terrorist chemical attacks.

In many cases it is necessary to decontaminate exposed victims. The decontamination procedure varies according to the contaminant. One general rule with many substances is that the exposed victim has to be washed and given uncontaminated clothing. The dead must be decontaminated externally and sometimes internally as well.

Victim Identification

There is no professional rule concerning the presence of forensic pathologists at the mass-casualty site. Most pathologists want to visit the site to gain a first-hand impression of what happened. Others rely on police reporting. In any event, the functions of victim identification teams at the scene are to photograph all bodies and property where they were found, then remove them to a forensic institute. Victim identification is not done on-site.

On-Site: Nonmedical

Communications

Communications gear should be accessible to all responders. Senior coordinators should have equipment enabling contact with counterparts in other agencies (for example, both fire to police, and fire from jurisdiction A to backup from jurisdiction B).

Studies show that the most significant problems in response almost always revolve around issues of communications.

Communications systems should have backups. Mobile phone lines notoriously become overloaded and nonfunctional. Batteries also fail. One communication possibility that should not be overlooked is a point-to-point landline telephone, from, for example, the command center to the commander on site (usually a short distance away). This provides excellent security of conversation while at the same time providing a line that is always available.

Equipment

A reality in disaster response is that available equipment rather than predetermined planning usually determines a unit's function.

One successful approach to organizing response equipment is advance packaging for a specific function, with an officer in charge of logistics for transporting the packages. In pragmatic terms, it is assumed that a police crime scene unit is responsible for handling the mass-casualty site (similar to their routine work). Their equipment would be divided into various suitcases – photography supplies, interrogation forms, etc. The unit logistics officer would be responsible for transporting the suitcases, either by individual police officers or in a larger shipment.

Mass-casualty equipment should be prepared in advance and checked periodically. An ambulance, whether in a single or mass-casualty response, generally deals with only one patient. Many other functions, however, deal with a situation much larger than routine and need appropriate equipment in larger quantities.

Responder Identification

It is helpful if all responders wear uniforms and/or vests to identify their function and command status (e.g., supervisor) at a mass-casualty response. Vests have the added advantage of being specially designed with pockets to carry essential equipment such as communications gear or writing tools.

At later stages of the incident it is recommended to use badges changed daily to control entrance into incident response facilities.

Volunteers

On-site volunteers can be classified according to groups. Other than individuals, professionals, or otherwise, who chance to be near a mass-casualty incident, there are volunteers who are members of nongovernmental organizations (NGOs), and those who are an auxiliary force within the framework of an official government group (e.g., volunteer fire). NGOs and official volunteers are often motivated to offer their services both from charity and excitement or importance.

Psychological Reactions

Posttraumatic stress disorder (PTSD) is a common psychological reaction to mass-casualty incidents. Its symptoms can start at the scene, but they are much more likely to develop afterwards. Some response agencies station a clinical psychologist at a mass-casualty site to monitor the behavior of personnel; this has both mental health and quality-of-work benefits. In any event, postincident debriefings are held several days later, after responders have pondered their actions. At these sessions psychologists can detect reactions beyond the norm.

Job burnout has some symptoms which are similar to PTSD, but the problem and its treatment are significantly different. It is important that a trained psychologist makes this differentiation.

Off-Site

Information Bureau

The purpose of an information bureau is to coordinate details about an incident and to provide relevant information to various customers. An information bureau is best staffed by representatives of numerous organizations, taking into account foreign-language requirements. When run properly, the information bureau will accept a maximum number of telephone and personal inquiries, so that other organizations can carry on routine and emergency functions as far as possible (e.g., an airline whose aircraft has crashed still needs to make other flights; an ambulance service needs lines free to accept emergency calls unrelated to the mass-casualty incident).

Casualty Bureau

A casualty bureau is a subset of the information bureau. It is set up to centralize the collection of personal information about the victims of an incident.

One specific function of an information bureau is to assist families to locate injured or missing relatives without overloading hospital telephones. This is done by centralizing all hospital patient lists and relieving hospitals of the burden of answering inquiries.

Sometimes a casualty bureau is confused with a fatality bureau. This happens because, after all hospitalized victims are identified and reunited with family, the emphasis of work turns to the identification of fatalities.

When dealing with fatality inquiries, telephone staff are equipped with forms to be filled out concerning the relationship and contact numbers of those making inquiries. This will later be of assistance to facilitate possible police requests for antemortem data.

Victim Identification

DVI is the positive comparison of antemortem and postmortem information that is of sufficient significance. An institute of forensic medicine is usually in charge of DVI, even when the identification is apparently "obvious." This is necessary for subsequent legal proceedings.

The most common organizational system for DVI is that advocated by Interpol. Antemortem information is collected on forms printed on yellow pages. Postmortem information is collected on pink pages printed with the same questions. Administrative correspondence is done on white paper. (The forms can be downloaded from the Interpol website: www.interpol.int.)

A large chart is usually prepared showing the mortuary body number in a center column. On the one side are the various types of antemortem information, with a check mark to show what has been collected. On the other side are similar columns for postmortem information. One can then see at a glance what further information must be collected. For example, if there are no postmortem fingerprints, no antemortem prints are necessary. Finally, there is a column for the victim's name when it has been determined. Using a wall chart can be a positive factor in sustaining morale, allowing responding workers to see progress in identifications.

There are numerous computerized information comparison programs available. These are primarily for dental information, but general programs are also to be found. Experience has shown that input time and uniform terminology usually render these programs impractical. One manual method to cope with information management is to divide files into groups (adult/child, male/female, etc.). Mistakes (such as age) can be corrected by periodic regrouping.

In some mass-casualty plans, a single significant type of identification (e.g., fingerprints or odontology) is sufficient to assign a name to the deceased. In other plans multiple types of identification are preferred to prevent possible error.

In the USA nine disaster mortuary operational response teams (DMorts) have been established under the disaster response plan of the Federal Emergency Management Agency (FEMA). These teams include victim identification capabilities ranging from forensic specialties to morticians and clerical support. They stand ready to give support to local jurisdictions or to assume responsibility in federally recognized disasters. The teams are modular; part or all of the DMort infrastructure can be activated as a situation requires.

Notification of Death

Notifying next-of-kin about the death is both a humanitarian and legal function. From the viewpoint of the latter, family should be requested to acknowledge receipt of the notification.

Some emergency plans call for the presence of first-aid personnel and equipment at forensic institutes when notifications are made. In many instances those notifications include viewing the body of the deceased, which increases psychological trauma.

Burial

Burial (or cremation) of the deceased is not a part of the incident response. Identified bodies are released into the custody of the legal next-of-kin, who are then responsible for making all further arrangements. After a body is identified and found to be not from the country of the incident, it is "repatriated."

Memorial Services

It is common for the incident command to arrange for nonsectarian or multifaith memorial services, as is deemed appropriate. According to circumstances of the incident, such ceremonies can take place relatively soon after the incident and subsequently on annual anniversaries.

See Also

Mass Disasters: Role of Forensic Pathologists; Principles of Identification

Further Reading

Auf der Heide E (1989) *Disaster Response: Principles of Preparation and Coordination.* St. Louis, MI: CV Mosby.

Dynes RR (1974) *Organized Behavior in Disaster.* Columbus, OH: Disaster Research Center.

Einolf DM (1998) *HAZWOPER Incident Command: A Manual for Emergency Responders.* Rockville, MD: Government Institutes.

Interpol (1992) *Disaster Victim Identification Guide.* Lyons, France: Interpol.

Levinson J, Granot H (2002) *Transportation Disaster Response Handbook.* London: Academic Press.

Mitchell J, Bray G (1990) *Emergency Services Stress.* Englewood Cliffs, NJ: Prentice Hall.

Poulton G (1988) *Managing Voluntary Organizations.* New York: Wiley.

Skertchly A, Skertchly K (2001) Catastrophe management: coping with totally unexpected extreme disasters. *Australian Journal of Disaster Management* 6(1): 23–33.

Walsh M (1989) *Disasters, Current Planning and Recent Experience.* London: Edward Arnold.

Principles of Identification

C M Milroy, University of Sheffield, Sheffield, UK

Introduction

Mass incidents may bring challenges to the investigating authorities. In addition to the issues of identifying the victims, the police may be faced with a homicide investigation and the handling of the scene, and the postmortem examination must proceed with the assumption that a criminal prosecution is a possibility. In performing an autopsy the pathologist must answer a number of questions, in particular who the deceased was and how he/she came to die. There are a number of methods by which a body may be identified, and these will be discussed in turn. These criteria apply whether the incident is a true disaster or brought about by humankind, such as conflicts or acts of terrorism.

At any major incident the person who has the duty to investigate the death legally – be it the coroner, medical examiner, procurator fiscal, or examining magistrate – will need to liaise with other experts in the process of identification. A supervising pathologist should be identified to act as the person who conducts and oversees the autopsies to be performed and to liaise with the coroner or equivalent. A senior identification manager (SIM), a senior police officer, should also be appointed. These people should all be part of the Identification Commission, a team that is standard in Interpol countries. The Commission includes the Incident Commander, SIM, supervising pathologist, coroner, or equivalent position and other police officers, such as family liaison officers, whose duty is to confirm the identity of the remains. Ideally the Commission should meet daily.

The International Committee of the Red Cross has drawn attention to the duty of governments to help identify the victims of wars and internal conflicts in its project The Missing. The principles that apply to the identification of the victims of an air crash also apply to the victims found buried in a mass grave.

Basic Procedures

Following any mass incident a system of logging bodies at the scene should be in place so the continuity of any body can be traced. The same applies to any body parts. The bodies are placed in a body bag with identification labels both inside and outside. The bodies are then brought to the mortuary, whether it is a temporary mortuary or an established facility, again

preserving continuity. The bodies are photographed with the identification label and the clothing removed and searched. Consideration for collection of trace evidence and/or radiological examination should be made before any clothing is removed, e.g., if explosives are suspected as a cause for the incident. The body should be cleaned down and re-photographed. Radiological examination can also be performed at this stage. The body can then undergo the autopsy, documenting features for identification as well as determining the cause of death. At the autopsy, samples for DNA analysis should be collected, as well as for other analyses such as histology and toxicology.

Once the autopsy is complete, the body can undergo fingerprinting and footprinting, if necessary. These procedures can, if desired, be carried out before the autopsy after any necessary trace evidence has been collected. Following the autopsy the odontological examination can also take place, including dental radiology. Once the body has been autopsied and other ancillary procedures have occurred, it can be reconstructed and embalmed if required.

Methods of Identification

Identification criteria can be divided into primary and secondary identification criteria. The traditional methods of identification have been visual. They cannot now be considered as the best methods and are prone to inaccuracy. These methods are now considered as secondary identification criteria.

Primary Identification Criteria

Fingerprints   Fingerprints, if not destroyed , are easy to obtain and allow for accurate identification. Therefore, fingerprints should always be collected. They then need to be compared with preexisting fingerprints. These can be obtained from records if present, or by obtaining latent fingerprints. Fingerprints are taken from all citizens in some countries and in others when they have committed a criminal offence. Other groups, such as military personnel, may have fingerprint records. In other cases latent fingerprints may be obtained. In these latter cases, where there is a presumed identity article known to have been used by the deceased such as a shaving can, deodorant can, the car driven to the station, or similar objects that are known to have been handled, this can be examined for fingerprints and then compared with those taken from the body. As fingerprints are considered a unique identifier, fingerprints are an objective primary identification criterion. Similarly, footprints could be used if for some reason a record is kept, as is the case with some military personnel, or latent footprints could be obtained. However, consideration must be given to the problems created when the victim's home has to be searched and examined for these latent prints, which may be distressing to the grieving relatives. One issue that arose in the "Marchioness disaster" in the UK (an incident where two boats collided on the river Thames in London resulting in the loss of many lives) and led to a judicial inquiry (the Clarke Inquiry) was how fingerprints should be obtained from a body. In the Marchioness disaster a number of hands were cut off and sent to a laboratory. When this was discovered, it caused a significant outcry from the relatives and led to the establishment of a public inquiry in England into how victims should be identified following major disasters. The removal of hands or digits should never be carried out unless there is no alternative method of identification.

Odontology   Odontological examination of every victim should be considered, including radiological examination. Teeth are the most resilient structures in the body and therefore can survive conditions where other features are destroyed, whether by trauma, fire, or decomposition. Odontological examination has been one of the most employed methods for identification for many years. Although DNA analysis has now come to be a key feature of mass incident identification, dental identification remains important. As with other methods of identification, antemortem data are required for comparison and the ability to obtain dental records will determine how useful the method will be in any disaster. Furthermore, with improvements in dental health, no dental treatment may have been carried out. Therefore it is possible that this method of identification may not prove as useful as might at first have been anticipated. The removal of the jaws from the body for odontological examination should be considered carefully before being undertaken, as it may be distressing to the relatives. At present with appropriate antemortem dental records, forensic odontology provides a rapid method of identification which does not require the laboratory time that DNA analysis currently takes. Forensic odontology can also provide anthropological data and age estimation from the eruption of teeth, or by histological examination.

DNA analysis   DNA analysis has made a significant contribution to identification since its development in the 1980s. At the autopsy, tissue should always be collected for analysis. Traditionally blood or muscle has been used but any tissue can be analyzed. In intact bodies a buccal scrape can be used; this is the standard method by which those arrested for criminal offences are analyzed. As has already been described,

teeth are often the least damaged of tissue and can be used to obtain DNA for analysis. DNA analysis has two roles in mass incidents. These are in primary identification and in allowing dismembered bodies to be reunited. This latter role shows the power of DNA analysis but also raises questions about how far investigation is required for the reuniting of remains. This may depend on cultural and religious requirements as well as legal duties. Mitochondrial DNA may be an available resource when nuclear DNA has degraded, though only the maternal line will be identified.

The ability to store material for DNA analysis now means that where there are victims who cannot be identified, particularly where there is disruption or fire damage of bodies, as in the terrorist incidents of September 9, 2001 in the USA, subsequent tests in the future may become possible. As DNA technology advances, degraded or damaged DNA-containing tissue may become identifiable.

Secondary Identification Criteria

Visual identification   Traditionally a relative or close acquaintance would carry out the legal process of identification. This is still the commonest method of identification in single deaths, where the issue of identification is not in real dispute. However, there are many problems with visual identification in mass incidents and it should not be considered a primary method of identification. Relatives or other people who knew the deceased may not be available, but even if they are, incorrect identification of victims is well recognized with visual identification. Visual identification must be considered as a subjective method of identification. Therefore, if visual identification is to be used it should be used alongside another objective scientific criterion. Viewing of the body for grieving purposes by relatives is a separate issue and may be possible following confirmed identification.

Clothing and other artefacts   The clothing and jewelry worn by the victim may be identifiable by a relative as those worn by the deceased. This provides clues, but should not be considered as an objective criterion. Fashions may be copied and at some incidents, such as where sports spectators are killed, many people may be wearing the same shirts in support of their team. Similarly there are problems with other possessions. Personal items may be duplicated and the possibility of someone carrying another person's possessions cannot be excluded. In at least one mass incident a pickpocket had stolen a number of wallets before he died in the incident. Personal possessions should only be considered as secondary identification criteria.

Body features The sex, height, weight, hair color, and eye color are all useful pointers to the identification of the victim, but cannot be considered primary objective scientific criteria. Body scars, deformities, and tattoos should also be considered as pointers to identification, but it will be unusual for them to be considered objective criteria. Tattoos are said to provide possible unique identification, because their exact structure and position on a body could not be replicated, but to confirm this requires firm corroborative evidence, such as a good-quality photograph or the tattoo artist's professional opinion that he/she carried out the tattoo and these data are unlikely to be available in a mass incident setting.

Autopsy findings The use of a full autopsy in mass incidents will vary between jurisdictions. As well as establishing the cause of death, the internal examination may provide clues to identification if previous surgical procedures have been carried out or implants such as cardiac pacemakers inserted. However, these cannot be considered primary identification criteria, unless they have a unique identifying number, in which case the number may be able to be checked with medical records or the manufacturer, when it can then be considered a unique identification criterion.

Radiology Radiological examination may be performed as part of the autopsy. Radiological features such as implants or frontal sinus structure may be present which allow for identification. This will require a comparison of antemortem records, which are required for objective identification and may not exist, or be difficult to obtain.

Forensic anthropology Where there has been disruption of bodies or the remains have partially or completely skeletonized, forensic anthropology can provide useful information. Examination of the skeleton can allow an estimation of stature, build, and age of the victim. Along with the determination of sex and ancestry, this allows for exclusion of some victims and inclusion of others, refining the search for victims. With disrupted or skeletonized bodies, commingling of remains is a common problem and examination of the skeletons can determine the minimum number of victims as well as refining the criteria for identification. Typically, examination of the skeleton will only provide secondary identification criteria, though unique features, such as a previous amputation or unusual pathology, may allow more definite identification, especially in a closed incident.

Conclusion

Many methods of identification are available. Traditional methods such as visual identification are unreliable. Secondary identification criteria provide useful intelligence to narrow down the number of potential victims to be related to an individual body, but formal identification should be based on fingerprints, odontological examination, or DNA analysis.

See Also

Court Systems: Law, Japan; **Crime-scene Investigation and Examination:** Recovery of Human Remains; **Terrorism:** Suicide Bombing, Investigation; **War Crimes:** Site Investigation

Further Reading

Busuttil A, Jones JSP, Green MA (2000) *Deaths in Major Disasters. The Pathologist's Role*, 2nd edn. London: Royal College of Pathologists.

International Committee of the Red Cross. The Missing. www.icrc.org.

Jensen RA (1999) *Mass Fatality and Casualty Incidents. A Field Guide*. London: CRC Press.

Lord Justice Clarke (2001) *Public Inquiry into the Identification of Victims Following Transport Accidents*. London: Stationery Office.

Vardon-Smith G (2003) Mass disaster organisation. In: Payne-James J, Busuttil A, Smock W (eds.) *Forensic Medicine. Clinical and Pathological Aspects*, pp. 56–578. London: GMM.

Mass Disasters, Aviation *See* **Aviation Accidents, Role of Pathologist**; **Injury, Transportation:** Air Disasters

---

Mass Disasters, Scene Investigation *See* **Crime-scene Investigation and Examination:** Major Incident Scene Management

MASS MURDER

A Aggrawal, Maulana Azad Medical College, New Delhi, India

Introduction

Mass Murder

The term "mass murder" may mean different things to different people. It has been applied to as diverse situations as Whitman Texas Tower shootings, the mass poisonings in Jonestown, Jack the Ripper's murders, the Holocaust, Bhopal industrial disaster, Oklahoma bombings, World Trade Center attacks, the practice of euthanasia, and even the current liberal abortion policy around the world. The Federal Bureau of Investigation (FBI) Academy's Behavioral Science Unit at Quantico, Virginia, however, defines "mass murder" as the killing of four or more victims in a "single location" and in a "single event," with no emotional cooling-off period in between. The event is typically unplanned and unexpected. Killings of lesser numbers of victims have been given separate terminologies. Thus, killing of one victim is called a "single homicide," two victims at one time in one location is called a "double homicide," and three victims at one time in one location is a "triple homicide." Most authorities now believe that triple homicide should be treated as mass murder too. A few would even include a double homicide among mass murders. Thus Dion Terres, who killed two people and wounded a third at a McDonald's restaurant in Racine, Wisconsin, USA on August 10, 1993, is frequently classified as a mass murderer by many authorities. Similarly, Steven Benson of Florida, who set up a bomb in his car to kill his mother and adopted brother, on July 9, 1985, is also classified as a mass murderer. It is often the intention that counts. Benson had intended to kill a third victim – his sister Carol Lynn – but she survived the explosion.

Typically a mass murderer walks into a government office, restaurant, shopping mall, school playground, or other such public place and begins randomly shooting innocent bystanders. He usually commits suicide after his killing incident, or puts himself in such a situation that the police have to kill him – the so-called suicide by cop. A typical mass murderer is a loner male, with chronic extreme anger, paranoid ideation, and depressed mood. He kills in order to gain a brief moment of control by controlling the fate of others.

Serial Murder

An emotional cooling-off period is what differentiates a mass murderer (and spree murderer) from a serial murderer. "Serial murder" is defined as the killing of three or more persons in three or more separate events in single (when the killer returns to the same place to kill) or multiple locations, with an emotional cooling-off period between homicides. This emotional cooling-off period may last from a few hours to years. The serial killer premeditates his crimes, fantasizing and planning the murders in detail. He also selects his victim, usually a targeted stranger he has been stalking before the murder.

A serial killer usually goes after strangers, but the victims tend to share similarities such as gender, age, or occupation. Though he prefers a certain look or background, if he can't find his intended target, he will often substitute it with another victim.

The minimum number of killings which would qualify for the cluster of homicides being classified as a serial murder is a matter of controversy. Many authorities believe that killing two people in two different events should be enough to constitute a serial killing.

Spree Murder

A third type of multiple murder is the "spree murder," which is defined as the killing of three or more people (the number of killings is also controversial here) in a single event with no emotional cooling-off period in between, but at two or more different locations. The single event can be of short or long duration. In the case of Howard Unruh (**Table 1**), all killings and woundings took place in about 20 min. Charles Whitman, in comparison, killed over a period of several hours. On the night of July 31, 1966, he went to his mother's apartment (location 1) where he shot her; then returned to his house (location 2) and stabbed his wife to death (on August 1 at about 3.00 a.m.). He left his house at 9.00 a.m. the same day, and climbed up a 92-m (307-ft) clock tower at the university of Texas (location 3), where he started firing at 11.45 a.m. and continued shooting till around 1.20 p.m. In the tower, he killed an additional 15 people. The homicidal event in this case lasted almost a day, but since there was no emotional cooling-off period between the killings, it is classified as a spree murder.

A kind of hybrid is also known to exist, the spree serial killer, where the murders occur within a shorter time span than is usually taken by serial killers.

Table 1 Differences between various forms of multicides

Type of multicide	Time of murders (variable 1)	Location (variable 2)	Typical example	Year/day	Persons killed
Mass murder	Same (no emotional cooling-off period)	Same	Crown Prince Dipendra (Nepal)	June 1, 2001	9 (including himself) + 3 injured
Serial murder	Different (emotional cooling-off periods, varying from a few hours to years, between homicides)	Same/different	Jack the Ripper (London, UK)	From August 31, 1888 (the date of first murder) to November 9, 1888 (the date of last murder)	5 prostitutes according to most estimates. However, estimates differ, from 4 to 9
Spree murder	Same (no emotional cooling-off period)	Different	Howard Unruh of Camden, NJ, USA. Randomly fired his loaded German Luger while walking through his neighborhood	September 6, 1949	13 + 3 wounded

The time span could perhaps be several days. The victims of a spree serial killer do not share similarities, as they do with serial killers.

Two most important variables that differentiate the three major forms of multicides are the cooling-off period in between homicides (variable 1) and location (variable 2) (**Table 1**).

The presence of an emotional cooling-off period between two consecutive killings in serial murders is an important variable. It is during this period that the killer has the opportunity to control his behavior and stop the act of murder. His failure to do so makes the serial killer a much more dangerous criminal. The absence of a cooling-off period in mass and spree murder precludes the possibility of the killer controlling his behavior.

Another distinction between serial killers and mass murderers is that, while a serial killer painstakingly tries to conceal his crime, a mass murderer has little interest in doing so and indeed may kill himself after the crime. It has been suggested that mass murderers are often suffering from a mental illness that may be associated with childhood trauma and sexual and/or physical abuse. In contrast, serial killers may show little evidence of mental disturbance, and outwardly they appear quite normal, despite the horrendous crimes they have committed. **Table 2** lists important differences between serial and mass murderers.

Multicide

Mass murder, serial murder, and spree murder (also double and triple homicides, if they are counted as separate categories) are species of the larger family "multicide," which means multiple killings.

Classification of Mass Murderers

A number of classifications of mass murders exist. Here are some of them.

Classification by Douglas *et al.*

Douglas and coworkers classify mass murderers into two broad types: (1) classic mass murderers; and (2) family mass murderers.

Classic mass murderers Typically a classic mass murderer is a single person, operating in one location at one period of time. He is a mentally disordered individual, whose problems have increased to such an extent that he acts out against groups of people who are unrelated to him or his problems. He unleashes his hostility through shootings and stabbings. George Hennard is a typical example. Hennard smashed a pickup truck through a restaurant window in Killeen, TX, USA on October 16, 1991 and fired on the lunchtime crowd with a high-powered pistol, killing 23 people.

Family mass murderers A family mass murderer kills four or more family members in a single incident. Family mass murderers are further subdivided into two subtypes: (1) those who commit suicide afterwards; and (2) those who do not. Crown Prince Dipendra of Nepal (**Table 1**) represents the former and John List the latter. On June 1, 2001, 29-year-old

Table 2 Important differences between a serial and mass murderer

Trait	Serial murderer	Mass murderer
Personality	Psychotic individual, who kills for pleasure. Some have termed this "mental orgasm"	A deranged individual who explodes suddenly and unpredictably due to extreme stress
Emotional cooling-off period between killings	Present	Not present. All killings take place at the same time
Planning/premeditation	Plans his murders carefully	No planning. Acts on impulses
Pursuit of publicity	Quite often a motive	Rarely a motive
Patterns	Displays very well-defined patterns and rituals which he uses in each killing	Shows no patterns or ritual to his killing
Selection of victims	Selects his victims carefully	Usually no selection of victims. Kills at random
Location	Crime is committed at secret places, in isolation	Usually in public places, in full view of everyone
Use of multiple weapons	Takes one or two weapons to the crime scene	Takes many weapons and an enormous amount of ammunition (even provisions, in some cases) to the crime scene
Concealment of crime	Tries to conceal crime. Does not want to be apprehended. Tries not to leave evidence	No attempt at concealment. Not worried about leaving evidence
Suicide committed after crime	No	Quite often
Motive for killing	Mentally disturbed	May be mentally disturbed, but often revenge motives prevail

Crown Prince Dipendra killed eight members of his family and injured three, before killing himself. On November 9, 1971, 46-year-old John List shot his 85-year-old mother, his 45-year-old wife, 16-year-old daughter, and two sons aged 15 and 13, and absconded. He was apprehended by the FBI in 1989.

Classification by Dietz

Park Elliott Dietz first classified mass murderers into three subcategories: (1) family annihilators; (2) pseudocommandos; and (3) set-and-run killers. In 1992, Holmes and Holmes offered two further categories: (1) disciples; and (2) disgruntled employees.

Family annihilators These are generally chronic alcoholic middle-aged males who kill their wife, children, pets, parents, and in-laws, often without warning. They are usually depressed, paranoid, intoxicated, or a combination of these. The family annihilator usually commits suicide after the killings, or may force the police to kill him, the so-called suicide by cop. A typical example is the murders carried out by Nepal's Crown Prince Dipendra.

Pseudocommandos These are young men obsessed with firearms, who start shooting indiscriminately in crowded places. They fancy themselves as military types, and frequently plan their offense with some detail. Their rampage usually ends in suicide. A typical example is 41-year-old James Oliver Huberty who, on July 18, 1984, killed 21 people and injured 19 at a McDonald's restaurant in San Ysidro, CA, USA.

Set-and-run killers These killers set up the stage, so to say, and then quit. Arsonists, bombers, and poisoners who plan their attack sufficiently to make good their escape belong to this class. The unknown Tylenol poisoner may be classified in this subcategory, but would perhaps be better classified under the category of mass poisoner. Steven Benson of Florida, already mentioned, who killed his mother and adopted brother with a car bomb on July 9, 1985, would be classified in this category.

Disciples These are people who are unduly influenced to kill by a charismatic leader.

Disgruntled employees These are the employees who retaliate for what they feel was bad treatment by their employer. Thirty-three-year-old Paul Calden was an employee of Fireman's Fund Insurance Company in Tampa, FL, from where he was fired. On January 27, 1993, about 9 months after he was fired, he carried a gun into the cafeteria of that company and opened fire, saying, "This is what you get for firing me." He killed three coworkers and seriously injured two others. After the rampage, Calden killed himself. He represents a typical example of this group.

This classification makes use of several bases, mixing together motivation, the specific relationship between the victim and the offender, and technique for killing. This leaves a system that is neither mutually exclusive nor exhaustive in describing cases of mass murder. While several offenders could fit into more than one category, there are a number of other offenders who would not fit into any of them.

Classification by Levin and Fox

Levin and Fox classify mass murderers using just one base – motivation. According to their model, all mass murderers could be categorized as one or more of the following types.

Motivated by vengeance These are the individuals who think they have been wronged and they want to "pay back in the same coin." Several mass murderers, like James Oliver Huberty and Dion Terres, have been heard saying before killings, "Now it's payback time." This theme was also seen in the 1993 destructive action of Gian Luigi Ferri, the 55-year-old business man whose murders in a San Francisco law office were apparently due to his nursed resentments about failed business schemes and anger at the legal system.

These revenge-based homicides have three subtypes:

1. individual-specific, where the offender targets particular people
2. category-specific, where particular groups of people are targeted
3. nonspecific, where the murders are precipitated by the offender's paranoia, and where the offender does not have specific targets.

Motivated by a warped sense of love Rarely, a mass murderer can be motivated by a warped sense of love, such as the murders committed by John List, who was a respected accountant and known to be a very religious man. He felt, for no sound reason, that "he could not keep his family happy, so they had to go."

Motivated by profit These are felony murders, which are purely for monetary gain, such as murders committed during a bank robbery.

Motivated by political considerations Suicide bombers would come under this category. But since these killings carry a political statement, most experts would include them separately under acts of terrorism, rather than as mass murders. Thus, cases like the US World Trade Center attack or the Akshardham temple killings in India, where 28 innocent people praying in a temple were indiscriminately gunned down on September 24, 2002, are clearly cases of terrorism.

Classification by Kelleher

Kelleher identified seven categories of mass murder, all motivated by different factors:

1. Revenge: this is essentially the same as that found in Levin and Fox's classification.
2. Perverted love: again, this is similar to Levin and Fox's "warped sense of love" category, involving the killing of family or loved ones.
3. Politics and hate: this category is ideologically motivated, and usually involves acts of terrorism.
4. Sexual homicide: this theme is most often seen in serial murders and rarely in mass murders.
5. Mass executions: this involves the contract murder of several people in a single incident.
6. The insane: these have no motivation other than mental illness.
7. Motiveless: no motivation can be found in these cases.

Classification by Petee *et al.*

Petee and coworkers in 1997 provided one of the most comprehensive classifications of mass murderers to date. Instead of taking just one criterion for classification, they took two: offender motivation and target selection. Based on these two selection criteria, they came up with nine categories. They are careful to provide at least one convincing example from each category.

Anger/revenge – specific person(s) target In this category, the offender is angry and wants to "get even" with the persons who "wronged" him. He has in his mind specific persons as targets. He does not shoot at random. The case which best fits this category is that of 28-year-old student Gang Lu, who, on November 1, 1991 killed five people in Iowa City, IA, because he was not nominated for a prestigious award for his doctoral dissertation. He thought he had been wronged by his professors, so he shot down three of them, including the departmental chairman. He also killed a university administrator, as well as a Chinese fellow-student Linhua Shan, who had been nominated for the award Lu coveted.

Anger/revenge – specific place target In this category, the motivation remains the same as in the above category, i.e., anger and revenge, but the target is a specific place instead of specific persons. The place is usually where the killer was "wronged."

The case of 33-year-old Edwin James Grace best illustrates this category. An employment agency had been unable to secure a job for him. On June 21, 1972 he reached the place where the agency was located (Cherry Hill, NJ, USA) and started shooting indiscriminately. Six people were killed and six were injured. It is important to note that Grace targeted the location, not specific people. In fact, he killed people who were not associated with the employment agency.

Anger/revenge – diffuse target Here again the motivation remains the same, but the target is diffuse. This group can be subdivided into two further categories: (1) cases where specific groups or categories of people are targeted; and (2) cases where people are just shot at random.

Cases where specific groups or categories of people are targeted In this subcategory, the killer vents his anger on a specific group of persons, such as members of a particular race. The target is diffuse in the sense that no particular person is aimed at. Instead, the target is a particular group or community. The case exemplifying this category is that of 35-year-old Colin Ferguson, who killed six passengers (and wounded an additional 19) on a Long Island commuter train on December 7, 1993. He was consumed by a hatred of white people. On December 6, 1989, 25-year-old Marc Lépine killed 14 women at École Polytechnic, Montreal, Canada, because he hated feminists. George Hennard also disliked females and most of his targets were females. In 1989, Patrick Purdy shot and killed five people because he hated Asians. Roland James Smith was moved by feelings of antisemitism. Baruch Goldstein disliked Arabs and killed 29 in 1994. James Oliver Huberty disliked Hispanics and targeted individuals of that group.

Cases where people are just shot at random In this subcategory, the killer aims at his victims at random. Neither specific persons nor specific groups are targeted. The target is truly "diffuse." The case of Dion Terres, who killed at random at a McDonald's restaurant, best typifies this subcategory.

Domestic/romantic This category is mainly based on the criteria of target selection. It can also be subdivided into two further subcategories:

1. Domestic type: the killer targets members of his own family for various reasons. The case of John List best typifies this subcategory.
2. Romantic type: the killer may have been spurned in a love affair. Richard Wade Farley had been rejected by his colleague Laura Black. So he shot seven employees of the defense firm where Black worked, including her.

Direct interpersonal conflict This category seems similar to category 1 above, except that the anger is more immediate in this category. In the first category, described above, the feelings of anger may have been simmering for a long time, and finally find expression at some unpredictable time. In mass murders involving direct interpersonal conflict, the feelings of anger are generated "on the spot." The case of Ray Ojeda best typifies this category. He killed three persons in San Antonio, TX, in 1991. Ojeda had been involved in a minor traffic accident He began to argue with the driver of the other vehicle. As the argument escalated, Ojeda went back to his car, pulled out a gun, and shot the other driver. When two bystanders tried to intervene, Ojeda killed them as well.

Felony-related mass murder Here murders are committed during the commission of another felony, usually robbery. The killer may feel that the situation is getting out of hand, and may resort to mass murder. There may also be a need to eliminate witnesses.

The case of Robert Melson and Cuhuatemoc Peraita best typifies this category. In 1994, they robbed a Popeye's Chicken restaurant in Gadsden, AL. After gathering up all the money, they herded the employees into a walk-in freezer and shot them all, killing three and seriously wounding one. This case is also representative of multiple offenders involved in mass murders. It is estimated that more than half of felony-related mass murders involve an accomplice.

Gang-motivated mass murder This category includes murders during gang confrontations. Usually there are multiple offenders. The dispute between two Vietnamese gangs in New York in 1990 is characteristic of this type of offense. After an argument in a Manhattan bar, David Tai, Tommy Tam, Peter Wang, and Ywai Yip followed the members of a rival gang into a parking lot, shooting and killing all three execution-style. The infamous Valentine day massacre, which occurred on the morning of February 14, 1929 in Chicago, IL, also belongs to this type. Seven people (five belonging to the rival Bugs Moran gang) were mowed down by Al Capone's killers.

Politically motivated mass murder This category involves acts of terrorism. The motivation is primarily ideological, usually for some political cause.

Other causes may include religious intolerance, or a campaign for political change. Since these acts carry a political or a religious message, they are best classified as acts of terrorism.

Although Petee *et al.* do not suggest a further subdivision of this category, it can be divided into two further subcategories: (1) when the perpetrators are not present at the scene; and (2) when the perpetrators are present at the scene.

The perpetrators are not present at the scene　In this category the offender is typically absent from the scene of the crime when the victims are killed. This category thus corresponds to the "set-and-run" category suggested by Dietz. The bombing of the Alfred P. Murrah Federal Building in Oklahoma City, OK, on April 19, 1995 by Timothy McVeigh and of the World Trade Center in New York on February 23, 1993 serve as examples of this form of mass murder.

The perpetrators are present at the scene　In the early morning of May 14, 2002, three persons aged 19–20 years boarded a Himachal Tourism bus at Vijaypur, India. They were dressed in combat uniforms and looked like army personnel. The bus was going from Pathankot to Jammu. At 06.15 a.m. the perpetrators stopped the bus near Kaluchak, shot the driver and the conductor of the bus, and opened fire indiscriminately on the passengers in the bus. They also opened fire on a number of army personnel and their families in the vicinity. By 10.00 a.m., when all three had been killed by army personnel, they had killed 31 people and wounded another 47. The suspected political message that they carried was the liberation of Kashmir.

Nonspecific motive　Petee *et al.* like to call this category the "residual" category. Here the offender's motivation is not clear. He may be psychologically deranged. As an example they cite the 1988 case of Clem Henderson that occurred in Chicago, IL. Henderson murdered four people in a space of less than 20 min.

Amok and Mass Murder

Amok is a culture-bound syndrome (CBS) strongly associated with mass murder. Though initially reported from Malaysia in the sixteenth century by European travelers, it is seen, with somewhat lesser frequency, all over the world. A CBS may be defined as a constellation of symptoms, which may have little medical basis, but which are strongly influenced by a society's social codes and mores and its cultural values. It is more or less a "learned behavior," which may be expressed subconsciously. Violent self-sacrificial behavior, coupled with an initial fanatical charge, indiscriminate slaughter, and a refusal to surrender, is often taught as part of the cultural training of Malays and Javanese. A common tactic among Malay warriors was to charge forward brandishing their daggers shouting, "Amok! Amok!" This was supposed to increase their courage, while at the same time terrifying the opponent. Young warriors were socially and culturally encouraged to emulate this behavior, often as an instrument of social protest, if a ruler became a tyrant and abused his power. This behavior was also useful as an act of religious fanaticism, whereby it became necessary to slay all "infidels" indiscriminately. Since this behavior had a strong social value, it was often condoned – even encouraged – by the society.

Gradually amok lost its social value, and became more personal in nature. If, for example, a person's ego was bruised by an insult, he would often take recourse to this behavior. Most often, however, the behavior appeared motiveless. Typically, the assailant, known as a pengamok, would brood for several days. Then suddenly, without any warning, he would leap up with his dagger in his hand, and kill everyone within reach. Dozens of people might be killed during an attack. The attack would last several hours until the pengamok was either overpowered or killed. If he managed to survive, he would pass into deep sleep or stupor for several days, followed by total amnesia of the event.

Generally four components of amok are recognized:

1. a variable period of prodromal depression, often running into days
2. a sudden and unpredictable homicidal drive, lasting for several hours
3. absence of personal motive
4. a subsequent amnesia of the event.

Psychiatrists are divided over whether the act is conscious or a manifestation of automatism. That the behavior might be a conscious act, rather than an act of automatism, becomes evident when we note that the number of cases dropped sharply after the UK took over the administration of Malaya, and it was ordered that all amok cases be captured alive and brought to the court.

A number of social, cultural, personal, and medical causes of amok have been described in the literature. **Table 3** summarizes some of the major causes of amok. A combination of two or more causes may be present in a particular case.

Table 3 Major causes of amok resulting in mass murder

Category	Cause
Social	(1) An instrument of social protest by subjects, when their ruler became a tyrant or abused his power
	(2) As an act of religious fanaticism, whereby it became necessary to kill all infidels
Cultural	(1) Cultural training for warfare, a war tactic, a concept of courage
	(2) Emulation of epic heroes who behaved in this way
Personal	(1) Escaping from distress, a tension-reducing device
	(2) Fragile ego coupled with threatened self-esteem
Medical	(1) Psychiatric disorders (e.g., schizophrenia)
	(2) Febrile delirium
	(3) Tuberculosis
	(4) Syphilis
	(5) Epilepsy
	(6) Consumption of psychoactive drugs such as cannabis or opium

Profile and Characteristics of a Mass Murderer

A study of mass murderers in the USA and Canada during the past 50 years suggests that such individuals are usually single or divorced males in their 40s with various axis I paranoid and/or depressive conditions and axis II personality traits and disorders, usually clusters A and B. The episode of mass murder is precipitated by a major loss related to employment or a relationship. A warrior mentality suffuses the planning and attack behavior of the subject. If the perpetrator is psychotic at the time of the offense, greater deaths and higher casualty rates are significantly more likely. Only 20% of all mass murderers directly threatened their victims before the offense. Alcoholism and the use of pornography are usually associated with a mass murderer. Death by suicide or at the hands of others is the usual outcome for the mass murderer.

A number of situations seem to motivate a mass murderer to act, and such situations are called "high-risk situations." Some are continuous unemployment (especially men), the loss of a job, loss of self-esteem as a breadwinner, guilty feelings for not being a good provider, and hatred because of presumed wrongs by other people. These people may be the employer, spouse, figure of authority, the police, or even the "system." Sometimes, a mass murderer is moved by feelings of racial rejection.

In several cases, the mass murderer initially may have only one target in mind, for example, an ex-wife, a former boss, or a friend. But once the killer enters the place where his intended victim is, he may start indiscriminate shooting to kill everyone in the neighborhood.

Mass murderers tend to have violent changes of temperament. They may be meek at one moment and livid the next. This may happen because the perpetrator has feelings of inadequacy or feels he is being duped by society.

An important characteristic of a mass murderer is that he displays "predatory aggression" rather than "affective aggression." Affective aggression is a rather normal form of aggression, which is aimed to reduce threat. It is a defensive mode of violence, which is accompanied by high levels of sympathetic arousal and emotion such as anger, and is a time-limited reaction to an imminent threat. In contrast, predatory violence is an attack mode of violence. It is planned and emotionless and is accompanied by minimum autonomic arousal. The person engaging in predatory violence (the mass murderer) often appears very calm and confident, with no signs of nervousness. While a person displaying affective aggression does so in response to a perceived threat, there is no immediate perceived threat in predatory aggression.

Future Trends

Despite the work that has been done to date, research on mass murder is clearly in its infancy. One major reason for this is the very small sample size that is available for research. Just about 100 mass murderers are known to date. This has perhaps dissuaded most clinicians, sociologists, criminologists, and forensic psychiatrists from taking up this subject for further research. But clearly this subject is teeming with endless research possibilities. There are many areas that need further exploration. One is the pathophysiology of the limbic system in such individuals. The limbic system comprises the cingulum, hippocampus, thalamic and hypothalamic nuclei as well as the basal ganglia, midbrain, and the amygdala. It is this area that is associated with uncontrolled rage, such as is displayed by mass murderers just before their acts. How does the physiology of the limbic system in mass murderers differ from that of normal individuals? Which factors trigger it and how? Or is it different at all?

Another area of research could be the possible effects of heredity and environment. There are many studies indicating that genetic makeup as well as environmental factors may influence violent conduct in a person. Some studies seem to indicate that there is a distinctly increased tendency towards violence in individuals having the XYY chromosomal configuration. Is it possible to find some commonality in the genetic makeup and environmental influences of mass murderers? If it is, interventional steps may be taken to reduce this phenomenon.

Selective serotonin reuptake inhibitors (SSRI) are known to inhibit the predatory aggression that is often seen in mass murderers. When a potential future mass murderer is isolated, a pharmacological treatment with SSRIs may be considered. This is another area where more research is needed.

See Also

Mass Poisonings; **Murder–Suicide**; **Serial Murder**; **Terrorism:** Medico-legal Aspects

Further Reading

Dietz P (1986) Mass, serial and sensational homicides. *Bulletin of the New York Academy of Medicine* 62: 477–491.

Douglas JE, Burgess AW, Burgess AG, Ressler RK (1997) *Crime Classification Manual – A Standard System for Investigating and Classifying Violent Crimes.* San Francisco, CA: Jossey-Bass.

Geberth VJ (1986) Mass, serial and sensational homicides: the investigative perspective. *Bulletin of the New York Academy of Medicine* 62: 492–496.

Hempel AG, Meloy JR, Richards TC (1999) Offender and offense characteristics of a nonrandom sample of mass murderers. *Journal of the American Academy of Psychiatry and Law* 27: 213–225.

Holmes RM, Holmes ST (1992) Understanding mass murder: a starting point. *Federal Probation* 49: 29–34.

Kelleher MD (1997) *Flashpoint: The American Mass Murderer.* Westport, CT: Praeger.

Kon Y (1994) Amok. *British Journal of Psychiatry* 165: 685–689.

Levin J, Fox JA (1985) *Mass Murder: America's Growing Menace.* New York: Plenum Press.

Levin J, Fox JA (1991) *Mass Murder.* New York: Berkeley Books.

Lindquist O, Lidberg L (1998) Violent mass shootings in Sweden from 1960 to 1995: profiles, patterns, and motives. *American Journal of Forensic Medicine and Pathology* 19: 34–45.

North CS, Smith EM, Spitznagel EL (1994) Posttraumatic stress disorder in survivors of a mass shooting. *American Journal of Psychiatry* 151: 82–88.

Petee TA, Padgett KG, York TS (1997) Debunking the stereotype: an examination of mass murder in public places. *Homicide Studies* 1: 317–337.

Rappaport RG (1988) The serial and mass murderer: patterns, differentiation, pathology. *American Journal of Forensic Psychiatry* 9: 39–48.

Time-Life (1992) *Mass Murderers.* Alexandria, VA: Time-Life Books.

MASS POISONINGS

A Aggrawal, Maulana Azad Medical College, New Delhi, India

Introduction

The term mass poisoning can be defined as poisoning – with or without a fatal outcome – of three or more victims in a single location and in a single event. When the poisoning takes place at different intervals, say over a period of months or years, it may be termed serial poisoning. Both forms will be considered together in the current discussion.

Classification

Mass poisoning can be classified as described below and is illustrated with historical examples.

Intentional

Homicidal

1. A specific victim targeted with a specific motive (e.g., Marie Besnard, who poisoned 12 of her relatives with arsenic in 1950s, so that she could inherit money)

2. No specific victim targeted (e.g., tylenol capsule murderer, who laced tylenol capsules with cyanide and caused the deaths of seven random victims in 1982)

3. Terroristic in nature, i.e., when the poisoner wants to make a political statement (e.g., Tokyo subway attack with the nerve gas sarin on March 20, 1995 by the members of the Japanese cult Aum Shinrikyo, in which 12 people were killed and 5000 injured)

4. Antiterroristic in nature, i.e., when a group or government intends to save hostages from terrorists (e.g., release of BZ gas by Russia on October 26, 2002, when Chechnyan rebels took more than 750 hostages. BZ gas killed 118 people, including mostly hostages)

5. Warfare (e.g., in the First World War (1914–1918), deliberate use of chlorine, phosgene, and mustard gas resulted in more than 100 000 deaths and 1.2 million casualties).

Suicidal Suicide pacts (e.g., the case of Jim Jones and his followers, who drank cyanide-laced grape Kool-Aid in Jonestown, Guyana, on November 14, 1978.

A total of 914 people died, including Jones. There were 638 adults and 276 children).

Unintentional

Accidental

1. Natural (e.g., eruption of Mount Vesuvius, near Pompeii, Italy, in 79 AD, releasing toxic gases. More than 2000 people were killed)
2. Caused by humans, or industrial (e.g., death of over 2000 people on December 2, 1984 in Bhopal, India, due to accidental release of methyl isocyanate from a small pesticide division of Union Carbide Company manufacturing carbaryl)
3. Related to medicinal drugs (e.g., the thalidomide, where this sedative and hypnotic drug was taken by thousands of pregnant mothers in Europe from 1958 until 1961. It only became apparent in 1961 that this drug was responsible for the congenital anomalies amelia and phocomelia; also in this category are variable responses to drugs)
4. Associated with illicit drugs (e.g., contaminated drugs used intravenously)
5. Related to food (e.g., there were several outbreaks of St. Anthony's fire in the Middle Ages due to infected rye containing ergot alkaloids)
6. Related to water (e.g., outbreaks of chronic arsenic poisoning amongst people who had been drinking ground water with very high arsenic levels. This is common in Calcutta, India, and Bangladesh)
7. Occupational (e.g., chronic lead poisoning occurring in professions dealing with lead (plumbers, potters, printers, pewters, and painters))
8. Related to poor standards of sanitation (e.g., any number of food- and water-poisoning cases occurring in various places).

History of Mass Poisoning

Criminal mass poisoning was not uncommon in Ancient Rome. Several factors accounted for this phenomenon. There was no effective law against poisoning. A reasonably vast variety of poisons were known and were easily available to all and sundry. Finally effective treatment against poisoning was not known. The first known episode of mass poisoning occurred in about 200 BC. The Roman historian Livy informs us that, after investigation, about 190 matrons, mostly of patrician birth, were finally executed for this episode.

A similar episode occurred again in Rome about two centuries later. About 150 women poisoners, again mostly patricians, were executed. But the supplier of their poisons – a woman known as Locusta – so impressed the then Emperor Nero (37–68 AD), that not only did he grant her a complete pardon, but he appointed her as a court poisoner! Nero took great interest in her poisoning activities. Nero and Locusta would often experiment on slaves together, trying out and testing their newfangled poisons.

One ally of Locusta was Queen Agrippina (16–59 AD), wife of Emperor Claudius I (10 BC–AD 54), and mother of Nero. In quest of power, she is thought to have assassinated a number of persons by poisoning, including her own husband Claudius.

The Italian School

In the Middle Ages mass poisoners returned when the ancient Roman art of mass poisoning was perfected by a Spanish family Borgias, living in Italy. (It is worth quoting Max Beerbohm: "I maintain that though you would often in the fifteenth century have heard the snobbish Roman say, in a would-be-off-hand tone, 'I am dining with the Borgias tonight,' no Roman was ever able to say, 'I dined last night with the Borgias'.") The main proponents of mass poisoning in this family were Rodrigo Lenzuoli Borgia (1431–1503), who became Pope Alexander VI in 1492, and his two illegitimate children, a son, Cesare Borgia (1476–1507) and a daughter, Lucrezia Borgia (1480–1519). Between them, they are reputed to have poisoned hundreds of political adversaries. The poison they used was a concoction known as "La Cantrella," which was believed to contain arsenic in high quantities.

"La Cantrella" was prepared elaborately. It is believed that a hog was killed with arsenic; its abdomen was opened and sprinkled with more powder, which contained more poison. Some historians think that the powder contained just arsenic, but it may have contained other poisons as well. The animal was then allowed to putrefy. The juices that trickled from the decaying corpse were collected and evaporated until only dry powder remained.

Such was the Borgias' reputation that people were afraid even to shake hands with them, as even the rings they wore were supposed to be laced with poison.

Two other Italian mass poisoners of note during this period were Heironyma Spara, an astrologer, sorceress, and a mass poisoner all combined in one, who was executed in 1659, and Madame Giulia Toffana (c. 1635–1719), also known simply as La Toffana.

Toffana – perhaps the most active mass poisoner of all time – was supposed to have been responsible for killing at least 600 people. Just as the Borgias' poison had a special name, Toffana's poison had one too; it was known by a number of names, such as aqua toffana, agua toffana, aquetta di Napoli, manna of St. Nicholas di Bari, or elixir of St. Nicholas of Bari, Bari being a town whose water had healing qualities. It was supposed to be a cosmetic (to keep the law at bay, presumably), but most buyers knew why they were buying it. They were instructed about its poisonous properties and its potential as a lethal weapon! La Toffana was finally caught and executed in 1719.

The French School

The Italian school of mass poisoning flourished through the fifteenth and sixteenth centuries. In the seventeenth century, the art of mass poisoning was brought to France by Catherine de Médici (1519–1589) of Florence. She married King Henry II (1519–1559) in 1533. Her main accomplices were the Florentines René Bianco and Cosme Rugieri. Catherine poisoned many of her adversaries, principally the Queen of Navarre, Jeanne d'Albert; Duc d'Anjou; a Marshall of France, Coffe, and finally, the Cardinal of Lorraine.

The French school of mass poisoners was undoubtedly typified by Marie Madeleine, the Marquise de Brinvilliers (22 July 1630 to 16 July 1676). She married Marquis de Brinvilliers at the age of 21 (1651). In 1660, she became friendly with one Chevalier Godin de Sainte-Croix. Her father had him thrown in the Bastille, where he met an inveterate poisoner Antonio Exili. Exili taught him the art of poisoning during the 7 weeks Sainte-Croix was in jail. After his release, Sainte-Croix teamed up with his lover and unleashed an era of indiscriminate poisoning, where people were poisoned for seemingly trivial reasons; for example, a person had to die because he had spilled coffee on Brinvilliers' dress. The Marquise de Brinvilliers perfected her art of poisoning by experimenting on hospital inmates. She used to pay visits to a hospital run by the Sisters of Mercy, the Hôtel-Dieu, carrying poisoned biscuits and preserved fruits for the inmates as gifts. As they deteriorated, she used to pay courtesy visits, but in fact she was taking down copious notes about their condition.

Sainte-Croix died in July 1672, apparently poisoned by Brinvilliers herself. Her reign of indiscriminate poisoning finally ended with her decapitation on July 16, 1676.

Another French mass poisoner of note at this time was Catherine Deshayes (1638–1680), also popularly known as Catherine Montvoisin, or La Voisine. She killed over 2000 infants, many as human sacrifices in the worship of Satan. Her end came 4 years after Brinvilliers'. She was burnt at the stake on February 23, 1680.

Table 1 gives information on these and other notable mass poisoners of history.

Medical Professionals as Mass Poisoners

Medical professionals such as doctors and nurses are in a special position to be able to administer poisons on a mass scale, since their relationship with their patients is that of belief and trust.

The first known case of a medical mass murderer is that of Dr. William Palmer, also known as "the Rugeley poisoner." Palmer is supposed to have killed as many as 15 persons during 1855–1856 with antimony (**Table 1**). That this phenomenon has not come to an end is typified by the modern case of Dr. Harold Frederick Shipman. Born on January 14, 1946, in Nottingham, UK, Dr. Shipman killed about 220–240 of his patients during a professional life spanning 24 years (at an average of 10 patients per year) by administering lethal doses of diamorphine (pharmaceutical heroin).

Nobody knows exactly what his motive may have been. In one case, however, he had forged one of his victims' wills so he would benefit financially. Finally on January 31, 2000, he was convicted at Preston, UK, of murdering 15 of his patients. He was sentenced to 15 concurrent terms of life imprisonment and was told by the judge that in his case life imprisonment would mean that he would remain in prison until his death. Shipman committed suicide in his prison cell on January 13, 2004, a day before his 58th birthday.

Several nurses are also known to have indulged in mass poisoning. Two who stand out among them are Van der Linden of Leyden, Germany, who is supposed to have killed 27 persons between 1869 and 1885 with arsenic; and Jane Toppan, who killed 30 patients with morphine and atropine in 1902. Mass-poisoning nurses have also had a modern representative in Genene Jones, who used to kill young children with succinylcholine. She is known to have killed at least two babies, but may have killed as many as 20.

Mass Poisoner Targeting Random Victims

John Harris Trestrail III, of the Regional Poison Center, Grand Rapids, Michigan, USA, has identified two types of poisoners: type S, who select a specific victim, and type R, who select random victims. Both categories have two subgroups, a subgroup S, where the poisoning is slowly planned, with a carefully selected poison, and a subgroup Q, where the poisoning is quickly planned. There are thus four categories of poisoners: type S/S (specific/slow), type S/Q (specific/quick), type R/S (random/slow), and type R/Q (random/quick). Mass poisoners generally belong to type R. It is more difficult to apprehend them, as no specific motives can be identified; their motives appear to be to experience power

Table 1 Twenty-five most notorious mass poisoners in history, and their poisons

S. no.	First name	Last name	Sex	Country	Year of activity/death[a]	Poison used	No. of victims	Fate
1	Locusta		F	Rome	1st Century AD (first known court poisoner, appointed by Nero)	Several including poisonous mushrooms and arsenic	Several hundred	No information about her death is available, but it is believed that she died a natural death in the court of Nero
2	Julia	Agrippina	F	Rome	(49–59 AD)	Poisonous mushrooms	Several hundred	Killed by her son Nero
3	Marie	Besnard	F	France	1947–61	Arsenic	12	Acquitted
4	Cesare	Borgia	M	Italy	15th Century	"La Cantrella," a secret potion containing arsenic	Several hundred	Killed in a skirmish with rebels in 1507, at the age of 32
5	Richard	Brinkley	M	UK	1907	Hydrocyanic acid	3	Hanged at Wandsworth prison on 13 August 1907
6	Marquise de	Brinvilliers	F	France	1660–76	Arsenic	100+	Decapitated
7	George	Chapman	M	UK	1897–1902	Antimony	3	Hanged on 7 April, 1903
8	Mary Ann	Cotton	F	England	1852–73	Arsenic	20	Hanged
9	Catherine	de Medici	F	France	1589	Arsenic	Many	Natural death
10	Catherine	Deshayes (La Voisin)	F	France	1680	Arsenic	+2000	Burnt at stake on 23 Feb, 1680
11	Mrs. Julius	Fazekas[b]	F	Hungary	1914–1929	Arsenic (obtained by boiling fly papers)	+100	Committed suicide
12	Johann	Hoch	M	USA	1905	Arsenic	15 (wives)	Hanged
13	Hélène	Jegado	F	France	1833–51	Arsenic	26	Guillotined
14	Genene	Jones (nurse)	F	USA	1984	Succinylcholine (Anectine)	2 children; suspected of killing at least 20 other babies in her care	sentenced to 99 years for the murder of one patient and 60 years for the attempted murder of a second
15	Christa Ambrose	Lehmann	F	Germany	1954	E–605 (Parathion)	3 (her husband, father-in-law, and the daughter of a neighbor).	Sentenced to life in prison

			Sex	Country	Year[a]	Poison	Victims	Fate
16	Van der	Linden (nurse)	F	Leyden, Germany	1869–85	?Arsenic	Attempted on the lives of 102 persons, of which 27 died	?Executed
17	Martha	Marek	F	Austria	1932	Thallium	3	Beheaded
18	Daisy de	Melker	F	South Africa	1932	Arsenic	3 (2 husbands and son)	Hanged
19	Dr. William	Palmer (a.k.a. The Rugeley Poisoner)	M	UK	1855–6	Antimony	15	Hanged outside Stafford Gaol on 14 June 1856. The Parliament had to pass the famous "Palmer Act," perhaps the only Act to be named after a convicted criminal, so he could be tried in London instead of his place of residence Rugeley, Staffordshire, where he could not get a fair trial because of rising resentment against him
20	Dr. Harold Frederick	Shipman	M	UK	1990s–2000	Diamorphine (pharmaceutical heroin)	240	Sentenced to life. Committed suicide in the prison cell on 13 January 2004
21	Hieronyma	Spara	F	Rome, Italy	1659	"Aquetta di Perugia" (containing arsenic)	+100	Publicly hanged
22	Giulia	Toffana	F	Italy	17th Century	Aqua Toffana (Composition unknown, but may have contained arsenic)	600	Executed in Naples
23	Jane	Toppan (nurse)	F	USA	1902	Morphine and Atropine	30 (may be as many as 100)	Sent for life to mental asylum
24	Graham	Young	M	UK	1971–2	Thallium	Several, of which two were proven.	Sentenced to life imprisonment
25	Anne Marie	Zwanziger (nurse) ('monster' of Bavaria)	F	Germany	1811	Arsenic	11	Beheaded

[a]In case where precise years of activities are uncertain, the year in which the poisoner was caught/died is given.
[b]She was a midwife by profession. Her cohort in crime, reputed to be a witch, was Susanna Olah, a.k.a., "Auntie Susi."

over helpless people. In addition, there is the curious case of a type S poisoner, who kills randomly (in addition to killing his specific target), in order to confuse the investigators. These are type S poisoners camouflaged as type R. These mass poisoners are also very difficult to apprehend.

The most typical example of a type R poisoner (or perhaps of a type S poisoner camouflaged as type R) is that of the tylenol capsule murderer, who laced tylenol capsules with cyanide and caused the deaths of seven random victims in 1982, in Chicago, Illinois, USA. No killer has ever been caught and no motive has been established. There was nothing common between the seven victims.

The series of mass poisonings started at 6 a.m. on September 29, 1982, when the first victim, a 12-year-old schoolgirl, died. Waking up with a sore throat in one of Chicago's peaceful northwestern suburbs, she had taken an analgesic at her father's suggestion before dropping lifeless to the floor. Over the next few days, until October 1, six more victims died in a similar way (**Table 2**).

The mass hysteria rose to such a pitch that frantic calls were being made to poison control centers from worried patients who had taken tylenol. Many people thought their toothpaste smelt oddly or their antacids tasted strangely in what pharmacists described as "over-the-counter fear" or the "tylenol syndrome." The mayor recalled all capsules, the public were warned not to inhale or even touch the capsules, the manufacturer offered refunds for the capsules and announced a $100 000 reward for any information that might solve the mystery. Investigators looked for disgruntled shop assistants, for fingerprints over the capsules, but nothing helped, and the case remains one of the biggest mysteries related to mass poisonings.

The Suicidal Mass Poisoner

Another strange case is that of a mass poisoner who instigates his followers to take poison on a mass scale.

The best-known example is that of Reverend Jim Jones, who founded the commune colony of Jonestown in Guyana. About 1000 of his followers moved there from San Francisco. When there were allegations of human rights abuses at Jonestown, Congressman Leo Ryan visited the colony on November 14, 1978 on a fact-finding mission. Just as he was about to leave, with three journalists and one of Jones' followers, some of the remaining followers opened fire on them and killed them all. Soon after this, Jim Jones "ordered" his followers to drink a cyanide-laced drink. A total of 914 people died, including Jones, who was found with a bullet in his head.

Mass Poisoning as a Result of Drug Misadventure

Rarely mass poisoning may occur in drug addicts who have used adulterated drugs. Sometimes the sample received may be "purer" than the one the addicts are used to, resulting again in mass poisonings by unintentional overdose.

Investigating Mass Poisonings

Whether mass poisonings are a result of homicide, compulsive poisoning, suicide, drug misadventure, or accident, a thorough forensic investigation is a must. Among the questions to be answered are:

1. Which chemical/poison was involved and was it actually the cause of death or injury?
2. Was the incident homicidal/suicidal/accidental in nature?
3. Who were the perpetrators?
4. How many victims were involved?
5. How could such incidents be prevented in future?

The Scene of Mass Poisoning

The first step in the forensic investigation of mass poisoning is a visit to the scene. The scene of mass poisoning poses special challenges, and its examination may require special precautions. Poisons may

Table 2 Seven victims of the Tylenol Capsule mass poisonings

S. no.	Victim	Sex	Date and time
1	A 12 year old schoolgirl	F	29 September 1982, 6 am
2	A young Polish born post-office worker, who had taken the day off to play with his children	M	29 September 1982, few hours later
3	Above man's wife	F	29 September 1982, in the evening
4	Above man's brother	M	29 September 1982, in the evening
5	A young woman suffering from headaches	F	30 September 1982
6	A young mother who had just given birth to her third child	F	30 September 1982
7	An air stewardess	F	1 October 1982

still be lurking in the air (as in the case of subway attacks by the nerve gas sarin and in the Bhopal gas tragedy), and this may pose serious dangers to the investigators. A few rules must be followed while investigating scenes of mass poisoning. These are:

- Never smoke, eat, or drink at the scene.
- Do not dispose of anything by throwing it in water.
- Do not pour water over anything.
- Have a qualified chemist with you to assist.
- Have personnel trained to handle potential explosive material.
- Use gas masks, protective suits, overshoes, and gloves.
- Do not shut off any mechanical or electrical apparatus (heaters, stirring motors, etc.).

Securing the scene   The scene of mass poisoning should immediately be cordoned off, with an inner and an outer cordon. Members of the general public should be kept outside the outer cordon. Representatives of the media and police personnel may be permitted to enter the outer cordon, but may not be allowed beyond the inner cordon. Only members of the forensic and rescue teams should be allowed to go inside the inner cordon. Appropriate clothing must be donned at the entry point of the inner cordon, and must be deposited back when coming out. This ensures that no toxicological evidence is inadvertently "carried in" or "walked out" of the scene.

Physicians accompanying the rescue teams within the inner cordon must look for signs of life in the victims lying there. If there are any signs of life, the victims should be immediately transported to the nearest hospital. Postmortem examination should be undertaken on all those who have died.

Collection of evidence   Much valuable toxicological evidence lies at the scene. Urgency is important as much of it may be evanescent. Toxic gases may not be there in the environment if inordinate delays are made. If mass poisoning has occurred because of a toxic gas or vapor (e.g., industrial gas disasters, terrorist attacks with toxic gases in subways), it will be appropriate to sample the toxic gas and vapor using a portable pump, and passing the air through a suitable adsorbent material, such as charcoal. Packets of unused poison and used syringes (e.g., in case of drug misadventure) should be collected, sealed, and sent for chemical analysis.

Samples of vomited material, feces, and urine found at the scene must be lifted, as they may contain the toxic material. Clothes soiled with vomit, feces, or urine must also be collected, packed in clean paper bags, and sent for chemical analysis.

The Forensic Autopsy in Mass Poisoning

In instances of mass poisoning, there is a tendency on the part of forensic pathologists to conduct the autopsy on only a few representative cases. This practice has caused insurance problems in the past as insurance companies have contested the cause of death in those cases where a postmortem examination was not carried out. It is thus a safe practice to conduct a thorough postmortem examination in every case of death due to mass poisoning.

Standard autopsy protocols are used. Internal organs such as liver, spleen, kidneys, lungs, brain, and spinal cord are preserved for chemical analysis. Body fluids such as blood, urine, bile, cerebrospinal fluid, and vitreous humor are preserved using standard protocols.

Screening tests for common drugs and poisons are employed. The ideal screening tests for poisons are rapid (a short turnaround time), highly specific (no cross-reactions with other drugs or poisons), sensitive (capable of detecting low levels of poisons/toxins), and reliable (one laboratory would derive the same results as another). Clearly such tests are not available for all agents. In addition, a screening test should be inexpensive and easily performed technically. Confirmatory tests include gas chromatography, high-performance liquid chromatography, gas chromatography–mass spectrometry, and immunoassay techniques. Finding a common toxin/poison in all victims makes the case for mass poisoning.

See Also

History of Toxicology; **Mass Disasters:** Role of Forensic Pathologists; **Mass Murder**; **Toxicology:** Overview; Methods of Analysis, Postmortem

Further Reading

Aggrawal A (1997) Poison, antidotes and anecdotes. *Science Reporter* 26–29 (also available online at: http://Prof_Anil_Aggrawal.tripod.com/poiso001.html).

Aggrawal A (2002) Poisons and antidotes through the ages, with special reference to Indian history and mythology. *Mithridata (Toxicological History Society Newsletter)* XII: 13–18.

Aggrawal A (2004) Agrippina, the first forensic odontologist and the greatest poisoner in ancient Rome. *Mithridata (Toxicological History Society Newsletter)* xiv: 6–11.

Pillay VV (2003) *Comprehensive Medical Toxicology.* Hyderabad, India: Paras.

Trestrail JH III (2000) *Criminal Poisoning.* Totowa, NJ: Humana Press.

Trestrail JH III (2000) *Mithridata: The Newsletter of the Toxicological History Society – The First Ten Years (Jan 1991–July 2000).* Grand Rapids, MI: Center for the Study of Criminal Poisoning.

MEDICAL DEFINITIONS OF DEATH

B Jennett, University of Glasgow, Glasgow, UK

Introduction

Recent medical technological developments have led to a need to extend the definitions of death to cover unusual and unnatural situations where the traditional criteria of death cannot easily be applied. In particular the concept of brain death has had implications for both medical and legal practice, which have given rise to considerable controversy in several countries. Although this account is written from the UK perspective, reference is also made to problems elsewhere.

History of Definitions of Death

This title might seem to imply that recognizing death, as well as recording its cause, has long been a medical matter. For centuries, information about deaths depended on entries in parish registers by clergymen, who relied on what families told them. These were the basis of the Bills of Mortality that feature in historical accounts of death rates in communities and of the frequency of different fatal diseases. The Registration Act of 1836 (for England and Wales, but not applied to Scotland until 20 years later) led to more formal recording of deaths. Books of death certificates were sent out to 10 000 medical practitioners in 1841 but how these recipients were selected is uncertain because there was no medical register to identify *bona fide* doctors until 1858. In 1874 an official recommendation requiring a medical certificate for registering a death was introduced. However, the doctor could certify the death without having seen the patient in the preceding 2 weeks or without verification of death by inspection and this holds good even now. Poor people or those who lived in remote areas often did not have a doctor and this led to registration of uncertified deaths in some places. Because of this a parliamentary investigation was initiated in 1893, in which one report indicated that 40% of registered deaths were uncertified in Inverness, compared with only 2% in Glasgow.

Since biblical times the conventional sign of death was the absence of respiration, as verified by no movement in a feather or no misting of a mirror held in front of the nostrils and mouth. The unreliability of this as a sign of death was widely recognized in the eighteenth century when fear of premature burial led to various types of ingenious devices to enable victims of a mistaken diagnosis of death to signal to the living that they were still alive. In 1740 a paper entitled "The uncertainty of the signs of death and the danger of precipitate internments" concluded that putrefaction was the only sure sign of death. Signs sooner than this that would have been available at that time include rigor mortis and the coldness of the body (given that the ambient temperature was reasonable).

The introduction of the stethoscope in the nineteenth century led to attention being focused on the heartbeat rather than respiration as a more reliable sign of life. Recently a professor of forensic pathology made recommendations on confirming recent death. These include listening to the chest with a stethoscope for 2 min, detecting lack of tension in the eyeballs, observing that the pupils are in midposition with no reaction to light, and viewing with an ophthalmoscope the segmentation of blood in the retinal veins, which occurs very soon after death (an appearance known as "railroading" or "cattle-trucking"). By no means all of these procedures (or indeed any of them) are routinely carried out in practice and occasional mistaken declarations of death do still occur, sometimes only recognized after removal to the mortuary. Circumstances that may lead to simulation of death, when special care should be taken to avoid such a mistake, include drug overdose, hypothermia, electrocution, and drowning. If an electrocardiogram is available in such a situation the presence of continuing heart action can be reliably detected or excluded and this may help in correct declaration.

Consequences of Recent Technologies

If the introduction of the stethoscope made the definition and recognition of death easier, the development in the early 1950s of certain resuscitation and life support technologies has confused the issue and has led to the need to redefine death under certain artificial conditions. For example, cardiac defibrillators are now widely available not only in hospitals but also in ambulances and other locations that deal with emergencies in public places. These may enable a heart that has stopped to be restarted – and if the intervention is timely the patient may recover adequately. During cardiac surgery the heart may be deliberately stopped for an extended period during which the circulation of the blood is maintained by an external pump (cardiac bypass). In such cases it may not be correct to suggest, except in an attempt to dramatize the event, that these patients have recovered after having been dead. The development of small portable mechanical ventilators to substitute for failed breathing has posed more of a problem, necessitating the emergence of a new definition of death – brain death. This concept and its practical implications are now widely accepted in many countries, albeit after some controversy. Together with the development of organ and tissue transplantation these technologies have led to the recognition that death is a process rather than an event because not all organs and tissues become nonviable at the same time. The World Medical Association Declaration of Sydney in 1968 stated that, from a medical viewpoint, the time of death of different organs and cells is less important in determining the death of the individual than the certainty that the process has become irreversible. Others have stated that it is not the death of the whole organism that matters, but the death of the organism as a coordinated whole. At what point during the process of dying an individual is regarded as having died is to some extent arbitrary. At different stages in this process it may be appropriate to abandon futile treatment, to remove organs for transplantation, to move the body to the mortuary, or to dispose of the body.

The Concept of Brain Death

The process of dying is most commonly initiated by the arrest of either the heart (i.e., the circulation of the blood) or, less often, of the breathing. The consequence of either event is that within minutes the brain also fails irreversibly from lack of oxygen and there is death of the brain. However, even an hour later kidneys may be removed and will survive if transplanted, and many hours later corneas or bone may be retrieved and preserved for later transplantation. When breathing has ceased a mechanical ventilator can restore respiratory function. If respiratory failure is due to spinal injury or disease, prolonged survival with full mental function is possible by continuing with mechanical ventilation. If a ventilator is needed because of failure of the respiratory drive from the brainstem, then provided this was started sufficiently quickly so that further irreversible brain damage did not occur from lack of oxygen, full recovery is possible if the brainstem failure

proves to be temporary. If, however, the brain failure proves to be irreversible (either from primary brain damage or as a result of delayed resuscitation), the ventilator may only serve to prolong the process of dying. It allows the heart to continue to beat and to maintain the blood circulation, which supports the function of other organs. This state of artificially maintained ventilation with the heart continuing to beat and the patient kept warm and pink, although the brain is dead, is termed brain death. This unnatural state is the price paid by these patients for the successful ventilation of other patients because, inevitably, those who initiate mechanical ventilation as an emergency resuscitation measure do not then know whether the brain can recover. After brain death it is usually only a matter of a few days before the heart stops, but during this time the brain may begin to decompose. Exceptionally, bodily survival after brain death may be extended for some weeks when special efforts are made in a pregnant woman to maintain the life of the fetus until it can survive delivery.

Controversies about Brain Death

These have centered on the motivation for recognizing this condition and on the reliability of criteria for its diagnosis. It was intensive care specialists who originally described brain death because they were anxious to avoid having to continue to ventilate comatose patients with irrecoverable brain damage. To do so was considered to deprive the patient of death with dignity, to prolong needlessly the distress of relatives, and to be an inappropriate use of scarce resources. However, organ transplantation emerged at about the same time as the concept of brain death and this led some to assert that brain death had been identified primarily in order to facilitate the provision of donor organs. In fact it was not until 10 years after brain death had been described that there was more than one kidney transplant per week in the UK. At that time most kidney donors were cadavers from whom organs were removed some time after the heart had stopped, while other kidneys came from healthy volunteers. Indeed, in an American review in 1971 more than half the transplants were from living donors. What the definition of brain death did for kidney transplantation was to remove from cadaver donation the sense of unseemly haste to remove organs once the heart had stopped, because there was now a window of several hours for discussion with relatives before kidneys had to be removed. By 1977 one British transplant unit reported that two-thirds of its kidneys came from brain-dead donors but

4 years later all came from such a source. Even so, a few units still use some donors declared dead only after the heart has stopped, whilst increasing numbers of kidneys now come from volunteer living donors. By contrast, the more recent development of heart and lung transplantation depends entirely on brain-dead donors because the heart has to be still beating when it is removed. But heart transplantation only became a frequent procedure after 1979, 20 years after the first description of brain death. In practice only a fraction of brain-dead patients become donors because some are unsuitable for medical reasons whilst for others permission is either unable to be sought or is withheld by relatives. If transplantation were ever to be superseded by alternative treatments there would still be several thousand brain-dead patients in intensive care units every year for whom a decision about whether to continue ventilation would have to be made.

The Diagnosis of Brain Death

Criteria for the diagnosis of brain death were first formally published in 1968, 10 years after the phenomenon was first described. The Harvard committee that developed these criteria included lawyers and theologians as well as anesthetists, neurosurgeons, and neurologists. The Harvard criteria required that there be absence of all motor activity and that the electroencephalogram (EEG) be flat – that is, showing no electrical activity in the brain. This implied the necessity for evidence that the whole of the central nervous system was no longer functioning – the cerebral cortex, the brainstem, and the spinal cord. It was subsequently observed that limb movements from spinal cord reflexes can persist after brain death, because the cord is less vulnerable than the brain to hypoxic insult. Although the brainstem is necessary for coordinated activity in the higher brain as well as for spontaneous breathing it has become apparent that residual physico-chemical activity with some electrical component can persist in some isolated cortical areas above a dead brainstem in some patients. As a result, the emphasis is now on the death of the brainstem rather than of the whole brain and this is a feature of the UK criteria. These were developed by a Health Department committee that included a coroner, a barrister, and a patient representative, and were subsequently agreed and published in 1976 by the UK Medical Royal Colleges. They require that certain preconditions should be met before embarking on tests to confirm brain death (**Table 1**). These are

Table 1 Preconditions before testing for brain death

- Deep coma persisting after correction of systemic hypotension and hypoxia, and attempts to reduce high intracranial pressure
- Apnea requiring continuous mechanical ventilation
- Evidence of severe structural damage to the brain, e.g., head injury, intracranial hemorrhage, or an episode of severe systemic hypotension or hypoxia
- Exclusion of causes of temporary brainstem failure, e.g., depressant drugs, muscle relaxants, hypothermia

Table 2 Tests for brain death (after preconditions have been satisfied)

- Absent corneal, papillary, and gag reflexes
- No eye movements in response to ice-cold caloric stimulation (oculovestibular reflex)
- No respiratory movements when $Pa\text{CO}_2 > 6.65$ kPa during ventilator disconnection while oxygen is delivered at $6 \, l \, min^{-1}$ via endotracheal tube (apnea test)

that the patient is in deep coma and has been on a ventilator since the arrest of spontaneous breathing (apnea), that the diagnosis of irreversible brain damage has been established, and that there are no confounding factors that could cause temporary depression of activity in the brainstem (such as depressant drugs or hypothermia). If these preconditions have been met the diagnosis can be made on the basis of simple bedside tests to exclude continuing function in the brainstem (**Table 2**). These must always include the important apnea test to establish without doubt that there is still absence of spontaneous breathing.

The UK criteria require that the tests be carried out on two occasions (without any specified time interval between the two tests) and that two experienced doctors should be involved. A further memorandum from the UK Colleges in 1979 asserted that if the brainstem is dead then the brain is dead and if this is so then the patient is dead. According to this it is therefore appropriate to declare death when the brain death tests are satisfied for the second time, and this should be recorded as the time of death for legal purposes. The subsequent withdrawal of the ventilator is then regarded as the removal of an inappropriate technological procedure from a person who is already dead, rather than an intervention to allow that patient to die. When two convicted prisoners claimed on appeal that their victims had died as a result of doctors withdrawing the ventilator after brain death, the Lord Chief Justice opined that it would be otiose to suggest that when medical treatment had failed to save the life of a patient the doctors who withdrew that treatment should be considered responsible for that person's death.

That legal case occurred in the aftermath of a challenge to the validity of the UK criteria in a notorious BBC Panorama program in 1980 entitled "Transplants – are the donors really dead?" This asserted that brain death was a concept that had emerged from the medical profession without proper discussion – in spite of the fact that it had been ratified on both sides of the Atlantic by committees that included nonmedical members. It also alleged that its emergence was primarily to satisfy the need for organ donors, although as already explained, that was not the case. But its most serious allegation was that the UK criteria were less reliable than those in other countries because there were no mandatory confirmatory tests, in particular the EEG. Doctors from the USA and France supported these allegations and there were interviews with patients who had been mistakenly declared to be brain-dead in the USA. After an unprecedented period of controversial discussion in the newspapers, medical journals, and in the House of Commons, the BBC exceptionally allowed a team of British doctors to make a reply program that answered the criticisms, with the on-screen support of other doctors from the USA. This program established that none of the patients alleged in the original program to have recovered from supposed brain death would have been declared to be brain-dead by the UK criteria. There has subsequently been no modification of the UK criteria, apart from a preference for the term "brainstem death." Indeed, many other countries as well as many institutions in the USA have subsequently adopted criteria for the diagnosis of brain death that are virtually identical to those published in the UK.

Brain Death Legislation

The UK has not considered it necessary to bring in legislation to deal with brain death: a patient is dead when a doctor declares this, and on what basis that was done is regarded as a medical matter. However, as early as 1970 the US state of Kansas enacted a brain death law and many other American states have since followed suit, as have several European countries. These laws stipulate that death may be declared by neurological criteria but do not specify these criteria, indicating instead that these should be according to the standards of the day – recognizing that these may change. The reason why laws are deemed necessary in some places is in order to protect doctors and to anticipate and thereby avoid futile appeals by

convicted assailants that they were not responsible for the subsequent deaths of their victims.

In many countries the concept of brain death and its practical implications are accepted without continuing controversy. However, in three countries active debate did continue long after the issue seemed to have been settled elsewhere. In Denmark in 1985 a transplantation committee recommended accepting brain death criteria but when the Ministry of Justice proposed a bill 2 years later there was strong opposition in the media. A Council of Ethics in 1989 proposed that organs could be removed during the death process but that the time of death should be when the heart later stopped. Copies of this were widely distributed to the public, 200 local debating groups were set up and a video film was shown to more than 500 local groups. The law, passed in 1990, was virtually identical to that proposed in 1987 before the public debate. In Germany, acceptance of brain death went unchallenged for over 20 years. However, draft legislation to formalize accepted practice in 1995 stirred up opposition coordinated by the Berliner Initiative Against Brain Death, but the proposed law was eventually passed in 1997.

In Japan the debate was much more contentious and prolonged. Over many years one pediatric neurologist organized steady opposition to brain death, maintaining that it was no more than an aid to transplantation. In 1988 the Japanese Medical Association voted to accept the concept, but divisions appeared between specialists, some of whom feared that the disabled might become unwilling donors. In 1992 a cabinet committee was deeply divided but the majority approved the acceptance of brain death, but this was rejected the next day by the Ministry of Justice and the police. Eventually a law was passed in 1997 accepting brain death but this was restricted to patients for whom permission had been given for transplantation. This thereby emphasized the connection between brain death and transplantation that other countries had striven so hard to play down.

The Present Situation

In 1999 an American book, *The Definition of Death*, suggested that there were unresolved controversies in the USA about brain death that some academics believed should be debated. In particular, the assertion that brain-dead patients were already dead was believed by some to be incoherent. It stemmed from the dead donor rule – the insistence of transplant surgeons that potential donors and their families should be told that their organs would be taken only after the death of the donor. It now seems to some that it would be more realistic to admit that there is a stage in the irreversible process of dying when it is appropriate to take organs without having to declare the patient already dead. This makes it no different from acknowledging that at an earlier stage in this dying process it may be appropriate to withdraw all active treatment. There is, however, no evidence that there is pressure in the public domain to enact such a change, particularly not in the UK where the long-standing diagnostic criteria and the present legal position have served so well.

An ethical dilemma does sometimes arise when relatives are unwilling to accept the diagnosis of brain death and object to the discontinuation of ventilation. Such denial may arise from confusion in the minds of relatives between the formal diagnosis of brain death and other states such as the persistent vegetative state and deep coma from which they have heard that patients declared irrecoverable do sometimes recover. They need to have it explained that these are quite different conditions and that the diagnosis of brain death with its formal protocol and involvement of two doctors is more reliable than any other medical diagnosis and implicit in that diagnosis is that the patient cannot recover. In such circumstances it is very helpful to be able to point out that legally the patient is already dead, and that legally it is only the doctor who can decide about the appropriateness of continued treatment. In such circumstances permission is no more needed to stop the ventilator than it is needed to move the body to the mortuary.

See Also

Coma, Definitions and Differential Diagnoses: Pediatric; Adult; **Head Trauma:** Neuropathology; **Legal Definitions of Death**; **Organ and Tissue Transplantation, Ethical and Practical Issues**; **Religious Attitudes to Death**

Further Reading

Conference of the Medical Royal Colleges and their Faculties in the United Kingdom (1976) Diagnosis of brain death. *British Medical Journal* 2: 1187–1188.

Conference of the Medical Royal Colleges and their Faculties in the United Kingdom (1979) Diagnosis of death. *British Medical Journal* 1: 322.

Cranford RE (1999) Ethical dilemma: discontinuation of ventilation after brain stem death – policy should be balanced with concern for the family. *British Medical Journal* 318: 1754–1755.

Health Departments of Great Britain and Northern Ireland (1988) *A Code of Practice for the Diagnosis of Brain Stem Death*. London: Department of Health.

Jennett B (1981) Brain death. *British Journal of Anaesthesia* 53: 1111–1119.

Jennett B (1999) Ethical dilemma: discontinuation of ventilation after brain stem death – brain stem death defines death in law. *British Medical Journal* 318: 1755.

Swinburn JMA, Ali SM, Banerjee DJ, Kahn ZP (1999) Ethical dilemma: discontinuation of ventilation after brain stem death – to whom is our duty of care? *British Medical Journal* 318: 1753–1754.

Wijdicks EFM (ed.) (2001) *Brain Death*. Philadelphia, PA: Lippincott/Williams & Wilkins.

Youngner SJ, Arnold RM, Shapiro R (eds.) (1999) *The Definition of Death*. Baltimore, MD: John Hopkins University Press.

MEDICAL MALPRACTICE

Contents

Overview

I Wall, Ruislip, UK

Litigation

Doctors are now facing an increasing risk of legal action by their patients. Consumer enfranchisement, an emergent "compensation culture" encouraged by a growing personal-injury "industry," and a disenchantment with modern medicine's inevitable inability to keep apace with public expectations have all been ascribed a role in this incipient litigiousness.

This phenomenon has reached full maturity in the USA, where a "crisis" of excessive liability premiums, dwindling professional entry into high-risk disciplines, and reduced patient access now afflicts healthcare provision.

While figures indicate that civil suits in the UK have in fact been falling over the last decade, this ignores the considerable contribution made by settlements outside the legal arena in calculating overall costs.

The growing economic burden of servicing clinical negligence litigation in the UK, with the attendant repercussions of diverting funds from other areas of patient care, has been the focus of increasing political attention.

The Law of Negligence

Medical error is a constant, if not inevitable, companion to clinical practice; however, where iatrogenic harm is the result of negligence in the delivery of healthcare it is actionable at law.

The law of negligence is an instrument of corrective justice and a means of policing the exercise of proper care. It is concerned with the protection of private interests from the careless and unreasonable interference of others, and with the provision of financial compensation where such infringements have resulted in personal injury.

The common-law tradition, rather than undertaking the task of disentangling the complexities of subjective states of mind, concentrates instead on an examination of wrongdoing from an objective perspective. Negligent conduct is thus punished by a failure to meet court-determined standards based on a test of "reasonableness." In this way, the link between the related concepts of legal fault, moral blame, and the duty to make reparation is purportedly maintained.

Liability in negligence depends on the existence of a duty of care between the parties based on a proximate relationship (the "neighbor" test, initially formulated in *Donoghue* v. *Stevenson* [1932] AC 562, a breach of that duty by one of the parties' failure to take reasonable care, and injury caused by this breach.

The elements of this legal formula overlap to a greater or lesser extent, and their individual conceptual clarity is further clouded by a degree of judicial contrivance, employed to satisfy often covert policy considerations directed at limiting liability.

In the majority of cases, clinical negligence litigation can be distilled into disputes arising over an issue involving a breach of duty or an issue of causation.

Clinical Standards and Legal Standards

The notion of the "standard of care" is a matter of law to be determined by the court. It serves to define how individuals ought to behave and is a measure of the acceptability of conduct. A failure to attain this required level of conduct is the essence of an actionable breach of duty.

The seminal judgment in *Bolam* v. *Friern Hospital Management Committee* [1957] 2 All ER 118 established the general standard required of a professional exercising a particular skill to be that of the reasonably competent or skillful practitioner.

A clinician holding him-/herself out as possessing specialist medical skill will be judged by the objective standards of a person exercising that particular skill and occupying that specialist post. Tort has traditionally eschewed a variable standard, so in judging the actions of the neophyte practicing in a specialist environment, the court will make no allowance for inexperience (*Wilsher* v. *Essex Area Health Authority* [1987] QB 730 CA).

When adjudicating on an individual clinician's conduct, the court will invite expert testimony as to what constitutes accepted and prudent practice within the appropriate specialty. Liability will then depend on whether the clinician's conduct has failed to conform to this requisite clinical standard.

A departure from "customary" practice is, however, defensible at law if a responsible body of professional opinion can be found to support the propriety of the purportedly negligent conduct. Under these circumstances, the court is bound to find in an accused clinician's favor (*Maynard* v. *West Midlands Regional Health Authority* [1984] 1 WLR 634), even if an opposing body of opinion exists that is critical of the conduct in question. The court's preference for one body of opinion over another is not sufficient grounds to infer negligence.

This protectionist quality of the Bolam test creates an uneven contest, as claimants are doomed to failure if practitioners are able to find sanction for their conduct, albeit via a minority school of thought.

The introduction of national evidence-based guidelines on patient care may serve to inject an apparent degree of objective clarity into the courtroom provided there is an appreciation of their status as policy rules to control clinical behavior, and not necessarily as guarantees of customary practice. "Guidelines" are not directly admissible in court due to the common-law rules on hearsay. They may be introduced in order to support expert testimony, but in these circumstances will be accorded the same weight as other evidence. Critics of the Bolam test point to the undue reliance courts place on medical judgment when determining the standard of care, and therefore ultimately the question of negligent conduct. By way of contrast, it has been suggested that expert witnesses, whose tendency is to focus on ideals of clinical practice, rather than the commonly accepted, have artificially elevated the standard of care to a level unachievable by the majority of practitioners.

English case law appeared to signal a departure from the traditional reliance it placed on the conclusiveness of peer opinion (*Bolitho* v. *City and Hackney Health Authority* (1993) 4 Med LR 381 (CA)). Courts may now evaluate evidence that purports to be representative of a reasonable and responsible body of medical opinion and reject it as "unreasonable" if it is incapable of withstanding logical analysis.

Such departures from Bolam are likely to be rare, however, as the "illogicality" test is restrictive, but this novel judicial skepticism may represent a nascent release from the constraints placed on claimants. Courts may now exercise this inherent entitlement to invalidate "illogical" minority (or even "maverick") opinion that may hitherto have provided a successful defense under the Bolam test.

Causation

There is no liability in negligence if a direct connection between the negligent act and the injury complained of cannot be established (*Barnet* v. *Chelsea and Kensington Hospital Management Committee* [1969] 1 QB 428), even where the particular example of behavior can be shown to be demonstrably negligent by any measure.

Success on the issue of factual causation depends on an injured party demonstrating that, but for the defendant's negligent act, on the balance of probability, the injury complained of would not have occurred.

The burden of proving causation, which lies with the injured claimant, often presents insuperable problems. Clinical interactions may be complex, and where causal associations exist, expert medical evidence may be either unable to support the causative link or do so in a form that is not readily accessible to legal analysis.

Such problems are particularly acute where injury has resulted from two sources or from one of a number of potential causative agents. In certain circumstances the court may be willing to bridge the evidential gap and infer causation as a matter of law where particular insult can be shown to have exerted a "material contribution" to the injury complained of.

Tort Practice and Theory

The continued existence of negligence law despite reformatory pressure is perhaps a testament to its robustness and its explanative, deterrent, and retributive role in society. The effectiveness of tort law's principal function as an instrument of compensation has, however, been undermined by empirical evidence that indicates only a small proportion of patients who suffer injury due to negligence instigate formal legal action, and where claims are pursued, only a minority proportion are successful.

Such inefficiencies are accentuated by the costs of a system of civil litigation where, in over one-half of actions that proved successful, the injured party received no compensation because legal costs had consumed the damages awarded.

Civil procedure rules introduced in the UK aimed at remedying endemic problems of delay, and consequentially inflated costs, which had previously becalmed the litigation process, now require the courts actively to manage cases to ensure their timely disposal, and, where possible, to encourage mediation. State-sponsored legal aid has been withdrawn for most categories of clinical negligence and contingency fees have been introduced in its place.

Equally implicit is tort's relative deficiency at identifying and holding clinicians accountable for substandard care and, by extension, failing to deter careless practices. Undoubtedly fears of the personal and professional consequences of litigation are real, though the existence of state underwriting of civil liability, and the laws on vicarious liability, serve to divorce notions of fault from negligent conduct, and the effect of any financial deterrence is mitigated because compensation payments are not directly met by the wrongdoers.

To Blame or Not to Blame

The punitive and "blame-based" ethos of civil litigation has long been recognized as a disincentive to open admission and reporting of errors. The limited scope of the civil inquiry is concerned more with attributing individual fault than a quest for truth and, despite some limited success, is ill-equipped to expose systemic failure.

In addition, the civil forensic process does not provide a conducive environment for a full elucidation of the circumstances in which harm has been caused. The confrontational climate has been commonly regarded as responsible for breeding distrust rather than promoting resolution, and as injurious to the doctor–patient relationship.

Other jurisdictions have examined the entire notion of the role of "fault" in clinical negligence and have introduced no-fault (or, more accurately, minimal fault, as most have eligibility criteria) schemes founded on principles of proof of injury rather than proof of fault, irrespective of whether or not negligence can be demonstrated.

New Zealand has taken legislative action to abolish the right to take common-law actions in respect of personal injury, substituting this with a right to access to an administrative compensation scheme where injury has been suffered as a consequence of "misadventure." In Scandinavian countries, compensation is capped, and recourse to the tort system is retained.

Despite frequent calls for the introduction of a comprehensive no-fault system in the UK, its general introduction has recently been rejected by proposals that instead favor a system of "redress." Under this scheme eligibility will be founded on the nebulous concept of "serious shortcomings in the standards of care," and access to the courts is likely to be retained in deference to the right to a fair-hearing provision under Article 6 of the European Convention on Human Rights.

The challenge facing any no-fault system is the need to retain an incentive to ensure that appropriate clinical standards are maintained.

Preventive Medicine

While some jurisdictions have sought to tackle the burgeoning litigation by legislative means such as capping damages and reducing the limitation period, the UK proposes to approach the problem from a different angle.

A growing awareness of the need to minimize the risks of negligence occurring in the first place, and an understanding that injury may be the result of systemic or organizational failures, has resulted in the UK government instituting an array of proactive quality assurance initiatives with an emphasis on protecting and promoting patient safety.

It is anticipated that adherence to principles of clinical governance, risk management, and meaningful audit will assist in detecting, addressing, and eventually remedying failing standards. This in turn will, it is hoped, reduce the circumstances in which clinical error can flourish and in turn reduce the incidence of clinical negligence.

A greater understanding of the anatomy of clinical errors would undoubtedly contribute to their reduction. Key to this is the establishment of a system of reporting and investigation that encourages candor by guaranteeing anonymity or offering amnesty from legal censure.

The existence of institutions that collect anonymized information relating to adverse events is certainly not a novel concept; their future success in reducing errors will depend principally on their ability to look beyond epidemiology and into etiology.

See Also

Medical Malpractice – Medico-legal Perspectives: Negligence, Standard of Care; Negligence, Duty of Care; Negligence, Causation; Negligence Quantum

Further Reading

Department of Health (2000) *An Organisation with a Memory.* London: The Stationery Office (www.doh.gov.uk/cmo/orgmem/).

Department of Health (2004) *Making Amends: A Consultation Paper Setting out Proposals for Reforming the Approach to Clinical Negligence in the NHS* (www.doh.gov.uk).

Merry A, McCall Smith A (2003) *Errors, Medicine and the Law,* chapter 6. Cambridge, UK: Cambridge University Press.

National Institute for Clinical Standards. *UK Clinical Guidelines* (www.nice.org.uk).

Report by the Comptroller and Auditor General HC 403. (2004) *Handling Clinical Negligence Claims in England.* London: The Stationery Office (www.nao.gov.uk).

Report on the Inquiry into the Management of Care of Children Receiving Complex Heart Surgery at the Bristol Royal Infirmary. Command paper CM 5207. Legal Systems and Public Enquiries (www.bristol-inquiry.org.uk).

Accident and Emergency

J Wyatt and R Taylor, Royal Cornwall Hospital, Truro, UK

Malpractice in Accident and Emergency in Context

Staff working in accident and emergency departments often face difficult challenges. These include attempting to treat a number of different patients with different conditions at the same time, but without the benefit of much background information and often with the added complication of patients under the influence of alcohol and/or drugs. Considering all of this, it is perhaps not surprising that on occasions, medical assessments and treatments do go wrong. Malpractice or negligence is relatively frequently claimed against those working in accident and emergency, when compared with other specialties – in one UK study, the two specialties quoted as being most at risk of receiving negligence claims were accident and emergency and obstetrics and gynecology. Historically, rates of claims have varied significantly between different countries, with those in the USA greatly exceeding those in the UK.

Malpractice Defined

The essence of malpractice (which for practical purposes may be regarded as being negligence) is that incorrect management resulted in definite patient harm. The term is understandably inextricably linked in a legal way to claims for (financial) compensation. The exact definition is therefore different in different legal systems and requires to be proved in slightly different ways. Under many legal systems, to prove negligence against a clinician, the patient needs to show the following:

1. the clinician had a duty of care
2. the clinician breached that duty
3. the patient suffered as a result.

Duty of Care

For those working in accident and emergency, there is often agreement that the clinician does have a duty of care to a patient. Difficulties arise when patients (for various reasons) refuse to comply with treatment, perhaps exhibiting aggressive behavior or leaving the hospital against medical advice. In these circumstances, other legal issues can cloud the simple issue of whether adequate care was provided.

Breach of Duty

A key component of proving negligence is showing that the clinician's care failed to reach minimum standards for the specialty. For some conditions, there are published and agreed national standards against which to compare treatment. However, most of the conditions that make up accident and emergency medicine do not have agreed standards. As a result, each case tends to be examined on its merits and the clinician may be judged or measured against what a similarly experienced and expert clinician would be expected to do. In the UK, the clinician will try to defend him/herself by showing that he or she "acted in accordance with a practice accepted as proper by a responsible body of medical men skilled in that particular art." This approach has underpinned the defense against negligence since the Bolam case in 1957.

Patient Harm Resulting

Having shown that a clinician did have a duty of care and that this care did not reach minimum standards, negligence did not occur unless the patient can be shown to have suffered as a direct consequence. In many instances, significant errors or omissions in management, whilst potentially harmful, do not actually result in any harm or damage to the patient.

The Background to Complaints and Claims

A significant proportion of patients and/or their relatives who complain about treatment are not primarily seeking financial redress. However, those who submit legal claims almost invariably are. There are common themes amongst published data relating to complaints and claims against accident and emergency departments. Complaints frequently relate to the attitude and failure of communication of accident and emergency staff, but claims for negligence more often cite failure to obtain X-rays or to interpret correctly those X-rays that have been obtained. Failures relating to obtaining or interpreting X-rays do not appear to cause serious problems frequently. However, claims relating to missed medical and surgical diagnoses are also quite common, and do frequently result in significant harm. For example, amongst patients discharged from accident and emergency after a failure to diagnose acute appendicitis, there were high rates of ruptured appendix and postoperative complications. Historically, a particular problem has been accident and emergency staff missing diagnoses of acute cardiac problems (myocardial infarction and unstable angina); with current pressures to discharge patients rapidly from hospital, this problem shows no sign of disappearing.

Risk Reduction

Improving care, resulting in a reduced number of claims, would benefit both patients and staff: the emotional cost of complaints being made against staff is not inconsiderable. There is some evidence

that training may reduce rates of malpractice claims. Analysis of previous claims reveals areas worthy of consideration. Rates of missed fractures on X-rays analyzed by junior doctors in accident and emergency in the UK are acknowledged to be high and justify special focused training. The problem has also been tackled by an almost universal system of rapid reporting of X-rays by an appropriately trained expert, enabling errors to be quickly identified and patient harm minimized. In the fast-moving field of management of chest pain, emergency physicians are searching for ways of providing evidence-based treatment, allowing rapid discharge without compromising care (or risking litigation). Chest pain observation units, where patient care is determined by strict protocols, are emerging as a useful way forward.

The process of deciding whether or not negligence occurred almost inevitably relies heavily upon exactly what was documented in the medical notes. These comprise the crucial legal document in any dispute. The importance of making good contemporaneous notes cannot be underestimated. When subjected to scrutiny, observations and interventions that have not been documented will be assumed not to have taken place: all accident and emergency staff need to be reminded of this.

See Also

Medical Malpractice – Medico-legal Perspectives: Negligence, Standard of Care; Negligence, Duty of Care; Negligence, Causation; Negligence Quantum

Further Reading

Branney SW, Pons PT, Markovchick VJ, Thomasson GO (2000) Malpractice occurrence in emergency medicine: does residency training make a difference? *Journal of Emergency Medicine* 19: 99–105.

Goodacre SW (2000) Should we establish chest pain observation units in the UK? A systematic review and critical appraisal of the literature. *Journal of Accident and Emergency Medicine* 17: 1–6.

Guly HR (2001) Diagnostic errors in an accident and emergency department. *Emergency Medicine Journal* 18: 263–269.

Gwynne A, Barber P, Tavener F (1997) A review of 105 negligence claims against accident and emergency departments. *Journal of Accident and Emergency Medicine* 14: 243–245.

Hulbert DC, Riddle WL, Longstaff PM, Belstead JS, Beckett MW (1996) An audit of litigation costs in four accident and emergency departments. *Journal of Accident and Emergency Medicine* 13: 400–401.

Kadzombe EA, Coals J (1992) Complaints against doctors in an accident and emergency department: a 10 year analysis. *Archives of Emergency Medicine* 9: 134–142.

Karcz A, Korn R, Burke MC, *et al.* (1996) Malpractice claims against emergency physicians in Massachusetts: 1975–1993. *American Journal of Emergency Medicine* 14: 341–345.

McCarthy BD, Beshansky JR, D'Agostino RB, Selker HP (1993) Missed diagnoses of acute myocardial infarction in the emergency department: results from a multicenter study. *Annals of Emergency Medicine* 22: 579–582.

Montague A (1996) *Legal Problems in Emergency Medicine*. Oxford, UK: Oxford University Press.

Pope JH, Aufderheide TP, Ruthazer R, *et al.* (2000) Missed diagnoses of acute cardiac ischaemia in the emergency department. *New England Journal of Medicine* 342: 1163–1170.

Powell PV (1995) An audit of the handling of medical negligence complaints by a health board. *Health Bulletin* 53: 196–205.

Redmond A (1987) Medicolegal aspects of accident and emergency medicine. *Archives of Emergency Medicine* 4: 71–72.

Rusnak RA, Stair TO, Hansen K, Fastow JS (1989) Litigation against the emergency physician: common features in cases of missed myocardial infarction. *Annals of Emergency Medicine* 18: 1029–1034.

Rusnak RA, Borer JM, Fastow JS (1994) Misdiagnosis of acute appendicitis: common features discovered in cases after litigation. *American Journal of Emergency Medicine* 12: 397–402.

Wyatt JP, Weber JE, Chudnofsky C (1998) The work of the American emergency physician. *Journal of Accident and Emergency Medicine* 15: 170–174.

Wyatt JP, Illingworth RN, Clancy MJ, Munro P, Robertson CE (1999) *Oxford Handbook of Accident and Emergency Medicine*. Oxford, UK: Oxford University Press.

Anesthesiology

T E J Healy, University of Manchester, Manchester, UK

Introduction

> Then the Lord God cast a deep sleep upon Adam and when he was fast asleep, He took one of his ribs and filled up flesh for it.
>
> Genesis, Chapter 2, verse 21.

In this article the processes involved in the practice of anesthesia and the associated common adverse events are described. Anesthesia is the discipline of pain relief. Pain may result from many different causes but the nonanesthetist immediately links the anesthesiologist with the relief of pain during surgery. Indeed, the relief of pain during surgery has made all the advances in surgery possible. It is therefore true to say that surgery stands on the shoulders of anesthesia. In this article the process of anesthesia is discussed and some of the common difficulties which may lead to litigation explained. Pain relief during surgery may be provided by general or regional anesthesia or by a combination of both.

General Anesthesia

General anesthesia may be considered in three sections: (1) induction; (2) maintenance; and (3) recovery.

Induction Induction is the start of anesthesia and may be by the inhalation of a gas such as nitrous oxide or of a vapor, classically ether or chloroform, but today the anesthetist may use sevoflurane, enflurane, or halothane. Halothane is now being used much less frequently as its use may result in a centrilobular necrosis of the liver and death. This occurs particularly when the patient has been "sensitized" by a recent exposure to halothane. Anesthetists are advised to avoid the use of halothane within three months of a patient's previous exposure to halothane. An important property of inhalation drugs used for induction, apart from an absence of side-effects, is that they should be nonirritant.

A significant advance was the introduction of the intravenous anesthetic induction drugs. The first of these were barbiturates. Thiopental, a thiobarbiturate, was introduced in 1935. Thiopental is still widely used but has been largely replaced by propofol, which was introduced in 1981. Members of the benzodiazepine family, initially diazepam but more recently midazolam, are also used to induce anesthesia.

Vasodilatation is an unwanted side-effect of intravenous anesthetic drugs. Great care is therefore required to avoid hypotension by introducing the induction drug slowly while monitoring its effect on the cardiovascular system. This is particularly relevant when a reduced blood volume can be expected, such as following a large-volume hemorrhage, or after heavy diarrhea or vomiting. Intravenous drugs are usually injected into veins in the back of the hand or in the antecubital fossa. The basilic vein in the antecubital fossa lies over the brachial artery, which is an end artery, that is, there is no collateral arterial supply to the tissues supplied by the brachial artery. The accidental injection of thiopental into the brachial artery has resulted in precipitation of crystals of insoluble thiopental in small vessels in the limb and impaired circulation to the tissues supplied by the brachial artery, causing permanent loss of the peripheral regions of the fingers. Some drugs including thiopental are very irritant when injected into the subcutaneous tissues outside the vein and, if this occurs, the injection must cease immediately and the drug in the tissues must be diluted by the injection of 10 ml N-saline into the tissues. Failure to do this may result in significant tissue damage, irritation, and ulceration, litigation has followed.

Maintenance Maintenance is the period during which surgery takes place. The drugs used during this time are similar to those used during the induction process. Maintenance may therefore be by the use of inhalation or by intravenous anesthetic drugs. Propofol is the first intravenous drug suitable for both induction and maintenance and it is widely used for both purposes. Drugs administered by inhalation include sevoflurane, isoflurane, enflurane, and desflurane. Halothane may also be used but it is now increasingly restricted because of its association with liver damage. Nitrous oxide (laughing gas) and oxygen are used as the carrier gases for the vapors of the inhalation agents listed above.

A combination of nitrous oxide with oxygen and one of the vapors, with the patient breathing spontaneously constitutes a standard anesthetic formula. Other drugs may be given at this time and these include a muscle relaxant. The use of a muscle relaxant paralyzes the patient and therefore makes controlled ventilation mandatory. Potent analgesics such as morphine, fentanyl, sufentanil, alfentanil, or remifentanil may also be given.

Recovery Recovery is the period during which anesthesia is withdrawn and consciousness returns. Other drugs may be given at this time. These include the muscle relaxant reversal drugs, analgesics, and other miscellaneous drugs, including anticholinergics. These drugs will be mentioned later.

Local Anesthesia

The practice of local anesthesia may also be considered, though less commonly, under three headings of induction, maintenance, and recovery. The techniques of local anesthesia, sometimes called conduction blockade, may be considered under three headings: (1) infiltration anesthesia; (2) regional anesthesia; and (3) intravenous local blockade.

1. Infiltration is the injection of the local anesthetic drug directly into the tissues in the surgical area or through which the nerve supply to those tissues passes. This is experienced when visiting the dentist who infiltrates local anesthetic drug around the mandibular nerve and into the gum around the tooth which is to be the subject of the treatment. A similar technique, that is, local anesthetic drug infiltration, may be used for the repair of a hernia or the removal of a ganglion or other lump.
2. Regional anesthesia is typified by blockade of a large but defined area, as in the case of epidural or spinal injection of the drug. The various plexus blocks such as the brachial, lumbar, or sacral plexus block are also included under this heading.
3. Intravenous local blockade involves injection of a large dose of the local anesthetic drug into a vein in the arm or leg. This is known as a Biers block. A tourniquet must be used to reduce the amount of the drug that may escape, from the intended area of block into the general circulation lest a generalized toxic reaction and, of course, loss of blockade occurs. Local anesthetic may nonetheless escape through intraosseous capillaries, therefore, the use of toxic local anesthetic drugs such as bupivacaine for intravenous local anesthesia is forbidden.

The Process of Anesthesia

Preoperative Assessment

Many patients who present for surgery have intercurrent disease apart from the pathology for which surgery is required. For example, the patient requiring hip replacement surgery may also suffer from hypertension and angina. The same patient is likely to be taking medication to control blood pressure. Some of the medications may interact with some of the drugs used during anesthesia. Beta-adrenergic receptor-blocking drugs may precipitate heart failure and the bradycardia associated with their use may limit the heart's ability to respond to hemorrhage. The prolongation of the action of suxamethonium by ecothiopate eye drops and the interaction between monoamine oxidase inhibitors and opioid narcotic analgesics and sympathomimetic amines are well-recognized examples, but there are many more.

The drugs that the patient is taking reveal some of the patient's intercurrent diseases, and therefore, some of the likely pharmacological difficulties that may occur during anesthesia. The preoperative discussion and examination may identify various other problems such as untreated or inadequately treated hypertension, angina, previous myocardial infarction, upper and lower airway disease, epilepsy, multiple sclerosis, or use of the contraceptive pill. Previous problems with general anesthesia include acute adverse reactions to drugs used during anesthesia (anaphylactic or anaphylactoid). A patient who suffered an anaphylactic reaction to pancuronium, but survived with slight brain damage, suffered a similar reaction to vecuronium and died. The similar chemical structures are illustrated in **Figure 1**. The life-threatening features of an anaphylactic reaction include bronchospasm, hypotension, and tachycardia.

Untreated or inadequately treated hypertension may result during anesthesia in a very unstable blood pressure, that is, marked rises or falls in blood pressure may occur. Furthermore, when hypotension occurs in a diabetic hypertensive patient, especially when associated with hemorrhage, ischemic optic neuropathy and associated blindness have resulted in litigation.

It is important to discuss the effect that anesthesia has had on other members of the patient's family, as some interactions with anesthesia are inherited. These include an inherited atypical cholinesterase that results in an unexpectedly prolonged paralysis following the muscle relaxant suxamethonium; some patients develop a malignant hyperpyrexia following injection of suxamethonium or inhalation of halothane; and patients with dystrophia myotonica are at very serious risk following the use of muscle relaxants. Sickle-cell anemia is a genetically linked condition common in patients with Afro-Caribbean roots. In this condition, hypoxia and hypothermia

result in a change in shape of the normally spherical red cells. The red cells become sickle-shaped and thrombosis, severe pain, and hypoxia result. Acute hemolytic crises include fever, rheumatic pains, and abdominal symptoms. There may be severe anemia. The anesthetist must therefore identify whether a blood transfusion is required before surgery.

The preoperative examination provides the opportunity to anticipate the likely need for an intraoperative transfusion and to arrange for an appropriate volume of blood to be cross-matched. It is a wise practice in the case of patients who are more than 55 years of age to arrange for an electrocardiogram and for some patients, that is, when disease is suspected, a chest X-ray should be performed. Relevant blood analyses must be available before surgery begins, for example, a hemoglobin estimation is essential when bleeding has occurred, or when there is clinical evidence that suggests that the patient is anemic.

It is important to be aware of loose teeth which may be inadvertently dislodged and inhaled during anesthesia. It is essential to identify the patient who will be difficult to intubate, and to plan how control of the airway patency can be assured. The anesthetist must nonetheless be prepared to deal with unexpected life-threatening airway obstruction. In **Figure 2** a large tumor which completely obstructed the airway can be seen rising from behind the tongue. The patient, who had no previous evidence of a tumor in her throat, was about to undergo surgery for a breast carcinoma.

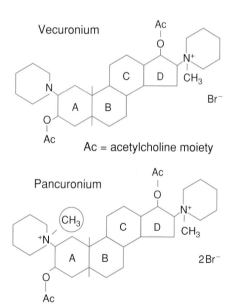

Figure 1 The chemical structures of vecuronium and pancuronium. A patient suffered an anaphylatic reaction to pancuronium and subsequently suffered a similar reaction to vecuronium and died.

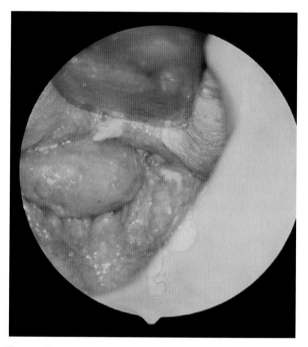

Figure 2 A large tumor can be seen rising up behind the tongue during attempted intubation.

The preanesthetic discussion can provide information that may be very important when planning postoperative care. Obstructive sleep apnea, a condition in which respiratory obstruction occurs during normal sleep, may occur following general anesthesia and lead to hypoxia and brain damage, or death. For these patients, great care must be exercised when selecting the dose and the drug to be used for postoperative analgesia and the analgesic drugs used during surgery, which affect the postoperative period. Indeed, in many cases postoperative care plans may be arranged before surgery starts. A patient with obstructive sleep apnea that required postoperative care in a high-dependency unit, but was sent back to the general ward, suffered respiratory obstruction, and died.

The examples given represent only the flavor of the investigations and clinical management required. The preoperative examination offers an important opportunity to identify the need for additional precautions. Nonemergency surgery for patients with uncontrolled hypertension, thyrotoxicosis, or an upper or lower respiratory tract infection should be postponed.

Premedication

Many patients desire sedation while others wish to remain fully awake during induction of general anesthesia, or during the injection of local anesthesia. Temazepam, an oral benzodiazepine, is an effective anxiolytic in a dose which has only minimal sedative action. Opioid drugs such as morphine or diamorphine may be used when the patient is in pain and to augment the analgesic effects of the anesthetic drugs.

Consent

Volenti nonfit injuria It is during the preoperative interview and examination that consent should be obtained. Great care is required to provide sufficient and appropriate information for the patient to make an informed decision. In providing information to the patient, it is necessary for the doctor to have identified those matters that are of maximum importance to each individual patient. Not all patients have identical priorities. Lawyers will know well the Australian case of Rogers and Whitaker. The patient, Mrs Whitaker, had only one sound eye but the surgeon suggested that he could give back the sight to the damaged eye. Mrs Whitaker requested that all care should be taken to protect her good eye. The surgeon failed to mention the possibility of sympathetic ophthalmia, a condition in which the eye that is not being subjected to surgery develops an inflammatory response in sympathy with the eye that has been the subject of surgery. This occurred in Mrs Whitaker's

case and she lost the sight in her good eye, without gain in the previously damaged eye. The surgeon had considered the likelihood of damage from this cause to be 1 in 14 000 and therefore unimportant and not worth mentioning. It was however the type of information that Mrs Whittaker needed. Her most important interest was her good eye, and she had made this quite clear. Consent is a state of mind!

The Induction of Anesthesia

General The drugs to be used, the anesthetic machine, the monitors, and other equipment must be carefully checked. The patient's preinduction blood pressure, pulse rate, and pulse oxygen hemoglobin saturation should normally be measured and recorded. It is a standard practice to activate a continuous electrocardiograph display. These activities make some patients, such as children, very anxious by these activities and it may not be appropriate to make all these measurements until the child is asleep, but they must be introduced as soon as possible.

It is essential that an intravenous cannula is in place, usually in a vein in the back of the hand, before intravenous induction drugs are administered. The administration of multiple drugs is made easier by this, but more importantly the established venous access makes possible an immediate corrective response when an adverse reaction occurs. There are a number of local anesthetic creams that can be used to reduce the prick sensation and these are particularly valuable for children.

The intravenous anesthetic drug is then given slowly, and the patient is observed continuously. If given too quickly, the induction drug may, in those patients who are compensating for a reduced blood volume, cause vasodilatation and grave hypotension and even death. After induction a face mask may be applied to the face or a laryngeal mask passed into the throat. When a face mask is used, the lower jaw must be held forward in order to lift the tongue off the posterior pharyngeal wall to avoid respiratory obstruction (**Figure 3**). The laryngeal mask is an alternative to the face mask. The laryngeal mask is placed to lie behind the tongue and over the glottic opening. The primary advantage of the laryngeal mask over the face mask is that the anesthetist has both hands free for other tasks. It has been observed that the laryngeal mask is ideal when the patient is breathing spontaneously, but that it should not be used for positive-pressure ventilation, that is, when the patient's breathing is controlled by a ventilator. This is because there is the ever-present risk of anesthetic gases passing into the stomach, with the increased possibility of regurgitation or active vomiting. This

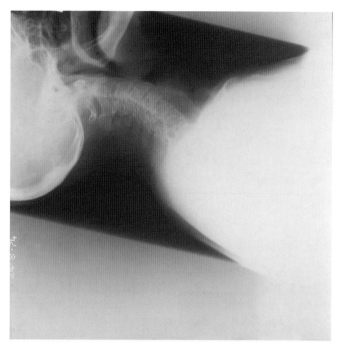

Figure 3 X-Ray neck shows the tongue obstructing the airway.

view has the support of many anesthetists, but by no means all. It seems to be a practice that may in due course require settlement by the judiciary.

The alternative approach is to intubate and ventilate the patient, that is, control the ventilation. Intubation involves placing a tube in the trachea, i.e., an endotracheal tube. An endotracheal tube with an inflatable cuff is usually used. When the cuff is inflated against the tracheal wall it forms an airtight fit. The tube may be passed through the mouth or through the nose. It is routine practice to paralyze the patient to facilitate intubation. The patient may also be intubated while breathing spontaneously under deep anesthesia, or if conscious, local anesthesia may be used. Intubation may be easy or exceedingly difficult. The anesthetist's view of the glottic opening during intubation can be seen in **Figure 4**. The tube can be seen lying in the trachea in **Figure 5**.

Before induction, the careful anesthetist will assess the degree of difficulty expected to achieve intubation by using a scoring system. The Mallampati system is most commonly used to identify the degree of difficulty that may be expected to achieve intubation.

When a difficult intubation is expected the anesthetist must be prepared to use a fiberoptic laryngoscope, or one of the special techniques such as passing a catheter through the cricothyroid membrane, just below the thyroid cartilage (the Adam's apple), up towards and behind the tongue and then passing the

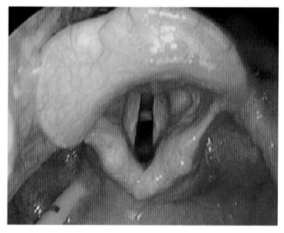

Figure 4 The anesthetist's view of the glottic opening during intubation. Reproduced with permission from Haslam N, Parker L and Duggan JE (2005) Effect of cricoid pressure on the view at laryngoscopy. *Anaesthesia* 60: 41–47. Copyright Blackwell Publishing 2005.

endotracheal tube over this and on through the glottis. The endotracheal tube may also be railroaded over a gum elastic catheter. It is absolutely essential, in all but emergency surgery, that the anesthetist confirms, using a face mask, that the patient can be ventilated before giving a relaxant drug. It must be remembered that the paralyzed patient cannot breathe; therefore, if the anesthetist cannot intubate

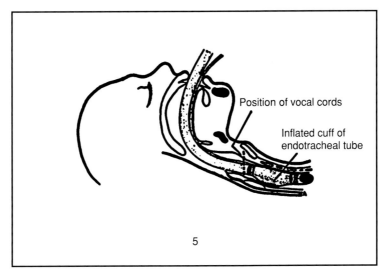

Position of vocal cords

Inflated cuff of
endotracheal tube

5

Figure 5 Endotracheal tube lying in the trachea.

and cannot ventilate using a mask, an immediate tracheotomy is required or the patient will die.

It is essential to confirm the correct placement of the endotracheal tube which is achieved most safely by the use of a capnograph to measure the expired carbon dioxide levels. Clearly, no anesthetic should be started until a capnograph has been tested and is included in the airway circuit. Unfortunately, while the use of capnograph is a requirement of the Royal College of Anaesthetists, in a recent anesthetic case no capnograph was used and this led to the death of a patient, a young healthy woman, following esophageal intubation. A failed tracheal intubation must be recognized immediately to avoid life-threatening hypoxia. The presence of breath sounds over the chest, while reassuring, may be heard when the endotracheal tube is in the esophagus. It is important nonetheless to auscultate over the chest after known correct intubation to confirm that the tube has not been passed in too far, that is, beyond the carina into the right main bronchus. This position would result in a hypoxic patient and, unless identified, a collapsed left lung (**Figures 6** and **7**).

The angles at which the main bronchi join the trachea are the reason why the right main bronchus is invariably the one that is entered by an endotracheal tube placed too deeply. Particular problems present when there is a partial laryngeal obstruction. In some cases, such as carcinoma of the larynx, it is essential for some patients first to perform a tracheotomy under local anesthesia to ensure that the airway is protected and the danger of a complete obstruction has been avoided. Deaths have occurred when this precaution has been ignored. Intubation may be used to prevent respiratory obstruction in young children with acute epiglottitis. In one case, it was agreed that

if the patient had been intubated, the cardiac arrest and brain damage that followed would have been prevented. The careful anesthetist will always ensure that when there may be difficulty, the surgeon is scrubbed and ready to carry out an emergency tracheotomy if control of airway patency is lost during the attempted intubation of these patients.

It is usual to require that the patient has been fasting from food and drink for at least four hours, preferably six hours, to ensure that the stomach contents are reduced as much as possible before induction of anesthesia. The danger is that, during induction of anesthesia, esophageal regurgitation of gastric contents and their inhalation may occur. Even following anesthesia, the glottic protective reflex may be inactive for around two hours. In an emergency, this ideal may not be possible, and the risk that the patient may inhale gastric contents, regurgitated up the esophagus into the pharynx, must be guarded against. This protection may be achieved in a number of ways. The patient may be turned on his/her side with a few degrees of head-down tilt. If regurgitation or active vomiting occurs, the material will pass out of the mouth and not pool in the posterior pharynx and overflow into the glottis.

Another common approach is to have the patient lying supine with the anesthetist's assistant pressing down on the cricoid cartilage. The pressure prevents passive regurgitation but not necessarily active vomiting. This technique is sometimes known as Sellick's maneuver. Failure to prevent the inhalation of gastric material, which includes hydrochloric acid, results in damage to lung tissue with pulmonary edema (**Figure 8**), developing into pneumonia and frequently death. This syndrome is known as pulmonary aspiration or Mendelson's syndrome.

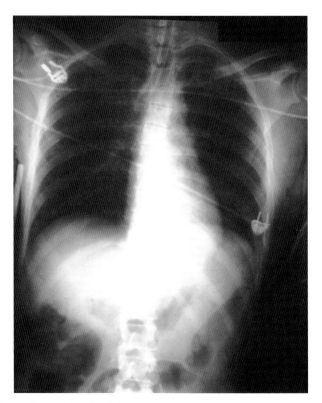

Figure 6 Endotracheal tube shown directed into the right main bronchus.

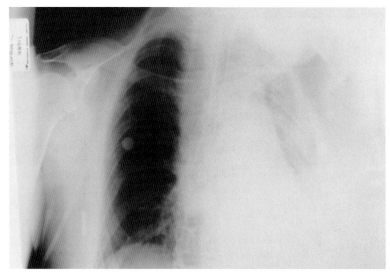

Figure 7 The endotracheal tube passing into the right main bronchus. The left lung is collapsed and airless.

Maintenance Naturally occurring opioid drugs such as morphine or diamorphine and synthetic opioids such as fentanyl, alfentanil, and remifentanil are frequently given to provide analgesia. These drugs are used in addition to the inhalation anesthetic drugs mentioned above or in addition to propofol during total intravenous anesthesia (TIVA). In patients whose breathing is controlled, a muscle relaxant is also used. Controlled ventilation may be without a muscle relaxant, though deeper levels of anesthesia are usually required. The muscle relaxant makes controlled ventilation easier at lighter levels of anesthesia. However, when the surgery is intraabdominal, muscle relaxation is essential to prevent

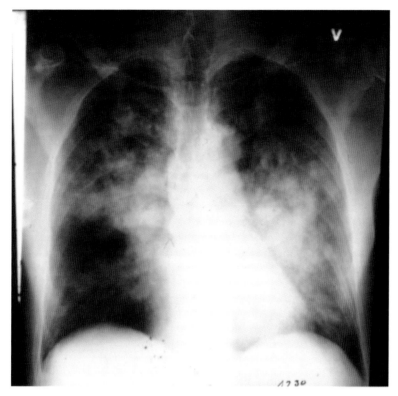

Figure 8   X-ray view of a patient's lungs following inhalation of gastric contents during intubation before cesarean section.

the abdominal contents from being forced out of the abdominal cavity and at the end of surgery to permit the easy closure of the anterior abdominal wall.

Nitrous oxide is usually used as the carrier gas for the anesthetic vapor. It also has strong analgesic properties. Patients are generally hyperventilated during the period of anesthesia. Hyperventilation ensures that the blood carbon dioxide does not rise and the patient gains from the analgesic effect of hypocarbia. Hypercarbia may result in vasodilatation with increased bleeding.

It is essential to monitor expired carbon dioxide continuously throughout surgery not only to ensure that the pulmonary ventilation is appropriate, but also to monitor anesthetic tubing disconnection. It is not surprising that ventilatory circuit disconnections occur, especially during head and neck surgery and when general changes in position are required. Of course, the anesthetist should confirm the security of the oxygen/anesthetic tubing connections, but disconnections can occur when least expected; hence, it is essential to use a capnograph. During a disconnection, no expired carbon dioxide reaches the capnograph, indicating that a disconnection has occurred.

Other standard monitors include an automated blood pressure-measuring device. Blood pressure may rise or fall during surgery. Falls in blood pressure

may be due to an increase in the depth of the anesthetic or an interaction between the various drugs used. It may also indicate a sudden or progressive loss of blood. Loss of blood is usually but not always obvious. It must be remembered that the circulation depends on the heart rate, the venous return flow, myocardial contractility, and the peripheral resistance. The heart rate may be affected by surgical activity such as stretching of the bowel. The venous return is affected by hemorrhage and vasodilatation. Myocardial contractility is affected by the depressant action of drugs, including the anesthetic drugs. The peripheral resistance depends on the degree of vasodilatation, which is affected by anesthetic drugs. Bleeding may occur deep in the peritoneal cavity, or indeed be hidden in the tissues and, while not seen by the anesthetist, should be anticipated. A fall in expired carbon dioxide may indicate that circulatory failure has occurred. Cardiovascular stability may also be disturbed by cardiac rhythm changes, which may signify other pathologies, including myocardial infarction. It is therefore essential to follow the blood pressure changes continually. The five-minute intervals are generally considered appropriate, though more frequent recordings may be required. The heart rate may reflect changes in blood pressure, inadequate analgesia, and a response to hemorrhage or to some drugs. In particular the anticholinergics increase heart rate, while the beta-blocking drugs slow the rate. Heart rate must therefore be monitored continuously.

Changes in cardiovascular performance influence excretion of carbon dioxide, hence the essential importance of capnography, but oxygenation may also be affected. Oxygenation also affects cardiovascular performance. It is essential therefore to display oxygen/hemoglobin saturation continuously. This is easily done by attaching a sensor to the finger or the earlobe. Gross changes in oxygen/hemoglobin saturation are visible in light-skinned Caucasians as a blue color of the skin and mucous membranes (cyanosis). The skin changes are not as visible in a dark-skinned people, but the mucous membranes and tissues inside the body such as the muscles show the same blue (cyanotic) changes in all peoples, as do the mucous membranes.

More sophisticated measurement of cardiovascular function includes central venous pressure (CVP) and pulmonary artery (PA) pressure measurements. CVP requires a catheter to be passed up a great vein such as the basilic vein in the arm, or the internal/external jugular veins in the neck, until the tip of the catheter is in the right atrium of the heart. The position is confirmed by the pressure waveform. The catheter is then withdrawn until the pressures fall, and changes in the pressure are related to breathing. Alternatively, a chest X-ray may be used to identify the position of the catheter tip. The CVP is frequently measured by passing the catheter into the subclavian vein. The common complication of this approach is a pneumothorax following penetration of the lung by the needle. Damage may also occur to the subclavian artery, leading to hemorrhage and hematoma formation. It is essential that both of these potentially serious complications are excluded by a chest X-ray following catheter insertion. Failure to X-ray the chest immediately has resulted in both hemorrhage and pneumothorax threatening the patient's life. The CVP pressures are, of course, much lower than the pressures in the atrium. CVP measurement should always be used when major hemorrhage is anticipated or is taking place and when cardiac failure is present or anticipated. The pressure measured is generated by blood returning to the heart and, while not a measurement of blood volume, it is an indication of over- or undertransfusion. It is therefore an indication that appropriate blood replacement has been or is being given. Rises in CVP may indicate overtransfusion or cardiac failure and therefore provide an invaluable window into cardiovascular function. PA measurement requires that the catheter be passed through the right atrium and right ventricle into the PA. This device provides extensive information about cardiac function.

It is now considered important to monitor continuously the inspired/expired anesthetic vapor concentrations. The term minimum alveolar concentration (MAC) of an inhaled anesthetic agent is used to describe the concentration of vapor in the alveoli at which only 50% of rats will remove their tails from a hot plate. The MAC value is obviously directly related to the brain concentration of the agent being used. The term, in clinical anesthetic practice, is used to describe the MAC value for any inhalation agent, that is, the alveolar concentration at which 50% of patients will be asleep. Clearly, at 2 MAC a greater percentage of patients will be asleep. The number of patients reaches 100% at 3 MAC. Other factors, such as the concentration of nitrous oxide used as a carrier gas and the doses of analgesics given, will alter the required MAC necessary to ensure that the patient is asleep. The measurement of the inspired and expired concentrations of the anesthetic vapor is therefore essential for good anesthetic practice. The measurement of the MAC value is not a measurement of the depth of anesthesia, nor even an indication that the patient is asleep, but it can be used with the measurement of other variables such as the pulse rate and an assessment of other patient social factors, such as alcohol intake and surgical stimulation, to judge the appropriateness of the anesthetic being given.

Position during general anesthesia is an important risk factor; in particular, avoidable nerve damage can result.

In the case of prolonged surgery, the patient's temperature, unless heat conservation or heating is used, is likely to fall. It is important in these cases to monitor core temperature. The use of skin temperature measurement is useless as vasoconstriction occurs in the skin during cooling and therefore skin temperature will not reflect core temperature. Esophageal or rectal temperature is therefore monitored. Intravascular temperature monitoring may also be used. Temperature may be maintained by infusion of warm fluid, blood, or crystalloid (salt solutions), by a water-heated mattress, and by blowing warm air around the patient. Hot-water bottles may cause skin burns and should not be used. Temperature measurement and control are essential for babies and small infants.

Recovery Essentially, recovery requires the anesthetic to be switched off and then breathed out, or in the case of a TIVA to be metabolized to nonanesthetic substances, or excreted to allow consciousness to return. It is important to reverse the residual action of the muscle relaxants and this is achieved by the injection of a drug with an anticholinesterase action.

The most commonly used drug is neostigmine and another is edrophonium. These drugs prevent cholinesterase, an enzyme present in the blood and in the region of the neuromuscular junction, from breaking down the acetylcholine. Acetylcholine is the substance secreted at the nerve endings, which activates muscle depolarization and contraction. The actions of acetylcholine are of two types: nicotinic and muscurinic. At the neuromuscular junction, acetylcholine is nicotinic, whereas it is muscurinic at the acetylcholine receptors in the heart and its action slows the heart. The muscurinic action of the acetylcholine is blocked by the use of anticholinergic drugs such as atropine or glycopyrollate. Failure to give the anticholinergic has resulted in a cardiac arrest. Bradycardia during surgery has also been treated, though not always effectively, by the use of an anticholinergic. Bradycardia which fails to respond to an anti-cholinergic drug is usually treated with epinephrine (adrenaline), isoprenaline or another inotrope and oxygen.

Following general anesthesia the glottic reflex may remain obtunded for about two hours and therefore following extubation the patient should be nursed on his/her side, at least until fully awake; otherwise vomiting or passive regurgitation, with the inhalation of gastric contents, and the serious complication of pulmonary aspiration syndrome are possible risks.

Patients may complain of pain during recovery and adequate pain relief must be given. Opioid drugs such as morphine are still the most commonly used analgesics, though there is an increasing use of nonsteroidal antiinflammatory drugs (NSAIDs), or combinations of an opioid and an NSAID. Diamorphine (heroin) is also widely used in the UK. It is common practice to inject a small dose of opioid drug intravenously to achieve a rapid onset of effect, but great care must be taken to avoid respiratory depression. Alternatively, the analgesic may be injected intramuscularly or administered rectally. The use of spinal and epidural anesthesia (analgesia) for postoperative pain relief is common practice, especially following lower abdominal and lower-limb surgery. A very popular technique is patient-controlled analgesia (PCA). This approach must be discussed with the patient. The patient is able to inject an intravenous bolus of analgesic in a preset dose by pressing a button when in pain. Lockout times are built into the computer program to prevent an overdose. The doctor may, when required and if judged safe, override the lockout and administer a separate bolus. The use of a PCA has proved to be one of the most significant recent advances in postoperative pain control. In some ways, it is analogous with the self-administration of a drug, by inhalation, such as nitrous oxide during labor. Care must be taken with elderly patients to differentiate between

confusion and pain. Analgesics are not appropriate when confusion is related to hypoxia.

It is the responsibility of the anesthetist to detail the postoperative care instructions, that is, the variables to be monitored and the limits before medical advice is sought, and the analgesia and intravenous fluid prescriptions, in addition to any other drugs taken routinely.

Regional Anesthesia and Analgesia

Regional blockade may be considered under two sections – central and peripheral – and may be described as the use of a local anesthetic agent to block pain sensation from a defined region of the body.

Regional blockade may be used in conjunction with general anesthesia. Controversy continues concerning the placing of the local block after the start of general anesthesia, in particular, when the local blockade is central, that is, subarachnoid (spinal) or extradural (epidural), including caudal. The passage of the spinal needle may, on impact with a nerve root or nerve, cause an unpleasant sensation in the distribution of the nerve concerned. This is the signal for the anesthetist to withdraw the needle slightly or completely and then recommence the placement at a different vertebral level. The anesthetized patient cannot communicate that the needle placement caused pain and may therefore suffer serious damage if the injection of the drug is started while the tip of the needle is within the nerve. Disruption of the nerve may result in permanent loss of motor power and sensation in the region supplied by the damaged nerve or nerve root. The potential for serious damage is so great that central blockade should be established, or the catheter must be in position and tested before general anesthesia is induced.

Central blockade Central blockade is widely practiced. Many patients undergo cesarean section under spinal or epidural anesthesia. Neurological complications may also follow spinal ischemia associated with hypotension or air embolism, the neurotoxic effects of the drug, compression of the nerve root or the spinal cord by hemorrhage, and abscess formation. Some authorities have expressed the opinion that one area of unwarranted complacency is the belief among many experienced anesthetists that they can identify intervertebral spaces accurately by palpation. This is not the case. The usual clinical method for identifying the interspace is by a line that joins the two iliac crests, but this depends on the line being at a constant vertebral level, which it is not. The line, Tuffier's line, crosses the vertebral column with a maximal incidence at the L4–L5 disk but it may be higher and, if a higher level coincides with an identification error, that is, a higher space is thought to be L4–L5, there is danger to the spinal cord. The lumbar subarachnoid space should be entered below the termination of the cord. Unfortunately, the spinal cord does not always end at or above the interspace L1–L2. Great care is therefore required in needle placement.

Other complications of spinal anesthesia include hypotension, bradycardia, spinal hematoma, nausea and vomiting, headache, urinary retention, and infection. An unexpected high block can result in respiratory difficulty and unconsciousness.

Other complications of epidural blockade include dural puncture; if this is unrecognized, a large dose of local anesthetic may be injected into the subarachnoid space, leading to hypotension and spinal ischemia, respiratory depression, unconsciousness, and convulsions following an intravascular injection. Even recognized dural puncture may, as a result of cerebrospinal fluid leak, result in a severe postdural headache. Hemorrhage may result in a spinal hematoma.

Peripheral blockade Peripheral blockade includes intercostal, intrapleural, paravertebral, inguinal, cervical, brachial plexus, and lumbar plexus anesthesia. Specific nerve blockade is also employed and includes ulnar, radial, and median nerve blockade, and the lower-limb femoral, obturator, and sciatic nerve blockade. Pneumothorax is generally considered to be the complication of an intercostal block, although this is not common. In the case of an intrapleural block, care must be taken to avoid a rapid injection of local anesthetic resulting in toxic blood levels. Paravertebral block may be associated with a pneumothorax, toxicity is associated with high volumes of drug, and damage to spinal nerves may arise from subarachnoid and extradural injection of local anesthetic drug. Great care is required for cervical blockade, which may result in vascular or dural puncture, leading to convulsions. In addition, the phrenic nerve, stellate ganglion, and the recurrent laryngeal nerve may be blocked depending on the approach to the brachial plexus. Intravenous regional blockade is a common blockade used for limb surgery but complications may occur, such as a toxic response to an overdose if the tourniquet cuff deflates. Anesthesia is limited by the duration of the circulatory arrest. Femoral blockade is associated with intravascular injection, hematoma formation and nerve damage. It is contraindicated in the presence of a femoral graft.

Conclusion

The term anesthesia is derived from the ancient Greek word "anaisthesia," which means "the want of consciousness or sensation." The possibility of operating without pain has been the most important step in the development of modern surgery, following the aseptic treatment of wounds. The desire to relieve pain is as old as human history but its consummation extended over many centuries, during which endless attempts were made to relieve human suffering. Such attempts were forcibly expressed by Hippocrates: "*Divinum est opus sedare dolorem.*" (It is divine work to relieve pain.)

The countless attempts and failures over the centuries led Velpeau to express his thoughts using these rather melancholic words shortly before the discovery of anesthesia: "*Eviter la douleur dans les opérations est une chimère, qui n'est pas premise de poursuivre.*" (To discover ways of avoiding pain during operations is an imaginary objective which it is not permitted "to us" to pursue.)

Anesthesia has been described as a reversible journey toward death, and it is for this reason that the evolution of modern anesthesia has been influenced by increasing concerns for safety. The immediate influence of the various agents on the cardiovascular and respiratory systems and their inherent toxicity, affecting hepatic and renal function, has influenced the direction and rate of progress. In spite of substantial advances, life-threatening anaphylactic or anaphylactoid responses still occur particularly during the induction of anesthesia. These require an immediate and correct response by the anesthetist to avoid serious damage or death. Surgery may be considered as minor or major depending on its complexity. However, anesthesia, both general and regional, always brings with it a threat to life or of serious damage.

The responsibilities of the anesthesiologist and the dangers through which he/she must guide the patient are well illustrated by the ancient words spoken by Hippocrates centuries ago: "Life is short – the art is long – opportunity is fleeting – experiment is perilous –decision is difficult."

See Also

Consent: Treatment Without Consent; **Medical Malpractice – Medico-legal Perspectives:** Negligence, Standard of Care; Negligence, Duty of Care; Negligence, Causation

Further Reading

Barontini F, Conti P, Marello G, Maurri S (1996) Major neurological sequelae of lumbar epidural anesthesia. *Italian Journal of Neurological Sciences* 17: 333–339.

Bolitho v. *City and Hackney Health Authority* (CA) (1993) 4 Med LR 381.

Britt BA, Gordon RA (1964) Peripheral nerve injuries associated with anaesthesia. *Canadian Anaesthetist's Society Journal* 11: L514–L536.

Broadbent CR, Maxwell WB, Ferrie R, *et al.* (2000) Ability of anaesthetists to identify a marked lumbar interspace. *Anaesthesia* 55: 1122–1126.

Dundee JW (1976) Intra-arterial thiopental. *Anesthesiology* 45: 610–621.

Fischer HBJ (1998) Regional anaesthesia – before or after general anaesthesia? *Anaesthesia* 53: 727–729.

Frerk CM (1991) Predicting difficult intubation. *Anaesthesia* 46: 1005–1008.

Haslam N, Parker L, Duggan JE (2005) Effect of cricoid pressure on the view at laryngoscopy. *Anaesthesia* 60: 41–47.

Healy TEJ, Knight PR (2003) *Wylie and Churchill Davidson's A Practice of Anesthesia*. Arnold.

Hogan QH (1993) Tuffier's line: the normal distribution of anatomic parameters. *Anesthesia and Analgesia* 76: 1004–1007.

Kulendran Y, Rahman S, Venkat N (1999) Long-term neurological complication following traumatic damage to the spinal cord with a 25 gauge Whitacre spinal needle. *International Journal of Obstetric Anesthesia* 8: 62–66.

Mallampati SR, Gatt SP, Gugino LD, *et al.* (1985) A clinical sign to predict difficult intubation: a prospective study. *Canadian Anaesthetist's Society Journal* 32: 429–434.

Moore DC (1975) Intercostal nerve block for postoperative somatic pain following surgery of the thorax and upper abdomen. *British Journal of Anaesthesia* 47: 284–286.

Reynolds F (2000) Logic in safe practice of spinal anaesthesia. *Anaesthesia* 55: 1045–1046.

Reynolds F (2001) Case report. Damage to the conus medullaris following spinal anaesthesia. *Anaesthesia* 56: 235–247.

Rogers v. *Whittaker* (HCAus) (1993) 4 Med LR 79.

Tomlin PJ, Howarth FH, Robinson JS (1968) Post-operative atelectasis and laryngeal incompetence. *Lancet* 2: 1422.

Child and Adolescent Psychiatry

J Jureidini, Women's and Children's Hospital, Adelaide, SA, Australia

Introduction

Medical misconduct (the kinds of behavior that bring doctors before medical boards) is more commonly a problem in child psychiatry than medical malpractice (the kinds of behavior that bring clinicians before civil courts). The limited available data suggest that child psychiatrists may be at greater risk of being disciplined than their adult colleagues. Disturbingly, child psychiatrists appear to be at least as likely to commit sexual indiscretions as their adult colleagues. In determining whether medical misconduct has occurred in child and adolescent psychiatry, the guiding principle is that the best interests of the child are paramount. Because the child is not regarded as legally responsible for actions, more responsibility resides with the clinician than is the case with adult patients. The child's minor status also introduces a third-party decision-maker (usually the parents, but sometimes the state), and it is not uncommon for issues of responsibility to be further clouded by the child psychiatrist developing a therapeutic relationship with the parent.

Definition

Medical malpractice occurs when there is "dereliction" of "duty of care" that is the proximate cause of harm to a patient.

Duty of Care

Although duty of care requires that a therapeutic relationship be established, face-to-face contact is not required, so that telephone advice to a parent can establish duty of care. There may also be a duty of care to nonpatients (e.g., Tarasoff requirements to warn those who may be at danger from a patient). Nor do all face-to-face contacts necessarily impose a duty of care. It is usually accepted that a discrete child psychiatric assessment for forensic purposes does not impose a duty of care provided the purpose of the assessment is made clear to the family (but forensic assessment does carry the same mandatory notification requirements).

Dereliction of Duty

This requires a deviation from the ordinary standard of care, by commission or omission. Expert testimony is required to demonstrate negligence, but not "intentional tort" (where there is judged to be deliberate intent to harm, or that the psychiatrist ought to have known that his/her behavior was wrong, for example, sexual misconduct). An error of judgment does not constitute negligence. There is an expectation of ordinary competence, ordinary being defined in terms of national standards. However, even where explicit practice guidelines are available, these are generally not regarded as binding and a "respected minority" approach is usually acceptable. In addition, special circumstances can be taken into account, for example, the requirement for an isolated practitioner to make decisions outside his/her core area of expertise because more expert services are not available locally.

Proximate Cause

To establish malpractice, the dereliction of duty needs to have made a substantive contribution to the harm done. Thus the child psychiatrist who provides a prescription that ultimately leads to a child's death by suicide would not be held responsible if it could be shown that the child was likely to commit suicide by some other means if the tablets had not been available.

In adult psychiatry, misconduct is sometimes mitigated by demonstrating that the patients themselves have contributed to their outcome by not suitably advising their psychiatrist of, for example, their suicidal intent. This mitigation would hold less in child psychiatry where children are not held responsible for their actions.

Harm

Malpractice claims usually involve compensatory damages for physical or psychological harm.

Malpractice in Child and Adolescent Psychiatry

There are no recent data, but surveys in the 1970s and 1980s suggested that fewer than 1% of medical malpractice claims concerned psychiatrists and of these only a small minority (5–20%) concerned child psychiatrists. These low survey figures get some confirmation from the fact that insurance premiums are low for child psychiatrists. There are few systematic data, but the commonest precipitants to litigation in child and adolescent psychiatry are probably suicidal behavior, physical or sexual assault by another patient in the inpatient unit, inadequate treatment, the commitment process (and, on the other hand, failure to hospitalize), diagnostic error, and failed supervision of a case.

Suicide

Guidance as to what constitutes malpractice in cases of attempted or completed suicide is compromised by the lack of a universal standard of care. It is important to document a history that identifies the severity of known risk factors, but this will provide only a limited guide to decision-making. There is a common assumption that hospitalization is the preventive response to suicidal intent but clinicians should bear in mind that hospitalization carries its own problems, both clinical and legal, and the aim should always be to respect individual freedom and offer the least restrictive alternative for care. What is sometimes forgotten is that death or injury are not the only dangers for a suicidal adolescent, and the risk of suicide needs to be balanced against the risk to the child of restrictive treatments such as inpatient care. Courts will support the decision to discharge patients from inpatient units even if they subsequently complete suicide provided that the discharge decision has been taken on sound clinical grounds. The clinician's position will be strengthened if:

- the decision-making process is well documented (thinking out loud)
- the case has been discussed with colleagues
- the duty to disclose possible risk to parents/guardians has been met
- appropriate care has been taken to minimize exposure to risky means
- a safety plan is in place which offers the child and parents clear pathways to gain further help and support if required
- documentation demonstrates that the clinician has more than a superficial understanding of what underpins the child's possible suicidal intent.

Inpatient Care

Medical negligence claims relating to harm done in an inpatient environment most commonly relate to failure to protect a child from adverse events in that setting. Seclusion and restraint are potentially risky activities, and must always be demonstrably in the patients' best interests. Inpatient units need to have explicit and conservative policies for the implementation, audit, and evaluation of restraint. Because it is common for admitted children to have been abused, and for this to affect their behavior, there is an increased risk of further abuse in inpatient units. Note that the treating psychiatrist will be responsible for the child's well-being even if care is primarily carried out by junior medical and/or nursing staff. Should an inpatient unit arrive at a wrong diagnosis and implement inappropriate and potentially harmful treatment, the nominated child psychiatrist could be held responsible even if he/she has not been actively involved in the inpatient setting.

Where one patient assaults another, action might be brought on behalf of the assaulted child against the psychiatrist managing the child who perpetrated the alleged assault. For such litigation to be successful, lawyers for the assaulted child are likely to need access to the medical record of the assailant. Courts will not always accede to such requests.

Drug Therapy

The most common drug involved in misconduct actions is methylphenidate (probably because of its image as much as its true dangerousness). However, with increasing acceptance of the view that newer antidepressants (perhaps particularly paroxetine) can increase the risk of suicide, more litigation about such drugs is expected. In obtaining informed consent from the guardian (and preferably also assent from the child) it should be borne in mind that the more experimental the drug, the more information needs to have been demonstrated to have been provided in gaining consent. Risk of litigation will also be lessened by proper monitoring of medication. Adverse events on a drug do not necessarily imply misconduct, and a clinician who has prescribed a damaging drug where no less disabling drug would have been as effective is unlikely to be held negligent. However, it is essential to show that prescribing has been for therapy and in the best interest of the child and not for others' convenience. This might particularly apply in children whose behavior is troublesome to others and prescribing could be argued to be for the benefit of those managing the child.

Confidentiality

Children rarely sue for unauthorized disclosure but the parents may, for example, for giving information without consent to a school. Care must be taken to ensure appropriate consent to use case histories and video recordings for research, teaching, or other publication. Some information has privileged status before the courts, that is, the psychiatrist may not be obliged to reveal information, even under subpoena. Conditions of privilege will vary according to the jurisdiction, and legal advice is recommended if the conditions are unclear to the psychiatrist.

There are situations in which confidentiality must be breached in order to protect some party, usually the child. These include: suspected child abuse; in some jurisdictions, access to firearms if there is suicidal intent; duty to warn others who are in danger from the patient; and unlawful sexual intercourse. Clinicians would generally be protected in making such notifications but care is required to ensure that mandatory requirements are not exceeded. For example, child abuse allegations by one parent against another should be reported to statutory agencies, but might not justify advice to that parent to withhold access from the alleged perpetrator.

Minimizing Risks

Good clinical practice is not driven by a preoccupation with reducing risks of litigation but rather is aimed at increasing opportunities for children and their families. Nevertheless, there are some principles that can be followed to reduce potential risk of litigation (these principles also apply to pediatric emergency physicians and community pediatricians, who play an increasing role in children's mental health):

- Ensure that all medical records contain a genogram (family tree) that clearly identifies living, custodial, and guardianship arrangements.
- Discuss patients with colleagues, and ask for second opinions (this is not an admission of lack of competence). Case conferences about difficult patients or families frequently enhance clinical outcomes as well as providing legal protection.
- Document thoroughly and preserve documents because the statute of limitations does not have force until the child reaches adult status. Note, however, that courts will accept a psychiatrist's recollection even if it is not documented. Data can be added to case notes at a later time (preferably before the notes are subpoenaed) but any additional entry should be clearly dated as to the time of the addition.
- Provide clear explanations of assessment (including uncertainties) and treatment plans, and clearly document informed consent. Where possible, also get consent (or at least assent) from the child.
- Provide clear (preferably written) guidelines for the use of medication and other treatments that the child is expected to engage in outside therapy sessions.
- Use safety plans; invite families to contact you again if they are concerned or if unexpected developments occur.
- Terminate treatment contracts if you believe that something unreasonable is being asked of you (but remember that you have continued responsibility for a patient after termination until the family sees another clinician, and terminating contracts unilaterally risks action for abandonment).
- Be mindful of conflict of interest. For example, the profit motive may influence admission and discharge decisions in inpatient units; managed care might pressurize premature discharge. Note that it is the psychiatrist who will be held responsible for the consequences of premature discharge if he/she cannot demonstrate that he/she has taken adequate steps to represent the child's needs for continued care.
- Avoid taking on a forensic role unless it is explicit to all parties that the purpose of the interview is court-related.
- In child protection cases, the responsibility of the child psychiatrist is to bring suspected abuse to the

attention of the appropriate authorities. Unless a child psychiatrist has had additional training in child protection, it is not appropriate to carry out any level of child protection investigation. In particular, Munchausen syndrome by proxy should be conceptualized as a form of child abuse so that the child psychiatrist has no investigative role except as coordinated by an appropriate child protection expert. The child psychiatrist should also avoid giving opinions about diagnosis in parents where they have not made a direct assessment of that person.

- Interactions with parents need to be documented at least as well as those with the child.

If litigation occurs or is thought to be likely:

- Notify insurer and seek advice early.
- A clinician who has little experience of court proceedings should seek supervision on how best to act in court. For example, learning that lawyers can be deliberately provocative can help clinicians respond more calmly to what seems to be unreasonable statements made in the court proceeding.
- Where a clinician believes that malpractice has occurred, he/she is required to advise the patient/ family of this possibility. Otherwise the clinician might be regarded as having perpetrated a fraud on the patient by withholding information about potential misconduct.

See Also

Forensic Psychiatry and Forensic Psychology: Assessment; Forensic Interviewing; Personality Disorder; **Munchausen-Syndrome-by-Proxy**

Further Reading

Armitage DT, Townsend GM (1993) Emergency medicine, psychiatry and the law. *Emergency Medicine Clinics of North America* 11: 869–887.

Ash P (2002) Malpractice in child and adolescent psychiatry. *Child and Adolescent Psychiatric Clinics of North America* 11: 869–885.

Geraty RD, Hendren RL, Flaa CJ (1992) Ethical perspectives of managed care as it relates to child and adolescent psychiatry. *Journal of the American Academy of Child and Adolescent Psychiatry* 31: 398–402.

Holder AR (1994) Legal issues in consultation and liaison child psychiatry. *Child and Adolescent Psychiatric Clinics of North America* 3: 629–637.

Nurcombe B (2002) Malpractice. In: Lewis M (ed.) *Child and Adolescent Psychiatry. A Comprehensive Textbook*, 3rd edn., pp. 1293–1304. Philadelphia, PA: Lippincott/ Williams and Wilkins.

Nurcombe B, Partlett DF (1994) *Child Mental Health and the Law*. New York: The Free Press.

Schetky DH, Cavanaugh JL (1982) Psychiatric malpractice. *Journal of the American Academy of Child Psychiatry* 21: 521–526.

Vernick AE (2002) Forensic aspects of everyday practice: legal issues that every practitioner must know. *Child and Adolescent Clinics of North America* 11: 905–928.

Colorectal Surgery

M M Henry, Chelsea and Westminster Hospital, London, UK

Introduction

Colorectal and anal diseases are extremely common, particularly in developed countries. Hemorrhoids are a frequent source of irritating symptoms, and colorectal cancer is one of the three most common cancers in these countries. As a direct result, the treatment of these conditions often results in complications, which may be life-threatening or disabling and sufficient to give rise to profound resentment in the patient who subsequently may seek retribution via various legal agencies.

The public are protected, to a significant degree, by public bodies such as (in the UK) the General Medical Council (GMC) and the Royal College of Surgeons (RCS), who seek to monitor the professional abilities of those who propose and eventually carry out as individuals various treatments for colorectal disorders. Specifically, the Association of Coloproctology (AoC) is a society to which all who propose themselves as specialists in colorectal surgery are invited to apply and will be accepted for membership provided they meet the required criteria. The GMC is more usually concerned with ethical and moral issues, but its judgment may be invoked if there are serious issues of professional and technical malfunction or misjudgment. The RCS is more frequently associated with educational commitments rather than disciplinary matters. To be removed from the association of this august institution would not bar the individual from clinical practice. Similarly, the AoC provides an educational forum in the specialty and also frequently, as a consequence of peer activity, guidelines on management of complex issues within the specialty. It is the author's opinion that any patient seeking colorectal advice from a specialist should ensure that he or she is a member of this society (information can be obtained from the *Medical Directory*).

Anal Disorders

Anal disorders are extremely common, the majority of adults in the western population experiencing symptoms at some stage in their lives. The most common underlying cause of symptoms is hemorrhoids, but there are other disorders, that can be confused with hemorrhoids, which can lead to potentially serious errors in management.

The symptoms commonly associated with hemorrhoids are: rectal bleeding, anal discomfort, anal swelling, prolapsing anal lump, perianal itching, and anal discharge. Of these, rectal bleeding is the most prominent and troublesome. It is also the most common symptom from which serious clinical errors in misdiagnosis can arise. Because rectal bleeding may also be a clinical feature of colorectal cancer, it is imperative that the clinician should exclude this possibility before undertaking treatment of hemorrhoids. The decision as to in how much detail to investigate a patient with rectal bleeding is a complex one. The younger patient can be generally assumed to be bleeding from hemorrhoids and can be spared complex and unpleasant investigations. The older patient, or the patient who has a family history of colorectal neoplasia, needs to be investigated in more detail, including full colonoscopy or by computer tomography (CT) scanning. All patients presenting with anal or rectal symptoms should be examined by digital examination of the anus/rectum and by sigmoidoscopy. The latter is a simple and safe procedure whereby the lining of the lower bowel can be visualized directly and a malignancy of the rectum readily excluded.

Other anal pathologies (e.g., anal cancer) can be confused with hemorrhoids. Wherever doubt exists, any macroscopic lesion should be biopsied and subjected to histological examination. This is usually a minor procedure causing little discomfort or morbidity.

Investigation of Rectal Bleeding

Colonoscopy is a relatively safe and highly skilled visual examination of the colon and rectum employing sophisticated (and expensive) fiberoptic instruments. The examination may be uncomfortable for the patient, but this can usually be circumvented by the use of intravenous analgesia. The procedure's chief advantages lie in the accuracy of diagnosis and ability to biopsy any pathology seen or in some cases removal of polyps. The chief disadvantage, apart from expense, lies in the small but real risk of colonic perforation during the procedure. If this complication occurs, there is a significant probability of fecal peritonitis developing, and the patient's life is placed at risk. Often emergency major abdominal surgery has to be considered.

Recently, CT pneumocolons have been well established as a noninvasive method to investigate the colon and rectum. This technique suffers from the disadvantage of involving large doses of radiation to the patient; for this reason, it is an investigation only considered in the older patient, i.e., beyond reproductive age. There is also the additional disadvantage that no biopsy is possible if pathology is visualized. Such patients may then have no alternative but to proceed to colonoscopy in addition.

Anal Trauma

The clinician must always be aware that anal injury may be consistent with anal rape or damage sustained during childbirth (third-degree perineal tear) and careful documentation of the injury may be required for subsequent medicolegal needs. Clinical examination would include simple inspection to assess damage to skin and digital examination to assess damage to the underlying anal sphincter musculature. At a later stage, objective documentation of the presumed injury would include visualization of the sphincter complex by anal ultrasonography and magnetic resonance imaging (MRI) and possibly would also include a physiological assessment of the anal canal.

Rectal Disorders

The most important disease which the clinician needs to exclude in a patient suspected with rectal disease is rectal carcinoma. Often the diagnosis can be achieved by simple digital examination of the anal canal: the majority of rectal cancers have been shown to be "within reach" of an examining finger. Following digital examination, sigmoidoscopy, which is a simple and safe examination of the rectum, is performed without anesthetic in the outpatient environment. This simple instrument allows examination of the entire rectum and some of the colon just beyond. At the same time, if any pathology (e.g., rectal carcinoma or polyp) is identified, a small biopsy can be safely taken for histological examination. In the author's opinion, it would be considered negligent not to carry out these two simple investigations in a patient suspected of rectal disease.

Colonic Disorders

Simple clinical examination including digital examination of the rectum and sigmoidoscopy is mandatory in all patients suspected of colonic disorders. Again, the most important disorder which needs to be excluded is carcinoma of the colon. Since the diseased area is likely to lie beyond the reach of the sigmoido-scope, more invasive methods are required, e.g., colo-noscopy, to make the diagnosis. At the time of the colonoscopy, as discussed above, any pathology seen can be readily and safely biopsied.

Specific Complication of Colorectal Surgery

As with all other forms of surgery, many of the pro-cedures employed to treat these diseases are invasive with attendant risks for the patient. For this reason, it is now mandatory to discuss the potential risks in detail with the patient (or relative) preoperatively and list the most important risks on the consent form prior to the patient's signing.

Anal Surgery

Hemorrhoidectomy is the most common performed procedure within this speciality and also is the most common procedure which may result in profound patient dissatisfaction and possible litigation. In most cases, the procedure involves excision of peri-anal skin which is rich in sensory-nerve endings. Hence, the operation is often associated with severe perianal pain in the postoperative stage, the pain being greatly aggravated by defecation. Because hemorrhoids have a rich blood supply hemorrhage is a common postoperative complication.

Because of these major problems, it is extremely important to counsel any patient undergoing anal surgery (even minor surgery, such as excision of an anal skin tag) that they must expect symptoms which can be severe and can only be partially countered by the use of powerful analgesics and local agents. The patient must be warned that they will require a suit-able period of convalescence and cannot expect to return to work after a short period.

In rare circumstances, the procedure may be performed negligently such that the anal sphincters may be damaged leading to permanent fecal in-continence. Under these circumstances, substantial damages are usually awarded against the surgeon concerned, justifiably.

The treatment of anal fissure is generally by local agents that carry no significant complications (e.g., dilitiazem, and glyceryl trinitrin). However, a small number of patients do not respond to these agents and require treatment by surgery: sphincterotomy. This procedure involves division of a small portion of the lower end of the internal anal sphincter. In some patients, this could lead to partial anal inconti-nence: namely, incontinence to liquid stool and to flatus. It is, therefore, vital to counsel such patients

prior to surgery and warn them of the risks involved. The risks are minimized if the surgeon is careful not to divide the entire length of the internal anal sphincter.

The treatment of anal fistula may involve division of a portion of both the internal and external anal sphincters in order to achieve adequate drainage of the sepsis. The skill of the surgeon lies in the under-standing of how much sphincter can be safely divided without rendering the patient fecally incontinent postoperatively. A preoperative MR scan of the perineum should be performed so that the fistula tract can be accurately mapped out preoperatively and a prognosis provided on the subsequent risk of functional problems resulting postoperatively. Where extensive division of the anal sphincter mech-anism appears necessary to achieve satisfactory drain-age (i.e., in high anal fistulas), it is sometimes possible to avert problems by the application of a ligature (seton) around the affected anal sphincter to promote drainage.

Rectal Surgery

Excision of the rectum, either total or partial, may be necessary in the treatment of malignant conditions of the rectum or in certain inflammatory disorders (e.g., Crohn's disease and ulcerative colitis). Dissection of the rectum may involve damage to the delicate sym-pathetic nerves which surround the rectum and sub-sequently innervate the bladder and penis (or vagina). Therefore, damage to these nerves may subsequently give rise to problems with micturition and/or sexual function (e.g., failure of ejaculation and failure of erection) postoperatively. It is therefore extremely important that patients are warned of the 5% risk of these complications developing. In the author's opinion, these complications are unfortunate and are not the result of negligence on the part of the surgeon.

Abdominal dissection of the rectum involves a pelvic dissection close to the anatomical site of the ureters and bladder. It is relatively common to dam-age either of these structures inadvertently. Wherever possible a preoperative CT and MR scan of the pelvis should be carried out so that the anatomical site of the ureters with reference to the rectum and relevant pathology (e.g., carcinoma) can be assessed so that the surgeon is prewarned if there is close proximity of the tumor to one of the ureters. During the operation, it is good practice to identify both ureters at an early stage and carefully exclude them from the dissection.

In the procedure of anterior resection of the rectum, the rectum is partially excised and an anasto-mosis constructed between the colon and lower rectum. If the portion of rectum remaining is of short length, the reservoir capacity of the rectum is much reduced, with the result that these patients may experience considerable functional problems postoperatively. Commonly, these patients experience marked urgency of defecation, soiling, and in severe cases, frank fecal incontinence. Patients must be warned preoperatively of these risks, and it should be discussed whether or not they would prefer to undergo total rectal excision with the provision of a stoma as a preferable line of therapy.

Colonic Surgery

As a consequence of colonic resection, either ureter may be damaged and during dissection of the right side of the colon the duodenum may be inadvertently damaged with the risk of a duodenal fistula developing postoperatively. As with rectal disease, it is vital to carry out a proper and full preoperative assessment including a detailed imaging, such as CT scanning. Hopefully, this will allow the surgeon to be prewarned of possible technical difficulties and permit measures to reduce the risk of inadvertent damage. For example, if the CT scan shows proximity of the tumor to either ureter the risk of damage may be reduced by asking a urologist to insert a ureteric catheter preoperatively.

Stomas, which can be created from either the terminal small bowel (ileostomy) or the colon (colostomy), are frequently performed in colorectal surgery. They can be fashioned either as a permanent measure such as in the treatment of a cancer of the lower rectum or as a temporary measure. In the latter instance, this may be a measure instituted to divert fecal matter away from a technically difficult anastomosis below the stoma. The stoma would then be closed when it is judged safe and the anastomosis demonstrated to be fully healed.

Stomas understandably cause great anxiety to patients and are the principal cause for delay in seeking advice where rectal cancer is suspected. In practice, they are rarely a major problem for patients, most of whom rapidly adapt to their management. It remains vitally necessary that any patient being considered for a stoma should be fully counseled both by medical staff and by fully trained stoma therapists. The counseling includes discussion on the most suitable siting of the stoma for the individual patient, as well as general management and possible cosmetic and sexual problems they may experience. Ideally, the preoperative workup should include the availability of a volunteer ileostomist or colostomist, who would be prepared to discuss the implications of a stoma with the patient.

Summary

The potential for surgical accident and litigation in this specialty is high, but fortunately rare. This is largely the result of intensive and closely supervised training of the junior grades followed by rigorous examination before the trainee is permitted to apply for the part of a consultant. The activities of the RCS and the AOC have done much to improve the quality of training and, thereby, the public remain, to a large extent, protected from incompetent clinical practice.

See Also

Medical Malpractice: Overview

Further Reading

Keighley MRB, Williams NS (1993) *Surgery of the Anus, Rectum and Colon.* London: WB Saunders.
Pemberton JH, Swash M, Henry MM (2002) *The Pelvic Floor.* London: WB Saunders.

Ear, Nose and Throat Surgery

D Gatland, Southend Hospital NHS Trust, Essex, UK

Introduction

Despite the importance of this topic there is a surprising dearth of related literature, no doubt due to the relative infrequency of complaints and litigation in the past. A Medline search revealed only ten articles related to informed consent or medical negligence in ear, nose, and throat (ENT) practice. However changing attitudes have led to an increasing number of complaints in recent years, while the scope of ENT surgical practice has broadened and encompasses facial plastic surgery as well as endoscopic and skull base surgery; dissatisfaction with the outcome of rhinoplasty and complications of endoscopic sinus surgery are common.

In this article a general consideration of malpractice in ENT surgery will be followed by specific problems in otology, rhinology, and head and neck surgery. All the outcomes described have resulted in complaints or litigation.

The term malpractice, like negligence, implies blame. The terms mishap or adverse event, however, do not necessarily imply surgical error. Many apparent errors originate primarily in system failures rather than solely in an individual's acts or omissions.

In ENT practice errors are common but few result in injury, and few of these lead to malpractice claims.

Good communication makes a claim less likely, as many complainants say they only want the truth and to ensure others are not similarly afflicted, rather than money.

Lack of time can lead to a failure of communication. The British Association of Otolaryngologists (BAOL) indicates that a 3-hour clinic should contain no more than 12–14 patients. In law being too busy is no defense, nor is fatigue.

Surgeons must ensure they are properly equipped, both technologically and personally, and have adequate trained nursing and ancillary staff. The tendency of some hospitals to lose medical records is lamentable. The records must be full, accurate, and contemporaneous.

Duty of Care

For a claim of negligence to succeed there must first be a duty of care. All medical practitioners are responsible for their acts or omissions, but consultant surgeons are also jointly liable for that which is done under their supervision. A consultant must ensure that appropriately trained or supervised individuals carry out all care. Trainees are more likely to err; for example, the incidence of adverse events after stapedotomy is less when only senior surgeons operate.

Training and Malpractice

Surgeons must be able to show that they have appropriate training for the work they do, otherwise an accusation of malpractice is difficult to defend. While most ENT surgeons undertake general ENT cases, subspecialist training is bringing greater experience and expertise to complex work. In pharyngeal pouch surgery for example, CEPOD (Confidential Enquiry into Perioperative Deaths) (UK) for 1996–1997 recommended that a single surgeon in each district should have responsibility.

The master and apprentice training model is applicable in head and neck surgery but in otology and rhinology much of the surgery is done single-handed, with the risk of error when the operator is inexperienced, even while the supervisor may be watching the monitor.

Otologists have always trained and practiced on human cadaver temporal bones; however these are now difficult to obtain. Regional temporal bone dissection courses are slowly evolving, and synthetic bones are now available. A recent British survey showed that an average ENT trainee comes to the end of six years of training with little experience of complex middle-ear surgery and is not therefore properly equipped to practice otology. Similar considerations apply to surgical residents in the USA and in other training programs. Subspecialism in the last two years of training should improve outcomes, and consultants wishing to take on subspecialist interests should undertake appropriate training or arrange supervision while performing new procedures.

Outcomes

On Florence Nightingale's wards, outcomes were measured as relieved, unrelieved, or dead. Nowadays any complaint is more defensible if surgeons can quote their own figures for outcomes rather than data published by others. A case series with limited numbers of a particular procedure or with poor results compared with the average can imply a poor standard of care. Such suppositions should however take into account the case mix: a series dealing with particularly complex cases is expected to have poorer results than those for routine or uncomplicated work. Currently data are routinely obtained for head and neck cancer outcomes but the continuing general failure to audit both in terms of quality of life and specific outcomes is surprising. It is however difficult to obtain meaningful data for such complex outcomes as those for ear surgery and basic data sets are now available to assist in this process, while similar data sets are evolving for rhinology.

How Errors Occur

Errors may be classified as an act of omission or commission.

Omission

- Failure to examine properly, investigate appropriately, or act upon the findings.
- Failure to refer either to a colleague in another specialty as appropriate or to a colleague with specific experience of the case in hand.
- Failure to institute mandatory treatment, for example, prophylactic antibiotics before neck surgery where the pharynx is opened. A fistula after this event would be grounds for a claim of negligence.
- Failure to monitor the facial nerve when it is at risk, for example, in mastoid surgery or parotidectomy. Surveys indicate, surprisingly, that this is not a standard practice.

Commission

- Lack of care or judgment in management, for example, taking on a case for which the surgeon is not adequately equipped.

Informed Consent and Negligence

Wide variations currently exist in the consenting process. It is clear that, unlike in the USA, UK law does not require a document describing the minutiae of every conceivable adverse event; however, worldwide it is negligent if common or serious complications are not discussed.

Complications may be regarded as avoidable and unavoidable. An example of the latter might be graft failure, while, of the former, a dislocated incus during a stapedotomy represents a poor standard of practice. In microsuction of the ear, it is unacceptable that a previously normal eardrum be perforated. Facial palsy during a straightforward superficial parotidectomy or mastoid exploration should not occur. In the USA and more recently in the UK, this event often leads to a successful claim for negligence. Consent does not necessarily exonerate surgical mishaps.

Patients should understand the normal postoperative course so that routine events, for example

bruising after rhinoplasty, are not misinterpreted as adverse events.

Figures 1 and 2 show the relative frequency of complaints in various areas of independent ENT practice derived from claims dealt with by the UK Medical Defence Union. These are now discussed under the specialty headings.

Head and Neck

An accurate and documented history and examination must be carried out.

Fiberoptic nasendoscopes must be available in globus sensation to exclude tumor. Failure to diagnose carcinoma of the larynx is not uncommon.

In glue ear in an adult, it is important to exclude nasopharyngeal cancer, particularly in Chinese patients.

Failure to Investigate

If a neck gland is removed that is subsequently shown to be a metastasis from a squamous carcinoma, then the patient has at best had an unnecessary operation or at worst has a worse prognosis. Fine-needle aspiration prior to parotid or thyroid surgery may indicate the need for more or less radical surgical treatment.

Foreign Bodies

These can be missed, particularly if radiolucent, such as dentures. Foreign bodies must be ruled out in the case of unilateral rhinorrhea or recurrent chest infection.

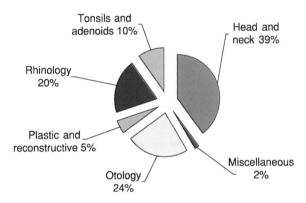

Figure 1 Complaints in ENT surgery (main area of practice).

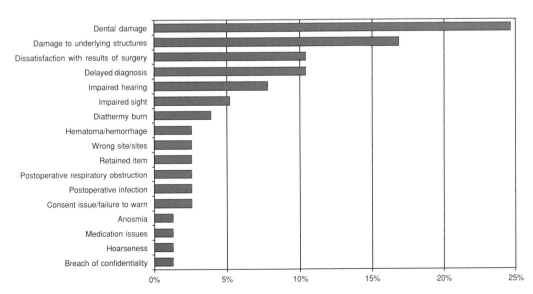

Figure 2 UK ENT settled claims in a 14-year period.

Failure to Stage Accurately

In head and neck cancer the existence of distant metastases must be investigated in addition to local staging and treatment.

Potential Neural Complications

Although always cut in a classical radical neck dissection, the spinal accessory nerve should be preserved in a conservative neck dissection unless it is close to involved nodes. Section of this nerve during a node biopsy is indefensible and is an occasional source of litigation.

The vagus and phrenic nerves are at risk, though they are rarely damaged.

With regard to the brachial plexus, it is essential to stay superficial to the deep fascia when dissecting in the root of the neck.

The facial nerve trunk is at risk if a neck dissection is taken very high to get above tumor, or during total parotidectomy.

The marginal mandibular nerve may potentially be injured at the time of a submandibular gland resection and will be sacrificed if forming part of a classical radical neck dissection.

The recurrent laryngeal nerves are at risk during thyroidectomy as well as the superior laryngeal nerves.

Frey syndrome and salivary fistula should be discussed before parotidectomy.

Dental problems are common sources of complaint following adenotonsillectomy as well as other transoral procedures. Secondary hemorrhage occurs in 5% of cases but is still a source of litigation.

Obstructed tube or displacements are potentially lethal complications of tracheostomy.

Operations in the floor of the mouth may result in airway obstruction due to edema: the UK Medical Defence Union has dealt with one death resulting in litigation from this cause.

Perforation should not occur in a straightforward upper esophagoscopy; it is debatable whether rigid endoscopes should be used in the lower esophagus where there is much greater risk. There is a risk of perforation when removing foreign bodies or dilating structures.

Otology

Failure to Examine

Attic disease may be missed if microscopy and suction clearance are not carried out.

Failure to Investigate

With regard to unilateral sensorineural hearing loss and tinnitus, a plethora of audiological techniques have been used to indicate the likelihood of a lesion in the cerebellopontine angle. However magnetic resonance imaging (MRI) is now the "gold standard;" failure of diagnosis where no MRI scan is requested is negligent.

Computed tomographic (CT) scanning in chronic suppurative otitis media is not yet mandatory, but CT shows erosions or fistulae, so that the patient can be advised of an increased risk of hearing loss or facial nerve injury.

The BAOL in the UK has published guidelines that ototoxic antibiotic eardrops may be used in discharging middle ears, however it is safer to use ciprofloxacin drops. These are licensed for that purpose in most countries but not in the UK, where eye drops can be used in the ear on a named-patient basis. Povidone-iodine solution is ototoxic and care must be taken when cleaning the skin prior to operations where the eardrum is perforated.

Ear syringing is usually carried out by general practitioners or their practice nurses. It is estimated that 1:1000 cause major complications. It is essential to rule out a history of preexisting ear disease and to adhere to protocols for safe practice.

In the surgery of chronic suppurative otitis media, patients must be aware of the failure rate in terms of a continued wet ear and worse hearing. The author has been involved with two medicolegal cases where sensorineural hearing loss and tinnitus have followed apparently straightforward myringoplasties. Cholesteatoma surgery does not necessarily avoid subsequent intracranial complications in chronic otitis media.

In stapes surgery, sensorineural hearing loss or tinnitus may result in a complaint. Facial palsy should not occur. Where a persisting stapedial artery is coagulated there is a small chance of blindness.

In corda tympani nerve section, contrary to traditional teaching there are more long-term symptoms if the nerve is cut rather than stretched. Corda symptoms are more likely in cases where there is no inflammatory disease.

It has traditionally been regarded as bad practice to operate on the only hearing ear; however, with conservative technique it is safe to operate in chronic otitis media on the only hearing ear where necessary.

In cases of congenital ear anomaly, unilateral canal atresia should not be operated. Bilateral disease should be managed in a specialist center.

Rhinology

While septal and turbinate surgery is within the province of the ENT generalist, the Hopkins rod endoscope has revolutionized the practice of sinus surgery.

With improved understanding of the pathophysiology of the sinuses, simple but invasive and traumatic procedures such as the Caldwell-Luc operation are rarely indicated. However, the advent of endoscopes and CT scanning has encouraged surgeons to take on more complex maneuvers close to the orbit and skull base with the potential for injury to the lacrymal apparatus, the optic nerve and ocular muscles, and the anterior ethmoidal artery or meninges. The incidence of complications is in fact no greater than before but the new litigation climate has led to an increase in the number of claims. It is important to stress that surgery is unlikely to help common complaints such as postnasal drip or facial pain.

Rhinoplasty is recognized by the medical defense organizations as an appropriate operation for the appropriately trained ENT surgeon. However, patient dissatisfaction with the results of this operation is relatively more common than for any other ENT procedure.

Failure of Diagnosis

Endoscopic examination in clinic is now mandatory for patients presenting with sinonasal symptoms.

CT scanning is mandatory prior to endoscopic sinus surgery.

Failure of Management

Training in endoscopic sinus surgery must include the avoidance and management of iatrogenic trauma to the skull base and orbit, including orbital hematoma.

Hyposmia may be present before surgery, although smell test kits are not customarily used and it is therefore difficult to defend an allegation that surgery has negligently resulted in this complication. The removal of the middle turbinate will by definition remove some olfactory fibers and an important landmark.

See Also

Drug-Induced Injury, Accidental and Iatrogenic; **Drugs, Prescribed:** Licencing and Registration; Product Liability; **Medical Malpractice – Medico-legal Perspectives:** Negligence, Standard of Care; Negligence, Duty of Care

Further Reading

Hawthorne M, Barker I (1997) Medical negligence in otolaryngology. In: Gleeson M (ed.) *Scott Brown's Otolaryngology, Basic Sciences* 1; 29: pp. 1–13. Oxford, UK: Butterworth-Heinemann.

Hinchcliffe R (2003) Ethics law and related matters. In: Luxon L (ed.) *Textbook of Audiological Medicine*, pp. 131–147. London: Martin Dunitz.

Maran A (2000) Otorhinolaryngology. In: Powers M, Harris N (eds.) *Clinical Negligence*, 3rd edn., pp. 1585–1607. London: Butterworths.

Ramadan MF, Roland R (2001) Medicolegal issues in ENT surgery. In: Roland N, McRae R, McCombe A (eds.) *Key Topics in Otolaryngology*, pp. 162–166. Oxford, UK: BIOS Scientific.

Rosenthal M, Mulcahy L, Lloyd-Bostock S (1999) *Medical Mishaps*. Philadelphia, PA: Open University Press.

Facio-maxillary Surgery

M F Patel, Royal Berkshire Hospital, Reading, UK

Definitions

The specialty of maxillofacial surgery is centered on the bones and soft tissues of the jaws and face but traditionally includes surgery from the clavicles to the skull vertex. Thus the specialty currently enjoys a position in the head and neck not dissimilar from that of the general surgery of yesteryear before subspecialization removed urology and vascular surgery from the generality of general surgery.

Maxillofacial surgeons might thus be viewed as the "general surgeons" of the head and neck region. Due to the dense complexity of the structures in the head and neck region, certain organs are excluded from this generality. The brain and cervical spine, globe and middle and inner ears are properly the domain of the neurosurgeon, eye surgeon, and ear, nose, and throat surgeon. However, inevitably, subspecialization within maxillofacial surgery is also possible with the evolution of cancer surgeons specializing in head and neck malignancy, orthognathic surgeons treating jaw disproportion, facial esthetic surgeons normalizing facial deformity, trauma surgeons dealing with head and neck damage, and even salivary gland surgeons.

Terms allied with maxillofacial surgery are "craniofacial surgery," in which serious facial deformity requires the combined surgical skills of the neurosurgeon and maxillofacial surgeon, or in which the maxillofacial surgeon facilitates the access of the neurosurgeon to the skull base by reflecting soft- and hard-tissue flaps. The term "head and neck surgery" tends to be used for major surgery in the region, particularly when malignancy is treated. The term "facial orthopedics" is occasionally used to describe the treatment of trauma to the facial skeleton or elective surgery to the facial bones due to disproportion.

The Nature of Maxillofacial Surgery

Maxillofacial surgery has a number of core areas of surgical interest and expertise. These include malignant diseases of the mouth, jaws, face and neck, orthognathic surgery, the surgical treatment of oral disease, orofacial trauma, salivary gland disease, surgery of the temporomandibular joint, orofacial reconstruction, and facial esthetic surgery.

Essentially, the specialty is concerned with investigation, diagnosis, and treatment of conditions of the head and neck. The work of senior surgeons will depend on their training and expertise in other specialties. While they will be competent to deal with most conditions within areas of core interests for the specialty, some surgeons will subspecialize and have greater competence in one discipline or another.

Malpractice

It is interesting that, despite the highly emotive nature of conditions around the face and mouth requiring treatment including surgery, the specialty of maxillofacial surgery is less beset by lawsuits than specialties such as neurosurgery or plastic surgery. In the case of neurosurgery, with its connotations of life and death, or more poignantly, life beset with tragic restrictions, it is perhaps understandable that legal redress will be sought for such major dissatisfactions. In the case of plastic surgery, the cosmetic element is frequently beset with litigation due to the highly charged and emotional nature of the expectations that are placed on such surgeries and the inevitable associated costs.

In this article maxillofacial surgical procedures most prone to malpractice suits are covered with a brief description of why the procedure might be required and how it is accomplished. The information and warnings that should be given in order to obtain valid consent are described along with common complications that might be associated with negligence or malpractice.

Surgical Procedures

It is important when dealing with surgical procedures that are of an intermediate or major nature to ensure that the information given to patients is not only what the surgeon feels is appropriate, but also what the patients need. Once the information is given, it is the responsibility of the surgeon to ensure that it is also understood and that patients have sufficient time within an encouraging atmosphere to ask further questions and explore their concerns. The development of a sympathetic relationship with both surgeon and patient should work toward the best possible outcome. It is also important for the surgeon to share with the patient his/her concerns with regard to the procedure and its possible complications. It is only in this atmosphere of mutual support and trust that best treatment will occur and that when problems arise, they may be understood by the patient to be unavoidable within a caring context, when this is the case.

Surgical Resection of Malignancy

The majority of malignant tumors in the head and neck region that require major surgery are squamous cell carcinomas. These tumors, in common with most cancers, are capable of metastasizing or spreading to other parts of the body. These secondary tumors, arising from a primary lesion from within the oral cavity or nasopharynx, spread via the lymph drainage system, blood, or directly through soft tissues.

Basal cell carcinomas of the facial skin are also commonly dealt with by maxillofacial surgeons, but these lesions characteristically do not metastasize and are usually dealt with by local resection and primary closure when small, although they may require large flaps and even free grafts on occasions.

Surgery is not the only option in the treatment of head and neck cancer, and in many cases, radiotherapy can offer an equally successful outcome, sometimes with a lower morbidity. Chemotherapy, although rarely curative for squamous cell carcinoma of the head and neck, can be a useful adjunct at certain stages of the disease. There are times when active treatment must give way to palliative care when a cure is impossible and further active treatment is unkind or inappropriate. It is therefore important that a maxillofacial surgery cancer patient is assessed on a combined clinic with a team of one or more surgeons with a special interest in head and neck surgery, a clinical oncologist, a radiotherapist, speech therapist, and dietician in order that the most appropriate treatment may be discussed with the patient.

Computed tomography or magnetic resonance imaging will usually be required to assess the stage of the disease which, with a detailed clinical examination, will be able to describe the disease by the TNM notation (tumor, node, and metastasis). The aim of cancer surgery is to resect the complete malignant lesion and reconstruct the surgical deficit in order to return the anatomy and function to as near normal as possible. When major cancer surgery has been carried out in the head and neck region, there is frequently some reduction in natural function and/or an orofacial deformity. The removal of an adequate and appropriate margin of healthy tissue around the carefully marked tumor is essential and unequivocal.

Once the resection has been carried out, the degree to which the patient is returned to a satisfactory cosmetic and functional state will depend upon the skills and experience of the surgeon, and thereafter, the further skills of the speech therapist and dietician. Potential complications of this type of surgery include: speech, swallowing, facial appearance, the presence of scars, and potential damage to nerves, including in particular, the lingual nerve providing sensation to the tongue, the inferior dental nerve providing sensation to the lower lip and chin, the hypoglossal nerve moving the tongue, and the facial nerve moving the muscles of facial expression, the patient should be warned of these in as supporting and caring a way as possible.

Despite the ravages of the malignant tumor and the inevitable destruction of the resection process, patients and their legal advisers are becoming increasingly concerned with the appropriateness of the surgery that has been provided and the quality of reconstruction. These are not as yet major sources of contention but may become so in the future.

Salivary Gland Surgery

The major salivary glands comprise the paired sublingual glands in the floor of the mouth anteriorly below the tongue, the paired submandibular glands in the submandibular fossae just below the horizontal rami of the mandible bilaterally, and the large parotid glands over and around the ascending rami of the mandible bilaterally.

The sublingual glands are removed due to the formation of ranulae or cysts associated with these glands which protrude into the floor of the mouth or due to concerns with tumors within the glands. The larger submandibular glands may require removal due to poor functioning associated with pain and swelling which may be occasioned by the formation of calculi or stones within the glands or ducts. The presence of a tumor within the gland will also necessitate its removal.

The parotid glands are frequently operated in order to remove a benign tumor known as a pleomorphic adenoma but may also require surgery if they are suspected of harboring other tumors or a malignancy or if the glands are functioning poorly with pain and swelling or prone to recurrent infection.

The sublingual salivary glands are usually removed by making an incision in the floor of the mouth and dissecting the gland free with its attachments. In contrast, the submandibular and parotid salivary glands require an incision in the neck for removal of the submandibular gland or an incision, usually anterior to the ear and extending into the neck, in order to remove the parotid gland.

Patients will be prone to soreness, swelling, and bruising after surgery. As well as warning patients of the relatively minor complications, it is important that they appreciate that the lingual nerve supplying sensation and taste to the tongue can be permanently damaged in the removal of the sublingual gland to which it is closely related. The lingual, hypoglossal, and lower branches of the facial nerve are closely associated with the submandibular gland and are at risk in its removal. Along with the damage to the taste sensation associated with the lingual nerve, the hypoglossal nerve allows movement of the relevant side of the tongue and the lower branches of the facial nerve control movement of the angle of the mouth and lower lip on the side of surgery. The trunk of the facial nerve closely abuts the parotid gland. All significant branches of the facial nerve pass through the parotid gland en route to the muscles of facial expression. Significant damage or transection of the trunk of the facial nerve will result in paralysis of the muscles of facial expression on that side, giving the appearance of a stroke. The great auricular nerve, which passes below and close to the parotid gland, frequently requires transaction, resulting in permanent numbness of parts of the external ear and, in particular, the earlobe.

It is important that the patient is warned of the important risks of nerve damage which, in the case of benign disease, are rare. Scarring on the face or neck is inevitable in removal of the parotid and submandibular glands, but the scars may be well disguised by the incisions being made into skin creases, as long as healing is uneventful. Temporary weakness after parotid gland surgery occurs in approximately one-third of operations but usually recovers within three weeks while numbness of the skin flap usually improves over four to six months. Frey syndrome (gustatory sweating of the face) can occur in up to 50% of parotidectomy patients. Sialocele and salivary fistulae can occur after parotidectomy and usually resolve spontaneously after some weeks. The removal of part or all of the parotid gland can result in an anesthetic hollowing of the facial profile.

When unwarned complications occur, or when the degree of complications is not commensurate with the level of disease, patient dissatisfaction and litigation are possible sequelae.

Orthognathic Surgery

This type of surgery to correct dentofacial deformity is so called as it straightens or normalizes the jaws and in so doing must also produce a balanced occlusion. It is usually necessary for realignment of teeth before such jaw surgery, and it may even be necessary to continue realignment after surgery is complete. It is important therefore that patients for whom orthognathic surgery is contemplated should be seen in a combined clinic between a maxillofacial surgeon and an orthodontist.

Although the surgery is primarily functional in nature, in order to improve disproportion and occlusion as well as jaw position, the esthetic element must not be ignored. "Normalizing" the tooth position by orthodontics followed by "normalization" of jaw position by orthognathic surgery tends to "normalize" facial appearance to a great extent. It is important that patients are aware of changes that will be occurring in their teeth, jaws, and facial appearance before treatment begins as it may affect their decision to have surgery. It may be that additional surgical procedures need to be carried out in order to create a harmonious facial appearance after the planned jaw movements, and these must be agreed with the patient.

X-rays, predictive drawings, and computer-predicted images can be of help in allowing the patient to imagine the appearance the surgeons and orthodontists feel is likely. It is important that the patient realizes that such predictions generally indicate a trend rather than an absolute appearance and no guarantees should be made. It should be the goal of the surgeon to carry out the minimum of surgery to attain the required and agreed result and osteotomies, or cutting of the jawbones. Osteotomies are usually described as segmental (where sections of alveolar bone, usually bearing teeth, are sectioned) as well as LeFort 1, 2, and 3 osteotomies of the upper facial skeleton, depending on whether the bone cuts are made at the low, middle, or high levels. In the lower jaw, segmental surgery is also feasible, although sagittal splitting or vertical subsigmoid osteotomies of the mandibular ramus are more usual with or without genioplasty procedures to adjust the chin point position.

Once jawbone osteotomies are carried out, the bone is secured in its new position either by direct wiring or plating with screws or indirectly by wiring teeth together for around six weeks. There is a strong trend toward the increasing use of plates and screws in order that patients may open their jaws, thus protecting their own airway and to allow communication, eating, and drinking, all of which are easier when jaws are not wired together. Common complications include pain, swelling, bruising, and modest weight loss in the immediate aftermath of surgery. Patients must be warned however that a degree of relapse of the new jaw position can occur, although this is usually modest. In conditions where the jaw is open anteriorly (anterior open bite) there is a greater tendency for relapse to occur.

The inferior orbital nerves providing sensation to cheek and nasal skin, including the upper lip and associated gum, the inferior dental nerve giving sensation to the lower lip and chin skin, and the lingual nerves providing tongue sensation, are all closely associated with the osteotomy cuts usually required in this type of surgery and are therefore at risk of damage. Authorities vary widely regarding the frequency and degree of nerve damage that occurs in such surgery, but permanent and noticeable numbness probably occurs in less than 5% of patients undergoing such surgery.

The catastrophic loss of large portions of osteotomized jawbone is recorded in the literature as occurring rarely and is probably more prevalent in patients who have experienced cleft-lip and palate repairs where scar tissue and possibly aberrant vascularization are present. This type of surgery is usually carried out electively and on young persons and, although considered functional, also has a strong esthetic element. For this reason such surgery is inevitably associated with optimistic expectations by the patient with reassurance, usually by the surgeon, that such surgery is normally "routine." It is therefore not surprising that when a desired result is not achieved or when a major complication occurs, dissatisfaction can deteriorate to litigation.

Facial Esthetic and Cosmetic Surgery

The surgical "normalization" of facial appearance when it falls significantly outside the mid-range might be considered as facial esthetic surgery while a convenient further division of surgery to improve facial appearance might be considered as "cosmetic" where surgery to mitigate the normal appearances of natural aging or to "improve" certain features already within the normal range is carried out. Such surgery, which is emotive, often patient-driven, and privately funded, will inevitably be associated with higher levels of dissatisfaction than when surgery is carried out to treat pathological processes. Such elective esthetic or cosmetic surgery includes blepharoplasty to improve the eyelids, rhinoplasty to adjust the appearance of the nose, rhytidectomy or facelift to mitigate the effects of aging on the facial skin, and a panoply of surgical procedures too numerous to mention here but amongst which are laser skin resurfacing, botulinum toxin injections to eliminate wrinkles, and collagen injections to bulk out lips.

There appears to be a trend toward lawyers and courts looking upon such elective and nonessential surgery as more a commodity than a medical treatment, and it is inevitable that litigation will increase and the test for surgeons to satisfy in court will also escalate.

Trauma A major commitment in maxillofacial surgery is the treatment of facial trauma, usually occasioned by either interpersonal violence or road traffic accidents. There is tacit acceptance by both patient and surgeon that the surgeon will do his/her best in difficult circumstances to repair the damage done to facial tissues, while accepting that the circumstances and the emergency nature of surgery would allow for certain compromises.

There is a trend in trauma, as in other areas of surgery, for patients who are now better informed and empowered to replace blind gratitude with a discerning and occasionally litigious demeanor. In fact, this only serves to highlight the necessity for all professional healthcare workers to be aware of the latest and best accepted treatment for surgical conditions and to carry this treatment out in the patient's interest. The employment of sound audit, regular clinical governance, and continuing medical education is important as it will ensure that patients receive the best and most appropriate care and that surgeons are professionally satisfied and, of course, protected.

Temporomandibular joint surgery The temporomandibular jaw joint is heir to degenerative, traumatic, and psychosomatic conditions. Osteoarthritis and rheumatoid arthritis can affect and damage the function of the temporomandibular joint, as may trauma to the jaw joint, particularly where the bony or cartilaginous elements are badly damaged. In addition, conditions such as arthromyalgia and temporomandibular joint dysfunction are common conditions affecting one-third or more of the population at some time according to some authorities, but are rare in childhood or old age. The condition appears to be due in part to stress or anxiety and may generally be treated conservatively with reassurance, bite guards, physiotherapy, and other physical treatments such as ultrasound, mega-pulse, and manipulation. It is rarely necessary for surgery to be carried out, although minimally invasive techniques such as lavage of the jaw joint, manipulation, and jaw joint arthroscopy can be helpful. Surgery to the bone of the joint or the meniscus/cartilage is occasionally required for pain, locking, or unpleasant sounds and sensations which emanate from the jaw joint.

In medicolegal terms, deterioration in long-standing temporomandibular dysfunction symptoms or the development of such symptoms *de novo* are

frequently the subject of litigation after road traffic accidents, particularly when there are whiplash injuries. Such claims must be dealt with on a patient-by-patient basis, although as a general rule if the condition has markedly deteriorated as a result of the alleged accident or assault or occurred as a new symptomatic condition, it would seem to form the basis for a valid claim.

Conclusion

In short, the maxillofacial region is an important and emotive part of the body and the surgeons who treat this region have, until recently, been spared the medicolegal attention given to their colleagues operating in different specialties. Although this is likely to change, it signals an excellent opportunity for the specialty to respond by ensuring that it is giving the best possible care and to continue to improve the healthcare partnership with the patient at the center.

See Also

Medical Malpractice: Ear, Nose and Throat Surgery

Further Reading

Fonseca RJ (2002) *Oral and Maxillofacial Surgery: Cleft/Craniofacial/Cosmetic Surgery.* New York: Saunders.

Harrison SD (2002) Temperomandibular joint pain. In: Zakrzewska JM, Harrison SDD (eds.) *Assessment and Management of Orofacial Pain*, pp. 191–208. London: Elsevier.

Patel MF (1998) *Medical Legal and Ethical Considerations in Cosmetic Surgery.* LLM thesis. Cardiff, UK: Law Library of Cardiff University.

Patel MF (1998) Trauma. In: Langdon JD, Patel MF (eds.) *Operative Maxillofacial Surgery*, pp. 317–352. London: Chapman & Hall Medical.

Posnick JC (ed.) (1999) *Craniofacial and Maxillofacial Surgery in Children and Young Adults.* New York: Saunders.

Reyneke J (2003) *Essentials of Orthognathic Surgery.* London: Quintessence.

Salyer KE, Bardach J (2000) *Atlas of Craniofacial and Cleft Surgery.* London: Lippincott/Williams and Wilkins.

Trenta GL (2003) *Atlas of Aesthetic Face and Neck Surgery.* New York: Saunders.

Urken ML, Buchbinder D, Costantino PD (2004) *Major Flap Utilization in Head and Neck Reconstruction: A Defect-Oriented Approach.* London: Lippincott/Williams and Wilkins.

Ward-Booth P, Schendel SA, Hausamen J-E (1999) *Maxillofacial Surgery.* London: Churchill Livingstone.

General Practice

S E Josse, Formerly University of London, London, UK

Introduction

This article describes the situation in the UK.

Negligence by a doctor in his/her professional capacity due to or following an action or inaction on his/her part is all too common. Substandard practice is unacceptable for general practitioners to the same degree as it is for any other doctor in medical practice. Because of the Bolam principle, albeit modified by Siddaway and Bolitho, the medical profession does appear to have a legal advantage over other citizens in the field of negligence. Negligent acts so carelessly and recklessly performed and leading to a criminal charge are rare. The Bolam principle is helpful to the medical profession by allowing the standards of care to be expressed as those exercised by the relevant medical peer group but at the same time other or minority views and opinions, if held by respectable peers, are acceptable. However, the opinions must be reasonable. In other words, the same legal rules apply to the general practitioner as to any other doctor. Negligence is governed by a duty of care to the individual concerned and a breach in that duty, which leads to damage that otherwise would not have happened. The civil system works on the balance of probabilities. If the probability is less than 50%, a claimant would not succeed.

General practitioners are expected to have a core of knowledge and skills common to general practitioners as a whole and be able to apply them in as effective and acceptable a manner as the next general practitioner, whether working in the National Health Service (NHS), that is the system of care provided largely through taxation and mostly free at the time in the UK, or privately, or both.

It has also to be recognized that complaints about a general practitioner's services may additionally be investigated by agencies outside the process of litigation, namely the contracting authority and subsequently the Health Service Commissioner and finally the General Medical Council (GMC). If a criminal charge involving negligence against a general practitioner is proven, this will be reported to the GMC.

The Problem

It has to be appreciated that changes in medical practice occur following new diagnoses or an increased understanding of disease and pathology, altering treatments and drug discoveries and changes in the natural history of disease. It is expected that doctors make themselves aware of these changes and modify their practice accordingly. Lord Donaldson in a judgment stated: "If a doctor fails to exercise the skill which he has or claims to have he is in breach of his duty of care. He is negligent."

For the general practitioner, the standard is that of other general practitioners, not specialists, but this holds whether the doctor is in year 1 or year 20 of practice. However, the general practitioner cannot or should not guarantee the results or outcome of his/her medical interventions as could an engineer building a bridge. Of course, even trained professionals make errors all the time but these tend to be trivial or easily reversible. Good training enables people to anticipate or quickly recognize problems so as to take evading action. The fact that general practitioners work in a medical environment that is uncertain and often at the early stages of the presentation of disease can create a climate where diagnostic errors may occur. It also has to be recognized that errors may occur not because of individual imperfections but because the system in which the practitioner works lacks processes or mechanisms that check organizational efficiency, detect errors, or provide sufficient resources.

Rules and Regulations

Technically speaking, self-employed general practitioners in the NHS do not have contracts with individual patients, be they registered under permanent, temporary, emergency, or other procedures. The general practitioner's own contract with a health authority is sufficient to establish a duty of care in respect of a registered patient, including those patients not registered with the general practitioner concerned whose conditions have to be considered in an emergency situation. The current General Medical Services Regulations (2004) make it clear that a practice providing general medical services under their contract is expected to act "with reasonable care and skill." This means in a like manner as would other practices under similar circumstances where partners or employees were exercising professional judgment requiring generally accepted knowledge, skills, and care but no higher. Of course, this would not prevent any general practitioner from exercising a higher standard. Clearly if the generality of general practitioners became more knowledgeable and skillful, this would affect the acceptable standard of care provided by increasing it.

Part 5, Section 12 of the General Medical Services Regulations sets out the general statement that the general practice shall provide essential medical services to their patients. There are separate contractual arrangements for other specific services such as intrapartum obstetrics and minor surgery involving cutting or injections, but whatever contract or contracts are held, a general practitioner is expected to have the relevant knowledge and skills to undertake the required care. Employed doctors, such as assistants or general practitioner registrars or other employees such as nurses, receptionists, or secretaries in undertaking their relevant tasks may do so in a negligent manner but the employing general practitioner(s) have to be ready to take legal responsibility for their acts (or omissions). However, all these employees are or should be covered by separate independent indemnity cover to that of the general practitioner principals themselves. The position regarding locum practitioners is not clear. However, an employing general practitioner could be held responsible if he/she engaged a locum without checking that the locum was competent for the purpose and subsequently the locum injured a patient, amounting to negligence. It has to be remembered that general practitioners in partnership are or may be equally liable.

Factors Leading to Claims

1. There may be problems of communication. The medical notes and records or telephone messages may be incomplete or illegible. Reliance on memory is no substitute for recorded information. Communication amongst members of the practice staff (or from a deputizing service that is an organization providing locum doctor services) may be poor. Incomplete information may be conveyed to other outside agencies, especially in relation to hospital referrals, e.g., a history of anaphylaxis to penicillin or other drug reactions. Clearly, medical records must not be changed falsely. If changes can legitimately be made, these should be made clearly, initialed, and dated.
2. If, following a consultation or other medical intervention, circumstances arise or are noted in which follow-up, treatment, or referral to other agencies would be desirable or necessary, then the relevant option should be discussed with the patient and acted upon. This would also include considering or carrying out treatment advised by hospital specialists. It would be especially important to note in the records a patient's refusal for treatment or referral. It may well be that the general practitioner's examination was deficient and this had a direct effect on a harmful outcome. However, given an acceptable examination, a mistake in making or considering a diagnosis would not necessarily be negligent. If the failure to make a

diagnosis is because an examination is not carried out, e.g., failure to visit and avoidable harm results, this may well lead to a claim being made. Telephone consultations do occur. There are advantages and disadvantages in relying on such proceedings but it has to be recognized that there may be avoidable risks in offering advice in the absence of a physical examination.

Problems may arise if the general practitioner does not act on abnormal results of investigations which he/she has initiated or ordered. It is wise for the general practitioner (or nurse) to ask the patient to contact or visit the surgery to obtain the results. Failure of the patient to do so may not exculpate the general practitioner if he/she fails or fails to attempt to contact the patient. Abnormal results derived from hospital clinics would be expected to be acted upon by the responsible hospital doctor concerned.

3. If a patient suffers from an adverse drug reaction (whosoever had originally prescribed the drugs), the general practitioner should note this clearly in the medical records. Represcribing a drug that had previously resulted in an adverse reaction may be deemed negligent. Blind prescribing of a drug little known to the general practitioner at the behest of a hospital doctor, especially if clinical control is maintained by the hospital, resulting in harm to the patient, may not be excusable. It must be remembered that the prescribing doctor is or may be legally responsible for any mishap. He/she is certainly legally responsible for writing the prescription and, in the best of all worlds, the doctor who has and retains clinical responsibility for the patient should undertake the prescribing. Joint responsibility may occur, as in obstetric care, but each doctor must know what the other one is doing and prescribing. In other words, a general practitioner cannot escape legal responsibility for any harm by stating he/she was merely carrying out the orders or request of a hospital doctor. The general practitioner should always have an up-to-date *British National Formulary* (a comprehensive book describing the drugs in use, their indications, doses, side-effects, contraindications, interactions, and dangers) at hand and use it. Family doctors in other countries would no doubt have a similar publication to which to refer.

In prescribing a drug or drugs, the general practitioner should do so in accordance with the manufacturer's data. Product liability may fall on the general practitioner if for example he/she mixes two incompatible liquid drugs in a syringe and harm results.

4. General practitioners must take care before or during procedures so as to minimize or avoid harm. Such measures include only using a single-use syringe once, sterilizing equipment, or properly taking a cervical smear so that abnormalities can be detected.

5. General practitioners would be expected to maintain their professional premises in such a way to safeguard the safety of staff and patients, e.g., safe electric wiring, correctly positioning carpets on stairs, or ensuring that drinking water does not become contaminated.

The Good and Bad Sides to the Equation

It is interesting to note that it is only within the past 15 years that the number of claims against general practitioners in the UK has risen dramatically. In 1992 Margaret Brazier in her book *Medicine, Patients and the Law* reported on the relative rarity of malpractice claims against general practitioners, citing as reasons that general practitioners were viewed with a high measure of esteem by patients (which is still the case), that long-standing personal relationships could lead to mistakes being overlooked, and that negligence could be more difficult to prove against general practitioners.

Furthermore, the NHS complaints procedures then in place could allow patients to have any problems concerning their doctor's services aired. Additionally, it was easy for a general practitioner to refer a patient into the secondary care system.

These factors still remain but the Medical Protection Society reported in 1999 that general practitioners were 13 times more likely to be sued successfully by their patients than in 1989 and were 33 times more likely to be pursued with what were described as "spurious" claims. Furthermore, the amounts paid in damages have risen considerably. Many reasons have been advanced for the increase in the number of claims, including the development of a compensation culture amongst members of society but this merely describes what has happened and does not provide reasons for it. Further consideration of this is outside the scope of this article.

The Proposed Solution

Problems can be minimized if the general practitioner listens, takes a proper history, conducts the required examination, makes full records in the correct folder (both of the consultation and other contact events such as phone calls), carries out any appropriate investigations advising the patient of options and outcomes, obtaining agreement for any actions, treats the patient, referring him/her to other agencies when necessary, and visits when required. He has a duty to keep up to date and now has to be prepared for reaccreditation.

The General Medical Council's advice is:

1. You must keep your knowledge and skills up to date throughout your working life. In particular, you should regularly take part in educational activities which maintain and further develop your competence and performance.

2. Some parts of medical practice are governed by law or are regulated by other statutory bodies. You must observe and keep up to date with the laws and statutory codes of practice which affect your work.

3. You must work with colleagues to monitor and maintain the quality of the care you provide and maintain a high awareness of patient safety. In particular, you must:

   a. take part in regular and systematic medical and clinical audit, recording data honestly. Where necessary you must respond to the results of audit to improve your practice, for example by undertaking further training

   b. respond constructively to the outcome of reviews, assessments, or appraisals of your performance

   c. take part in confidential enquiries and adverse event recognition and reporting to help reduce risk to patients.

Carrying out these activities is likely to reduce the possible danger to the health of patients (and others for whom the general practitioner bears a responsibility). General practitioners will still make mistakes, but hopefully ones that will not lead to litigation.

See Also

Medical Malpractice – Medico-legal Perspectives: Negligence, Standard of Care; Negligence, Duty of Care; Negligence Quantum

Further Reading

Brazier M (1992) *Medicine, Patients and the Law*. London: Pelican Books.

Carey D (1998) *Medical Negligence Litigation*. Sutton Coldfield, UK: CLT Professional.

General Medical Council (2001) *Good Medical Practice*. London: General Medical Council.

Harpwood V (2001) *Negligence in Healthcare*. London: Informa.

Hughes C (1995) *Law and General Practice*. Beckenham, UK: Publishing Initiatives.

Irwin S, Fazan C, Allfrey R (1995) *Medical Negligence Litigation: A Practitioner's Guide*. Great Britain: Lag Education and Service Trust.

Jackson JP (1991) *A Practical Guide to Medicine and the Law*. London: Springer-Verlag.

Jones MA (1996) *Medical Negligence*. London: Sweet and Maxwell.

Kennedy I, Grubb A (2000) *Medical Law*. London: Butterworths.

Lewis CJ (1998) *Medical Negligence, A Practical Guide*. London: Butterworths.

Medical Defence Union (2002) *Clinical Negligence*. London: MDU.

Montgomery J (1997) *Healthcare Law*. New York: Oxford University Press.

NHS (2004) NHS (General Medical Services) Regulations. London: HMSO.

Phillips AF (1997) *Medical Negligence Law: Seeking A Balance*. Aldershot, UK: Dartmouth Publishing.

Powers M, Harris N (2000) *Clinical Negligence*. London: Butterworth.

Intensive Care

G Park, Addenbrooke's Hospital NHS Trust, Cambridge, UK

Introduction

Critically ill adults are amongst the most vulnerable patients in the hospital. They suffer from serious diseases that in combination with the treatment render them defenseless and completely dependent on their carers. In addition, they are often unconscious or confused. The complete physical dependence along with mental incompetence makes them vulnerable to injury caused by criminal, accidental, or negligent acts.

Criminal Acts – Murder

All parts of society have their mad, bad, sad, and misguided members and the medical and nursing profession has its share. Unfortunately, attempts to murder patients continue to occur. Most, but not all, episodes of murder in the critically ill are performed by nurses and are usually multiple. The reason for this is the amount of time spent with patients alone. Nurses have the opportunity because they are alone with patients for long periods. They are also responsible for making up drugs and adjusting ventilators. Doctors are rarely alone with patients, drawing up or giving drugs, and so do not have the opportunity. When a doctor does look after a patient alone, a single death may be viewed as bad luck, two deaths are really bad luck, but three deaths would be suspicious. Conversely, nurses look after patients all the time and with the high mortality (about 20% in most intensive care units (ICUs)) death is not unexpected and this may allow murder of patients to go unnoticed for a long period.

Attempts at murdering patients may be from the omission of drugs. For example, the doctors may have prescribed a catecholamine infusion, such as epinephrine (adrenaline). The nurse making up the prescription may omit the drug from the infusion, i.e., just put saline in the syringe, but still sign to say the drug is in the syringe. The absence of the drug results in hypotension. This is more common than might be thought.

In one postal survey of American critical care nurses, Asch found that 17% of nurses had received requests from the patient or family for euthanasia or help with suicide. Euthanasia (most often using high-dose opioids) had been engaged in by 16% of the nurses. A much smaller percentage (4%) had pretended to give essential treatment ordered by a doctor.

Directly harmful acts do occur. Nurses have been known deliberately to give muscle relaxants to patients who are not on mechanical ventilators, thus paralyzing their respiratory muscle. Similarly, they may make up antibiotics and other drugs for doctors to give with potassium rather than sodium chloride. If the doctor is careless and fails to check all the ampoules, then injection will cause sudden cardiac arrest. Administering a large dose of morphine is a further way of killing patients. The other way that nurses can murder patients is by adjusting the ventilator so it delivers insufficient oxygen or malfunctions in some other way.

The motive for these criminal acts varies. For some, a cardiac arrest after injection of potassium chloride generates excitement as the cardiac arrest team is called, and perhaps the patient's life is saved, or not. Others may want to see an improvement in the service. One pediatric nurse gave the reason for administering suxamethonium (a muscle relaxant) to children as a means of increasing the mortality rate so that services could be improved to reduce it. More commonly, it is a desire to see suffering stop in a dying patient. In this case there may be poor leadership by the medical staff: dying patients are not recognized and futile treatment withdrawn, so the nurse decides to take matters into his/her own hands. This may be by giving unprescribed doses of morphine, omitting drugs, or adjusting the ventilator improperly. Sometimes there is proper leadership, but the nurse just decides to end the patient's life because the patient is suffering.

Proving there was misdoing is very difficult. With this type of crime it is only after many patients have died that colleagues become suspicious. After that there is usually further delay while the hospital authorities decide what course of action to take. More delay occurs when the police decide whether or not to investigate. The patient is dead, there are usually no witnesses, and the ventilator has been used on many other patients. Toxicology is occasionally useful, but more often than not it proves impossible to interpret. The drugs that may have been used to commit a crime have been used therapeutically, their elimination is abnormal, and tolerance develops. Because of this tolerance high serum concentrations may not mean that poisoning has occurred. It should also be remembered that the high death rate may mean that clusters occur purely by chance, leading to a crime of just "being there" or "having a bad run."

Surprisingly, the patient record can be of value in investigating whether unprescribed opioids have been used. To give these drugs special records are needed and nurses often continue to complete the forms meticulously, even if the drugs are not prescribed. Other drugs are much more difficult. In one case, the author looked through nearly 200 records completed by one nurse who had allegedly killed patients. There were multiple differences between the prescription and the administration of all types of drugs. Multiple nurses had made these errors.

There are much rarer cases of doctors being accused of murder. In a Canadian case it was alleged that a consultant gave large doses of first an opioid (hydromorphone $500 \, mg \, h^{-1}$) to relieve a dying patient's suffering, which is perfectly proper. However, the patient continued to live and the physician gave a large, intravenous undiluted dose of a vasodilator (nitroglycerine) and then went on to give undiluted, intravenous potassium chloride. Both drugs were injected through the same femoral venous catheter. The patient died. The police were subsequently informed, and the doctor tried. The doctor was acquitted because there was doubt that the venous catheter was in the vein.

Negligence

Negligent acts in the critically ill appear to be more common amongst doctors than nurses. This is simply because doctors do more invasive procedures and prescribe drugs. In many countries a reduction in

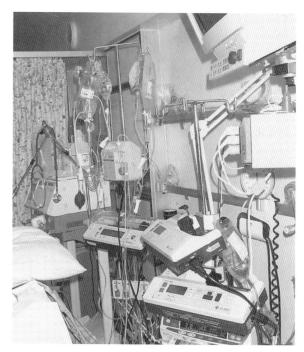

Figure 1 Multiple pieces of equipment in an ICU.

doctors' working hours has led to the nursing staff doing more both in the ICU and on the wards. As they take on extended roles, they will be more likely to encounter these allegations.

In the UK, litigation for negligence was rare in the critically ill, since most patients and their relatives were glad to have survived such an illness. This sentiment is now changing, and there has been a dramatic increase in litigation. However, because litigation was uncommon, medical note-taking was not as good as it is in other areas. Indeed, it is still common to find a medical intervention not recorded in the medical notes but recorded in the nursing record.

There is an adage that the more you do to a patient, the greater the risk of something going wrong. As a body fails, more and more needs to be done to the patient, increasing the risk of something going wrong. The ICU is a very technical environment and the complexity of the equipment makes it even more likely for equipment to malfunction or be misused. As the equipment becomes more complex, the corresponding level of experience in both the junior medical and nursing staff is decreasing. This is not just a UK problem, but a global one (**Figure 1**).

Some of the technologies and problems are described below.

Central Venous Lines

Central venous lines are one of the commonest causes of attempted litigation. Puncture of the carotid artery when the internal jugular vein is catheterized is an accepted risk of about 2%, with a range of 0–30%. Usually, this leads to a hematoma and little else. Unfortunately, this type of accident is also associated with complete occlusion of the artery and the development of a stroke. So long as the central line was needed and inserted using the proper technique this is not negligent. Unfortunately, the situation has been complicated in some cases by the doctor using the line to infuse drugs that are irritant or cause thrombosis, and failing to remove the line for many hours. This method is not considered acceptable practice.

The National Institute for Clinical Excellence (NICE) has recently published guidelines indicating that these types of lines should only be inserted (except in emergencies and the like) using ultrasound guidance. Since monies have been made available for the purchase of this expensive technology; in the future if there is a complication during insertion, failure to use ultrasound may be considered substandard.

Perforation of the heart is another complication that may arise from this procedure. If the line ends above the heart, then perforation of a great vein results in a hydrothorax as fluids are infused. However, if the line tip is below the pericardial reflection, then perforation into the pericardium will result. If fluids are infused, they will cause tamponade, which may result in death. To prevent this complication a chest X-ray needs to be taken to confirm correct positioning of the tip before it is used for infusion, except in an emergency.

Nerve injuries may also occur as a complication. The recurrent laryngeal nerve may be injured after an internal jugular approach and similarly the femoral nerve after femoral vein catheterization.

Positioning

The critically ill patient is often semiconscious, either from illness or from the sedation and analgesia given to help the patient tolerate the interventions needed in the ICU. The resulting immobility, perhaps coupled with the need to use unusual positions and reduced arterial blood pressure, renders the patient more likely to suffer a pressure injury. These are varied and range from peripheral nerve entrapment through pressure sores to necrosis of the breast from turning the patient prone and pressure on a breast implant. It can be difficult to determine if the injury is caused by substandard care.

Peripheral nerve injuries in isolation most likely result from a failure to protect a vulnerable part of the body. However, the ulnar nerve may be injured, even if all precautions are taken, if its anatomy is unusual and it is outside the ulnar groove at the elbow. Multiple neuropathies occurring during a

period of intensive care are usually caused by something other than poor positioning. These other causes may include critical care neuropathy or preexisting illness such as excessive alcohol consumption.

Pressure areas, such as the heel, may also be damaged if there is a prolonged period of immobility. Usually, there are other confounding factors, such as the use of catecholamine infusions causing poor skin perfusion in combination with hypotension. Some unusual pressure-relieving methods, designed to help, may worsen the situation. Diarrhea, a common complication of critical illness, may exacerbate a sacral sore.

Misuse of Drugs

As many as 20 drugs may be used in a critically ill patient at any one time. The potential for straying outside the recommended dose, duration of treatment, drug interactions, and adverse events is enormous. However, there are some relatively common problems with drugs of which both doctors and lawyers need to be aware and illustrations of these are given below.

Nonsteroidal antiinflammatory drugs (NSAIDs) These drugs are good at relieving some forms of pain, especially those where there is an element of inflammation. In addition, in severe pain they reduce the amount of opioids needed to treat severe pain. They have therefore found widespread usage in many areas of medicine. In the critically ill, two of their side-effects cause concern. The first is their effect on renal function. Because they all inhibit prostaglandin synthesis they prevent renal vasodilatation. In conditions of poor renal blood flow, such as shock, they add to the renal vasoconstriction and may precipitate renal failure after multiple doses (rarely one or two). If they are prescribed to the critically ill, then the renal function must be known and observed for toxicity of these drugs. Since the Royal College of Anaesthetists has published guidelines on their use (www.rcoa.ac.uk), failing to follow these guidelines in a critically ill patient may be considered substandard care if the patient develops renal failure as a consequence.

Deep-vein thrombosis (DVT) Immobility increases the risk of a DVT and a subsequent pulmonary embolus. The incidence of DVTs in the critically ill is between 13% and 30% and can lead to pulmonary embolism and death. In many areas of medicine, such as orthopedics, there is proven benefit from DVT prophylaxis. Some lawyers have suggested that failure to give DVT prophylaxis has resulted in avoidable pulmonary embolism and death. However, many trials exclude the critically ill and only a few have shown benefit in some patients. The lack of this information makes it difficult to construct guidelines on which patients should receive prophylaxis.

Failing to give a drug   The advent of life-saving, very expensive drugs has opened up a whole new era of potential negligence. In 2002, activated protein C (aPC: Xigress: Lilly Products) was introduced into clinical practice for the treatment of life-threatening sepsis. It has been shown to produce a 6% reduction in mortality from this condition. Its great expense (£5500) and the frequency of sepsis means that the cost pressure on some hospitals is large. Some have responded by not using it at all, arguing it has not been through the NICE procedure and recommended by NICE. (Once a drug has been approved by NICE, central funding to cover its cost is made available. It is also a requirement that the drug is introduced.) Others have introduced a system of rationing. There is no doubt for the majority of clinicians that this drug works, and it will be interesting to see if failure to give it will be considered unacceptable.

Starch solutions   It is not just drugs that have adverse effects: common, everyday intravenous fluids also have adverse effects. Some fluids have a maximum amount that can be infused in a certain time. Starch solutions are used to replace intravascular volume, depleted either from sepsis or hemorrhage. Unfortunately, some starches interfere with blood clotting, causing an acquired lack of von Willebrand factor. This interference can increase the risk of hemorrhage in a susceptible critically ill patient.

Professional Problems

Doctors and nurses are expected to practice to the highest possible standards and failure to do so may result in allegations of professional misconduct. There are some common problems that affect ICU staff.

Sexual Hallucinations

About a quarter of patients suffer from abnormal dreams or hallucinations while they are in the ICU. Almost half of these abnormal dreams disturb the patient; many involve violence, death, attempted murder, and physical harm to him/her. It is easy to explain to the patient that this did not happen since he/she has no physical signs of violence. Much more difficult are the hallucinations that involve sexual assault such as rape and sodomy. A careful history and examination of the record may show precipitating events such as a vaginal examination or the insertion of a rectal temperature probe. Unfortunately, sometimes the patient will complain to the police or other authority first and an investigation may be started. Usually this is very damaging to the person against whom the allegation is made.

Patient Autonomy

Respect for the patient's autonomy is also expected. This becomes difficult when faced with an unconscious critically ill patient whose prognosis is poor. Issuing a do-not-resuscitate (DNR) instruction without consulting the patient or the family (as a surrogate) is expected of doctors. The same is true of a do-not-escalate (DNE) instruction. If the patient is competent then his/her wishes should be respected. As the case of Mrs. B in the UK showed, even if the patient wants life-supporting measures (such as mechanical ventilation) to be withdrawn, he/she has the right to that treatment being removed. However, it is important to draw the distinction between refusal of treatment and assisted euthanasia.

Organ Donation – Money for Organs

Transplantation of the heart, lung, and liver is life-saving. Unfortunately, the advances in this area have made it a victim of its own success. These organs can only be obtained from heart-beating cadaveric organ donors. This type of donor is only found in ICUs. There are organizations worldwide that offer transplants where the cost is many more times the cost of a transplant in the UK or elsewhere. Caution is needed by ICU doctors not to become involved in any trade of organs. It is strictly forbidden in most societies, although the matter is under debate.

Reporting of Deaths

Many of the deaths in an ICU need to be reported to a coroner, procurator fiscal, or medical examiner. Rules vary between countries and even regions of the same country (including within the UK) as to who should be reported. We have shown that directors of intensive care can be unaware of some of the regulations; but then the same study also showed that so were some of the coroners.

Record-Keeping in the Critically Ill

As in many areas of medicine, the patient record may be a central piece of evidence in a court case. The critically ill are often of interest to coroners, compensation lawyers, as well as criminal and civil lawyers. It is worth remembering that what you write in the notes may be read out in court. If you fail to record something, then you are unlikely to remember it later.

Do not criticize your colleagues and their treatment of the patient unless you are prepared to justify your criticisms later.

If you do find yourself giving evidence in court, always read the notes in advance of your appearance.

See Also

Complaints Against Doctors, Healthcare Workers and Institutions; Expert Witness: Medical

Further Reading

Asch DA (1996) The role of critical care nurses in euthanasia and assisted suicide. *New England Journal of Medicine* 334: 1374–1379.

Balasubramaniam B, Park GR (2003) Sexual hallucinations during and after sedation and anaesthesia. *Anaesthesia* 58: 549–553.

Bernard GR, Vincent JL, Laterre PF, et al. (2001) Efficacy and safety of recombinant human activated protein C for severe sepsis. *New England Journal of Medicine* 344: 699–709.

Booth SA, Norton B, Mulvey DA (2001) Central venous catheterization and fatal cardiac tamponade. *British Journal of Anaesthesia* 87: 298–302.

Booth SA, Wilkins ML, Smith JM, Park GR (2003) Who to report to the coroner? A survey of intensive care unit directors and Her Majesty's Coroners in England and Wales. *Anaesthesia* 58: 1204–1209.

Burdet L, Liaudet L, Schaller MD, Broccard AF (2001) Bilateral breast necrosis after prone position ventilation. *Intensive Care Medicine* 27: 1435.

Delmonico FL, Arnold R, Scheper-Hughes N, et al. (2002) Ethical incentives – not payment – for organ donation. *New England Journal of Medicine* 346: 2002–2005.

Elkind P (1983) *The Death Shift.* New York: Viking Penguin.

Geerts W, Selby R (2003) Prevention of venous thromboembolism in the ICU. *Chest* 124: 337S–363S.

Geerts W, Cook D, Selby R, Etchells E (2002) Venous thromboembolism and its prevention in critical care. *Journal of Critical Care* 17: 95–104.

Harris J, Erin C (2002) An ethically defensible market in organs. *British Medical Journal* 325: 114–115.

Martin D (1989) Nurses who murder. *Nursing Standard* 3: 19–20.

Michiels JJ, Budde U, van der Planken M, et al. (2001) Acquired von Willebrand syndromes: clinical features, aetiology, pathophysiology, classification and management. *Best Practice and Research Clinical Haematology* 14: 401–436.

National Institute for Clinical Excellence (2002) Guidance on the use of ultrasound locating devices for placing central venous catheters. Technology Appraisal No. 49, London.

Park GR (1996) Molecular mechanisms of drug metabolism in the critically ill. *British Journal of Anaesthesia* 77: 32–49.

Park GR, Khan SN (2002) Murder and the ICU. *European Journal of Anaesthesiology* 19: 621–623.

Park GR, McElliot M, Torres C (2003) Outreach critical care – cash for no questions? *British Journal of Anaesthesia* 90: 700–701.

Rocker G (2003) End of life care in Canada after a murder charge in an ICU. *Intensive Care Medicine* 29: 2336–2337.

Rosen M, Latto P, Ng S (2004) The internal jugular vein. In: *Handbook of Percutaneous Central Venous Catheterisation*, pp. 115–153. London: WB Saunders.

The Allitt Inquiry 1994. London: HMSO.

Neonatology

N K Ives, University of Oxford, Oxford, UK

Introduction

The pediatric subspecialty of neonatology has advanced to a degree that public expectation of intact newborn survival, fostered by press coverage of "miracle" babies, could be considered unrealistic. Recourse to legal action following adverse outcome may have been suppressed in the past by the strong emotional ties that a family forms with their pediatrician during an infant's critical illness. Nowadays, neonatal death or complications with long-term sequelae are being increasingly subjected to medicolegal scrutiny. Claims of this nature are a justifiable means, and presently the only route in the UK, to securing large sums of money necessary to support a disabled individual appropriately for life. In as many as a quarter of such cases clinical negligence can be identified. That is not to say that all clinical negligence claims are successful, as the link to causation of an injury is often complex. Much neonatal morbidity is multifactorial in origin.

When considering any intervention in medicine the risk-to-benefit ratio has to be taken into account. This is no more so than when dealing with the fragility of life of a baby born 4 months prematurely and weighing between 500 and 750 g. Intact survival is possible but cannot be guaranteed. The parents have the right to be fully involved with decisions regarding viability and resuscitation at this early gestation. They must be aware that many of the innate complications of prematurity cannot be prevented, and that interventions carry the risk of iatrogenic injury.

Malpractice in neonatology covers failure of a medical or nursing professional to provide an accepted level of duty of care through reprehensible ignorance or negligence or through criminal intent, especially when injury or loss follows. Negligence is a breach of duty of care, which causes damage. A doctor is in breach of his/her duty of care if he/she fails to provide a reasonable standard of care. Pediatricians, as in other specialties, can only be judged according to the state of advancement of their clinical field at the time of the plaintiff's injury. By contrast, deliberation on causation may benefit from discussion of the latest science. Recent therapies such as prenatal steroids to promote fetal lung maturation and postnatal surfactant replacement therapy for respiratory distress have halved mortality from severe hyaline membrane disease in the newborn. For a clinician to deprive a patient of the benefits of such treatments would constitute negligence if the breach of duty of care resulted in damage, such as death, chronic lung disease, or other complications attributable to the greater severity of lung disease.

In contrast to an adult patient of sound mind who is obliged to make a claim with respect to personal injuries within 3 years, limitation in the case of a child damaged by an injury in the newborn period is extended to his/her 21st birthday, or beyond. If the injured party remains incapable of managing his/her own affairs he/she is regarded by law as "being under a disability." In such cases, the right to sue continues throughout life and up to 3 years after death for the benefit of the claimant's estate.

Unlawful Killing and Manslaughter

Collective decisions on the withholding or withdrawing of care are regularly made by senior clinicians, parents, and nurses on delivery suites and neonatal units in the UK. The majority of deaths on neonatal units are directly attributable to withdrawal of care, in circumstances where the baby may or may not have succumbed to the underlying illness. The situation is unique to the newborn and only applies in cases of extreme prematurity, gross malformations, and in the context of profound brain damage. These difficult events need to be fully documented and second opinions should be provided. Approached with sensitivity, understanding, and flexibility according to parental wishes, it should be possible to act in the patient's best interests and prevent exposure of the parents or doctor to criminal law or the media. In legal terms, this remains a "gray area." Technically, the doctor who switches off a ventilator is committing a positive act that results in unlawful killing and is guilty of murder. Omitting to act where there is a duty to do so, such as at resuscitation, could legally be interpreted as manslaughter. The UK courts are

sometimes used in individual complex cases to grant one-off "declarations of legality" to make lawful the decision to withdraw care.

The complexity of these issues is highlighted by a case in the USA where the medically qualified father was acquitted of manslaughter after taking his daughter (a 25-week gestation baby, weighing 780 g) off the ventilator on day one, despite the neonatologist's conviction that intensive care should be continued. In an era when babies born at 23 and even 22 weeks gestation are surviving, the majority of UK tertiary-level neonatologists would feel it appropriate to offer intensive care to a baby delivered at 23 weeks gestation, weighing more than 500 g, and born in a viable condition. They would do so in the knowledge that they hold joint responsibility with the parents for considering stopping intensive care if profound brain damage was identified, or a severe clinical deterioration meant that death was inevitable.

Iatrogenic Disorders in Neonatology

The invasive nature of neonatal intensive care and the fragility of many of its recipients result in a higher proportion of disorders arising from complications of procedures and treatment than in most other fields of medicine. These iatrogenic disorders are in many cases unavoidable despite optimal care. They should, however, be anticipated, recognized, and promptly treated. Malpractice occurs when there has been an unacceptable delay in recognizing or treating these disorders, or when the complication results from an unacceptable standard of care, such as a drug error or incorrect ventilatory settings (e.g., pneumothorax). Examples of conditions with potential iatrogenic causes or components are listed in **Table 1**.

Many drugs used in neonatology carry the risk of significant side-effects. For example, indometacin, used to encourage a patent ductus arteriosus to close, may cause gastrointestinal hemorrhage or perforation. The same complications can occur with the steroid dexamethasone when used to treat chronic lung disease, although this use of postnatal steroids

Table 1 Conditions with potential iatrogenic causes

Pneumothorax
Chronic lung disease
Subglottic stenosis
Retinopathy of prematurity
Necrotizing enterocolitis
Intestinal perforation
Gastric rupture
Conjugated hyperbilirubinemia
Periventricular hemorrhage
Periventricular leukomalacia

has been dramatically curtailed in the light of mounting evidence of an association with an increased risk of cerebral palsy.

Indwelling arterial lines placed either peripherally in the radial or posterior tibial arteries or centrally via the umbilical artery are invaluable for continuous blood pressure monitoring and atraumatic blood sampling. They do, however, carry the risk of hemorrhage and devastating ischemic injuries involving digit and limb loss (**Figures 1** and **2**). Umbilical artery catheters may also be associated with thrombotic or embolic obstruction of the renal arteries leading to renal failure, the mesenteric arteries causing gut perforation, and the lumbar arteries resulting in paraplegia. Buttock necrosis and sciatic nerve damage have also been described. As with intravenous infusions, regular nursing observations of arterial lines are essential for early detection of perfusion-related complications. As soon as there is evidence of compromised tissue perfusion an arterial line must be

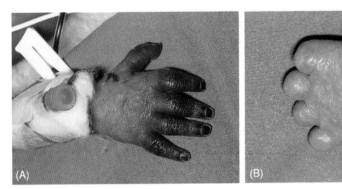

Figure 1   (A) Gangrenous fingers following radial arterial catheterization. (B) Subsequent loss of fingers and thumb. Reproduced with permission from Rennie JM, Roberton NRC (eds.) (1999) *Textbook of Neonatology*, 3rd edn. Edinburgh, UK: Churchill Livingstone.

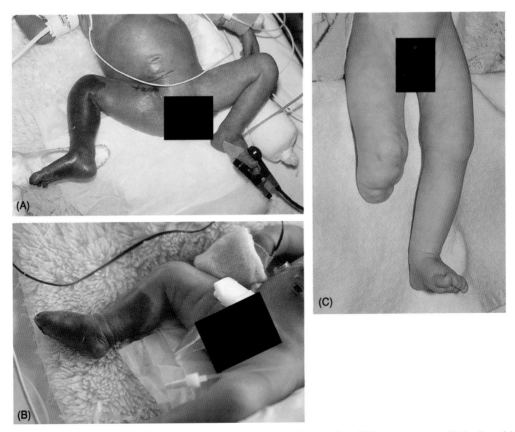

Figure 2   (A) Acute ischemia to the right leg following insertion of a femoral artery line. (B) Some recovery with the line of demarcation below the knee. This resulted in a below-knee amputation (C). Reproduced with permission from Rennie JM, Roberton NRC (eds.) (1999) *Textbook of Neonatology*, 3rd edn. Edinburgh, UK: Churchill Livingstone.

removed, and supportive measures to improve the circulation should be started. These measures may extend to thrombolytic therapy and surgical referral for embolectomy. In terms of malpractice, it is rarely the arterial line insertion technique that is open to question, but more often it is the delay in managing the complication that prompts legal scrutiny. When any arterial line is being used it is essential that pressure alarm limits are correctly set to alert staff to hypotension. This may be the first indication that hemorrhage is occurring from a line. Umbilical venous catheters carry complications of their own, such as hepatic necrosis and portal vein thrombosis when sited in the liver or cardiac tamponade if the tip perforates the right atrium. The ideal position for an umbilical venous catheter is at the junction of the inferior vena cava and the right atrium.

The incidence of iatrogenic injuries and errors in drug prescription and administration will tend to increase at times when a neonatal unit is at its busiest and the medical and nursing staff are overstretched. Monitoring of clinical incident reports and equating

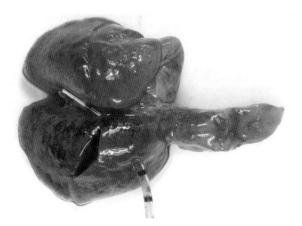

Figure 3 A postmortem specimen showing perforation of the lung by a chest drain that had been inserted with the intention of draining a pneumothorax. Photo courtesy of SJ Gould.

adverse events to staffing levels and staff mix has become an essential tool in risk management. In cases of injury that come to legal attention, some allowance is made for the grade of the doctor involved. However, it is to be expected that a junior doctor performing a neonatal procedure should be sufficiently experienced and competent to perform an allocated task, and to be able to recognize complications (*Wilsher* v. *Essex Area Health Authority* 1987. Queen's Bench 730). Perforation of the lung during chest drain insertion for a pneumothorax (**Figure 3**) may be considered clinical negligence if the operator was untrained and unsupervised.

Malpractice in Neonatal Medicine

Examples of conditions that are most frequently cited in claims of neonatal clinical malpractice are listed in **Table 2**. The majority of perinatal litigation is centered on hypoxic–ischemic encephalopathy and the question as to whether obstetric malpractice was to blame for the suboptimal or depressed state of the newborn infant and subsequent cerebral palsy. Occasionally the brain insult in such cases may be compounded by or entirely result from inadequate neonatal resuscitation. There may also be comorbidity from failure to treat associated complications such as hypoglycemia or hypotension.

The forms of brain injury that are more likely to occur postnatally and in the preterm population are periventricular hemorrhage (PVH) and periventricular leukomalacia (PVL). Even in the context of high standards of obstetric and neonatal care, these potentially devastating cerebral lesions can occur unpredictably as complications of prematurity. There is increasing awareness that many cases of PVL result from chorioamnionitis (*in utero* infection). A claim of malpractice may be invoked in cases of PVH if, for instance, a malplaced endotracheal tube (ventilation tube) or a pneumothorax had not been recognized

Table 2 Conditions frequently cited in cases of neonatal malpractice

Condition	Context
Hypoxic–ischemic encephalopathy (HIE)	Standard of resuscitation
Periventricular hemorrhage (PVH)	Standard of ventilatory support
Periventricular leukomalacia (PVL)	Hypotension or hypocarbia
Retinopathy of prematurity (ROP)	Hyperoxia. Failure to monitor/treat
Chronic lung disease (CLD)	Standard of ventilatory support
Hypoglycemia	Monitoring and treating risk groups
Neonatal infection	Delays in diagnosis and treatment
Extravasated infusions and scarring injuries	Delays in recognition and treatment
Severe jaundice leading to kernicterus	Failure to recognize and treat
Hemorrhagic disease of the newborn	Failure to provide vitamin K
Drug errors	Failure to take remedial action

and promptly corrected. Similarly, in a case of PVL, it can be shown that there was a failure to recognize or sufficiently promptly treat known causes such as hypotension and severe hypocarbia (resulting from overventilation).

Infection in the newborn (e.g., pneumonia, septicemia, necrotizing enterocolitis, and meningitis) can be rapidly overwhelming even when antibiotics and supportive therapy are commenced as soon as clinical suspicion is raised. Neonatal malpractice arises in such cases when there has been a failure to recognize risk factors for infection and there has been an unacceptable delay in treatment.

The majority of newborns will develop mild jaundice in the first week of life, but in a small proportion the level of the jaundice pigment bilirubin will reach potentially brain-damaging levels that can lead to cerebral palsy. This form of cerebral palsy, referred to as kernicterus, is preventable with phototherapy and exchange blood transfusion. Failure to recognize cases of severe jaundice or to intervene with treatment at published recommended levels represents malpractice.

Retinopathy of prematurity is a complication usually confined to infants born at extreme low birth weight (less than 1.0 kg). Whilst strict monitoring of oxygen therapy may reduce the incidence of this condition, there are several etiologies at play and the retinal disease cannot always be avoided. What can be prevented in the majority of cases is progression of the disease to its end-stage of macular disruption, retinal detachment, and blindness. There are national guidelines for screening preterms with eye checks and for instituting timely treatment with laser or cryotherapy. Failure to provide such a service constitutes a breach of duty of care.

Hypoglycemia, defined for newborns as a blood sugar level less than $2.6 \, \text{mmol} \, l^{-1}$, is not an uncommon finding. Otherwise, healthy term infants usually have alternative brain fuel supplies that prevent them becoming symptomatic. Higher-risk groups, such as preterms, growth-retarded babies, infected babies, infants of diabetic mothers, and some cases of inborn errors of metabolism are at greater risk of developing signs such as convulsions, coma, and apnea from which they may go on to develop neurological sequelae. Failure to assess and maintain the blood sugar adequately in these at-risk categories to the extent that a baby develops neuroglycopenic symptoms would be considered clinically negligent.

Unfortunately, some scarring injuries are an inevitable hallmark for graduates of neonatal intensive care. Intravenous lines, blood sampling, and chest drain insertion are all inclined to leave their mark. The injuries from infusions occur when extravate is aggravated if they contain hypertonic solutions or toxic drugs and electrolytes (**Figure 4**). It is a fact that drip extravates do not reflect negligent practice, but if this event, which signals the need for a replacement cannula, goes unheeded for more than 1 hour, the nursing care can be called into question. Nursing observation charts provide for hourly documentation of the condition of intravenous sites, and the perfusion of limbs and extremities if indwelling arterial lines are being used. In the case of extravasation injuries, malpractice occurs if there has been inadequate surveillance of the infusion site and a consequent delay in recognition of the injury. Since it is now a textbook-recommended practice that in cases where there is ischemia of the overlying skin, the tissues should be flushed as soon as possible with a hyaluronidase solution, it may be considered malpractice if there is a failure to offer such treatment.

Skin preparation with concentrated iodine and alcohol solutions will reduce invasive sepsis during procedures, but if not rinsed off with milder solutions, and particularly if a baby is allowed to lie in a pool of such agents, chemical burns may ensue.

Prior to being discharged home, babies born in hospital should receive a routine screening examination.

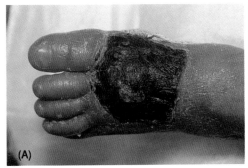
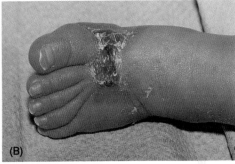

Figure 4 (A) Tissue damage to the dorsum of the foot following extravasation of total parenteral nutrition. (B) Healing, with a time interval between (A) and (B) of 5 weeks, has resulted in an extensor contracture. Reproduced with permission from Rennie JM, Roberton NRC (eds.) (1999) *Textbook of Neonatology*, 3rd edn. Edinburgh, UK: Churchill Livingstone.

Table 3   Failures leading to potential neonatal malpractice

Failure to detect an obvious and significant abnormality on newborn examination
Failure to follow up appropriately an abnormality found on newborn examination
Failure to adhere to published guidelines for the management of neonatal jaundice
Failure to maintain the blood sugar in babies at risk of symptomatic hypoglycemia
Failure to give vitamin K at birth as prophylaxis against hemorrhagic disease
Failure to screen for or treat progressive retinopathy of prematurity

Whilst this is designed to pick up significant conditions (such as heart disease, developmental dysplasia of the hip (DDH), or head growth abnormalities), a number of conditions can be understandably missed. For instance, it is recognized that up to half of DDH is not detected on clinical examination of the hips. Similarly, it is not always possible to detect the milder forms of cyanotic congenital heart disease. But, as Roberton points out in his *Textbook of Neonatology*, there is no legal defense if the examination has not been performed and DDH is subsequently detected, or if an abnormal finding on routine neonatal examination is inadequately reviewed. These are examples of failures leading to potential neonatal malpractice, as listed in **Table 3**.

Conclusion

Neonatology encompasses a wide spectrum of ethics, the law, and clinical situations with heightened potential for malpractice. Decision-making on withholding resuscitation or withdrawal of care places neonatologists in a legal "gray area," bordering on unlawful killing and manslaughter. Successful outcome of neonatal intensive care can be hindered by complications, and a large proportion of these will be iatrogenic. Conditions with potential iatrogenic causes are highlighted in this article, along with complications frequently cited in cases of neonatal malpractice. Also emphasized are omissions of disease detection and treatment provision that constitute breach of duty of care.

See Also

Medical Malpractice – Medico-legal Perspectives: Negligence, Standard of Care; Negligence, Duty of Care; Negligence, Causation; Negligence Quantum

Further Reading

Brain AJL, Roberton NRC, Rennie JM (1999) Iatrogenic disorders. In: Rennie JM, Roberton NRC (eds.) *Textbook of Neonatology*, pp. 917–937. Edinburgh, UK: Churchill Livingstone.

Ives NK (1999) Neonatal jaundice. In: Rennie JM, Roberton NRC (eds.) *Textbook of Neonatology*, pp. 715–732. Edinburgh, UK: Churchill Livingstone.

Leigh MAMS (1999) Neonatology and the law. In: Rennie JM, Roberton NRC (eds.) *Textbook of Neonatology*, pp. 1351–1355. Edinburgh, UK: Churchill Livingstone.

Limitation Act (1980) London: Her Majesty's Stationery Office.

Paris JJ (1996) Manslaughter or a legitimate parental decision. The messenger case. *Journal of Perinatology* 16: 60–64.

Roberton NRC (1999) Frequent medico-legal problems. In: Rennie JM, Roberton NRC (eds.) *Textbook of Neonatology*, pp. 1357–1365. Edinburgh, UK: Churchill Livingstone.

The Royal College of Ophthalmologists, British Association of Perinatal Medicine (1996) Retinopathy of prematurity: guidelines for screening and treatment. *Early Human Development* 46: 239–258.

Wall SN, Partridge JC (1997) Death in the intensive care nursery: physician practice of withdrawing and withholding life support. *Pediatrics* 99: 64–70.

Whitelaw A (1986) Death as an option in neonatal intensive care. *Lancet* 8502: 328–331.

Neurosurgery

P Marks, The General Infirmary at Leeds, Leeds, UK

Introduction

Neurosurgery is undoubtedly a high-risk surgical discipline, but shares a number of common medicolegal problems with other branches of medicine. It also has a number of problems peculiar to itself. This article deals with malpractice in its broadest sense, outlines areas where medicolegal problems may develop in neurosurgical practice, and suggests strategies for their avoidance.

Frank Furedi, an academic sociologist at the University of Kent at Canterbury, has coined the term "litigation culture." Essentially he described the concept that, if a person gets hurt, it must be the fault of somebody rather than being just a chance event to which no culpability should be attached or, in other words, bad luck. Moreover, within this mindset the injured party assumes that compensation will not only be due, but will be his/her inalienable right, and there is often an expectation of a large payout, along the lines of the damages payable in various cases in the USA.

Often, the desire for pecuniary gain may be veiled behind apparently altruistic motives, such as a desire to "stop it from happening to someone else," but the bottom line is invariably financially driven.

In the USA, litigation culture has, in fact, brought about a national crisis in medical practice. This has been encouraged by a legal system in which conditional fees operate, under which as much as 50% of any award may go to the lawyer. Furthermore, US juries, in addition to awarding economic damages, can award "punitive damages" and can use their powers to inflate awards in the knowledge that if they do so, the plaintiff will still receive a substantial sum, in spite of the legal top-slicing of the award.

The mean award for damages from malpractice in the USA is $3.5 million. It is therefore no surprise to find that malpractice insurance premiums have risen by as much as 45% in certain high-risk specialties, such as neurosurgery, obstetrics, and orthopedic surgery.

The effect of this is for some practitioners in these disciplines to retire early, move to another location (state), or to confine their practice to low-risk procedures, e.g., neurosurgeons not undertaking intracranial surgery and only performing carpal tunnel decompressions.

The ripples of this litigation culture have spread out from the USA. In the UK, litigation culture currently costs 1% of the gross domestic product, which equates to approximately £10 billion per annum.

Neurosurgery is a relatively new discipline and seeks to diagnose and treat disorders affecting the central and peripheral nervous systems. Many of the disorders that fall within its compass are life-threatening and may require emergency surgery of a highly skilled and specialized nature.

Malignant cerebral tumors are associated with a poor prognosis and their surgical treatment may be associated with the risk of death or the production or worsening of a neurological deficit. Similarly, benign skull-base neoplasms such as meningiomas, which may have an intimate relationship to important neurovascular structures, demand the highest degree of surgical skill yet their removal may be associated with neurological deficit.

The management of aneurysmal subarachnoid hemorrhage is another area where the poor natural history of the disease has to be set against the not inconsiderable management morbidity and mortality. Even if a technically perfect operation is performed, the patient may still die or be disabled because of delayed ischemic neurological deficit consequent upon vasospasm. In such circumstances, criticism of the treatment received by the patient may follow, despite there being no grounds for complaint.

Communication and Consent

A recent study examined the reasons why doctors were sued and concluded that communication is an important reason. Adverse events are inevitable in medical practice but should not necessarily result in litigation. Factors that tend to result in litigation are, for example, a preexisting adversarial relationship between doctor and patient, or the development of one following the occurrence of such an event. It has been shown that litigation tends to occur when the patient or his/her family believe that the doctor has been economical with the truth and may have "covered up" important information.

It has also been shown that the surgeon's tone of voice may be a deciding factor in the decision to complain or seek redress at law when outcomes have been perceived as being adverse. If the surgeon does not sound concerned or is imperious, litigation is more likely to follow.

It will thus be readily appreciated that good communication skills are vital for good practice. Good communication skills should be seen as one of the important building blocks of good medical practice. They can be used to build a framework for dealing with patients when it comes to obtaining consent for treatment.

Consent is now a complex topic but one with which the neurosurgeon must be familiar. The simple rule for consent laid down in 1914 by Judge Cardozo has had to be developed to suit an enquiring and well-informed society as well as for the protection of the medical profession against individuals who would take the opportunity to sue.

Missen in 1992 proposed that "consent" is inadequate, as it implies that the patient is "doing the doctor a favor" by signifying agreement. In this era of patient participants, Missen felt that the term should be replaced by "request for treatment." The request for treatment emphasizes that there may not be a "cure," but that a "treatment" may be all the doctor can ultimately provide. Understanding that a definite cure may not be forthcoming may facilitate a move away from the bitter disappointments and legal actions that patients do take when their expectations are not fulfilled.

A recent investigation into the practice of obtaining consent sought to establish the frequency with which potential complications were discussed with the patients. The results indicated that a wide range of discussions took place with some surgeons emphasizing every conceivable complication, while others emphasized very few. The authors concluded that a "checklist" should be drawn up emphasizing the informed aspects of consent that were discussed. There should be a clear explanation of the indications for the proposed surgery and that an open discussion of the principles and risks of the procedure should take place. They also recommended that an honest discussion of the consequences of not undergoing treatment should take place. Furthermore, a discussion about alternative treatments should occur.

There is clearly a dichotomy between enumerating all the risks of surgery and failing to obtain informed consent. The naming of all possible complications will increase the anxiety and stress levels of a patient, but balanced against this is the duty of the doctor to explain the nature of the disease, the available treatments, as well as the risks and benefits of the proposed procedure.

In neurosurgical practice, litigation is likely to be caused by lack of informed consent, delays in the definitive diagnosis being made, and unrealistically high expectations on the part of the patients and relatives. McManus and Wheatley suggest that the consent should be more patient-centered, as it is in Australia with the patients demanding more information before undergoing surgery. They imply that there is a simple equation in which the higher the amount and quality of information the patient receives, the lower will be his/her level of anxiety. They conclude that hospitals should design skeleton websites and leaflets, clearly setting out the risks and benefits of various procedures in order to help patients make informed decisions about their treatment.

In neurosurgical patients, the problems of obtaining informed consent can be greatly exacerbated by difficulties in communication due to dysphasia or impaired consciousness. Furthermore, the complications from intracranial surgery can be so devastating that it may be difficult for patients to make a clear judgment about the benefit of undergoing a procedure, if the natural history of the disease from which they are suffering is particularly unfavorable and the risks of complications are high. Particular attention must be given to ensuring that there is a match between the explanations given to the patient and his/her ability to understand them. It is vital in neurosurgical practice to explain the nature and consequences of serious complications, even if the likelihood of their development is remote. In the Australian case of *Rogers* v. *Whitaker* (Australian Law Reports (1992); 109: 625–637), an Australian ophthalmologist was found to be negligent of not warning his patient of a 1 in 14 000 chance of the development of sympathetic ophthalmitis. This judgment clearly suggests that there is a case for warning patients about devastating complications even if the risk of their development is very small.

The principal way in which problems centering on consent can be avoided is to spend time with the patient and his/her relatives and enter into a frank and meaningful discussion with them about the proposed treatment, the natural history of the disease in question, and alternative therapeutic strategies. Time should be allowed for questions to be asked and the doctor obtaining consent should in general be the person performing the procedure.

Withdrawal of Treatment

Issues of consent and the patient's autonomy are highly pertinent when considering the question of withdrawal of treatment. Advanced techniques of resuscitation and life-preserving technology that allow the life of a patient to continue in the presence of devastating neurological deficit now exist. Dilemmas arise when patients, doctors, and relatives struggle to decide whether to prolong and sustain life where the life in question is of very poor quality and there is no prospect for spontaneous recovery.

The ethical problem of deciding whether the quality of life for the patient in a persistent vegetative state (PVS) is worth continuing is highly contentious. It is impossible to know exactly what someone else is experiencing and doctors cannot merely impose their own values on those of an incompetent patient. A recent review entitled *Withdrawing of Life Sustaining Treatment* attempts to address this problem and points out that a patient's autonomy and values can conflict with the responsibility of the attending clinicians.

The case of Miss B, who had a hemorrhage into a cavernous hemangioma in the upper spinal cord in 1999, is particularly pertinent (*Ms B* v. *an NHS Hospital Trust* 2002 EWHC 429 (Fam)). She recovered from this hemorrhage but rebled in February 2001 and became tetraplegic. She was dependent on artificial ventilation and was unable to do anything for herself. She had no control whatsoever of her limbs and sphincters and had no hope of recovery. Miss B felt her life was intolerable and wanted to be removed from her ventilator.

Dame Elizabeth Butler Sloss found that Miss B was competent to decide upon her treatment and stated *inter alia*: "a mentally competent patient has an absolute right to refuse to consent to treatment for any reason, rational or irrational or for no reason at all, even where that decision may lead to his or her own death." Her judgment also emphasized that "the right of the competent patient to request cessation of treatment must prevail over the natural desire of the medical and nursing professions to keep her alive."

Competent patients have the right to decide on the benefits, burdens, risks, and overall acceptability of treatment. They have the right to refuse treatment, even if this results in death.

Good surgical practice published by the Royal College of Surgeons of England in September 2002 also endorses this policy and advises surgeons to consider advanced statements or living wills very carefully.

Negligence

Negligence is defined very aptly by Alderson in the case of *Blyth* v. *Birmingham Waterworks Company* ((1856); 11 Exch 781). "Negligence is the omission to do something which a reasonable man, guided upon those considerations which ordinarily regulate the conduct of human affairs, would do or doing something which a prudent and reasonable man would not do." Emphasis is placed upon the reasonableness and the ordinariness of the "prudent man," although experts are expected to be skilled and competent in their work.

In medical cases, the appropriate standard of care is determined by a legal standard ratified by the courts and not by the medical profession.

Thus, McNair J summarized the question of the standard of care in his speech to the jury during the *Bolam* v. *Friern Barnett Hospital Management Committee* case of 1957 (2 All ER 118):

A doctor is not guilty of negligence if he has acted in accordance with the practice accepted as proper by a reasonable body of medical men skilled in that particular art. Putting it the other way around a doctor is not negligent if he is acting in accordance with such a practice, merely because there is a body of opinion which takes a contrary view.

It is important to consider some of the general legal principles that cover the tort of negligence. For an action of negligence to succeed, three components must be present, and the burden of proof rests upon the plaintiff. First, he/she must show, on the balance of probabilities, that there exists a duty of care which was owed to him/her by the defendant. Second, he/she must show that the defendant was in breach of that duty. Finally, that damage resulted to the plaintiff as a result of that breach.

One of the more difficult concepts to appreciate is that of causation. Although it can be established that a duty of care existed and that the defendant was in breach of that duty of care, the outcome may have been the same even if that breach had not taken place. Medical negligence cases can be extremely complex and there may be competing reasons why a particular problem develops which may have nothing to do with the alleged negligent act of the defendant.

Thus, the relationship between a hypoxic perinatal event and the subsequent development of learning difficulties or deafness may be far from clear and there may be other competing causes which could equally explain the problems later experienced by the child.

Again, the plaintiff must be able to prove, on the balance of probabilities, that the alleged negligence was the cause of the subsequent problem or that it made a material contribution to the extent of the disorder. In many medical negligence cases, the defendants may admit liability but deny causation. The seminal case on causation is *Bolitho* v. *City and Hackney Health Authority* (4 Med LR 381 (1993) and 39 BMLR 1 (1998)).

Two illustrative cases demonstrating the problems associated with causation in neurosurgical practice are now outlined.

Case 1

A 68-year-old woman presented to an Accident and Emergency department with a two-week history of headache and unsteadiness. She received a cursory examination, and a diagnosis of a viral infection was made. Her relatives were concerned when she was allowed to go home without investigation. Her condition deteriorated and she returned to the same hospital 5 days later. Again, she was told that she was suffering from a viral infection, but now her relatives insisted that she should have a computed tomography (CT) brain scan, but this was refused. Three days later, following increasing headache, she represented to the same hospital but on that occasion was seen by a different doctor. A CT head scan was performed: it showed a mass lesion in the right cerebellar hemisphere, the radiological appearances of which were suggestive of metastasis. Further investigation showed the presence of a right upper-lobe bronchogenic carcinoma with hepatic and adrenal metastases. She died 3 days after palliative resection of her cerebellar lesion. Her relatives issued legal proceedings against the hospital.

Although it was conceded that the hospital was in breach of its duty of care to this woman, causation could not be established, as expert evidence held that, even if a scan had been performed at the time of her first attendance, the outcome would still have been the same, as her disseminated carcinoma was incurable and rapidly fatal.

Case 2

A 38-year-old man, who had not previously suffered from headaches, developed a headache of sudden onset associated with a brief loss of consciousness. His general practitioner was called and a diagnosis of wry neck was made. His headache failed to improve over the next few days and he attended his general practitioner's surgery; he was sent for an X-ray of his cervical spine and prescribed diclofenac.

Six days later, he had a further episode of headache, this time associated with aphasia and a right hemiparesis. He was taken to hospital where a CT head scan was performed that showed diffuse subarachnoid blood and an intracerebral hematoma within the left sylvian fissure.

He was transferred to a neurosurgical unit where cerebral angiography was performed. This revealed a left middle cerebral artery aneurysm which was treated by craniotomy and clipping.

He remains disabled with impairment of fine movement in his right hand and has some speech difficulties.

Expert advice suggested that no reasonable general practitioner would have failed to consider the diagnosis of subarachnoid hemorrhage when confronted with headache of sudden onset associated with loss of consciousness. Moreover, if the diagnosis had been made at that stage, on the balance of probabilities, he would have been investigated and found to have a left middle cerebral artery aneurysm. This would have been treated before a second hemorrhage occurred, producing a profound neurological deficit.

The case thus succeeded not only on the grounds of breach of duty of care and liability, but also on causation. These cases are relatively straightforward examples of the problems of causation, but in neurosurgical practice it is not uncommon for the issues of causation to be extremely complex and, in analyzing a case, several experts with specific subspecialist skills may need to be instructed.

Although the burden of proof in negligence cases lies with the plaintiff, the legal principle known as *res ipsa loquitor* may be applied, in which case the burden of proof is lightened. The expression means "the thing speaks for itself." When invoked, the argument on negligence shifts to the defendant and he/she has to explain how the matter in question could have occurred in the absence of negligence. Typical instances where this legal maxim might be applied would include matters such as operating on the wrong side of the head or doing the wrong level in a spinal procedure without taking steps to ensure that the correct level was treated.

It should be remembered that negligence can occur as a result of poor communication between medical experts. In neurosurgery, the telephone has been said to be the most commonly used "instrument" and instructions between referring clinicians and neurosurgeons must be absolutely explicit and irrefutable. Furthermore, adequate arrangements should be made for the safe discharge or transfer of patients back to referring hospitals once neurosurgical intervention has taken place.

Good Practice

Good practice in medicine is a fine balance between providing the absolute best service for each patient and providing a cost-effective service that is financially supportable. Economic stringency puts pressure on doctors and governments alike. Centrally funded health services are constantly put in the position of having to make compromises as expensive medical technology and drugs evolve. Financial restrictions on centrally funded health providers who are forced to economize inevitably mean that there will be cuts in training new doctors, as well as in research and development.

A large amount of medical practice is now protocol-driven, as purchasers of medical care believe that this provides an efficient use of resources. The obverse of this is that clinical freedom is limited and litigation is encouraged in cases where there are even minor departures from the protocol.

In this rapidly changing environment in which surgeons are now working, what constitutes good surgical practice and how can this be achieved? It is established that good surgical practice is not merely dependent upon the technical or clinical skills of the surgeon, but also upon effective team-working and appropriate use of time and resources. The General Medical Council highlighted seven core headings in its document *Good Medical Practice* which set out the standards required of all doctors. Observation of these principles would certainly decrease the likelihood of a doctor becoming the subject of a serious complaint. In the context of surgical practice it is important for surgeons to realize that they are responsible for the standards of clinical care they offer patients and should bring to the attention of their employing authority any deficiencies in resources that impact upon the safety of their patients. Patients should be treated according to the priority of their clinical problems. When providing emergency care for patients, neurosurgeons should carry out procedures that lie within the range of their routine practice.

Unfamiliar procedures should only be performed if there is no clinical alternative, or a more experienced colleague is unavailable, or transfer to an alternative specialist unit is considered to be a greater risk. Surgeons working in private practice should demonstrate a high level of probity and transparency. They should have the same indications for treating patients in the public sector as in the private sector and should not "invent the need to operate because there is a fee." Furthermore in private practice, surgeons should not

Table 1 Problems that may occur in neurosurgical practice: errors in diagnosis

1. Headache of sudden onset – missed aneurysmal subarachnoid hemorrhage
2. Cauda equina syndrome – delay in diagnosis and treatment of central disk protrusions
3. Subdural empyema
4. Epilepsy of late onset with apparently normal scan with subsequent development of a glioma
5. Failure to appreciate that neck pain may be a presenting symptom of a posterior fossa space-occupying lesion
6. Remember that bilateral leg weakness can be due to a parasagittal meningioma in the presence of normal spinal imaging
7. Remember to obtain informed consent when dealing with patients who have had an aneurysmal subarachnoid hemorrhage. The relative merits of craniotomy and clipping and GDC therapy should be discussed
8. Particular care should be exercised when dealing with psychosurgery. Consent is vital, as is collaboration with the referring psychiatrist

Table 2 Potential problems that may occur during surgery

1. Operating on the wrong side of the head
   Avoid by checking the side of the lesion on the scan with a colleague and ensure that the surgeon operating is the person positioning and draping the patient. Do not make an incision on a patient who has been draped by an assistant without being absolutely certain about the side
2. Operating on the correct patient but using the wrong patient's scan
   Always ensure that the patient's name, date of birth, and hospital number are the same as those on the scan
3. Operating on the wrong level in spinal procedures
   Always take preoperative and intraoperative marking films and retain these in the patient's notes. With disk surgery, an X-ray with a marker in the disk space is irrefutable evidence that the correct level has been treated
4. Do not delegate operative procedures to trainees inappropriately
   Always ensure that an appropriate degree of supervision occurs at all times
5. Never let "the sun set" on a blocked shunt
   If a diagnosis of shunt failure is made, it should be operated on as soon as possible. The possibility of respiratory arrest and death should never be forgotten in cases of shunt blockage
6. Do not forget that aspirin can cause problems with hemostasis
   Unless the problem is immediately life-threatening, defer surgery for 10 days

carry out unusual or complex procedures that they would not normally perform in the public sector.

Neurosurgeons who are involved in medicolegal work should keep their clinical and medicolegal practices separate. They should not treat a patient who has been referred for a medicolegal opinion. Moreover, surgeons would be advised not to operate on patients in personal injury litigation at the expense of the defendant's insurers.

Finally, **Tables 1** and **2** suggest some obvious pitfalls that may occur in neurosurgical practice and some strategies for their avoidance. Remember, the majority of problems can be circumvented by paying "attention to detail" as well as by effective communication.

See Also

Medical Malpractice – Medico-legal Perspectives: Negligence, Standard of Care; Negligence, Duty of Care; Negligence, Causation; Negligence Quantum

Further Reading

Balderston RA, An HS (1991) *Complications in Spinal Surgery.* WB Saunders.
Dimon B (2003) Legal Aspects of Consent. *British Journal of Nursing Monograph.* Quay Books.
General Medical Council (2001) *Good Medical Practice.* General Medical Council.
Harris N, Powers M (eds.) (2000) *Clinical Negligence*, 3rd edn. Butterworths.
Jennett B (2002) *The Vegetative State, Medical Facts, Ethical and Legal Dilemmas.* Cambridge University Press.
Leadbeatter S (ed.) (1997) *Limitations of Expert Evidence.* London: Royal College of Physicians of London.
Machin V (2003) *Medicolegal Pocketbook.* Churchill Livingstone.
Royal College of Surgeons of England (1996) *Code of Practice for the Management of Jehovah's Witnesses.* Available on line: www.rcseng.ac.uk/services/publications.
Royal College of Surgeons of England (2002) *Good Surgical Practice.* Royal College of Surgeons of England.
Schloendorff v. Society of New York Hospital, 103 NE 92 (1914) at 93-94.

Nursing Issues

J Smith, Southend-on-Sea, UK

Introduction

Given that there is wide variation in nursing practice and procedure worldwide, this discussion centers on nursing practice in the UK. Malpractice can be defined as "any unjustified act or failure to act upon the part of a doctor or other healthcare worker which results in harm to the patient." When reading current media and professional journals, one could be forgiven for believing that professional misconduct, malpractice, or negligence amongst healthcare professionals is of epidemic proportions. Investigation of official facts and figures suggests that, for nursing in the UK at least, this is not the case. There were 632 050 nurses registered to practice in the UK as on March 31, 2001. At some point in their professional career most will make a potentially serious mistake. The Nursing and Midwifery Council (NMC) received 1240 (0.002%) allegations of misconduct against registered nurses in 2001, 221 (18%) of which were referred to the Professional Conduct Committee (PCC). This resulted in 104 (47%) nurses being found guilty and removed from the register – 0.0002% of the total registered. It is clear that most cases of nursing malpractice do not reach the NMC. However, should a nurse be reported to the NMC, and find himself or herself facing the PCC, there is an almost even chance that the right to practice will be removed.

In recent years the UK government has paid specific attention to the increasing rates and costs of medical negligence litigation. Annual expenditure for clinical negligence in the National Health Service (NHS) has risen from £1 million in 1974–1975 to £446 million in 2001–2002. This increase in costs is not reflected in the number of nurses disciplined by the NMC. Does this mean that malpractice is not an issue for nurses? Malpractice is an issue for everyone, but the prevention of malpractice should be the overriding issue for all healthcare professionals.

Widely publicized scandals such as Shipman (a general practitioner) and Allitt (a hospital nurse) have led to the formalization of clinical governance principles throughout the NHS. There is a strong focus on both the individual and collective accountability of all healthcare practitioners. All cases of medical negligence claims have to be reported to the NHS Litigation Authority, all cases of Serious Untoward Incidents – including "near-misses" – have to be

reported to the National Patient Safety Agency (NPSA). A great deal of work has been undertaken to try and understand the conditions that lead to adverse events, to minimize them through risk management processes, and to deal with them fairly and effectively when they arise. The aim of this activity is to move toward a "fair blame" culture where people are accountable for their acts and omissions, and learn from their mistakes.

In the light of clinical governance, nurses now face two distinct issues with regard to malpractice: (1) personal professional accountability and (2) from the nursing Code of Professional Conduct: A duty "to act quickly to protect patients and clients from risk if you have good reason to believe that you or a colleague, from your own or another profession, may not be fit to practice for reasons of conduct, health or competence."

In short, now all nurses are the keeper of their fellow healthcare professionals.

Professional Conduct and Accountability

It is accepted that nurses deliver the greatest part of healthcare to individual patients and clients. The nurse today, can give traditional basic bedside care or continue their professional development to become nurse anesthetists or endoscopists, for example. The range and scope of nursing intervention is potentially limitless and certainly complex. Regardless of the nursing role undertaken, a nurse's professional conduct in the UK is governed and regulated by the NMC. This regulatory body was created under the Nursing and Midwifery Order 2001 and is governed by statute (see **Table 1**).

In the USA, Nursing Practice Acts are laws in each state that are instrumental in defining the scope of nursing practice, and each nurse must practice according to the rules and regulations of the State Nursing Board.

The International Council of Nurses has issued general guidelines for nurses and states: "Nurses and their organizations, such as national nurses associations (NNAs), must understand the legal context within which they work."

The NMC issued a new Code of Professional Conduct in June 2002. It is a clear and concise document

Table 1 UK legislation and legal cases relating to nursing

Bolam v. *Friern Hospital Management Committee* [1957] 2 All ER 118
Bolitho v. *City and Hackney Health Authority* [1997] 4 All ER 771
Mental Health Act 1983. Section 2(2) (b)
Nursing and Midwifery Order 2001
Public Interest Disclosure Act 1998. Chapter 23

that outlines the principles that govern all nursing practice in the UK. It is explicit in terms of professional accountability – no one else can answer for the actions of a nurse:

> You are personally accountable for your practice. This means that you are answerable for your actions and omissions, regardless of advice or directions from another professional.

The highly skilled, professional nurse has long since replaced traditional images of the nurse as the doctor's handmaiden. A nurse can now make decisions, and take full responsibility for the care and treatment that is delivered. As a nurse is also personally responsible for her own professional development and continuing education, it is now imperative that nurses are competent in their own right:

> To practice competently, you must possess the knowledge, skills and abilities required for lawful, safe and effective practice without direct supervision. You must acknowledge the limits of your professional competence and only undertake practice and accept responsibility for those activities in which you are competent.

Clearly any idea of a nurse simply carrying out instructions from a senior colleague or doctor does not negate her or his personal responsibility for the care delivered. This differs from the medical profession where a consultant can be held accountable for the actions of a junior doctor in certain circumstances.

When things go wrong and, inevitably at some point they will, much depends on the outcome of the event. If no harm is done, there is no requirement for a legal remedy; however, this does not mean that malpractice has not taken place. A nurse can face disciplinary proceedings from both an employer and the NMC. The flow chart (**Figure 1**) outlines the various routes, within the UK, to sanctions for nursing malpractice which are not mutually exclusive.

As stated above, it appears that relatively few nurses are reported to the NMC. Anyone can report a nurse, although in reality the majority of reports come from employers. Directors of nursing in NHS Trusts (primary, community, or secondary care) have a duty to report nurses who, in their opinion, present a danger to patients and the public. Whilst there is a certain amount of discretion involved in the decision to refer a nurse, a director of nursing, who fails to report a nurse who then subsequently causes harm, will find that they too will be subject to professional disciplinary proceedings. The police also have a duty to report a nurse who has been convicted of a criminal offence, including driving offences, regardless of whether the offence has any relation to professional conduct. Where there is a potential for public confidence to be undermined, the NMC will take a view. Cynically, the more high profile the event, the more likely a hearing before the PCC.

However, being reported does not mean a nurse will face the ultimate professional sanction of being removed from the nursing register. It is actually very difficult to be struck off; malpractice has to be of a high and dangerous level. It can be both professional and personal; a conviction for rape or assault, for example, will justify removal from the register.

In the USA, complaints against registered nurses are investigated by the State Nursing Board. An assessment is made, by a sworn police officer, whether a crime has been committed or not and the case can be referred to the District Attorney. In cases of "minor" violation of the Nursing Practice Act, "a nurse can be personally fined"; in more serious cases a nurse can be placed on probation and be monitored through an

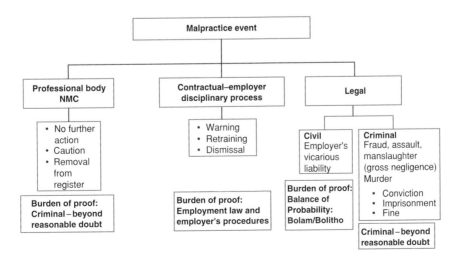

Figure 1 Malpractice – routes of accountability.

enforcement program. Ultimately, a nurse could lose the license to practice.

It is apparent that a nurse has a clear code of professional conduct to follow; however, nurses like other healthcare professionals are human beings and they do make mistakes. In the current climate of litigious claims for medical negligence, a nurse requires, as a minimum, thorough knowledge and clear understanding of the Code of Professional Conduct.

Professional Accountability for Others

It is clearly stated in the code of conduct that the behavior of other healthcare professionals is a nursing issue. If a nurse suspects that a colleague is "unfit" to practice, there is an obligation to report it in the interests of patient safety. This appears to be a reasonable diktat – patient safety must come above all other considerations. However, the reality of reporting a colleague is a far more personal dilemma, involving sensitive moral, ethical, and ultimately painful decisions. There is a contradiction in the current national drive within the NHS for a "fair blame culture" to encourage open and honest disclosure of genuine mistakes, and the unpalatable policy of "whistleblowing." Doctors are also expected, through their own codes of professional conduct, to whistleblow on their colleagues where there are concerns for patient safety. However, disclosure is a difficult decision to make and despite protection offered by the Public Interest Disclosure Act 1998, which a nurse is under a duty to be aware of, making serious allegations against colleagues is not an easy issue. It is, however, an issue that nurses increasingly have to face. It is the nurses who are in the unique position in relation to the whistleblowing expectations of the NHS. They work exclusively in the front line seeing and delivering the daily activity of the wards and clinics. It can be argued that they have far more direct contact with patients and other healthcare professionals than any other discipline, and as such are in a position to monitor, evaluate, and "police" professional standards of healthcare.

The introduction of the National Institute of Clinical Excellence (NICE) has formalized the test of reasonableness established by Bolam, and subsequently by Bolitho, with the publication of clinical guidelines that healthcare professionals are expected to follow (**Table 1**). NICE guidelines have yet to be tested in law, but there is an expectation that they will be implemented nationally into all clinical practice. Therefore, healthcare professionals now have publicly defined standards of care and treatment, established by a body of professional opinion by which to

judge the actions or omissions of themselves and their colleagues. As implementation of such guidelines now forms part of the NHS assessment process through the Commission for Health Improvement (CHI), they will become an important aspect of everyday clinical care and eventually medical law. NICE guidelines apply to nurses and they are expected to identify and deliver evidence-based care.

Malpractice: The Nurse and the Law

Nurses are subject to the same laws of the land, any land, as other citizens. They do have statutory powers in some areas of healthcare that effectively protect them from prosecution in certain circumstances, such as the power to detain under the UK Mental Health Act 1983. Other recent legislation, such as the Human Rights Act 1998, also impacts on nursing practice in areas such as consent and withdrawal of treatment. Whilst a nurse cannot be appraised of every aspect of the law, there is an expectation that nurses will be aware of the legal implications of their practice.

In English law, there are two routes that can be taken in response to malpractice that causes harm – civil and criminal. It is rare for criminal action to be taken against a healthcare professional, especially a nurse. Whilst indictments for manslaughter by gross negligence have increased in the UK in recent years, these cases have been brought against doctors, not nurses. There have been cases where a nurse has been convicted of manslaughter, but these are rare.

When a nurse murders, or attempts to murder, the criminal justice system is activated and, if found guilty, the nurse will be punished accordingly. Manslaughter charges are far more difficult to ascertain, the most difficult issue being the intention (*mens rea*) behind the event. Risk is inherent in all aspects of healthcare, and there will be times when risks materialize through human error, as well as malpractice. In some cases the result will be the death or serious injury of a patient. The level of malpractice required for a criminal case to be brought is that of gross negligence and/or recklessness – the action has to be so reckless that intent to do harm (*mens rea*) can be implied. Thankfully, to date this is a rare occurrence in nursing. Therefore, the legal remedy in most cases of malpractice where harm results is the civil justice system. The burden of proof in a civil case is that of the balance of probability and the injured party must prove three conditions:

1. There was a duty of care owed – this is largely taken as established in the case of NHS treatment.

2. The duty of care was breached.
3. The breach of duty either directly led or substantially contributed to the injury sustained.

In the majority of cases, the nurse is protected by the vicarious liability of the employer. It is wise to ensure that the hospital where one practices has adequate professional liability insurance. American nurses have found, to their cost, that in some instances they are not covered by their employer's insurance.

It is difficult to establish how many cases have been brought specifically against nurses, as law reports cite cases against hospital trusts rather than individuals. This does not mean that a nurse can afford to dismiss the possibility of repercussions of malpractice; the emotional impact of being involved in a civil case for medical negligence should not be underestimated.

Conclusion

In conclusion, malpractice is difficult to define and can occur at many levels, all of which are serious, but not all of which will result in harm to a patient or sanctions against a nurse. An awareness of professional and legal responsibilities, effective risk management processes, and potential sanctions should now be part of every nurse's daily activity and education wherever they work. As with all aspects of the law, ignorance is no defense.

Further Reading

California Board of Registered Nursing. www.rn.ca.gov

Chief Medical Officer, England and Wales (2003) *Making Amends: Consultation Document*. London: Department of Health.

Ferner RE (2000) Medication errors that have led to manslaughter charges. *British Medical Journal* 321: 1212–1216.

International Council of Nurses. www.icn.ch

Nursing and Midwifery Council (2002) *Code of Professional Conduct*. London: NMC.

Nursing and Midwifery Council (2002) *Statistical Analysis of the Register, 1.4.02–31.03.02*. London: NMC.

Professional Conduct Committee (2001) *Annual Report 2000–2001*. London: NMC.

Secretary of State for Health (2000) *NHS Plan: Modern, Dependable*. London: Department of Health.

Stauch M, Wheat K, Tingle J (2002) *Sourcebook on Medical Law*, 2nd edn. London: Cavendish.

The Student Nurse Forum. Nursing Law. http://kcsun3.tripod.com

World Health Professions Alliance. www.whpa.org

Oncology

V Barley, National Patient Safety Agency, London, UK

Introduction

Oncology is the study and treatment of cancer, including research, surgery, radiotherapy, and treatment with drugs, including chemotherapy. Since different medical specialties and professions are involved, the diagnosis and treatment of cancer are usually managed by specialized multidisciplinary teams. In the UK, clinical oncologists have expertise in both radiotherapy and drug treatment, whereas medical oncologists specialize in chemotherapy and other medical treatments. When cancer becomes incurable, care is often provided by specialists in palliative medicine, in collaboration with general practitioners.

This article concentrates on the diagnosis of cancer and its treatment with drugs, and it should be seen in the context of the overall management of patients with cancer (including the support of other clinicians who may contribute, for example, in medicine, surgery, palliative care, and general practice).

Natural History of Cancer

Cancer develops as a result of a harmful mutation (change) in a chromosome of a cell, which continues to multiply out of the control of the host and eventually causes death if untreated. Tumors grow undetected for many months until they are about 1 cm in diameter, when they contain approximately 100 000 million cells. Therefore, many cancers have spread before the primary tumor is diagnosed, although the metastases may not become evident until several months or years later. As a result, it may be difficult to demonstrate that a delay in diagnosis has altered the eventual prognosis.

In the following sections, the diagnosis and staging of cancer are explained, and two important medicolegal issues in oncology are considered: (1) the consequences of a delay in treatment of cancer; and (2) the harm caused by errors in chemotherapy.

Diagnosis

It is important to discover as much as possible about the nature and extent of cancer in order to be able to advise on treatment. The size and spread of a tumor can usually be determined by physical examination supplemented by X-rays, scans, and blood tests. Computed tomography (CT), magnetic resonance imaging (MRI), and ultrasound scans provide cross-sectional images that show the cancer in relation to other organs as well as any metastasis more than 1 cm in diameter. A bone scan uses radioactively labeled chemicals to detect spread to the skeleton, and positron emission tomography scans help to determine if a mass shown on CT or MRI scan is likely to be active cancer.

Histological examination is very important because the optimum treatment will depend on the type of cancer. A biopsy should be taken from the edge of the tumor if possible because the center may be necrotic (dead tissue). Alternatively, a core of tissue may be obtained for histology using a wide needle, or cells may be withdrawn by a fine needle for cytology. Malignant cells may also be found by cytological examination of scrapings, brushings, or washings from the site of the tumor or fluid (sputum, urine, or fluid from chest or abdominal cavities).

Staging and Grading

Cancer is described by its histological appearance and extent. Internationally standard classifications are helpful when considering treatment based on past experience, and they enable a valid comparison of the results of treatment in different hospitals.

The TNM (tumor, node, metastasis) staging is commonly used for solid tumors. The exact definition of each stage is different for each cancer, but **Table 1** summarizes the general principles. The grade or degree of histological or cytological abnormality seen under the microscope also influences prognosis (**Table 2**).

Table 1   Tumor, node, metastasis (TNM) staging

T is	Noninvasive, premalignant, carcinoma-in-situ
T1	Superficial, small, early, usually less than 2 cm diameter
T2	Early, but beginning to invade more deeply, 2–4 cm diameter
T3	Moderately advanced, invading deeply, but confined to the organ
T4	Locally advanced, invading adjacent structures and organs, fixed
N0	No detectable spread to lymph nodes (glands)
N1	Spread to immediately adjacent lymph nodes
N2	Regional lymph nodes involved
N3	Extensive involvement of fixed nodes, or more distant nodes affected
M0	No distant metastases detected
M1	Distant metastases present
Alternatively, a simpler system of four stages may be used.	
Stage I	Local disease only (T1 N0 M0)
Stage II	Spread to local lymph nodes (T1–2 N1 M0)
Stage III	Locally advanced (T3 N1–2 M0)
Stage IV	Disseminated (M1) or locally extensive

Table 2   Grading of tumors

Grade I	Tumor cells mostly appear differentiated, similar to normal
Grade II	Both differentiated and undifferentiated (abnormal) cells
Grade III	Mostly abnormal undifferentiated (anaplastic) tumor cells

When the staging has been confirmed after surgery by histological examination, the letter "p" is inserted (e.g., pT1, pN0) to show that this is the pathological and not just clinical stage. If it is not possible to determine the stage, "X" is inserted (e.g., T1, NX, MX).

Effect of a Delay in the Treatment of Cancer

Cancer growth and spread are uncontrolled, and it is therefore important to avoid unnecessary delays in diagnosis and treatment. Since tumors have been growing for many months or even several years before diagnosis is possible, it may be difficult to show that a delay of a few months has affected the prognosis or outcome of treatment. The effect of the delay will depend on the overall curability of the tumor (e.g., the majority of lung cancers have spread before the diagnosis can be made) and its rate of growth. A rapidly growing cancer, such as in the head and neck, may progress considerably within 3–6 months to a higher stage and become more difficult to cure. On the other hand, bowel cancer usually grows more slowly, and it is often not possible to prove that a delay of 6–12 months affects treatment or prognosis. Nevertheless, it is important to consider each patient individually to decide whether or not, based on probabilities, the delay has had a detrimental effect using published evidence about the rate of growth of tumors and what is known about the natural history and treatment of different cancers.

Treatment

Until the end of the nineteenth century, surgery was the only treatment available. Since many cancers spread before they are detected, the majority of patients with cancer died of metastatic (disseminated) disease.

Following the discovery of X-rays and radium, treatment with ionizing radiation has been developed and has become important in the cure and palliation of many cancers. Drug treatment for cancer has developed rapidly in recent years; it is the primary treatment of some malignant diseases, and is used in conjunction with surgery and radiotherapy in other cancers.

Surgery is the initial treatment for the majority of localized cancers (e.g., cancer of bowel, breast, and skin) and may be followed by radiotherapy (breast, head, and neck) or chemotherapy (ovary and breast). Treatment is usually based on nationally standard guidelines, developed with the benefit of clinical trials.

Chemotherapy

Cytotoxic (cell-killing) drugs affect cells that are multiplying, for example, in the bone marrow, skin, intestine, and other proliferating tissues as well as the cancer. Cytotoxic chemotherapy must therefore be given in such a way as to poison the maximum number of cancer cells while allowing the normal tissues to recover from the inevitable damage. Fortunately, normal tissues are stimulated to regenerate after chemotherapy, whereas malignant tumors lack the normal regulatory mechanisms. Therefore, drugs are usually given in pulses every 3 or 4 weeks to allow sufficient recovery of the normal cells (bone marrow in particular).

Some forms of cancer are cured by chemotherapy, such as leukemia, lymphoma, testicular teratoma, and choriocarcinoma (a rare tumor of placental tissue). Breast, ovarian, and bowel cancer are moderately sensitive, and although not curable by chemotherapy alone, the prospects of cure may be improved when chemotherapy is added after the complete surgical removal of the tumor. Although many other tumors are relatively resistant to chemotherapy, such as the majority of lung and prostate cancers and melanoma, selected patients may benefit and a trial of treatment may be considered. Chemotherapy may therefore be recommended to relieve symptoms due to advanced, incurable cancer without a prospect of increasing survival.

Risks Associated with Chemotherapy

Excessive Dose

In order to achieve the most benefit, the maximum dose that can be tolerated is given, calculated according to the patient's weight, height, general medical condition, and age. Some patients are more sensitive than the average patient (especially the elderly and frail), and doses have to be adjusted according to the response to treatment (e.g., as judged by its effect on the full blood count). Some patients will experience serious side-effects even if the correct protocol has been used, but too high a dose will increase the chance of serious problems and can prove fatal. For example, one patient died after double the correct dose of chemotherapy was prescribed in error. Another patient was given repeat prescriptions by his general practitioner for a drug that should have been taken for only 4 days. By the time the mistake was recognized 6 weeks later, his bone marrow was severely suppressed and he did not recover.

Extravasation

Most cytotoxic chemotherapy is given into a vein by a short (bolus) injection over 10–15 min or by slow infusion over several hours, days, or even weeks. If chemotherapy leaks outside the vein, it may cause serious damage to the local tissues. Some drugs, such as vincristine and Adriamycin, are particularly "vesicant."

Sometimes, extravasation, leakage of the drug outside the vein, occurs and the infusion should be stopped immediately it is noticed. The harmful effect of concentrated chemotherapy on the tissues may be ameliorated by medical treatment (such as the injection of steroids), but sometimes tissue destruction leads to the formation of an ulcer at the site of injection. For example, an elderly woman developed a large ulcer on the inside of the elbow after an injection of Adriamycin. Veins at the elbow should not be used for chemotherapy because it is difficult to check the cannula. Moreover, vesicant drugs should be given via a fast saline drip so that it dilutes the drug (and it is apparent if the cannula is misplaced).

Organ Failure

The serious toxic effects of chemotherapy include kidney failure (e.g., cisplatin), lung fibrosis (e.g., bleomycin), heart failure (e.g., Adriamycin), and nerve damage (e.g., vincristine and taxol). It is important to monitor organ function carefully in order to be able to modify treatment appropriately.

For example, a patient receiving Adriamycin for breast cancer had an abnormal ultrasound heart test after three doses, and Adriamycin should have been stopped. After a fourth dose, the patient developed severe heart failure and died.

Wrong Diagnosis

Sometimes, patients receive chemotherapy for what is presumed to be a malignant tumor but that is later found to be benign, and they have therefore suffered the side-effects of treatment unnecessarily. For example, following a liver scan that showed multiple cystic areas (thought to be due to the spread of cancer), chemotherapy was given to a patient without further scans or a biopsy. After several months of treatment, a more detailed scan confirmed that the cysts were benign.

Wrong Site

There are more than 20 reports of the injection of vincristine (instead of another less toxic drug) into the spinal canal, resulting in fatal outcomes. Guidelines have been issued to ensure that this error is prevented. The UK National Patient Safety Agency has carried out research on the use of a unique connector for spinal injections to prevent the injection of drugs designed for intravenous use.

Conclusion

Treatment of cancer requires accurate diagnosis and prompt treatment. However, since many tumors spread early, it may be difficult to demonstrate that delays of a few months affect the outcome. Chemotherapy is a potent treatment for cancer, but failure to take appropriate precautions may lead to unnecessary serious harm.

See Also

Medical Malpractice: Radiotherapy

Further Reading

Barley VL, Coleman R, Dunlop D, Sikora K, Stewart A, Wardley A (eds.) (2004) *MIMS Handbook of Oncology*, 4th edn. London: Medical Imprint.
Cassidy J, Bissett D, Spence RAJ (2002) *Oxford Handbook of Oncology*. Oxford, UK: Oxford University Press.
De Vita VT, Hellman S, Rosenberg SA (2001) *Cancer: Principles and Practice of Oncology*, 6th edn. Philadelphia, PA: Lippincott, Williams & Wilkins.
Neal AJ, Hoskin PJ (2003) *Clinical Oncology: Basic Principles and Practice*, 3rd edn. London: Arnold.
Spratt JS, Meyer JS, Spratt JA (1996) Rate of growth of human neoplasms. *General and Surgical Oncology* 61: 68–83.

Oral Surgery

M F Patel, Royal Berkshire Hospital, Reading, UK

Definitions

For the purposes of this article, oral surgery may simply be considered to include the diagnosis and surgical treatment of diseases of the oral soft and hard tissues, including the lips and teeth and their supporting structures. The surgery will normally be at a minor or intermediate level, usually conducted as an outpatient procedure, under local analgesia, or as a day-stay procedure under general anesthesia, rarely requiring an overnight stay in hospital.

Included within the ambit of oral surgery here are entities such as dentoalveolar surgery, minor oral surgery, and surgical dentistry.

Oral surgery may be undertaken in independent dental practices, community clinics, and within hospitals. Practitioners of oral surgery will be dentally qualified with additional expertise and training in oral surgical procedures. Increasingly, further qualifications and the requirement to be included on specialty lists are required.

The normal patient anxieties associated with routine dentistry and other procedures within the oral cavity make oral surgery a particularly challenging discipline when conducted under local analgesia. In view of the restricted access and the inevitable intimate juxtaposition of important structures, it is a form of surgery requiring meticulous and skilled practice in all its forms. When practiced on the conscious patient it is also the branch of surgery requiring the highest level of patient support and management skills.

The Nature of Oral Surgery

Oral surgery may be considered to be essentially a subspecialty of dental surgery and more broadly of surgery generally.

The subspecialty concerns itself primarily with the diagnosis and treatment of diseases of the oral cavity and associated structures. Whilst oral surgeons can be involved in the diagnosis and treatment of oral infections and oral lesions, they can equally become involved in the diagnosis and treatment of orofacial pain. However, most of the surgical procedures carried out will involve the surgical removal of teeth and roots, surgical endodontics, and the removal of oral lesions, usually for diagnosis.

Some oral surgeons will also become involved with orofacial trauma, particularly when working within hospitals, and will repair facial lacerations and facial bone fractures. They may also become involved in orthognathic surgery to realign jaws. The treatment of orofacial trauma and orthognathic surgery is dealt with in elsewhere.

Malpractice

Malpractice in oral surgery, in common with other medical specialties, is usually due to an omission to obtain valid consent, for whatever reason, or due to the commission of negligence. Malpractice in general will be dealt with elsewhere in this encyclopedia and in numerous medicolegal texts.

In this article, the common oral surgery procedures will be covered, including a brief description of why the procedure might be required and how it is accomplished. Importantly, the information and warnings that should be given to obtain a valid consent will be discussed and the common complications, which might be associated with negligence or malpractice, detailed.

In hospital practice generally, and no less in oral surgery, it is apparent that allowing junior or inexperienced members of staff, who may be incapable of actually undertaking a surgical procedure, to take consent is a potential reason for invalidating the consent. Such a practitioner can neither be relied on adequately to appreciate and explain the general benefits and disadvantages of a procedure nor be reliable in adapting this information to a patient's particular situation, let alone answer a patient's detailed question or concerns. The lack of appropriate and relevant information about a surgical procedure and a failure to allow patients adequate time to fully understand the implications of that information are areas of concern when attempting to obtain valid consent.

Surgical practice is inevitably contextual, and the context will include the complexity and vagaries of surgery and the interaction between the patient and clinician on a background of what is considered good practice. Damage to the inferior dental nerve and subsequent permanent anesthesia of half of the lower lip would be considered malpractice in the simple surgical removal of a mildly impacted wisdom tooth far from the nerve bundle. The same complication would be considered acceptable in the complicated removal of a deeply buried wisdom tooth, intimately associated with the nerve bundle and perhaps with related bony pathology, if the patient had received adequate warning.

The principal areas for malpractice in oral surgery are incompetent diagnosis or incompetent conduct of a surgical procedure, particularly where it needlessly damages adjacent structures.

Radiography

There is heavy reliance on X-ray imaging in oral surgery in order to assess dental and bony structures and associated pathology. Numerous radiographs are employed, including periapical and bitewing small films, occlusal medium-sized films, and those larger films that are used for rotational tomography to examine the jaws. Meticulous labeling of such radiographs with regard to patient name, side, and even the individual tooth (on smaller films) is required to

prevent mistakes happening. It is important that radiographic images are of good quality in order that an accurate diagnosis may be made and an appropriate procedure may be properly planned and carried out efficiently. Poor inappropriate radiographs or even the total absence of radiographs provide fertile ground for the growth of litigation.

Surgical Procedures

It is not possible or desirable to cover all procedures carried out by the oral surgeon.

The common procedures, which encompass the majority of the work done, will be covered along with a description of the procedure, why it is necessary and, briefly, how it is done. The appropriate warnings and common complications, which will form the basis of most putative suits in negligence, will also be covered.

Surgical Removal of Teeth or Roots

Symptomatic or unrestorable teeth and roots retained in the jawbone once the crowns are lost frequently require removal in order to prevent symptoms (usually pain and infection), but may also be removed to facilitate the restoration of a deficient occlusion.

The removal of impacted and symptomatic third molars (wisdom teeth) is one of the most common operations undertaken by oral surgeons and advice on the indications for this surgery is offered by the National Institute for Clinical Excellence (NICE) in the UK, and similar bodies in other countries. The guidelines for removal include pain and infection, tooth decay, and any other associated pathology that the removal of the third molars would obviate.

Clinical and radiographic assessment is required along with treatment planning prior to reflecting gum flaps, removing bone with drills or chisels, and removing the teeth or roots with elevators or forceps sometimes after surgical division of roots. These procedures may be carried out under local analgesia or general anesthesia where the patient or the procedure demands it.

It is usual to warn the patient routinely prior to these procedures of pain, swelling, bruising, and a transient limitation in mouth opening due to muscle spasm in the aftermath of surgery. In the case of the removal of wisdom teeth it would be considered normal practice also to warn of a risk of permanent anesthesia or paresthesia of the inferior dental and lingual nerves. In the event of a higher risk, this should be indicated to the patient and this may be due to an intimate association of the tooth with the inferior dental canal, for example, or due to the presence of associated pathology such as a large cyst.

Although the risks of damage to the inferior dental or lingual nerves are frequently bundled together, as was made clear in the UK court case *Heath* v. *Berkshire Health Authority* (1991), coincidental surgical damage to the lingual nerve during lower wisdom tooth surgery will generally be considered to be negligent. In addition, if an intimate relationship exists between the surgical site and the inferior dental nerve, along with evidence of having appraised the patient of this, a charge of negligence should be avoided.

Fracture of the lower jaw during removal of teeth or roots, although the subject of much apocryphal concern, is rare and would be likely to form the basis for a charge of negligence, unless the presence of an atrophic or pathological mandible had been drawn to the patient's attention.

Damage to adjacent teeth or restorations (crowns, bridgework, fillings) during the removal of teeth or roots when an especial vulnerability had not been drawn to the patient's attention would be likely to lay the surgeon open to an accusation of malpractice.

The displacement of teeth or portions of teeth during surgery into the pharynx, pterygoid space, or antrum, although rare, is a common cause for concern and precaution. It would depend on the exact circumstances as to whether negligence would be apportioned.

The risk of creating a communication between the mouth and antrum in removal of an upper tooth (oroantral communication) closely associated with the floor of the antrum (usually upper premolar and molar teeth) should be signaled to the patient prior to surgery. It is likely that many such occult communications occur and heal uneventfully, with both patient and surgeon blissfully unaware. On the occasions that such communications continue and the communication epithelializes to form a persistent fistula, a patient unaware of the risk might understandably become aggrieved and pursue compensation for the inconvenience of requiring a second surgical procedure to close the communication.

The likelihood of patient bewilderment deteriorating to dissatisfaction and on to litigation will be greatly influenced by their relationship with the surgeon and the support that they receive in the aftermath of any problems.

Surgical Endodontics

Conventional or orthograde endodontics (root canal therapy) is frequently required when the pulp of a tooth becomes inflamed and undergoes necrosis due to a carious lesion or thermal or chemical damage. Removal of the necrotic pulp tissue with debridement of the pulp chamber and root canal followed by obturation of the chamber and canal with a filling material will allow conservation of the tooth in the majority of cases.

On the occasions when an infection involving the apex of the tooth persists or recurs despite a satisfactory orthograde root filling, the procedure known as surgical endodontics or apicectomy with retrograde apical seal is carried out. The apices of teeth are accessed via a mucoperiosteal flap or, when possible, via a less intrusive semilunar incision over the root apex. The tooth apex is exposed by removal of overlying alveolar bone, usually from the buccal aspect, any soft-tissue lesion curetted, and the apex of the tooth is prepared minimally to receive a retrograde apical seal. The procedure is carried out in the expectation that discomfort or bony pathology associated with the tooth will resolve and the tooth remains functional. It would be normal to warn the patient that the procedure is not invariably successful and is frequently associated with some pain, swelling, and occasional bruising.

It is likely that the tooth will be uncomfortable for a week or so after surgery and that the use of a flap bordering the cervical margin of the tooth could be associated with a small element of gum recession in the healing process. The patient should be warned that this can expose the margin of a prosthetic crown, giving a less pleasing esthetic appearance than before surgery.

There is a risk of apicecting the wrong tooth root in a situation where roots of adjacent teeth are closely clustered together, but this is rare. Gum recession and the risk of the procedure failing should be mentioned to the patient.

An apicectomy and apical seal without a satisfactory orthograde root filling in place is more likely to fail and would only be contemplated in exceptional circumstances when the patient has been entirely appraised of the poor chance of success.

The technique and materials utilized in surgical endodontics have developed and improved in recent years, and the failure to use magnification (loupes or an operating microscope) during the procedure or a failure to use up-to-date techniques and materials might be grounds for concern. As always, damage to adjacent structures, including nerve bundles, adjacent teeth, and the antra, without adequate presurgical warning and good reason will make the surgeon vulnerable to an accusation of malpractice.

Dental Implantology (Osseointegrated Dental Implants)

The development of dental implants has revolutionized the concept of dental and occlusal reconstruction over the last 30 or so years. Missing or lost tooth units may now be replaced with implant-borne suprastructures (crowns, bridges, or dentures), which attach to dental implants that are firmly fixed in the bone. The implants are usually similar in length and width to the tooth roots they replace and are usually cylindrical and constructed of titanium, although other shapes and materials have been used. The success rate of dental implants can be very high and, if they are carefully placed and well maintained, can last for in excess of 30 years, although the suprastructure may require replacement every 7–10 years. Dental implants are therefore capable of providing rigid support for the replacement of single teeth, several teeth as a fixed bridge, or even overdentures, which are attached less rigidly but can be removed for cleansing.

Dental implants may be placed under local analgesia or general anesthesia and constitute intermediate surgery. A mucoperiosteal gum flap is reflected, a hole is carefully made within the bone to receive the implant, and the flap is closed for up to 6 months to allow osseointegration. The implant will usually become rigidly fixed due to the close apposition of bone with the implant. At this time a further minor surgical procedure is made to expose the head of the implant, followed by abutment placement, which will culminate in placing the definitive suprastructure.

This treatment will have been planned and agreed between the patient, oral surgeon, and restorative dentist (who will construct the suprastructures). It is important for the oral surgeon to discuss all the various restorative options with the patient before embarking on implant surgery. The patient should be aware of the advantages and risks of this treatment modality along with cost and timescale.

In view of the complexity and length of treatment allied with high cost and a number of surgical procedures, it is most important that the patient is aware of the implications of this form of treatment and that the restorative dental practitioner, as well as the oral surgeon, have the necessary experience and skills to be likely to produce a good result. Thorough planning, along with any necessary presurgical treatment, X-rays, study models, implant placement templates, or computed tomography scans should be carried out in order to give implant placement the best chance of success. Failure to discuss other treatment options such as dentures and bridgework or the cost or timescale will lay the oral surgeon open to criticism.

It is most important to plan the patient's implant treatment adequately with the restorative dentist and the dental laboratory in order that implant positioning and loading minimize disadvantage to the patient and maximize function and esthetics.

In the event that bone grafting is required to provide a sufficient foundation for dental implants, this requires detailed discussion and agreement with the patient, particularly if products derived from animals rather than inorganic materials are used.

Failure to use a high standard of sterile technique in surgery and to have available good-quality X-rays and planning templates will lay the practitioner open to accusations of malpractice on the occasions when a procedure does not proceed as it should.

Biopsy/Excision of Oral Lesions

Careful explanation with valid consent, albeit frequently verbal, allied with careful competent treatment minimizing damage to adjacent structures will make claims for negligence unlikely. Patients must be warned of pain, swelling, bruising and the placement of sutures, and any risks of recurrence.

General Considerations

The removal of a wrong tooth or fracture of the jaw during routine surgery or damage to adjacent teeth and restorations are complications likely to lead to accusations of malpractice.

Although discomfort from the temporomandibular joints, even when allied with clicking noises, can come to the patient's attention after oral surgery, it is usually an acute exacerbation of an underlying temporomandibular joint dysfunction. There does not appear to be good evidence that routine oral surgery causes temporomandibular joint dysfunction.

Great care should be taken not only to protect structures immediately adjacent to the surgical site but also the lips, face, and eyes: the eyes should usually be protected with safety spectacles during surgery.

An oral surgeon would be considered culpable if, whilst treating a patient for one condition, a more serious pathology was ignored. The efficient removal of a wisdom tooth in ignorance of a carcinoma on the lateral border of the tongue would be difficult to defend. The oral surgeon would also be expected to take adequate precautions with regard to providing antibiotic cover for those patients who require it (e.g., those with heart valve lesions) and to assess and treat correctly those patients on anticoagulation.

As a general maxim, an oral surgeon who practices the standard of care required by professional colleagues and hoped for by patients and who combines this care with humanity and gentle humor is least likely to disturb the repose of legal colleagues.

See Also

Medical Malpractice: Facio-maxillary Surgery

Further Reading

Andreasen JO (2003) *Traumatic Dental Injuries: A Manual.* London: Blackwell.

Babbush CA (2001) *Dental Implants: Principles and Practice – The Art and Science.* New York: Saunders.

Dimitroulis G (2001) *Handbook of Third Molar Surgery.* London: Wright.

Fonseca RJ (2002) *Oral and Maxillofacial Surgery: Anaesthesia/Dentoalveolar Surgery. Office Management.* New York: Saunders.

Forman GH (1998) Maxillofacial implantology. In: Langdon JD, Patel MF (eds.) *Operative Maxillofacial Surgery,* pp. 305–316. London: Chapman and Hall Medical.

Harris M (2003) *Outline of Oral Surgery and Medicine.* London: Butterworth Heinemann.

Heath *v.* Berkshire Health Authority (1991) *Butterworths Medico-Legal Reports,* 8, pp. 98–102. London: Butterworth.

Howe LC, Palmer PJ, Palmer RM, Smith BJ (2001) *Implants in Clinical Dentistry.* London: Taylor and Francis.

Kwon P, Laskin D (2001) *Clinician's Manual of Oral and Maxillofacial Surgery.* London: Quintessence.

Robinson P (2000) *Tooth Extraction: A Practical Guide.* London: Wright.

Plastic and Cosmetic Surgery

A Khanna, Sandwell General Hospital, West Bromwich, UK

Introduction

Plastic and cosmetic surgery covers a wide range of surgical procedures. There has been a significant increase in litigation against surgeons performing such procedures, and it is likely that this trend will continue. Cosmetic surgery is different from other surgical specialties as the benefits of surgery are mostly psychological rather than functional. This difference raises ethical issues and vulnerability of plastic surgeons to litigation. The causation and genesis of plastic and cosmetic surgery claims are discussed, including issues of consent before surgery. The pros and cons of plastic surgeons using computer-generated images and the internet for marketing and communication are also discussed.

The Scope of Plastic and Cosmetic Surgery

Plastic surgery can be defined as the branch of surgery concerned with restoration of form and function by reconstruction of congenital, traumatic, and acquired conditions. Plastic surgery covers a very large field and deals with patients with congenital conditions such as breast and chest-wall defects, cleft lip and palate, and other facial deformities, including craniofacial defects, hand defects, skin defects, and urogenital defects. It also deals with patients who have sustained burns, face, hand, and lower-limb trauma, scars, and tattoos. Plastic surgeons also deal with patients requiring reconstruction following mastectomy for breast cancer, head and neck conditions, patients with benign and malignant skin conditions, pressure sores, venous ulcers, degenerative hand conditions, and patients requesting cosmetic surgery. Variable amounts of reconstructive surgery are carried out in collaboration with other surgical disciplines, for example orthopedic, ear, nose, and throat (ENT), and maxillofacial surgeons.

Plastic surgery means the molding of the surface and sometimes deep structures of the human body. Techniques developed in plastic reconstructive surgery have been adapted for the purpose of rejuvenation and esthetic enhancement of the patients. Cosmetic surgery includes surgery to improve, alter or change the appearance in the absence of disease, trauma or congenital deformity. Cosmetic surgery has developed rapidly since the 1970s and involves surgery for facial rejuvenation such as facelifts; blepharoplasty; rhinoplasty; body-contouring procedures such as liposuction and abdominoplasty; esthetic breast surgery, including breast reduction and enhancement; and laser surgery. Cosmetic surgery is carried out not only by plastic surgeons but also by ENT surgeons, maxillofacial surgeons, and dermatologists.

Trends in Medical Malpractice in Plastic and Cosmetic Surgery

In the USA, there has been a significant increase in claims related to medical malpractice in plastic, reconstructive, and cosmetic surgery. In the 1950s one claim per every 100 doctors was filed. By the early 1990s that figure had increased by 1000% to more than ten medical malpractice claims being filed per 100 doctors. Physicians have seen their medical malpractice insurance premiums increase by as much as 500% since the 1970s. The likelihood of an incident for a plastic surgeon has been estimated at once every 2.5 years.

The Medical Defence Union (MDU) in the UK in a recent 12-year period settled 241 claims that arose from plastic, cosmetic, and reconstructive surgery (**Figure 1**). This resulted in expenditure of just under £6.7 million (US $12 million). This included

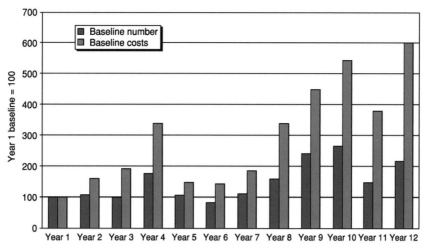

Figure 1 Number and cost of plastic and reconstructive surgery claims settled in a 12-year period. Reproduced with permission from the Medical Defence Union.

legal costs and the indemnity awarded to the patient. The size of claims ranged from £200 to £250 000 (US $360–450 000). This figure does not include those cases that were dropped by the claimant or won by the MDU. It also does not encompass the advisory matters that arose from this type of surgery such as complaints or referrals to the General Medical Council. The majority of these claims arose from consultations in the private sector and not from the National Health Service (NHS) as the NHS indemnity scheme was introduced in 1990.

Cosmetic Surgery: A Specific Problem?

As compared to other surgical specialities, cosmetic plastic surgery is one of the specialties most vulnerable and prone to litigation. This may be due to several reasons; for example, people who tend to seek cosmetic surgery are so concerned with enhancing their appearance that they may be less likely to tolerate imperfections, some patients may be receiving less than adequate care, and some patients are more willing to sue. There is also a growing emphasis on personal gratification and youth and a tendency on redress if things go wrong. People are requesting cosmetic surgery not only to look younger and sexier, but also because of dissatisfactions with life that are vague and diffuse.

The benefits of cosmetic surgery tend to be psychological, not necessarily functional, and difficult to evaluate. This form of surgery therefore raises the ethical problem of balancing risks and benefits of operations without functional benefit. If a patient has an injury such as a broken arm, the expected benefit of operative intervention is obvious whereas in cosmetic surgery the benefit is somewhat harder

to assess. It is therefore necessary to weigh the risks and complications of the procedure including that of the anesthetic against a benefit for the patient that may be difficult to evaluate. Unlike other surgical specialists, the plastic surgeon assessing a patient who requests esthetic surgery is not trying to make a sick patient better but rather a well patient better. This not only puts a much heavier burden of responsibility on the operating surgeon, but also subjects him or her to a much broader range of possible reasons for unhappiness. Sources of dissatisfaction can range from a catastrophic result to something as unpredictable as a patient's hidden agenda.

Causes of Malpractice in Plastic and Cosmetic Surgery

A survey of claims in the USA has shown in 700 cases over 15 years that esthetic breast surgery, both augmentation and reduction, has been responsible for most claims. Approximately 37% of all elective esthetic surgery claims involved breast augmentation surgery. The main complaints of dissatisfaction have been encapsulation with distortion and firmness, wrong size (too little or too much), infection, repetitive surgery and attendant costs, and nerve damage with sensory loss. For breast reduction surgery, complications included unexpected ugly scars; too little or too much breast tissue being removed; partial loss, distortion or misplacement of nipples; and dissatisfaction with the resulting breast shape. If the primary complaint was back and shoulder pain and those complaints were relieved postoperatively, the dissatisfaction quotient lessened considerably (**Figure 2**).

Facelift surgery and blepharoplasty cases accounted for 19% of claims in this series, and the complaints

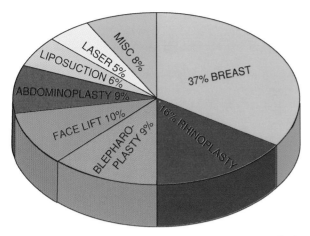

Figure 2 Total percentage of claims for elective esthetic surgery. Reproduced with permission from the Medical Defence Union.

with blepharoplasty included excessive skin removal, resulting in a starey look, dry eyes, the inability to close the eyes, and ectropion or scleral show, with resultant exposure keratitis. Visible scars, real or alleged visual impairment, and change of expression were also causes for complaint. In the rare but devastating postoperative blindness cases, the typical expanding hematoma commonly were not diagnosed and decompressed immediately.

Complaints with facelift surgery included visible or hypertrophic scars, sloughs or wound disruption (most often in smokers), facial nerve damage, inadequate result from insufficient or excessive tightening, persistent pain or numbness, and skin slough resulting in excessive scarring.

Rhinoplasty cases accounted for 16% of claims. Complaints with this procedure included unhappiness with disappointing results, airway obstruction, visible irregularities and scars, asymmetry, and emotional distress.

Abdominoplasty with or without suction-assisted liposuction represented 9% of claims with allegations of skin loss with poor scars, nerve damage, inappropriate surgery, and infection with or without appropriate postoperative management. The combination of liposuction and abdominoplasty increases the morbidity as this can affect skin circulation, leading to skin sloughs.

The most common allegations following liposuction were waviness, lumpiness, asymmetry, irregularities, disappointment with the degree of changes achieved, persistent numbness and pain, and the attendant cost of revision. In the techniques that entail superficial subcutaneous liposuction, skin circulation may be impaired. This can lead to major sloughs requiring extensive revisional surgery with substantial scarring. There were a number of undetected

abdominal wall and intestinal perforations that led to major secondary operations and in several cases death. Tumescent liposuction procedures have also produced problems secondary to volume exchanges, leading to profound physiological disturbances and pulmonary edema. There were also cases involving overdoses of local anesthetic. The necessity for revisional surgery with its attendant costs was a common theme in all categories.

Chemical peels/laser resurfacing accounted for 5% of claims, allegations included blistering or burns with significant scarring, infection, and permanent pigmentary changes. Approximately 8% of all complaints against plastic and reconstructive surgeons have to do with miscellaneous allegations such as untoward reaction to medications or anesthesia and improper use of pre-op or post-op photos.

There is a continual flow of avoidable claims that are directly linked to smoking. In surgery involving wide tissue undermining, such as facelift and breast surgery, the patients who were heavy smokers suffered sloughs or poor wound healing which subsequently caused poor scars. These problems could have been predicted preoperatively.

In the UK, the MDU in a recent 12-year period found that the largest group of claims settled (100 cases = 42%) was related to surgery performed on the face. Thirty-five of these claims resulted from rhinoplasty procedures and 27 from facelifts. Common themes in the expert reports for rhinoplasty claims were the lack of pre- and postoperative photographs and establishing the specific patient requirements during the counseling stage. There were numerous other types of procedures involving the face, including blepharoplasty, cheek and chin implants, chin reduction, and chemical face peel (**Figure 3**).

There were also a number of lip augmentation claims resulting in successful litigation. Of the cases arising from breast surgery, over half arose from breast augmentation procedures, mainly as a result of dissatisfaction with the cosmetic result. Approximately a quarter arose from breast reduction procedures. A vast majority of these procedures were performed purely for esthetic reasons, although some arose following reconstruction after mastectomy for breast cancer. The claims that arose from abdominal procedures followed either liposuction or abdominoplasty. Those citing the thigh were, apart from one case, related to liposuction. Claims where the site of operation was the arm were mostly related to tattoo removal, either by surgical excision or by using laser treatment.

The group marked "others" encompassed several types of procedures, none of which led to more than

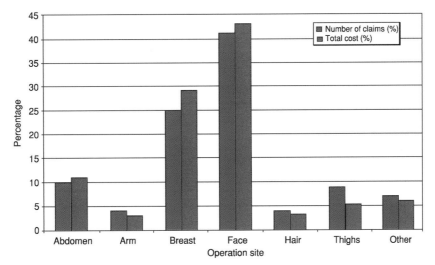

Figure 3 Distribution of claims by operation site. Reproduced with permission from the Medical Defence Union.

a handful of claims over the period. Sclerotherapy for veins on the face and leg was the only type of surgery in this category that gave rise to more than five claims over this period. There were three involving phalloplasty. This group included some of the less commonly performed procedures, including gender reassignment.

The most expensive claim resulted from dissatisfaction with the results of liposuction and fat transfer to the face. Breakdown of cost by anatomical region shows that claims resulting from breast surgery have been more expensive, although there is very little difference between those to the face and abdomen.

The Genesis of Malpractice Claims in Plastic and Cosmetic Surgery

There are certain issues that lead to malpractice claims against plastic and cosmetic surgeons. These include unexpected scarring, general dissatisfaction, and lack of adequate explanation or discussion that is not appropriate for the patient's level of understanding, resulting in poor consent. The patient's expectations may have been unrealistic. The patient's expectations may not have been known preoperatively and subsequently not have been met, or the patient's expectations may have been known preoperatively and were still not met. There are also patients who are more likely to pursue litigation claims in cosmetic surgery. These are patients with great expectations, excessively demanding patients, and those who may be indecisive, immature, and secretive. Patients who lack familial approval, those who have repeated cosmetic surgery procedures, and patients with psychological problems are also more

likely to sue. It is therefore important to know the patient before surgery and to screen out those patients with unrealistic expectations. If the patient has such unrealistic expectations the procedure will not be successful even if it was performed well, and the doctor may be blamed for a perceived poor result. A condition that is important for plastic surgeons performing cosmetic surgery to be aware of and assess patients for is dysmorphobia. Dysmorphobia is a psychological condition in which the patient suffers from a subjective feeling of ugliness despite having a normal appearance or a minimal cosmetic defect. Patients requesting cosmetic surgery may also suffer from psychiatric problems such as eating disorders for which surgery would not be indicated. It is essential for the surgeon to identify these traits preoperatively. Informing patients in great detail of the potential complications of the procedure as part of the consent process will not be enough if the expectations of the patient were unrealistic. Insisting on a referral from the patient's general practitioner, a cooling-off period before surgery and, if appropriate, referral to a psychiatrist may be helpful to deal with these issues.

The survey of claims in the USA showed evidence of the same generic problems in esthetic surgery claims such as substandard documentation with missing or poor preoperative photographs, inadequate informed consent, poor patient selection, and substandard operative results. The genesis of claims implicates improper patient selection or overly enthusiastic treatment. A trend was found among plastic surgeons to try to combine several procedures at one sitting. It is not appropriate to perform several major procedures combined in one long surgery in an office facility. Staged treatment sessions are

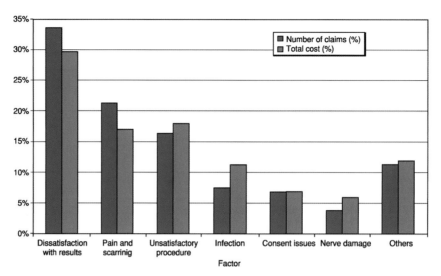

Figure 4 Factors leading to settled claims. Reproduced with permission from the Medical Defence Union.

preferable to trying to do as much as possible in one session. There were also a rising number of malpractice claims in which it was clear that economic consideration was put ahead of sound surgical judgment. This includes cases in which the patient did not need the proposed procedure, he/she was the wrong patient on whom to perform the procedure, and the surgeon was inexperienced.

The actual reason why patients pursue litigation is complex. Around half of all settled claims in this specialty by the MDU resulted from either dissatisfaction with the result of surgery and/or unsatisfactory procedures (**Figure 4**). Although similar, there is a subtle difference between the two groups. Claims arising from dissatisfaction with the results of surgery tend to arise from unrealistic patient expectations, and a successful claim will often result from deficiencies in preoperative counseling and poor clinical record-keeping. The unsatisfactory procedure group refers to problems arising directly from the surgical procedure and includes deficiencies in the surgical procedure, surgical technique used, or inadequate arrangements for postoperative follow-up. Another reason is where the main allegation was performing the procedure without the express consent of the patient. The "others" category includes a number of uncommon reasons, ranging from retained liposuction tubing and diathermy burns to brain damage resulting from hypotensive anesthesia. Interestingly, while dissatisfied patients have the largest number of successful claims, the most costly average claims arose from problems such as nerve damage and infection. The value of successful claims arising from pain and scarring was small.

Surgeons with lower claim rates may be more likely to manifest exemplary modes of professional peer relationships and responsible clinical behavior. A study has shown that the personal, educational, and professional characteristics of surgeons may contribute substantially to the incidence and outcome of malpractice claims. Common denominators of malpractice claims regardless of underlying cause are surprise, disappointment, and anger, followed by a breakdown in communications.

Issues Surrounding Consent and Basic Medical Legal Principles

Many malpractice claims are preventable. Most are based on failure of communication and poor selection criteria rather than on technical faults. Regardless of the technical ability of a surgeon, someone who appears distant or arrogant is far more likely to be sued than someone who has the ability to communicate well. Similarly, a surgeon who has a warm, sensitive, and caring personality is much less likely to be the target of a claim for negligence. An issue that may precipitate a complaint against a surgeon may not be a technical error made during the procedure but a failure by the surgeon to establish a reasonable rapport with the patient at the time of consultation. Exemplary surgical skills and good clinical judgment by the surgeon may be obscured in the patient's mind by what is felt at the time of consultation to be an offensive and arrogant attitude. The role of informed consent in cosmetic surgery is to try to ensure that patients know and understand what lies ahead if they want surgery to improve their appearance.

Surgeons should, as part of the informed-consent process, before any invasive procedure is performed explain to the patients the details of what is proposed, its purpose, potential risks, and any reasonable alternatives that may include no treatment at all. At the time of consent patients should not only be adequately informed but also should be capable of assimilating that information and thereby be competent to consent, and should be able to give that consent voluntarily without coercion, manipulation, or constraint on the part of the surgeon.

At the end of a comprehensive and detailed consultation it is difficult to know to what extent the patients have understood the details and potential complications of the procedure in question. A study performed 20 years ago has shown that simple written information increases the proportion of patients who understand their diagnosis from 31% to 70%. This was not at a level that matches the detail that applies to the consultation on cosmetic surgery today. A more recent paper has reported the outcome of a prospective randomized trial of patients' recall of verbal versus written preoperative warnings. Patients given verbal warnings were less able to recall them than those with written warnings.

Although a detailed consultation supplemented with written information, such as patient information sheets and copies of correspondence to the patients' general practitioner, would seem to be comprehensive, patients may still not assimilate the information that has been provided. It is therefore prudent to allow a cooling-off period during which the patient has the opportunity to dwell on the issues that have been raised. Patients should also be given the opportunity and encouraged to attend for further consultations to discuss any further issues that may arise.

In the UK, consent is based on a professional standard of disclosure or what a doctor believes a patient should know, whereas in the USA, consent is more patient-centered: the doctor owes a duty to disclose not only the inherent potential risks of treatment, but also any alternatives to that treatment and the likely consequence of nontreatment. Surgeons should, in respect for patient autonomy, give information over and above that required simply to protect them from the liability of battery. The physician must adhere to an applicable standard of care. In general this standard of care is that which would be rendered by a reasonable physician under like or similar circumstances. In order for a valid claim of negligence to be proven the physician must have owed a duty of care to the patient, the standard of care must have been violated by the physician, this violation of the standard of care must have proximately

occurred, and a loss or injury must have occurred for which the patient can be compensated. The standard of care is evaluated in light of the state of medical knowledge and skill available at the time of the allegedly negligent conduct. In a medical malpractice case, the standard of care will be delineated by the medical experts' testimony. Therefore, the defendant's and plaintiff's medical experts play a crucial role in any medical malpractice case.

Issues Surrounding the Use of the Internet and Computer-Generated Pictures

Computer imaging allows surgeons to manipulate digital photographs of patients to project and predict possible surgical outcomes. Some of the benefits these techniques provide include improving doctor–patient communication, improving the education and training of residents, and reducing administrative and storage costs. Despite the many advantages that these computer imaging systems may offer, surgeons are concerned that these imaging systems may expose them to legal liability. Surgeons may face possible claims of implied contract, failure to instruct, and malpractice from their use or failure to use computer imaging. A study, however, has revealed that surgeons who use computer imaging carefully and conservatively and adopt a few simple precautions substantially reduce their vulnerability to legal claims.

It is recommended that computer imaging be used primarily as a tool for improved communication between physician and patient. Its use for the selling of an operation and marketing of various procedures is not appropriate. A computer image cannot exactly replicate an image based on the surgeon's technical abilities and patient's preexisting conditions. The digital projected result should therefore be understated and patients should also be shown images of the possible unexpected and unfavorable outcomes of the procedure. The computer images should be used to enhance the informed-consent process and consent should be documented such that the imaging session is only a simulation and is in no way meant to be a guarantee or warranty of a surgical result.

Over the last few years many plastic surgeons have set up their own personal website pages to provide information about themselves and to inform prospective patients of the range of procedures they may provide. Also included is usually an electronic mail link to communicate with and educate prospective patients. These services are provided without actually meeting patients face to face. Some of the positive aspects of personal website pages revolve around their use as a marketing tool and as a tool in patient education. Physicians can advertise procedures that they commonly perform and this will probably expand their patient base. From a patient education point of view, one can depict actual procedures and place pre- and postoperative instructions for a procedure on the site.

It is recommended that a broad disclaimer of liability is used when posting medical information on a website. One should also not use information on the Internet in place of standard consent procedures. Surgeons should be aware of the implications of intellectual property/copyright infringement in the set-up of their website. If photographs of patients having undergone a surgery are used, then appropriate consent should be taken. It should be emphasized that the results depicted in the photographs may not represent the result another patient may achieve following the same procedure. An e-mail link on a personal website should be used for administrative tasks such as patient scheduling. Changes in medical information on privacy confidentiality laws and guidance from the General Medical Council on advertising should be followed.

Regulation of Cosmetic Surgery in the UK

Cosmetic surgery overlaps with a number of specialties in the UK, and it has no minimum standards of training leading to a certificate of completion of specialist training. The government was facing a problem in regulating this rapidly expanding market and responded by enacting the Care Standards Act following its response to the Health Committee's fifth report on the regulation of private and other independent healthcare, published in December 1999. This created a new body – the National Care Standards Commission (NCSC), which, with effect from April 1, 2002, took responsibility for the regulation of private healthcare throughout the UK in place of local authorities and health authorities.

In cosmetic surgery certain national minimum standards have been set, to which surgeons need to adhere. Some of these standards are that patients should always be given full details of the treatment they are to receive, they must not be admitted for treatment on the same day as the initial consultation, and referral for psychological counseling is available if clinically indicated. Surgeons performing cosmetic surgery must belong to the relevant professional body, which provides continuing medical education and adheres to the principles of the General Medical Council's good medical practice. They

must maintain a comprehensive outpatient service; and must assess the appropriateness for receiving cosmetic surgery and record that in the patient's health record. There should also be written procedures for the safe use of equipment for cosmetic surgery within the hospital and all staff using the equipment should have completed training in the safe clinical use of this equipment and have demonstrated competence documented to this effect. In April 2004, the role of the NCSC was taken over by a new body, the Healthcare Commission, which is now responsible for reviewing the quality of care with reference to national minimum standards in the NHS and private sector.

See Also

Complaints Against Doctors, Healthcare Workers and Institutions; **Consent:** Confidentiality and Disclosure; **Medical Malpractice:** Ear, Nose and Throat Surgery; Facio-maxillary Surgery; **Medical Malpractice – Medico-legal Perspectives:** Negligence, Causation

Further Reading

Adamson TE, Baldwin DC Jr, Sheehan TJ, Oppenberg AA (1997) Characteristics of surgeons with high and low malpractice claims. *Western Journal of Medicine* 166: 37–44.
Armstrong AP, Cole AA, Page RE (1997) Informed consent: are we doing enough? *British Journal of Plastic Surgery* 50: 636–640.
Chavez AE, Dagum P, Koch RJ, Newman JP (1997) Legal issues of computer imaging in plastic surgery. *Plastic and Reconstructive Surgery* 100: 1601–1608.
Gorney M (2002) Claims prevention for the aesthetic surgeon: preparing for the less than perfect outcome. *Facial Plastic Surgery* 18: 135–142.
Gorney M (2003) Truth and consequences, their truth our consequences. *Plastic and Reconstructive Surgery* 111: 2099–2101.
Koch RJ, Chavez A (1999) Medico legal aspects of imaging and internet communications. *Facial Plastic Surgery* 15(2): 139–144.
Macgregor FC (1984) Cosmetic surgery: a sociological analysis of litigation and a surgical specialty. *Aesthetic Plastic Surgery* 8: 219–224.
Meningaud JP, Servant JM, Herve C, Bertrand JC (2000) Ethic and aims of cosmetic surgery: a contribution from an analysis of claims after minor damage. *Medicine and Law* 19: 237–252.
Ward CM (1994) Consenting to surgery. *British Journal of Plastic Surgery* 47: 30–34.
Ward CM (1998) Consenting and consulting for cosmetic surgery. *British Journal of Plastic Surgery* 51: 547–550.

Police Surgeon

G A Norfolk, Association of Forensic Physicians, Bristol, UK

Introduction

In today's increasingly litigious world, doctors are only too aware of their vulnerability to claims of alleged medical malpractice. Forensic physicians are not exempt from these risks and, indeed, are exposed to certain particular dangers because of the unique nature of their work. Although this article considers medical malpractice in relation to forensic physicians in the UK, many of the principles and considerations are equally applicable to other jurisdictions.

The Role of the Independent Forensic Physician

Forensic physicians (also known as forensic medical examiners and police surgeons) are usually general practitioners who provide clinical forensic medical services to the police in the UK on a part-time basis, although in busy metropolitan areas doctors may work exclusively as forensic physicians.

The doctors are self-employed and contract independently with the police to provide medical care to detainees and to conduct forensic assessments of both suspects and victims of crime. Thus, by the very nature of their work, forensic physicians are more likely than most doctors to end up in court giving professional or expert evidence. However, when things go wrong, forensic physicians may also find themselves as defendants in civil and even criminal proceedings.

Negligence and the Forensic Physician

Just as in any area of medicine, forensic physicians are expected to exercise proper care in their work. If they neglect to do so and their patients are harmed as a result, they can expect to be criticized and may face claims for compensation arising out of alleged clinical negligence. In a series of 100 consecutive files that were opened by one of the UK medical defense organizations to advise and assist forensic physicians, there were a total of 28 such claims of negligence. The vast majority (81%) of these cases were in relation to a delay in diagnosis, usually a fracture, while the remaining (19%) related to a prescribing error. A breakdown of these cases is shown in **Table 1**.

Alcohol intoxication is extremely common amongst detainees in police custody, and the anesthetic effect of the drug may explain some of the difficulty in establishing an early diagnosis of a fracture sustained during the commission of an alcohol-related offense. Intoxication may also adversely affect an individual's demeanor and this can lead to delays in diagnosis because of difficulty in establishing effective communication. However, problems with delayed diagnosis can also arise because of a failure on the part of the doctor to take a careful history and conduct a comprehensive examination. In particular, an uncritical acceptance of police assertions that a detainee is feigning illness has been highlighted as an important factor in a number of cases where delayed diagnosis has resulted in a death in police custody.

Deaths in police custody are hugely expensive both in terms of the emotional cost for the individuals and families involved and also financially, in relation to the formal inquiry that inevitably ensues. Research evidence has shown that the main causes of deaths in police custody in the UK involve deliberate self-harm, substance misuse, and delayed diagnosis of medical problems, particularly head injuries. Unfortunately, justifiable criticism is occasionally leveled at the standard of care provided to the deceased by the forensic physician involved and, rarely, the doctor may face a charge of manslaughter following a death in police custody. To reduce the numbers of these deaths, it is important to recognize clinical forensic medicine as a distinct medical specialty and ensure that doctors practicing the craft are properly trained and forensically aware.

Gross Negligence Manslaughter

When a patient dies as a result of alleged gross negligence on the part of a doctor, the UK Crown Prosecution Service may consider that a charge of

Table 1   A breakdown of 28 consecutive claims against forensic physicians

Reason for claim	Number of cases
Delayed diagnosis	23
Fracture of hand	5
Fracture of skull	2
Other fractures and trauma	6
Myocardial infarction	3
Suicidal depression	3
Diabetes	1
Other	3
Prescribing error	5
Total	28

Data from Schutte P (2000) Pitfalls in police work. *The Journal of the MDU* 16: 16–18.

manslaughter is justified. The threshold for determining criminal liability was established by the Court of Appeal in a case involving Dr. Percy Bateman, who was convicted of manslaughter in the 1920s after the death of an obstetric patient in his care. The Court of Appeal stated that:

> To establish criminal liability the facts must be such that, in the opinion of the jury, the negligence of the accused went beyond a mere matter of compensation between subjects, and showed such disregard for the life and safety of others as to amount to a crime against the State, and conduct deserving of punishment.

The suggestion that, to establish criminal liability, a jury must be satisfied that the doctor's actions were criminal, is somewhat tautologous. Fortunately, greater clarity can be found from the case of Dr. Adomako, where the Court of Appeal listed four states of mind, any one of which may be grounds for a finding of criminal negligence. These states of mind are:

1. indifference to an obvious risk of injury to health
2. actual foresight of the risk, coupled with the determination nonetheless to run it
3. appreciation of the risk, coupled with an intention to avoid it, but also coupled with such a high degree of negligence in the attempted avoidance as a jury may consider justifies conviction
4. inattention or failure to advert to a serious risk which went beyond mere inadvertence in respect of an obvious and important matter which the defendant's duty demanded he/she should address.

The number of doctors actually charged with and convicted of manslaughter increased appreciably in the 1990s, and there is strong anecdotal evidence that the police now routinely consider the potential criminal liability of forensic physicians involved in the care of individuals who die in custody.

Medication errors appear to be the single most common cause for a charge of medical manslaughter, whether in relation to deaths in police custody or elsewhere. A review of all medical manslaughter cases occurring in the UK between 1970 and 1999 revealed a total of 17 deaths involving 21 doctors. Only two doctors were charged in each of the first two decades during this period, compared to 17 in the decade 1990–1999 (this eightfold increase in cases of gross negligence compares to only a twofold increase in cases of civil negligence between 1990 and 1998). Forensic physicians appear to be disproportionately overrepresented, accounting for three (14%) of all doctors charged.

One of these cases involved a 23-year-old prisoner who was transferred to a provincial police station after having spent eight weeks in custody elsewhere. During this period, he had been weaned off heroin and, on transfer, was considered to be "fit and healthy." Notwithstanding this, two forensic physicians prescribed an alarming cocktail of drugs to him over the next 11 days, including temazepam (160 mg at night), diazepam (80 mg a day), chlorpromazine (300 mg daily), and methadone (30 mg daily). The man "was changed into a zombie-like figure" and subsequently died from drug toxicity.

In the other case, a forensic physician was charged with manslaughter after prescribing what was alleged to be a "lethal dose of methadone" to a 22-year-old man who, it transpired, was intoxicated with benzodiazepines at the time.

Although these are the only three reported instances of forensic physicians being charged with manslaughter, the author is aware of several other cases where similar charges have been considered. Taking a careful history, conducting a thorough examination, and keeping meticulous contemporaneous notes are the readily identifiable means of ensuring that such a charge cannot be substantiated.

Malpractice and the Expert Witness

Forensic physicians frequently appear in court as either professional or expert witnesses. When doctors come to court to give evidence, they have the benefit of absolute immunity. This immunity is regarded as necessary in the interests of the administration of justice and is granted to doctors, and indeed all witnesses, as a matter of public policy. It extends to anything said or done by them in the ordinary course of any proceeding in a court of justice and protects them from any action that may be brought against them even if things that are said or done are false, malicious, or negligent. The case of *Darker* v. *Chief Constable of West Midlands* appears to extend this immunity to reports and statements that may be produced by forensic physicians in the knowledge that, if proceedings were brought, the report would form part of the evidence in those proceedings.

Not only do doctors have immunity from civil action in relation to the evidence they give in court, but, also it seems that they have only a limited duty of care to the victims of crimes that they examine during the course of their work. Thus, the Court of Appeal ruled that Dr. Agrawal, a forensic physician who examined an alleged rape victim, owed the victim no duty of care to attend as a prosecution witness at the alleged rapist's trial, even if the failure to attend court resulted in the collapse of the trial and an exacerbation of the victim's psychiatric trauma. In such circumstances, the court ruled, the doctor is carrying out an examination on behalf of the police and does not assume any responsibility for the victim's psychiatric welfare. The doctor's duty was simply to take care in the course of the examination not to make the patient's condition worse.

Whether the apparent immunity of forensic physicians to actions brought against them in relation to their work as professional and expert witnesses is as watertight today is open to debate. Certainly, in one recent landmark case, the Court of Appeal has ruled that children (but not their parents) can sue healthcare trusts and local authorities that wrongly conclude that they have been the victims of abuse. The three judges hearing the case held that the public policy considerations barring claims of wrongful diagnosis have been swept away by the Human Rights Act, which came into force in the UK in October 2000. It seems probable that this ruling will lay individual doctors, as well as healthcare trusts, open to negligence claims for wrongful diagnoses made in the course of legal proceedings.

Conclusion

Detainees in police custody represent a particularly vulnerable group of individuals by virtue of the high prevalence of substance misuse, mental illness, and previous episodes of deliberate self-harm amongst their number. Because of this vulnerability, forensic physicians involved in the clinical care of detainees expose themselves to an increased risk of civil and even criminal claims of medical malpractice if they fail to apply especial vigilance in the course of their examination and treatment of these individuals. Furthermore, it seems that forensic physicians may also be at risk of civil claims if they fail to exercise proper care when formulating forensic advice for the courts, if this advice is subsequently shown to be wrong.

See Also

Custody: Death in, United Kingdom and Continental Europe; Death in, United States of America; **Detainees:** Care in Police Custody, United Kingdom; Care in Prison Custody, United Kingdom

Further Reading

Darker, others v. *Chief Constable of West Midlands* (2000) UKHL 44.
Dyer C (2003) Judges rule that children can sue for wrongful diagnosis of abuse. *British Medical Journal* 327: 305.
N v. *Agrawal* (1999) Times Law Report June 9.
Norfolk GA (1998) Deaths in police custody in 1994: a retrospective analysis. *Journal of Clinical Forensic Medicine* 5: 49–54.
R v. *Bateman* (1925) 19 Cr. App. R 8.
R v. *Sullman, Prentice, Adomako* (1993) 15 BMLR 13 CA.
Schutte P (2000) Pitfalls in police work. *Journal of the Medical Defence Union* 16: 16–18.
Stark MM (2000) The medical care of detainees and the prevention of tragedy – the role of the forensic medical examiner. *Clinical Risk* 7: 15–19.

Psychiatry

J W Thompson, J Artecona, and B Bora, Tulane University School of Medicine, New Orleans, LA, USA

Introduction and Definitions

Psychiatric malpractice falls under the general heading of medical malpractice and the same principles of tort law apply. The USA is the forerunner of psychiatric malpractice litigation with other industrialized countries lagging behind. Since the USA is farther along in legal malpractice evolution, the US system will be the focus of this article.

The physician who engages in a doctor–patient relationship owes a duty to the patient to provide care within the acceptable national standard, that is, what an average or competent psychiatrist would have done in similar circumstances. A breach or dereliction of this duty resulting in direct causation of damages to the patient is considered malpractice. These four malpractice elements must be proved by a preponderance of the evidence (i.e., tilting the scales) for the plaintiff to obtain a monetary award from the physician. Medical expert testimony is almost always needed in malpractice litigation.

Psychiatric malpractice claims in the USA and in other countries have been steadily rising over the past 30 years. Traditionally psychiatrists were less likely to be sued since they had fewer patients and closer relationships with them than other specialties. As practice patterns have changed and society has became more litigious, the number of malpractice cases is likely to continue to rise.

There are many potential causes of action against psychiatrists, including breaches of confidentiality, lack of informed consent, inadequate medication management, negligent psychotherapy, inadequate suicide assessment and prevention, duty to warn or protect third parties from harm by psychiatric patients, and doctor–patient boundary violations.

These areas are the focus of this article since they are the most common causes of action.

Breach of Confidentiality

Psychiatrists, with some exceptions, are expected to protect patient confidentiality. Confidentiality is an ethical obligation imposed on psychiatrists by themselves and their professional organizations. Specific statutes and case law may also require certain patient information to remain confidential. Many federal and state statutes have codified this obligation. Some courts have held that protection of confidentiality is an inherent part of the therapist–patient relationship.

The most common bases of recovery for breach of confidentiality are breach of contract, invasion of privacy, negligent infliction of mental distress, and loss of employment. Recovery for invasion of privacy generally requires a public disclosure of a private fact, not a disclosure to an individual or small group such as spouse or family. Recovery in breach of contract suits is limited to economic losses that were a direct result of the breach and does not include losses stemming from subsequent mental suffering or loss of employment.

Defenses for breach of confidentiality are dependent on valid consent for the release of information. To be valid, the consent must be knowing and voluntary. It is prudent to have patients sign release forms or document their oral consent in progress notes. Physicians should consider having patients sign progress notes where the consent to release information is documented. Another defense is that the breach was necessary due to an overriding public interest. This usually involves warning third parties about potential harm such as violence. State law may require some notifications, such as warning sexual partners about human immunodeficiency virus (HIV) status or reporting child abuse.

When treating adolescents aged 14–16 years, psychiatrists should not generally release information to families without their consent. An exception is the protection of the basic welfare of the patient or family members.

Lack of Informed Consent and Inadequate Treatment with Psychotropic Medication

Claims involving psychotropic medication comprise a significant portion of malpractice claims against psychiatrists. Reasonable care should include a thorough medical history, physical and psychiatric examinations, past medication history, history of adverse reactions to medications, and appropriate laboratory testing. It is the psychiatrist's responsibility to explain the risks and benefits of medication, alternative treatments, and risks of no treatment so that a patient can give informed consent. Informed consent should be obtained whenever a new medication is started and may be required whenever dosages are changed. Proper documentation of informed consent and treatment decisions is an essential component of malpractice prevention.

There are many different causes of action in cases involving medications. In addition to the areas mentioned above, selected areas of potential litigation include: prescriptions of improper dosage or of improper duration; failure to recognize drug–drug or drug–food interactions; creating a dependence on prescribed drugs; failure to recognize, monitor, and treat side-effects; and improper record-keeping.

The decision for off-label (not approved by the Food and Drug Administration) use of drugs or exceeding recommended dosages of drugs should be based on reasonable medical judgment and supported by available literature. The rationale for the decision should be clearly documented, and informed consent should also be heightened.

Tardive dyskinesia (TD) is an area of particular concern with the use of psychotropic medication. Several large judgments have been awarded in the USA for malpractice involving TD. The American Psychiatric Association has developed guidelines for the prevention and management of TD, and these may be helpful to clinicians.

Negligent Psychotherapy

Negligent psychotherapy has historically been difficult to prove due to the lack of established practice standards. There are hundreds of schools of psychotherapy. Successful claims of negligence have been raised in cases where there has been evidence of physical assault by the therapist, inadequate referral upon termination (abandonment), or failure of the therapist to offer pharmacological treatment as an alternative to psychotherapy.

A therapist has a duty to reassess or terminate treatment that is harmful or ineffective. When therapy ceases to be beneficial, the therapist should get a second opinion from a colleague or seek supervision. If this does not work, the therapist should offer to refer the patient to another colleague after processing termination with the patient. If a psychiatrist is concerned about dangerous behavior upon termination, such as suicide, he/she should consider transferring the patient to another psychiatrist in a hospital setting. Patients may claim negligence if their therapy has been terminated without adequate referral options. Adequate procedures for termination should include providing the patient with reasonable notice of decision to terminate, assistance in finding another psychotherapist, emergency contact information, and an adequate supply of medication.

A psychiatrist has a duty to offer patients both psychotherapeutic and pharmacological treatment. Patients should be told that medication might hasten their recovery. They should also be given the option of psychotherapy without medication. Patients may claim negligence if they receive extended psychotherapy without a response and then improve soon after starting medication if they were not offered medication at the beginning of treatment.

Suicide Assessment and Prevention

Half of the patient suicides in the USA will result in malpractice litigation. Inpatient suicide carries the greatest liability, because the patient is in a controlled environment. Most *Diagnostic and Statistical Manual*, 4th edition (DSM-IV-TR) Axis I disorders, as well as some of the personality disorders, are associated with increased suicide risk. Suicide risk evaluation is a difficult task that involves the identification of specific risk factors for a given patient. Suicide prevention involves designing a treatment plan to address and minimize the patient-specific dynamic risk factors (**Table 1**).

The law recognizes that there are no absolute standards for the prediction of suicide because suicide results from a complex array of risk factors. Courts assume that a suicide is preventable if it is foreseeable; however, foreseeable does not equate with preventable in clinical practice. The term foreseeable is a legal term with no clear clinical equivalent. An action is foreseeable if there is reasonable anticipation that harm or injury is a likely result from certain acts or omissions. The standard of care for patients at risk for suicide includes the reasonable physician's ability to make a thorough assessment, to recognize relevant risk factors, and to design and implement a treatment plan that decreases the risk of suicide. No assessment is foolproof, and the patient determined to complete suicide may succeed despite a comprehensive prevention plan.

When a lawsuit is filed, the chart will be examined to determine whether the physician recognized the risk factors and considered limiting the risk by exerting greater control over the patient through hospitalization or other means. Documentation of encounters with actively suicidal patients should include a psychiatric evaluation with risk factor analysis, attempted discussions with family members, and a treatment plan with recommendations for ways

Table 1 Suicide risk factors

Epidemiological (static)
- Males > females
- Age: adolescents and geriatric population (males peak at 75 years, females peak at 55 years)
- Race: Caucasian and American Indian
- Marital status: single > divorced; widowed > married

Psychiatric (dynamic)
- Mood disorders, alcoholism, drug abuse, psychotic disorders, personality disorders
- Family history of suicide
- History of previous suicide attempt: assess lethality of intent
- Medical diagnosis of terminal illness (cancer, acquired immunodeficiency syndrome (AIDS)), chronic intractable pain, chronic and disabling illness (renal dialysis patient)
- Hopelessness

Psychosocial (dynamic)
- History of recent loss (loved one, job)
- Loss of social supports
- Important dates (holidays, birthdays, anniversaries, etc.)
- Access to weapons or lethal means
- Suicide plan: assess lethality of intent

The key to a favorable course and prognosis is early recognition of risk factors, early diagnosis and treatment of psychiatric disorder, and appropriate interventions for specific dynamic risk factors

to reduce the risk of suicide. Liability may also result from unforeseeable suicides if there is failure to assess suicide risk properly.

Injury to Third Parties

If a psychiatric patient poses a potential risk to a third party, it may be incumbent on the psychiatrist to manage the patient via notification or hospitalization. This principle was demonstrated in the case of *Tarasoff* v. *the Regents of the University of California* (529 P.2d 553 (Cal. 1974) 551 P.2d 334 (1976)). The Tarasoff decision made physicians in California responsible not only for warning potential victims of their patients, but also for protecting them. Psychiatrists may be expected to protect third parties and society at large by hospitalizing patients or petitioning for commitment. The patient should remain hospitalized until he/she is no longer considered imminently dangerous.

Psychiatrists have also been found liable to protect society when their patients injured third parties while driving automobiles (*Naidu* v. *Laird* 538 A.2d 1064 (Del. 1988)). The holdings in these cases contradict the American Psychiatric Association, which took the position that psychiatrists have no special expertise to assess driving ability. Such cases put psychiatrists in a precarious position since they have been found liable in situations where they have no special training.

Another area where psychiatrists have been found liable to third parties is in recovered-memory cases. In *Ramona* v. *Ramona*, a father was awarded a $475 000 settlement when his daughter's therapists had negligently induced false memories that her bulimia was a result of being sexually abused by her father (*Ramona* v. *Ramona* (judgment on jury verdict), no. 61898 (Napa City Superior Ct, July 11, 1994). The therapists had told the patient that the abuse was confirmed during an amobarbital interview. The Ramona court felt that Mr. Ramona was a direct victim of the therapist's negligent psychotherapy.

Doctor–Patient Boundary Violations

The concept of boundaries between psychiatrist and patient initially developed in the context of the psychotherapeutic relationship and has subsequently been influenced by ethical principles set forth by mental health professional organizations, legal statues, and case law. These principles apply to all psychiatrist–patient relationships. Boundaries in the doctor–patient relationship provide a set of rules and expectations that allow the patient to develop trust in the physician and to know what to expect from the relationship. It is the responsibility of the psychiatrist to establish clear and consistent boundaries. The basic principle of these limitations on physician behavior is that physicians have a fiduciary duty to their patients. This duty is to put the best interests of the patient above the physician's interests.

Boundary violations involve clear-cut transgressions of the accepted relationship between psychiatrist and patient. Examples include having sex or sexualized conduct with patients, exploiting patients for financial gain, and engaging in social relationships with patients.

Physician–patient sexual contact and other forms of patient exploitation may be the basis for discipline by physician regulatory bodies. The American Psychiatric Association has adopted ethical guidelines which declare it unethical for a psychiatrist to have a sexual relationship with a former or current patient. Even when patients engage in behaviors that may be considered seductive, it is the physician's responsibility to maintain appropriate boundaries. In the USA, a number of states have enacted laws that make it a criminal offense to have sexual relations with patients. The first state to enact such a law was Wisconsin, followed by Minnesota, North Dakota, Colorado, and Maine, as well as a growing list of states. Criminal charges may include sexual assault, rape, and adultery. Some states, such as Minnesota, Wisconsin, California, Illinois, and Texas have civil statutes that incorporate a standard of care that makes malpractice easier to pursue by finding a civil cause of action for the sexual exploitation of patients by therapists. Some insurance companies have refused to pay for defending physicians in sexual boundary violation cases. Professional sanctions may include ethical complaints, expulsion from professional organizations, and loss of licensure.

Summary

Psychiatric malpractice litigation is a growing field and will likely continue to grow as society becomes more and more litigious. The claims against psychiatrists fall into several general categories, including lack of confidentiality, lack of informed consent for treatment, inadequate medication management, inadequate suicide assessment and prevention, injury to third parties, and doctor–patient boundary violations.

Psychiatrists should recognize that the best protection against malpractice litigation is the provision and documentation of good care. The physician who takes an adequate medical and psychiatric history, performs an adequate physical/mental status examination of the patient, renders diagnoses, and prescribes medication or psychotherapy in a reasonable manner is at much less risk for successful malpractice litigation. Finally, all physicians should be aware that the documentation of the above care is essential for communication with other physicians and to create a record of the appropriate care provided. The best defense against a malpractice claim is a well-written record documenting treatment plans and rational decision-making.

See Also

Forensic Psychiatry and Forensic Psychology: Suicide Predictors and Statistics; **Medical Malpractice:** Child and Adolescent Psychiatry; **Medical Malpractice – Medico-legal Perspectives:** Negligence, Standard of Care; Negligence, Duty of Care; Negligence, Causation; Negligence Quantum

Further Reading

American Psychiatric Association (1992) *Tardive Dyskinesia: A Task Force Report of the American Psychiatric Association.* Washington, DC: American Psychiatric Association.

American Psychiatric Association (1998) *The Principles of Medical Ethics with Annotations Especially Applicable to Psychiatry.* Washington, DC: American Psychiatric Association.

American Psychiatric Association (2000) *Diagnostic and Statistical Manual of Mental Disorders,* 4th edn., text revision. Washington, DC: American Psychiatric Association.

Appelbaum PS (2001) Third party suits against therapists in recovered memory cases. *Psychiatric Services* 52: 27–28.

Appelbaum PS, Jorgenson L (1991) Psychotherapist–patient sexual contact after termination of treatment: an analysis and a proposal. *American Journal of Psychiatry* 148: 1466–1473.

Appelbaum PS, Zoltek-Jick RA (1996) Psychotherapists' duties to third parties: Ramona and beyond. *American Journal of Psychiatry* 153: 457–465.

Bisbing SB, Jorgenson LM, Sutherlans PK (1995) *Sexual Abuse by Professionals: A Legal Guide*. Charlottesville, VA: Michie.

Cannell J, Hudson JI, Pope HG (2001) Standards for informed consent in recovered memory therapy. *Journal of the American Academy of Psychiatry and the Law* 29: 138–147.

Felthous AR (1999) The clinician's duty to protect third parties. *Psychiatric Clinics of North America* 22: 49–60.

Gutheil TG (1994) Risk management at the margins: less familiar topics in psychiatric malpractice. *Harvard Review of Psychiatry* 2: 214–221.

Malmquist CP, Notman MT (2001) Psychiatrist–patient boundary issues following treatment termination. *American Journal of Psychiatry* 158: 1010–1018.

Monahan J (1993) Limiting therapist exposure to Tarasoff liability: guidelines for risk containment. *American Psychologist* 48: 242–250.

Resnick PJ (2003) *Forensic Psychiatry Review Course*. San Antonio, TX: American Academy of Psychiatry and the Law Annual Meeting.

Simon RI (1992) *Clinical Psychiatry and the Law*, 2nd edn. Washington, DC: American Psychiatric Press.

Simon RI (1999) Therapist–patient sex – from boundary violations to sexual misconduct. *Psychiatric Clinics of North America* 22: 31–47.

Simon RI (2003) Treatment boundaries in psychiatric practice. In: Rosner R (ed.) *Principles and Practice of Forensic Psychiatry*, 2nd edn., pp. 156–172. London: Arnold.

Simon RI, Sadoff RL (1992) *Psychiatric Malpractice: Cases and Comments for Clinicians*. Washington, DC: American Psychiatric Press.

Slovenko R (1999) Malpractice in psychotherapy: an overview. *Psychiatric Clinics of North America* 22: 1–15.

Wettstein RM (2003) Specific issues in psychiatric malpractice. In: Rosner R (ed.) *Principles and Practice of Forensic Psychiatry*, 2nd edn., pp. 249–260. London: Arnold.

Psychology

R J Edelmann, University of Roehampton, London, UK

Introduction

In many countries the term psychologist is not protected by law – in other words, anyone practicing "therapy," even if they have no qualifications, can effectively refer to themselves as a "psychologist."

However, those with appropriate qualifications, that is, a psychology degree and in many instances a postgraduate qualification in an academic or applied aspect of the discipline, choose to belong to their national society and hence to abide by the rules of conduct of that society. In countries where the term "psychologist" is not protected, as long as those using the term are reasonably accurate in their claims relating to expertise and experience and assuming they abide by the normal rules of everyday relationships, seeking redress in relation to perceived incompetent practice or poor record-keeping may be difficult to achieve. The only route for complaint would be directly through the legal process, and the only possible redress would be financial compensation, assuming that real and quantifiable harm has been suffered by the complainant. As practitioners in this instance would not be licenced or registered, there is no professional body from which they can be removed.

In many countries then, it remains incumbent upon the person seeking psychological therapy to ensure that the therapist they approach is a *bone fide* member of the regulating society within that country and, ideally, to verify the credentials that the person holds.

Codes of Conduct

Psychologists who are members of their national society are then bound by the rules of conduct of that society. For example, in the USA this is the American Psychological Association's (APA's) Ethical Principles of Psychologists and Code of Conduct (2002). In the UK it is the British Psychological Society's (BPS's) Code of Conduct, Ethical Principles and Guidelines (2000). Much of the material presented in this article will be drawn from their codes of practice.

Core principles relate to questions of competence, the advertising of services, confidentiality and record-keeping, personal conduct and interpersonal relationship issues, the conduct of research, assessment, and the use of test results. Each of these areas will be addressed in the following sections. Unfortunately, both legal action in relation to malpractice by psychologists and complaints made to psychological societies are increasing. In spite of this there is a striking absence of research relating to psychological malpractice in a general sense. However, there is an abundance of research relating to specific aspects of professional practice, particularly "dual and exploitive relationships" and a substantive literature relating to ethical dilemmas faced by psychologists, including issues of confidentiality and competence to practice.

Competence

Psychologists work within a variety of settings, which include educational, healthcare, and occupational environments. Many also hold various postgraduate qualifications, including neuropsychological and clinical, counseling, health, occupational, educational, and forensic psychology, which provide them with the necessary background to gain the expertise in order to practice in such contexts. As the APA code of conduct states: "Psychologists provide services, teach, and conduct research with populations and in areas only within the boundaries of their competence, based on their education, training, supervised experience, consultation, study, or professional experience." As such they should "recognize the boundaries of their own competence and not attempt to practice any form of psychology for which they do not have an appropriate preparation or, where applicable, specialist qualification."

In short, psychologists should only provide services for which they have obtained appropriate training and/or of which they have appropriate experience or expertise. It is also important to recognize that competence can erode over time. It is thus incumbent on the psychologist concerned to ensure standards of practice are maintained through continuing professional development. Psychologists offering services for which they are not appropriately qualified or for which they do not have suitable experience may be liable for malpractice.

Advertising of Services

As with issues relating to competence, advertising should reflect the qualifications and expertise of the psychologist concerned; advertisers should endeavor to present a truthful and accurate picture of themselves and their work. In any such advertisement, as a matter of principle, psychologists should not denigrate the services of other psychologists, should not make claims about the certainty of a "cure," nor should they offer to make a refund in the event that the "cure" fails, nor should they play on clients' fears in order to seek to generate work. Any psychologist so doing would be open to a complaint of malpractice.

Confidentiality

As a guiding principle, psychologists are expected to keep and maintain adequate records of any consultation or meeting with those to whom they provide services. Steps should also be taken to ensure the confidentiality of any information obtained or stored in any medium. Issues relating to confidentiality should be explained to the recipients of the service at the outset and any limitations of confidentiality made explicit. In certain instances, for example within criminal justice settings, the psychologist's duty is to the service rather than the inmate, and hence information obtained from the latter cannot be confidential. However, institutional guidelines should make clear how information obtained would be handled. Similarly, when a psychologist prepares a report for, or provides evidence to, a court he/she will be expected to divulge information within such a context that has been obtained from the litigant. However, if information has been obtained from a third party, such as relatives, spouse, friends, or colleagues, then the consent of the litigant must be obtained.

A further issue central to the question of confidentiality concerns risk assessment, that is, an assessment of the likelihood that a particular behavior will occur and a consideration of the consequences of such an occurrence. This can refer to a variety of behaviors, including sex offending, violence, or suicide. In criminal justice settings both open reporting and monitoring of the client's behavior are likely to occur. It is of interest to note that the disclosure of previous offenses increases according to the degree of confidentiality offered. However, if a client is seen in a mental health setting rather than a criminal justice setting, then care should be exercised when establishing with the client the boundaries of confidentiality. It would not be good practice to promise absolute confidentiality to a client when it then becomes apparent during the course of the assessment that the client poses a serious risk either to the client or to others.

Confidentiality issues are a frequent dilemma for psychologists, and in many instances it can be unclear whether confidential information should or should not be disclosed. Disclosure to appropriate others may be necessary, for example, when there are serious safety concerns either about the recipient of the service or those with whom they may come into contact or in instances of child abuse reporting. In relation to malpractice issues, it is clearly important to make the correct decision about revealing confidential information. If there is any doubt, it is incumbent upon the psychologist concerned to seek appropriate advice from colleagues or their professional body.

Issues pertaining to confidentiality apply across a variety of domains, from clinical practice to research settings. In the latter context, information should be stored and communicated in a way which will not allow identification of any one individual. The same is true in relation to material used in lectures or published material.

Personal Conduct and Interpersonal Relationship

As a general rule, the only relationship the psychologist should have with the recipients of the psychologist's services is a professional one. This applies to both personal nonsexual as well as sexual relationships. While this is true of professionals in general, many psychologists have longer periods of contact with their clients, often on a one-to-one basis, than is true of many other practitioners. Blurred, conflictual, dual, or multiple relationships may, however, present problems of varying magnitude. A blurred or conflictual relationship is one where professional and personal boundaries are not absolutely clear. Dual and multiple relationships are those in which the psychologist is in a professional role with a person while either at the same time being in another role with the same person, with a person closely associated with or related to that person, or if the psychologist promises to enter into another relationship in the future with the person or a person closely associated with or related to the person.

At one end of the continuum it may not always be possible to avoid blurred or dual nonsexual relationships with clients or former clients. For example, there are occasions when the psychologist may have a remote relationship with the client outside his/her professional contact, perhaps as acquaintances in small, rural communities. Whether this is a perfect situation is a matter of debate but may be inevitable in certain instances. However, there are other occasions when boundaries become blurred which can and should be avoided. As a general rule, professionals should not invite clients to social events at which they will be present, lend them personal possessions, focus on nontreatment-related issues during therapy, or allow the treatment session to become a "social event."

At the other end of the continuum are instances of therapist–patient, supervisor–supervisee, and lecturer–student sexual involvement. Research studies suggest that between 0.9% and 3.6% of male therapists and between 0.2% and 0.5% of female therapists self-report sexual involvement with their patients. There is some indication that the incidence of such behavior has declined over the years. This may be due in part to the efforts of professional bodies and in part to a number of highly publicized multimillion-dollar malpractice awards. In one case in the USA a plaintiff was awarded $1 million despite the psychologist's defense that he had waited until after termination of therapy to engage in sexual relations and that he had then married his former patient and remained married to her for five years!

It is generally recognized that patient–therapist, supervisor–supervisee, and lecturer–student sexual involvement is damaging for patients/supervisees/students. Most cases involve a male therapist/supervisor/lecturer and a female patient/supervisee/student with intimacy occurring during therapy, training, or study. However, patients engaging in sexual relations with the treating psychologist after the termination of therapy also report being harmed by the relationship. Negative effects can involve a range of problems, including feelings of ambivalence, guilt, emptiness and isolation, sexual confusion, impaired ability to trust, emotional lability, suppressed rage, increased suicidal risk, and problems with attention and concentration.

The Conduct of Research

There are a number of guidelines that psychologists should apply in relation to the use of participants in research. Participants should be informed about the purpose of the research, their right to withdraw from participation or to decline to participate and, should they choose to do so, that there will not be any implications with regard to their treatment, education, and so on. Particular consideration should be given to the deception of prospective research participants. If deception is felt to be scientifically justifiable, then care should be exercised to ensure that it does not result in undue emotional distress for the participants concerned. The study should be followed by prompt debriefing to inform participants about the nature of the study and to discuss any concerns that might arise.

Although it is almost always necessary to secure ethical approval for research, either from one's own institution or the institution from which the participants are to be recruited if it differs from the former, this does not *de facto* imply that participants are protected from unethical practice.

Unethical practice includes not only that which might be directed toward research participants, but also behavior relating to one's peers, for example, claiming someone else's work as one's own or failing to give appropriate credit to others who have contributed substantially to the work.

Use of Test Results

Assessment provides the cornerstone for much professional practice in a range of settings, including forensic contexts. As a guiding principle, psychologists, including those working in forensic settings, should only administer tests for which they have been trained, should be competent in the use of standardized tests, should use tests which fit the task and which fit the individual, should administer them correctly, should make appropriate use of computers in assessments, and should assess and report on factors which may affect the meaning of the test findings. In short, psychologists should administer only those tests that are appropriate for the task and whose validity and reliability have been established with the population to be tested.

Normal practice would be to provide the test-taker or other authorized person with feedback about the results in a manner which allows that person to understand the meaning of the results. If it is deemed that such release may cause harm or that the results may be misused or misrepresented or if confidentiality were to be compromised, then the psychologist may withhold the results unless required to do so by law.

Conclusion

Codes of conduct provide a set of minimum standards with which chartered or registered psychologists are required to comply. These professional codes are designed to protect the public from poor or incompetent practice and from those who misuse their professional status. The ideal is that "psychologists shall conduct themselves in a manner that does not bring into disrepute the discipline and profession of psychology." Unfortunately, there will always be a small minority who lay themselves open to complaints of malpractice.

See Also

Forensic Psychiatry and Forensic Psychology: Forensic Psychology, Education, Training and Certification; Ethics

Further Reading

American Psychological Association (2002) Ethical principles of psychologists and code of conduct. *American Psychologist* 57: 1060–1073.

Bersoff DN (ed.) (2003) *Ethical Conflicts in Psychology*, 3rd edn. Washington, DC: American Psychological Association.

British Psychological Society (2000) *Code of Conduct, Ethical Principles and Guidelines*. Leicester, UK: British Psychological Society.

Butcher JN, Pope KS (1993) Seven issues in conducting forensic assessments: ethical responsibilities in light of new standards and new tests. *Ethics and Behavior* 3: 267–288.

Cross HJ, Deardorff WW (1987) Malpractice in psychotherapy and psychological evaluation. In: McNamara JG, Appel M (eds.) *Critical Issues, Developments, and Trends in Professional Psychology*, vol. 3. *Professional Psychology Update*, pp. 55–79. New York: Praeger Publishers.

Hankins GC, Vera MI, Bernard GW, Herkov MJ (1994) Patient–therapist sexual involvement: a review of clinical and research data. *Bulletin of the American Academy of Psychiatry and the Law* 22: 109–128.

Lazarus A, Zur O (eds.) (2002) *Dual Relationships and Psychotherapy*. New York: Springer.

Pipes RB (1997) Nonsexual relationships between psychotherapists and their former clients: obligations of psychologists. *Ethics and Behavior* 7: 27–41.

Pope KS (1990) Therapist–patient sexual involvement: a review of the research. *Clinical Psychology Review* 10: 477–490.

Pope KS (1994) *Sexual Involvement with Therapists: Patient Assessment Subsequent Therapy, Forensics.* Washington, DC: American Psychological Association.

Pope KS, Bouhoutsos JC (1986) *Sexual Intimacies Between Therapists and Patients.* New York: Praeger.

Pope KS, Vetter VA (1991) Prior therapist sexual involvement among patients seen by psychologists. *Psychotherapy: Theory, Research, Practice, Training* 38: 429–438.

Pope KS, Vetter VA (1992) Ethical dilemmas encountered by members of the American Psychological Association. A national survey. *American Psychologist* 47: 397–411.

Radiotherapy

V Barley, National Patient Safety Agency, London, UK

Introduction

Radiotherapy, or radiation oncology, is the use of ionizing radiation (usually X-rays) to treat cancer and a few benign conditions. This article gives a brief outline of the nature of radiation and how it is used in treatment. The patient pathway is used as a basis for illustrating how problems can arise at any time during preparation and treatment.

Radiation

X-rays and radium were discovered just over 100 years ago and treatments of both benign and malignant tumors were developed during the first half of the twentieth century.

At first, only relatively low-energy radiation was available, which penetrated the tissues poorly and gave the maximum dose to the skin. Since the 1950s, high-energy "megavoltage" radiation has enabled the treatment of deep-seated tumors with a relatively lower dose to the overlying skin. Radioactive sources can also be inserted into accessible tumors, such as the cervix, to give a high dose of radiation locally, with a much smaller contribution to the adjacent normal tissues than from external treatment.

Effect of Radiation

Ionizing radiation damages the DNA and hence may affect the vital genetic code of the cell, causing it to die when it tries to multiply. With low levels of radiation, the damage may be repaired by the nucleus of the cell, and cells killed by radiation may be replaced by multiplication of the undamaged cells. Normal tissues have a greater ability to regenerate than malignant tissues, therefore radiotherapy is usually given in small doses daily over 4–6 weeks, which allows recovery of the normal cells. This gives a high total dose to eradicate the tumor while allowing the adjacent organs to survive.

Modern Techniques

Radiation oncology has become a sophisticated and highly technical specialty using the latest diagnostic methods and computerized planning and delivery of treatment.

Computed tomography (CT) and magnetic resonance imaging (MRI) scans have enabled oncologists to localize the tumor and adjacent organs accurately in three dimensions. Precise treatment plans can be prepared using this information to focus the radiation on the cancer and minimize the dose received by the adjacent normal tissues. Subsequent positron emission tomography (PET) scanning allows the metabolism of tissues to be studied, and helps to establish more accurately the extent of the cancer to be treated. The improved accuracy in planning treatment has permitted the safe delivery of higher doses of radiotherapy, resulting in a better chance of cure, without increasing the risk of damage to normal tissues.

The delivery of radiotherapy has also become more precise, as the penumbra at the edge of the radiation beam of a "linear accelerator" is relatively narrow. The correct localization can be checked by simulation and verified by images taken during treatment. Techniques and doses have been improved through experience, particularly by clinical trials which compare a new treatment with the current standard. In view of these continuing improvements, it is important to consider what techniques were in use at the material time when considering a standard of care.

The Patient Pathway

The treatment of cancer usually involves several medical specialties and professional disciplines and the majority of patients are cared for by a multidisciplinary team of doctors, nurses, radiographers, and other paramedical staff.

First an accurate diagnosis and staging is essential, including biopsy and histological examination of the tumor tissue to discover its type and likely behavior. A detailed picture of the extent of the cancer is derived from physical examination and imaging using X-ray, CT, MRI, or ultrasound scans. The results of all investigations are often reviewed by the experts in a meeting of the multidisciplinary team and a treatment plan discussed with the patient and relatives.

Patients who are to receive radiotherapy are seen in a planning clinic where the details of treatment can be explained and preliminary steps taken, such as making a mask for accurate localization in the head and neck region, or CT scans for pelvic tumors. A simulator (a diagnostic X-ray machine that can show the area to be treated) is often used to delineate the radiation field or check that the prepared plan is accurate.

Many radical (curative) treatments now require complex calculations by medical physics technicians using elaborate computer planning systems and it is therefore usual for treatment to start several weeks after the planning clinic.

Treatment normally lasts only a few minutes each day, Monday to Friday, and most patients will not notice any immediate effect. There are both early (acute) and delayed effects of radiotherapy. Early effects, beginning in the first few weeks after starting treatment, include tiredness, occasionally sickness, temporary soreness of the skin (in the area being treated), and diarrhea if the abdomen is included. The acute effects last for several weeks after the end of radiotherapy and may require treatment.

The delayed effects of radiotherapy, more than 6 months later, include thickening of the tissues under the skin (radiation fibrosis), a reduced blood supply (which may not be apparent unless there is a need for surgery), and bowel damage (permanent diarrhea and/or narrowing of the bowel in 5–10% following pelvic irradiation). Since delayed effects are irreversible, the problems persist and are often difficult to treat. It is therefore important to keep the dose of radiation below what is known to be the tolerance level for that particular organ or tissue.

Errors in Radiation Oncology

Incorrect Diagnosis

Radiotherapy is sometimes given before the diagnosis of cancer has been confirmed. In an emergency this could be life-saving, but may lead to unnecessary harm. For example, in 1986 a 63-year-old woman, who had completed chemotherapy and radiotherapy for lung cancer 2 months previously, developed weakness and tingling in her legs. This was thought to be due to the tumor pressing on the spinal cord, but at that time it was not possible to arrange an immediate MRI scan to confirm the diagnosis. Radiotherapy was given urgently to prevent deterioration, but the MRI scan subsequently showed no evidence of cancer. The radiotherapy given to the lung cancer 2 months previously had probably caused the symptoms, and the additional radiotherapy sadly caused further damage to the spinal cord.

Delayed Diagnosis

Sometimes the failure to make a diagnosis of cancer or a premalignant condition can result in extra treatment and its consequent side-effects.

A 58-year-old auctioneer suffered from hoarseness for 5 years before an advanced cancer of the vocal cords was discovered, necessitating urgent surgery. If he had been referred for investigations about a year previously, it is likely that an early cancer could have been cured by radiotherapy alone, thus avoiding the loss of his larynx.

A 32-year-old woman had an abnormal cervical smear, which was erroneously reported normal. Three years later she had abnormal bleeding during pregnancy, and a month before her first baby was due, cancer of the cervix was found. After cesarean section, she had a course of radiotherapy combined with chemotherapy, which cured the cancer but resulted in troublesome bladder and bowel symptoms. If the original smear had been reported correctly, the abnormal areas on the cervix could have been ablated, thus preventing the subsequent development of cancer, and avoiding the side-effects of radiotherapy and chemotherapy.

Failure to Obtain Informed Consent

It is important to discuss the treatment options and side-effects, warning a patient of any serious consequences of treatment (even if very uncommon).

A 70-year-old man developed an ulcer on his lower lip and biopsy showed cancer. There was no evidence of spread and he was advised to undergo surgery, which left an unsightly scar. Radiotherapy would probably have given a better cosmetic result with an equal chance of cure, but this alternative was not discussed when seeking his consent for surgery.

Some tissues are particularly sensitive to radiotherapy; for example, low doses of radiation enhance cataract formation in the eye and sterilize the testes and ovaries.

Informed consent should include a signed statement indicating that the patient has understood the potentially harmful consequences of radiotherapy.

When a new afterloading device was installed for giving radiation internally to the cervix, the dose rate was higher than the previous manual system. To compensate for the higher dose rate (which would be expected to have a greater effect than low-dose-rate radiation), the total dose was reduced by 20%. However, a careful study of the patients treated on the new machine showed that their side-effects were greater than had been expected, and the dose was later reduced further. Patients who were being treated first on the new machine should have been warned about the possibility of worse side-effects when signing a consent form.

The risk of developing cancer in the future may be increased by radiotherapy, especially in children and young adults. For example, it is important to warn young women of the increased risk of developing breast cancer following radiotherapy to the chest (for example, in the treatment of Hodgkin's disease).

Errors in Planning

Since planning involves several members of the multidisciplinary team (oncologist, radiographer, physicist, technician), mistakes by one member are usually noticed by another. A plan to treat the left tonsil was incorrectly marked on the right-hand side of the scans, but this error was recognized by the physicist before starting planning.

The medical records of one patient were not available while she was being prepared to receive a second course of radiotherapy. Fortunately, before radiotherapy was given, it was noted that there was an overlap with the previous treatment which could have led to a serious overdose.

Misidentification

Patients may sometimes come forward when another name is called. As in any other branch of medicine, it is important to confirm the identity of a patient so that the prescribed treatment is given to the right area of the correct patient.

A single dose of radiation to the wrong patient or wrong area may do little harm during a 6-week course of radiotherapy, but if a single large treatment is given incorrectly there may be more serious consequences.

Errors in Dose

The accuracy of the planning calculations on computer depends on using the correct information. After a new planning system was installed, a member of staff used an incorrect method for calculation, which meant that doses were about 25% lower than intended, resulting in a failure to cure some patients.

In another center, the radiotherapy equipment was incorrectly calibrated, which resulted in over 100 patients receiving 25% more radiation than prescribed.

Calculations and doses should be carefully checked by at least two qualified members of staff. Sometimes an overdose is due to a poor technique, which may have been the standard at the time.

A 55-year-old man with lung cancer was treated in 1988 with six large fractions of radiotherapy, as this was standard management in several centers. Radiation damage to his spinal cord caused paralysis a year later. It was subsequently recognized that the risk of damage was greater with large fractions compared with smaller fractions, and such treatment would now be regarded as negligent.

Over 100 women given radiotherapy for breast cancer suffered damage to the nerves in the armpit, since a technique being used until the late 1970s resulted in an overlap between radiation fields. Although it was recognized that the women had severe problems due to excessive radiation, their claims failed since the technique and doses were in common use at that time. Improved accuracy in positioning the treatment now avoids this problem.

Superficial radiation is sometimes used for benign skin disorders. A 75-year-old man was given low-energy radiation to the front and back of his hands, but no correction in dose was made for the radiation penetrating through the skin. He effectively received nearly double the dose intended, and suffered severe burns and damage to his fingers.

An accurate diagnosis and careful planning of treatment will optimize radiotherapy and reduce the risk of harmful effects. Improvements in equipment and techniques have reduced the likelihood of harm. Careful checking by at least two qualified staff usually identifies any potential errors.

See Also

Medical Malpractice: Oncology

Further Reading

Barley VL, Coleman R, Dunlop D, et al. (eds.) (2004) *MIMS Handbook of Oncology*, 4th edn. London: Medical Imprint.

Cancer information website, www.cancer.gov.

Cassidy J, Bissett D, Spence RAJ (2002) *Oxford Handbook of Oncology*. Oxford, UK: Oxford University Press.

De Vita VT, Hellman S, Rosenberg SA (2001) *Cancer: Principles and Practice of Oncology*, 6th edn. Philadelphia, PA: Lippincott, Williams and Wilkins.

Neal AJ, Hoskin PJ (2003) *Clinical Oncology: Basic Principles and Practice*, 3rd edn. London: Edward Arnold.

Pazdur R, Coia LR, Hoskins WJ, Wagman LD (2003) *Cancer Management: A Multidisciplinary Approach*, 7th edn. New York: SCP Communications Inc (also available at www.cancernetwork.com/handbook/contents.htm).

Rheumatology

M G Wright, London, UK

Definition

Rheumatology is the study and management of disorders and diseases of the joints and surrounding tissues – muscles, tendons, and ligaments. There may also be involvement of blood vessels and other organs, such as eyes, gastrointestinal system, kidneys, lungs, nervous system, and skin.

Rheumatology may be divided into two broad fields: (1) the diagnosis and management of inflammatory diseases that affect the joints and surrounding tissues. These are conditions that may also affect the rest of the body, constituting generalized disorders; (2) osteoarthritis, mechanical and degenerative spinal disorders, and soft-tissue conditions affecting the muscles, tendons, and ligaments around joints.

Neurologic conditions such as carpal tunnel syndrome and other nerve entrapments may fall into either of these groups.

Noninflammatory Disorders

These conditions constitute the bulk of rheumatologic practice, affecting virtually all the population at some time in their lives.

A rheumatologist should know the natural history of such disorders and their relationship to trauma; be able to comment on treatment and the likelihood of symptom relief; and know the potential for adverse effects of drugs and physical means of treatment.

Inflammatory Disorders

In clinical medical practice, inflammatory disorders are considered more important than noninflammatory disorders, as they have a significant effect on mortality and morbidity. An expert rheumatologist should be able to provide information on the natural history and variability of these conditions, and on their prognosis.

Litigation

An expert may provide a report after interviewing and conducting appropriate examinations on a claimant. This clinical assessment would usually be supplemented by examination of medical records.

In cases of work-related trauma, the occupational records may give further information about pre-accident performance and capabilities. These are sometimes important when assessing car crash or medical negligence claims.

In medical negligence claims it is sometimes necessary to give an opinion after examining the records. This opinion may form part of a preliminary assessment but also happens when there is a claim of failure of care from surviving relatives when the patient has died.

In the field of litigation, rheumatologists can provide information and opinion about the effects of trauma on the disease process. They can give an opinion on drug treatment and its likely consequences, including adverse effects.

Rheumatologists will be able to give an opinion on the standard of care; give expert guidance on disability; and recognize the potential for rehabilitation and methods used. The rheumatologists should also be well informed about physical means of treatment and the techniques of therapists providing it.

Rheumatologic Experts

Most consultant rheumatologists have a special interest, which may be broadly divided into conventional rheumatology and musculoskeletal medicine. Conventional rheumatologists may give expert opinions on more generalized disorders, such as rheumatoid disease and systemic lupus erythematosus and vasculitis. Musculoskeletal medicine specialists concentrate on noninflammatory disorders, in particular road traffic and work-related accidents producing neck or other spinal injuries and work-related upper-limb disorders (repetitive strain injury). Either group may have an interest in sports medicine or pain relief treatment.

Rheumatologists with a special interest in musculoskeletal medicine (and musculoskeletal physicians) should have expert knowledge in the field of spinal manipulation and injection. They often have personal experience in using these methods of treatment. Therefore, they may be ideally suited to prepare reports on physical methods of treatment such as

physiotherapy, osteopathy, and chiropractic. Rheumatologists who use these methods of treatment may be preferred to consultants in pain relief for preparing reports on claimants with chronic musculoskeletal pain, as they are trained in diagnosis as well as treatment. Pain relief consultants have considerable skill in treatment, but many do this based on the diagnosis made by others.

Most rheumatologists who act as expert witnesses should provide an appropriate report on inflammatory diseases. However, some experts will have a particular interest and experience in the more complex disorders. These include systemic manifestations of rheumatoid arthritis, systemic lupus erythematosus and pregnancy, and the relationship between trauma and arthritis. Other connective tissue diseases and vasculitis may be complex and sometimes require an expert with particularly specialized knowledge.

There are differences of opinion among experts on the relationship between trauma and arthritis. A significant number of rheumatologists do not accept the diagnosis of fibromyalgia. Posttraumatic fibromyalgia is even more contentious. It is reasonable in such cases to request an expert opinion on these subjects before instruction.

In medical negligence cases it may be preferable to instruct an expert working in a similar unit to the defendant.

Virtually all physical complaints have a psychological component. Rheumatologists are trained to recognize the effects of injury and disease on a person's psyche. They should also be informed about the effects of preexisting or concurrent psychological and psychiatric disorders on physical problems.

A rheumatology expert would be expected to comment on the likelihood that psychological or psychiatric factors could contribute to symptoms and disability. In particular, the expert should comment if there are complaints or physical signs that cannot be explained on a physical basis. Sometimes the rheumatologist may be able to differentiate between a psychological component or overlay, and deliberate exaggeration or malingering. Usually, this is a matter for judgment under legal examination. The rheumatologist may recommend appropriate management such as cognitive behavioral therapy. However, the expert does not provide detailed expert reports on either diagnosis or detailed management of psychiatric conditions.

Special Investigations

In noninflammatory disorders, there are no blood tests that assist with diagnosis. However, tests may be done to exclude other conditions. Failure to test

Table 1 Conditions appropriate for rheumatologic expert reports

Accidents
Ankylosing spondylitis
Arthralgia
Behçet's syndrome[a]
Brachial neuritis
Bursitis
Carpal tunnel syndrome
Cervical spondylosis and disk disorders
Complex regional pain syndrome (CRPS)[a]
CREST (Calcinosis, Raynaud's, Esophagus, Sclerodactyly, Telangiectasia)
Dermatomyositis in children[a]
Fibromyalgia
Gout
Hughes disease in pregnancy[a]
Intervertebral disk prolapse
Joint hypermobility
Juvenile arthritis[a]
Lumbar spondylosis and disk disorders
Osteoarthritis
Osteoporosis
Polymyositis
Pseudogout
Psoriatic arthritis
Raynaud syndrome
Reflex sympathetic dystrophy (RSD) – Sudeck atrophy
Rheumatoid arthritis
Road-crash injuries
Sarcoid arthritis
Sciatica
Septic arthritis
Shoulder capsulitis (frozen shoulder)
Spinal injuries
Spondylolisthesis
Spondylolysis
Sprains and strains
Systemic lupus erythematosus in pregnancy[a]
Systemic sclerosis
Tendinitis
Ulnar neuropathy
Vasculitis[a]
Wegener granuloma[a]
Work injuries
Work-related upper-limb disorders (WRULD)[a]

[a]Need for expert with special interest.

may be appropriate, but in some cases indicates negligence. The results of blood testing may be significant in inflammatory conditions. They are important in diagnosis and for monitoring disease progress and drug treatment.

There are guidelines suggesting which tests are appropriate and frequency of testing for monitoring drug therapy. These should not be taken as absolute, but a clinician would need clear reasons for not adhering to them.

Radiology may include simple X-ray films, isotope scan, computed tomography, and magnetic resonance imaging scans. Radiologists provide definitive expert reports on these investigations.

A rheumatologist interprets the findings in the clinical context. Normal films do not exclude disorder or dysfunction. Abnormalities shown may be irrelevant or even misleading.

Conditions Appropriate for Rheumatologic Expert Reports

Rheumatologic expert reports might be necessary for the conditions listed in **Table 1**.

Further Reading

Aceves-Avila FJ, Ferrari R, Ramos-Remus C (2004) New insights into culture driven disorders. Best practice and research. *Clinical Rheumatology* 18: 155–171.

Bingham SJ, Buch MU, Tennant A, *et al.* (2004) The importance of escalating conventional therapy in rheumatoid arthritis patients referred for anti-tumour necrosis factor-alpha therapy. *Rheumatology* 43: 364–368.

Harris EC, Budd RC, Firestein GS (2005) *Kelley's Textbook of Rheumatology*, 7th edn. Philadelphia, PA: Saunders.

Hutson MA (1997) *Work-Related Upper Limb Disorders*. Oxford, UK: Butterworth-Heinemann.

Maddison PJ, Isenberg DA, Woo P, *et al.* (1998) *Oxford Textbook of Rheumatology*, 2nd edn. Oxford, UK: Oxford University Press.

Ombregt L, Bisshop P, *et al.* (2003) *A System of Orthopaedic Medicine*, 2nd edn. London: WB Saunders.

www.rheumatology.org.uk (publications/library – guidelines; information on drug monitoring).

Vascular Surgery

W B Campbell, Royal Devon and Exeter Hospital, Exeter, UK

Introduction

Vascular surgery is the discipline which deals with peripheral arteries and veins. Throughout the world it is largely distinct from cardiac surgery, but vascular surgeons vary in the extent to which they deal with blood vessels in the thorax. In many countries, general surgeons still undertake small numbers of vascular procedures. There is a well-documented trend for poorer results from low-volume practice, which is likely to present a higher risk of medicolegal problems, particularly for surgeons working outside specialist groups.

Variation in the practice of vascular surgeons with regard to venous disease is important, because this is a major area for medicolegal activity. Many vascular surgeons deal largely with arterial work, which has traditionally been regarded as more serious and more challenging. This is reflected in the jargon "peripheral vascular disease," which is commonly used to refer only to arterial disease. Varicose veins (which are very common) have therefore often been dealt with by somewhat reluctant arterial specialists, by their trainees, and by nonspecialist general surgeons. This kind of approach is not universal and is gradually changing, but it has contributed to the high rate of medicolegal actions for treatment of varicose veins.

The margins and scope of vascular surgery as a specialty have become increasingly blurred by rapid dissemination of minimally invasive techniques such as angioplasty, stenting, and stent grafting. These techniques demand either a team approach (with interventional radiologists) or the acquisition of new skills: they can also precipitate "turf wars" between different specialties (including some cardiologists who engage in peripheral arterial work). All this can provide fertile ground for controversy and medicolegal problems.

Difficulties in Describing the Frequency of Medicolegal Claims

There are a number of difficulties in describing the numbers of medicolegal claims in any medical specialty, particularly for an international readership.

- Terminology varies, from the American use of "malpractice" to the fundamental British legal principle of "negligence." In this article the term "claim" will be used for a legal action against a doctor or hospital.
- Medicolegal claims may be initiated (or notified) but subsequently discontinued because they have no merit; they may be settled without admission of negligence or liability; or (in a minority) there may be a judgment that the responsible clinicians were indeed negligent. Any collation of claims must make clear which of these categories is being described.
- Some countries have seen considerable changes in the organizations dealing with claims. In the UK, for example, claims in private practice are dealt with by three defense societies. National Health Service (NHS) claims (the majority) were handled similarly until 1990; then at regional level until 1995; and since 1995 by a central litigation authority (even then, many smaller claims were still handled locally).

- There is no central database of claims in many countries so doctors have no way of knowing the details for their specialty.
- The scope of "vascular surgery" may be poorly defined in any review of medicolegal activity (does it include vascular surgeons only, general surgeons, arterial work only, amputation, varicose veins?).

Vascular Surgery Compared with Other Specialties

Arterial and amputation surgery is often required for patients who are elderly, who have multiple comorbidities, and whose arteries present difficult technical challenges. The incidence of adverse events is therefore high: 16% in the Harvard Medical Practice Study – higher than any other specialty. Aortic aneurysm repair and lower-limb bypass grafting had higher adverse event rates than any other operations in a study of 15 000 hospital admissions in Utah and Colorado, which judged 8% and 11%, respectively, of the adverse events to have been preventable. The Australasian Quality in Healthcare Study judged 49% adverse events in vascular surgery to be preventable. By implication, clinicians might be liable medicolegally for these events, but the Harvard study considered only 18% of the adverse events in vascular surgery to be due to negligence – a lower proportion than any other specialty studied.

Vascular Claims in the UK

The first collation of vascular claims in the UK was done in collaboration with the NHS Litigation Authority (using the data since its inception in 1995) and the Medical Defence Union (which handles the majority of private practice claims, using its data since 1990). The number of notified claims (claims notified to the defense organizations, but not settled or closed) was higher for varicose veins (244: 58%) than for treatment of arterial disease (174: 42%). Other data from the Medical Defence Union have shown that claims relating to varicose veins outnumber those for any other condition dealt with by vascular or general surgeons. Reasons for claims relating to varicose veins are shown in **Table 1**. The main reasons for claims relating to treatment of arterial disease are shown in **Table 2**.

The Medical Defence Union also indemnifies general practitioners (primary care physicians) and had on record 299 notified claims relating to vascular surgical problems during 1990–1999. Two-thirds alleged that mismanagement of limb ischemia resulted in amputation (80%) or death (16%) and one-third

Table 1 Notified claims (legal actions initiated) against surgeons in the UK relating to treatment of varicose veins. Surgeons were classified as "vascular" or "general" on the basis of the information they gave when notifying each claim. These claims cover the period 1990–1999, when much vascular surgery was done by "general surgeons with a vascular interest." The subdivision does, however, give some indication of the degree of specialization, and the proportions of claims contrast with those for arterial work (**Table 2**)

	Vascular surgeons	General surgeons	Total
Nerve damage	22	54	76
Incorrect/inadequate/ unsatisfactory surgery	11	25	36
Discoloration/scarring after sclerotherapy	5	16	21
Femoral vein damage	2	14	16
Infection	0	15	15
Femoral artery damage	3	10	13
Deep-vein thrombosis	5	6	11
Tourniquet damage	4	1	5
Miscellaneous	11	40	51
Total	63	181	244

From Campbell WB *et al.* (2002) Medicolegal claims in vascular surgery. *Annals of Royal College of Surgeons of England* 84: 181–184. Copyright the Royal College of Surgeons of England. Reproduced with permission.

Table 2 Claims relating to management of arterial disease notified by surgeons in the UK during 1990–1999 (see additional information in the legend to **Table 1**)

	Vascular surgeons	General surgeons	Total
Complications of aortic surgery	24	21	45
Failure to recognize/treat ischemia	27	9	36
Bypass grafting problems	22	6	28
Nerve damage at operation	9	7	16
Failure to diagnose/treat aneurysms	2	8	10
Miscellaneous/unclear	23	16	39
Total	107	67	174

From Campbell WB *et al.* (2002) Medicolegal claims in vascular surgery. *Annals of Royal College of Surgeons of England* 84: 181–184. Copyright the Royal College of Surgeons of England. Reproduced with permission.

alleged misdiagnosis of aneurysms. Vascular specialists therefore receive a significant number of referrals in which diagnosis has been delayed and this prompts legal action. Even though the underlying delay was not theirs, their management of the patient may be scrutinized aggressively during legal proceedings.

Treatments for Cosmetic Problems and "Lifestyle" Symptoms

Vascular surgery provides a good example of treatments for a range of conditions of different severity,

with inherently different medicolegal risks. At one extreme many patients with varicose veins request treatment for cosmetic reasons only. Even minor complications may therefore cause dissatisfaction and lead to legal action. The most common is sensory nerve damage – specifically damage to the sural nerve during short saphenous surgery. Very thorough explanation and counseling about the likely benefits and potential risks are essential (and this ought to include written information). Trainees are taught two aphorisms: "The patient's expectations should be the same as yours" and "The smallest veins can cause the biggest problems."

Treatment of intermittent claudication is a major part of the work of vascular specialists: it restricts walking ability, which is inconvenient but not medically dangerous. Use of bypass grafting to relieve symptoms carries a risk of significant complications, including failure or infection of grafts and limb loss. If these possibilities are not dealt with thoroughly during decision-making, there may be great difficulty defending a legal action if one occurs. In addition, medical control of risk factors is fundamental for patients with arterial occlusive disease, and vascular surgeons should beware of failing to advise patients about medical measures to prevent myocardial infarction or stroke. In an increasingly litigious world they may face legal action if they do not do so and a patient goes on to suffer such an event.

Treatments to Save Life or Limb

At the other extreme, patients with leaking aortic aneurysms are often in great pain, hypotensive, and, without an operation, they will die imminently. Any kind of detailed counseling is out of the question, and discussion of the many risks of surgery is both medically and pastorally inappropriate. Involvement of relatives is important, and this may include discussions about palliative care.

Patients with critical limb ischemia need limb salvage procedures or major amputation. Some of them are frightened, elderly patients who do not want to know about all the risks. That is their right (under British law) but it should always be assumed that they want to be informed until they state otherwise. If patients have asked specifically not to be told about the risks of treatment then the situation must be clearly recorded in their case notes.

Some patients with unsalvageable limbs or leaking aneurysms may be treated most humanely with good analgesia and terminal care. The cultural approach to this decision varies between countries, as do the medicolegal implications. In the USA, for example, relatives more often expect heroic treatment for the dying than in the UK. In a survey of UK vascular surgeons only 22% were influenced by medicolegal concerns when making the decision not to operate on a patient with a leaking aortic aneurysm.

Prophylactic Interventions

Many vascular interventions (in particular, elective treatment of aortic aneurysms and treatment of carotid artery stenoses) are prophylactic. They guard against serious risks – aneurysm rupture causing death or cerebral embolism causing stroke – but nevertheless, procedures are done on people who feel quite well and who are usually asymptomatic. These procedures have potentially very serious risks and absolutely clear discussion (accompanied by written information and well recorded) is essential to defend subsequent claims for negligence if adverse outcomes occur. It is particularly important to involve relatives in discussion, not least because it is they who may sue if the patient dies or suffers a disabling stroke.

Involving Relatives

Involving relatives is always good practice and helps to protect against legal action, as described in the sections above, but there are national differences in the legal requirements to do so. In the USA relatives have some legal rights to be informed and to participate in decision-making. This contrasts with the UK, where only the patient can give consent. If the patient is incapable, then it is the duty of doctors to act in the patient's best interests. The relatives have no legal right to participate in the consent.

Special Aspects of Risk Management in Vascular Surgery

Written Information and Records

These tenets are basic, but so important they are worth rehearsing. Written information, including a thorough description of benefits and risks, should be given to all patients considering vascular interventions. This information must be recorded in the notes and copies of the information must be archived for future legal use. Explicit letters about decision-making can be copied to patients. Letters are helpful in the consent process and provide a good record that the patient was well informed. These considerations are particularly important when the patient is being managed by more than one discipline – for example, vascular surgery, vascular radiology, vascular medicine, and anesthesiology. Comprehensive medical and nursing notes and prescription charts are indispensable as evidence.

Guidelines and Protocols

Guidelines and protocols are common in some countries, but less so in others. They are particularly important for ward-based treatments such as thrombolysis, in which a variety of staff are involved, some of whom may be unfamiliar with management. It is worth pointing out, however, that guidelines and protocols are not legally binding. There may be good reasons to depart from them for particular patients, but this should always be clearly recorded.

Prophylaxis

Omission of prophylactic antibiotics (to protect against graft infection) or of prophylactic anticoagulants (to reduce the risk of thrombosis) are particular matters which feature in medicolegal proceedings. There is little defense for having neglected antibiotics if a graft becomes infected, but scientific evidence is poor about the requisite number of doses.

Clear evidence is still more elusive about anticoagulant prophylaxis, and this may cause legal argument. There is no compelling evidence that heparin protects against arterial thrombosis during or soon after procedures, although it is usual practice and would be recommended by most experts. Anticoagulant prophylaxis against venous thromboembolism in varicose vein surgery is also a dilemma. Varicose veins feature in national and international guidelines as a risk factor for deep-vein thrombosis, but thrombosis after varicose vein surgery is uncommon and use of prophylaxis varies considerably. It is in areas like this that the results of large surveys of surgical practice may help to provide evidence which can be used in legal proceedings.

Summary

Vascular surgery is associated with many adverse events and has great potential for medicolegal action. Treatment of varicose veins is particularly prone to litigation. The keys to risk management and robust defense are thorough counseling of patients and their relatives; attention to detail (such as routine prophylaxis against infection); and meticulous record-keeping.

See Also

Medical Malpractice – Medico-legal Perspectives: Negligence, Standard of Care; Negligence, Duty of Care; Negligence, Causation

Further Reading

Adamson TE, Baldwin DC, Sheehan TJ, Oppenberg AA (1997) Characteristics of surgeons with high and low malpractice claims rates. *Western Medical Journal* 166: 37–44.

Brennan TA, Leape LL, Laird NM, *et al.* (1991) Incidence of adverse events and negligence in hospitalized patients. *New England Journal of Medicine* 324: 370–376.

Campbell WB, Ridler BMF (1995) Varicose veins and deep vein thrombosis. *British Journal of Surgery* 82: 1494–1497.

Campbell WB, France F, Goodwin HM, on behalf of the Research and Audit Committee of the Vascular Surgical Society of Great Britain and Ireland (2002) Medicolegal claims in vascular surgery. *Annals of the Royal College of Surgeons of England* 84: 181–184.

Gawande AA, Thomas EJ, Zinner MJ, Brennan TA (1999) The incidence and nature of surgical adverse events in Colorado and Utah in 1992. *Surgery* 126: 66–75.

Hewin DF, Campbell WB (1998) Ruptured aortic aneurysm: the decision not to operate. *Annals of the Royal College of Surgeons of England* 80: 221–225.

Michaels J, Palfreyman S, Wood R (2001) Evidence-based guidelines for the configuration of vascular services. *Journal of Clinical Excellence* 3: 145–153.

Wilson RM, Runciman WB, Gibberd RW, *et al.* (1995) The quality in Australian health care study. *Medical Journal of Australia* 163: 458–471.

MEDICAL MALPRACTICE – MEDICO-LEGAL PERSPECTIVES

Contents

Negligence, Standard of Care

M Flynn, Nova Southeastern University, Fort Lauderdale, FL, USA

Introduction

Medical malpractice is the term commonly used to describe negligence on the part of a doctor, hospital, or other medical care provider. Although medical malpractice may also include the legal liability of medical care providers for intentional misconduct, medical malpractice usually refers to medical negligence. Negligence is the legal doctrine that imposes liability for failing to use adequate care. Therefore, medical negligence can be defined as the failure to exercise adequate care in the delivery of medical care and treatment.

Negligence in General

Any discussion of medical malpractice, medical negligence, must begin with defining the tort of negligence. Tort, taken from the French word *tortum*, means a wrongful act. The tort of negligence refers to the type of wrongful act that falls below the standard of care required to protect others against an unreasonable risk of harm. There are four requirements to make a legal claim for negligence against a potential defendant:

1. The potential defendant must possess a duty to exercise reasonable care
2. The potential defendant must breach the duty to exercise reasonable care
3. The potential defendant's breach of the duty to exercise reasonable care must be the proximate cause of injury to another – the potential plaintiff
4. The potential plaintiff must sustain a legally cognizable injury.

The potential plaintiff in a negligence claim has the burden of proving all four of these elements in any kind of negligence claim. The potential plaintiff's burden of proof requires that all four elements of negligence be proven by a preponderance of the evidence. The preponderance of the evidence burden requires that the potential plaintiff introduce enough proof to show that it is more likely than not that each of the four elements of a negligence claim is true. Failure to prove with a preponderance of the evidence each of the four elements of a negligence claim will be fatal to that negligence claim.

The four elements of a negligence claim and the burden of proof requirement for a negligence claim apply equally to a medical negligence claim.

The Application of Negligence to Medical Care and Treatment

The application of the legal elements of a negligence claim to medical care and treatment requires a specific application and analysis of the duty, breach of duty, proximate cause, and injury elements.

The Existence of a Duty to Exercise Reasonable Care

In a medical negligence claim, "duty" refers to the obligation imposed by law on a medical care provider to act or refrain from acting in such a way that a patient is exposed to an unreasonable risk of injury. This "duty" element is akin to that portion of the Hippocratic oath, which states, "First, do no harm." It is important to note that the law imposes a duty on a medical care provider to protect a patient from an unreasonable risk of injury. This is particularly important because medical care and treatment often involve some risk of injury or harm to the patient. It is only the unreasonable risk of injury that the law of medical negligence concerns.

The law imposes a duty on a medical care provider upon proof of the existence of the medical care provider–patient relationship. In the absence of the establishment of the medical care provider–patient relationship, the law will not impose a legal duty on a medical care provider.

The medical care provider–patient relationship can be established in a number of ways. A consensual agreement, either oral or written, between a medical care provider and a patient to furnish medical care and treatment will establish the medical care provider–patient relationship. This describes the classic relationship established between a doctor or hospital and a patient who seeks medical care and treatment under a health insurance contract. Likewise, even in the absence of an expressed agreement, the medical care provider–patient relationship can be established when the medical care provider undertakes to render medical care and treatment to a patient. This describes the myriad of circumstances, including medical care and treatment dispensed in an emergency department of a hospital, in which

a medical care provider offers medical care and treatment to a patient.

The trademark of a medical care provider–patient relationship is that it is a voluntary professional relationship. In the absence of some other legal obligation imposed by statute or otherwise, a medical care provider can refuse and a patient can decline to enter into a medical care provider–patient relationship. In addition, the medical care provider–patient relationship is not everlasting; it may be terminated by mutual agreement of the medical care provider and the patient or may just end because the medical care and treatment concluded.

Upon the establishment of the medical care provider–patient relationship, the law imposes a duty on the medical care provider to protect the patient from an unreasonable risk of harm. To do this, the law then characterizes the medical care provider's duty as a duty to exercise reasonable care. The rationale is that if a medical care provider uses reasonable care in dispensing medical care and treatment, then the patient might not be exposed to any risk of harm or at worst, only the reasonable risk of harm intrinsic to the medical care and treatment supplied.

The Breach of the Duty to Exercise Reasonable Care

While the existence of a duty to exercise reasonable care is a question of law, whether a medical care provider breached the duty to exercise reasonable care is a question of fact.

The standard of care   The standard of care by which medical care providers will be judged is what a reasonably prudent, similar medical care provider would do in the same or similar circumstances. It is important to note that the standard of care described does not measure a medical care provider by what a "preeminent" or a "foremost" or even an "excellent" medical care provider would do. Rather, the standard of care looks to the "reasonably prudent" medical care provider. The reasonably prudent medical care provider is not unerring or infallible but also is not careless or incompetent. The standard demands a medical care provider to be ordinary – an ordinary, competent, attentive professional. Note also that ordinary does not mean the same thing as average – average would mean that half of the medical care providers breach the standard of care daily. On the contrary, all medical care providers, theoretically, can comply with the standard of care of a reasonably prudent medical care provider daily. For example, a reasonably prudent medical care provider may decide that a patient's leg needs to be amputated but a reasonably prudent medical care provider would not amputate the wrong leg.

The standard of care is an objective, not a subjective standard. A medical care provider's "good faith" in attempting to furnish medical care and treatment is not dispositive. Likewise, the fact that a medical care provider was well intentioned or performed the best he/she could is not relevant. The conduct of a medical care provider will always be judged by the standard of what a reasonably prudent similar medical care provider would do in the same or similar circumstances.

The objective standard of care raises another analytical issue. For example, what effect does "customary" medical care and treatment have on this standard? U.S. Justice Oliver Wendell Holmes perhaps expressed it best when he wrote that custom may describe what ought to be done, but what ought to be done must always be judged by what a reasonably prudent person would do under the circumstances. Translated and applied to medical negligence, this means that customary medical care and treatment may satisfy the standard of care, but only if the customary medical care and treatment are what a reasonably prudent medical care provider would do under the same or similar circumstances.

Another feature of this objective standard of care is that conduct of a medical care provider takes into account the same or similar circumstances in which the medical care and treatment is provided. At first blush, this "same or similar circumstances" language may appear to permit the subjectivity of the circumstances to impact the standard of care. However, this language precisely defines the parameter within which the objective standard of care will be analyzed. Therefore, rather than creeping subjectivity into the standard of care for medical care providers, this provision sharpens the objectivity of the standard of care.

Finally, historically, the geographic location of the medical care provider would seem to qualify as a "circumstance" that needs to be accounted for in the standard of care. In fact, many statutes specifically state that a medical care provider should be judged by the standard of a reasonably prudent medical care provider in the same locality. The "locality rule" is a vestige from the time when rural doctors, isolated from the latest medical treatment breakthroughs and medical facilities, needed relief from being judged by the standard of care applicable to doctors who had access to the latest and best medical treatment and facilities. At least in the USA the need for the locality rule has somewhat evaporated because of the speed at which information and people and facilities can be accessed. However, in those places where the locality rule retains some vitality, it further defines the parameter of the objective standard of care applicable to medical care providers.

Proof of the applicable standard of care   The applicable standard of care for medical care providers divides into two categories: the standard applied to medical care specialists and nonspecialists. The line between these two categories can be blurry, especially since general practitioners and family practitioners may now be considered "specialists." However, this distinction still holds in many instances. For example, a doctor trained in organ transplant surgery engages in a very different kind of medical practice to a primary care physician.

In either the instance of a medical care provider who is a specialist or a nonspecialist, proof of the standard of care is required before determining if there has been a breach of the standard of care. Proof of the standard of care comes in many forms. Usually such proof must come from an expert; another similar medical care provider. However, in some circumstances, proof of what a reasonably prudent similar medical care provider would do under the same or similar circumstances does not require expert testimony at all. Proof of the standard of care may be a matter of common knowledge. For example, perhaps expert testimony is not required when the medical care provider's alleged breach of the standard of care amounts to a failure to apply an antiseptic to an open cut. It may just be a matter of common knowledge that part of the required treatment for an open cut is the application of some kind of antiseptic to prevent infection.

Another instance where expert testimony may not be needed to establish the standard of care is when an authoritative medical reference book states the standard of care. Proof acceptable to a court that the medical reference book relied on is authoritative permits the court to consider the standard of care applicable to a medical care provider is as stated in the text. In other instances, the standard of care for a medical care provider may be stated in a statute or other legislative or administrative enactment. Here, the court will be bound to adopt this statutory enactment as the standard of care applicable to a medical care provider.

Aside from these instances where common knowledge or a medical text or a statute prescribe the standard of care, the testimony of an expert witness is critical to establishing the standard of care applicable to the medical care provider. This "expert" is more than likely also a medical care provider with the same or similar training, experience, and knowledge as the medical care provider who is the target of the medical negligence claim. In fact, if the expert does not closely mirror in training, experience, and knowledge the medical care provider who is the subject of the medical negligence claim, most courts will disqualify the expert from testifying as to the standard of care. Yet, even if the expert qualifies to testify, there is a professional reluctance to act as an expert witness in a medical negligence case against a colleague. This reluctance, referred to as a "conspiracy of silence," stems from a feeling of not being disloyal to fellow medical care providers and from being blacklisted by colleagues. However, it is not as difficult to convince a colleague to act as an expert witness in the defense of a medical negligence claim. Despite this reluctance, there are medical care providers whose entire medical practice consists of acting as expert witnesses in medical negligence lawsuits. Therefore, the tough task for the plaintiff-patient is to find not only an expert, but a credible expert.

The final method of proving the standard of care applicable to a medical care provider uses the legal doctrine of *res ipsa loquitur*. The doctrine of *res ipsa loquitur*, Latin for "the thing speaks for itself," infers a breach of duty from what happened. The remarkable aspect of a *res ipsa loquitur*-based claim is the lack of evidence that explains how the person was injured. Rather, in a *res ipsa loquitur*-based case, the injury cannot be explained except that such an injury does not ordinarily occur unless someone breached the duty to exercise reasonable care.

Application of the *res ipsa loquitur* doctrine is a question of law decided by the judge. The three requirements for the doctrine of *res ipsa loquitur* to apply are:

1. The injury that occurred to the plaintiff does not ordinarily occur unless someone breaches the duty to exercise reasonable care
2. The occurrence or instrumentality that apparently caused the injury was within the exclusive control of the potential defendant
3. The plaintiff did not contribute to the occurrence that produced the injury.

The doctrine of *res ipsa loquitur* can apply in a medical negligence claim. For example, suppose a patient undergoes abdominal surgery only to find out later that a piece of surgical material, like a sponge, was left inside the patient's body. Without direct evidence, a patient would be able to argue that: (1) a sponge or, for that matter, other surgical material is not ordinarily left inside a patient's body after surgery unless somebody breached the duty to exercise reasonable care; (2) the surgeon was in control of the surgery; and (3) the anesthetized patient did not contribute to leaving the sponge or other surgical material in the patient's body. In this instance, the patient could use the *res ipsa loquitur* inference to prove the surgeon's breach of duty.

The effect of proving a medical care provider's breach of duty through the use of the *res ipsa loquitur* inference is that a judge or jury has the option to accept or decline to accept the inference of the breach of duty. Proof of the breach of duty of a medical care provider by use of the *res ipsa loquitur* inference is not conclusive or binding on the jury or judge in a medical negligence lawsuit.

Although proof of the existence of a duty to exercise reasonable care and that a medical care provider has breached that duty to exercise reasonable care is commonly referred to as negligence, such proof is only half of a negligence claim.

Proximate Causation

To medical malpractice lawyers, the issue of causation, that is, whether the medical care provider's breach of duty is the proximate cause of injury to a patient, is the most critical requirement of a negligence claim. A medical care provider may violate the standard of care but if such breach does not cause injury, then the medical care provider's violation of the standard of care is not legally blameworthy – no harm, no foul!

The legal concept of proximate cause is really two causes in one: (1) cause in fact; and (2) legal cause. Both of these concepts are designed to ensure that the medical care provider's breach of duty is a substantial factor in the patient being injured.

Cause in fact is the legal term for cause and effect. The key to cause in fact is to show that "but for" the medical care provider's breach of the duty to exercise reasonable care, the injury to the patient would not have occurred. This test for cause in fact ensures a close connection between the injury to the patient and the breach of duty by a medical care provider. Although the statement of the legal test for cause in fact seems simple, proof of cause in fact in a medical malpractice claim is anything but simple.

Just as in the requirement of proof of a breach of standard of care, and perhaps even more, the proof of cause in fact rests in the hands of an expert witness. There may be some instances when proof of cause in fact may not require expert testimony, but this is rare. Therefore, the task of the plaintiff-patient is to find a qualified medical care provider to testify against a fellow medical care provider and have that expert say that more likely than not, but for the breach of duty by the fellow medical care provider, the injury to the patient would not have occurred. This can be a daunting task, not only because the medical analysis may be difficult, but also because finding a willing expert may be troublesome.

Even if a plaintiff-patient is successful in meeting the burden of proving cause in fact, the plaintiff-patient must also prove that the medical care provider's breach of duty is the legal cause of the patient's injury. Proof of legal cause hinges on establishing that the patient's injury falls within the foreseeable risk created by the medical care provider's breach of the standard of care. This kind of inquiry considers the "zone of danger" created by the medical care provider's breach of the standard of care. Questions of remoteness of time and space and distance can remove a patient's injury from the foreseeable "zone of danger" created by the medical care provider's breach of the duty to exercise reasonable care. For example, the existence of a preexisting condition or injury may mitigate proving that the current condition or injury suffered by the patient was caused in fact and legally caused by the medical care provider's breach of duty.

If a plaintiff-patient can successfully prove that, more likely than not, the medical care provider's breach of the standard of care is the cause in fact and legal cause of the patient's injury, then the medical care provider is the proximate cause of the patient's injury.

Legally Cognizable Injury

The last requirement of a negligence claim is proof of a legally recognized injury to the plaintiff-patient caused by the medical care provider. The sole purpose of a successful medical negligence claim – for that matter all tort claims – is for the "at fault" defendant to pay adequate money damages to the injured plaintiff. Tort law is not equipped to do anything else. In the context of medical negligence, an at-fault medical care provider may never be able to undo the physical and emotional harm suffered by an injured patient. Therefore, tort law in general and medical malpractice law in particular relies on the proposition that compensation awarded to a injured patient will provide some reparation for the loss suffered from the medical care providers who are at fault.

Money damages awarded to an injured patient can be divided into three types: (1) damages for economic loss; (2) damages for noneconomic loss; and (3) punitive damages.

Damages for economic loss include past, present, and future out-of-pocket expenses that a patient has incurred and will incur. These include medical expenses and wage or other income loss. Damages for noneconomic loss include past, present, and future damages for physical pain, emotional, and mental suffering, disfigurement, disability, and impairment of a patient's ability to enjoy life. Punitive damages, sometimes called exemplary damages, are damages awarded to punish an at-fault defendant. Although they are not authorized in all states, the assessment of punitive damages against a defendant is designed to act as an incentive to the defendant and other similarly situated potential defendants to refrain from engaging in certain kinds of conduct. Punitive damages are only awarded for conduct that goes beyond ordinary negligence.

Conclusion

Controversy abounds over the efficiency, effectiveness, and fairness of the tort law system in the USA, and medical malpractice claims are at the center of this debate. The rising cost of medical care and treatment impacts the amount of money awarded in successful medical malpractice lawsuits, the cost of medical malpractice insurance for medical care providers, and the profits of insurance companies. Tort reform proposals have focused on capping noneconomic damage awards and making it more difficult for injured patients to sue medical care providers. However, any reform of the tort system, especially medical malpractice litigation, must be careful not to abandon or disadvantage patients injured by the negligent act of a medical care provider. No system will be efficient, effective, and fair if the medical care provider who is at fault is not required to take the full amount of responsibility for injuring a patient.

See Also

Medical Malpractice – Medico-legal Perspectives: Negligence, Duty of Care; Negligence, Causation; Negligence Quantum

Further Reading

Dobbs D (2000) *The Law of Torts*. St. Paul, MN: West Group.

Furrow B, Greaney T, Johnson S, Jost T, Schwartz R (2001) *Health Law*, 4th edn. St. Paul, MN: West Group.

Jacobs H (1978) *The Spectre of Malpractice*. New York: Nationwide Press.

McClellan F (1994) *Medical Malpractice*. Philadelphia, PA: Temple University Press.

Prosser W, Wade J, Schwartz V (2000) *Torts*, 10th edn. New York: Foundation Press.

Weiler P, Hiatt H, Newhouse J, *et al.* (1993) *A Measure of Malpractice*. Cambridge, MA: Harvard University Press.

Zobel H, Rous S (1993) *Doctors and The Law*. New York: W.W. Norton.

Negligence, Duty of Care

M Flynn, Nova Southeastern University,
Fort Lauderdale, FL, USA

Introduction

Medical malpractice is the term commonly used to describe negligence on the part of a doctor, hospital, or other medical care provider. Although medical malpractice may also include the legal liability of medical care providers for intentional misconduct, medical malpractice usually refers to medical negligence. Negligence is the legal doctrine that imposes liability for failing to use adequate care. Therefore, medical negligence can be defined as the failure to exercise adequate care in the delivery of medical care and treatment.

Negligence in General

Any discussion of medical malpractice and medical negligence must begin with defining the tort of negligence. Tort, taken from the French word *tortum*, means a wrongful act. The tort of negligence refers to the type of wrongful act that falls below the standard of care required to protect others against an unreasonable risk of harm. There are four requirements to make out a legal claim for negligence against a potential defendant:

1. the potential defendant must possess a duty to exercise reasonable care
2. the potential defendant must breach the duty to exercise reasonable care
3. the potential defendant's breach of the duty to exercise reasonable care must be the proximate cause of injury to another – the potential plaintiff
4. the potential plaintiff must sustain a legally cognizable injury.

The potential plaintiff in a negligence claim has the burden of proving all four of these elements in any kind of negligence claim. The potential plaintiff's burden of proof requires that all four elements of negligence be proven by a preponderance of the evidence. The preponderance of the evidence burden requires that the potential plaintiff introduce enough proof to show that it is more likely than not that each of the four elements of a negligence claim is true. Failure to prove with a preponderance of the evidence each of the four elements of a negligence claim will be fatal to that negligence claim.

The four elements of a negligence claim and the burden of proof requirement for a negligence claim apply equally to a medical negligence claim.

The Application of Negligence to Medical Care and Treatment

The application of the legal elements of a negligence claim to medical care and treatment requires a specific application and analysis of the duty, breach of duty, proximate cause, and injury elements. This article will focus on the duty of care element of a medical negligence claim.

The Existence of a Duty to Exercise Reasonable Care

In a medical negligence claim, "duty" refers to the obligation imposed by law on a medical care provider to act or refrain from acting in such a way that a patient's medical condition is appropriately diagnosed and managed so that a patient is not exposed to an unreasonable risk of injury. This "duty" element translates into a duty to exercise reasonable care. Therefore, by law, a medical care provider bears the burden of the duty to exercise reasonable care in dispensing medical care and treatment. The key inquiry is to pinpoint, as well as possible, when this duty of a medical care provider to exercise reasonable care arises and what exactly is meant by the duty of a medical care provider to exercise reasonable care.

The Duty of Care – When the Duty of Care Applies

In a traditional negligence claim, the duty to exercise reasonable care arises upon proof that the potential defendant's conduct creates a foreseeable risk of harm. The risk of harm necessary for the law to impose the duty to exercise reasonable care requires proof that the likelihood and severity of the harm from the potential defendant's conduct are greater than the cost to the potential defendant to refrain or prevent the harm from occurring. Although it is a somewhat formalistic approach to the analysis of when a duty of care arises, this formula accurately highlights the key factors courts look at to determine as a matter of law if a duty of care applies.

In the context of a physician's duty to exercise reasonable care, this formula gives way to an analysis of the physician–patient relationship. The physician's duty to exercise reasonable care arises on establishment of the physician–patient relationship. It is this relationship that imposes or creates the physician's duty to exercise reasonable care.

When the physician–patient relationship is established can be a somewhat tricky question. Usually, the physician–patient relationship is based on an agreement by a physician to provide medical treatment to a patient. This agreement or contract between a physician and a patient can be expressed in some kind of written document or implied by the physician's act of providing medical treatment to a willing patient. The hallmark of a physician–patient relationship is privity of contract; that is the physician's agreement to provide medical treatment to a specific patient and the patient's willingness to accept medical treatment from a specific physician. However, this privity of contract can also be established by implication. For example, when a patient shows up at the emergency room of a hospital or visits a medical clinic or keeps an appointment at a physician's office, the physician, without a formal written contract to provide medical care to the patient, who then provides medical treatment to that patient creates a physician–patient relationship.

Advancement in technology, especially teleconferencing and internet websites, offers other opportunities for the physician–patient relationship to be created. The expert surgeon who is teleconferenced into the operating room from another part of the world and who offers medical advice and consultation during the surgical procedure establishes a physician–patient relationship with that surgery patient. In addition, the physician who operates an interactive or a passive website may create a physician–patient relationship with visitors to the website.

Complicating this seemingly simple question of establishing the physician–patient relationship is the rise of managed healthcare and the health maintenance organizations (HMOs). These contract-based health insurance programs provide a list of physicians from which patients enrolled in the program can select for medical treatment. Whether a physician–patient relationship is established just by the listed physicians and enrolled patients contractually agreeing to this managed healthcare arrangement, especially in the case where a listed physician refuses to treat an enrolled patient, is just another layer of issues surrounding the establishment of a physician–patient relationship.

The key factor in resolving these questions is to remember that the purpose of looking at when a physician–patient relationship is created is to pinpoint when the law will impose upon a physician the duty to exercise reasonable care. Most likely the mere signing of a contract or accepting a patient's request for an appointment will not create a sufficient physician–patient relationship to saddle a physician with a legal duty to exercise reasonable care. In addition, even in the absence of a contract or a patient appointment, as soon as a physician "lays hands" on a patient or provides other medical treatment, the physician–patient relationship will be established, with the accompanying legal duty, on the part of the physician, to exercise reasonable care.

The law of medical negligence has carved out some exceptions to the traditional privity of contract requirement needed to establish the physician–patient relationship. Most notably, these exceptions cover the physician who is providing psychiatric care to a patient or treating a patient with a contagious disease. In the context of psychiatric care, the physician will not only possess a legal duty to exercise reasonable care to the patient being treated but also to other third parties in certain circumstances. Many state laws and judicial opinions extend this physician's duty of care to identifiable third parties who may be harmed by the patient receiving psychiatric care. In this kind of circumstance, the physician may have the legal duty to warn persons identified by the patient as targets for physical injury. Likewise, the physician who is treating a patient for a contagious disease, like hepatitis or a sexually transmitted disease, may also have a legal duty to warn persons known to the physician to have been exposed to the disease. The reason for extending the physician's duty beyond the patient being treated in these circumstances is a concern for public health and well-being.

In summary, determining when the physician–patient relationship exists is not a particularly difficult question – it exists when the physician and patient either expressly or implicitly agree to enter into the physician–patient relationship. However, technological advancement in the delivery of medical treatment and public health and welfare concerns do impact and will continue to impact the establishment of the physician–patient relationship.

The Duty of Care – The Physician's Duty to Exercise Reasonable Care

Once the physician–patient relationship is established, from which the law will impose on the physician the duty to exercise reasonable care in dispensing medical treatment to the patient, the next inquiry is to determine what exactly is the reasonable care required of physicians. The classic answer to this legal question is, "it depends." The kind of physician and the nature of the medical treatment provided will dictate what amounts to reasonable care.

The law of medical negligence, either in statute or judicial opinion, is incapable of defining with particularity the duty owed a patient by a physician. Therefore, most state laws and judicial opinions define the physician's duty of care to be what a reasonably prudent physician with the requisite training and skill would do in the same or similar circumstances.

In determining what a reasonably prudent physician would do in particular circumstances, the type of physician makes a difference. Most state laws divide physicians into two categories: the specialist physician and the general practice physician. Consequently, the duty of care attached to a specialist physician would be the level of care of a reasonably prudent physician with the requisite training and skill in a specific medical specialty. Likewise, the duty of care connected to a general practice physician would be the level of care of a reasonably prudent physician with the requisite training and skill in the general practice of medicine. For example, an orthopedic surgeon or a neurologist would be considered a physician specialist while a primary care physician may not.

However, with the advancement of medical education, this distinction between the physician specialist and the general practice physician has become blurred. Many medical schools not only train students in the traditional medical specialties but also offer specialized training in family or general practice medicine. This merger of the distinction between physician specialists and general practice physicians clouds the analysis of the duty of care required of a particular type of physician. To handle this breakdown of physician categories, many state laws focus on the type of treatment provided by a physician rather than the type of physician providing the treatment. For example, if an orthopedic surgeon is not performing orthopedic surgery but rather is providing the medical treatment of a pediatrician, then the orthopedic surgeon's duty of care must match the level of care provided by a reasonably prudent pediatrician in the same or similar circumstances. Likewise, the family practice physician who is performing orthopedic surgery will be judged by the duty of care required by a reasonably prudent orthopedic surgeon in the same or similar circumstances.

By adapting the duty of care to medical treatment provided by the physician, state laws insure that a patient will receive the appropriate level of care for the medical treatment provided. In addition, because of this adaptation of the duty of care required of a physician, many physicians are hesitant, with good reason, to provide medical treatment that is outside their medical training. Consequently, patients can take some comfort in knowing that the physician who is providing medical treatment will be legally measured against a reasonably prudent physician providing treatment in the same or similar circumstances. Moreover, physicians will be reluctant to treat patients for medical conditions for which they are not qualified to provide medical treatment.

Duty of Care – Proof of the Physician's Duty of Care

Because the physician's duty of care depends on the type of medical treatment provided by the physician,

the proof of the level of care needed for the physician to satisfy this duty usually involves expert medical testimony. Most state laws set out specific requirements for a person to testify in court as a medical expert on the duty of care required for a physician. Again, these state laws divide medical expert witness qualifications into experts testifying about the duty of care of a physician specialist and experts testifying about the duty of care of a physician who is not a medical specialist. In any context, the key is that the expert medical testimony must come from a qualified medical professional and concern the medical treatment provided by a physician in the particular circumstance.

The qualifications for a person to testify as a medical expert usually require that the expert received a medical education degree from an accredited educational institution along with experience, in a clinical, research or academic setting in the medical treatment provided by the physician. In this way, the person testifying as a medical expert about the duty of care brings to the testimony not only educational qualifications, but also practical experience in the medical treatment provided by a physician.

Traditionally, many state laws also circumscribe the duty of care of a nonspecialist physician to that level of care provided by a reasonable prudent physician in the same or similar circumstances in the specific geographic location in which the physician provides medical treatment. This "locality" rule was designed to insure that rural physicians would not be judged by the level of care required of other physicians who have access to a wider array of medical treatment options. For example, a physician who practices in the remote regions of Alaska will not have immediate access to the kind of medical treatment advances that a physician practicing in a research hospital in New York City would have. Although advancement in communication and standardized medical education and the ease of travel have alleviated some of the need for this "locality" rule, it will still apply in appropriate circumstances.

The fundamental point of state laws that require medical expert testimony to be introduced by only those experts who are qualified in both educational background and practical experience related to the type of medical treatment provided to a patient, even in a unique location, is fairness. Potential defendant physicians are assured that by requiring medical expert testimony from qualified experts, their medical treatment will be judged by their physician peers and in the context within which the medical treatment was provided. Further, the necessity for qualified medical expert opinion to prove the duty of care required for a potential defendant physician in a medical malpractice case acts as a buffer to frivolous medical malpractice lawsuits.

Conclusion

The legal requirement that an injured patient in a medical malpractice lawsuit must prove that a defendant physician possessed a duty to exercise reasonable care and what that duty of care entails presents a prime example of the adversary legal system at work. In the context of medical malpractice lawsuits, it is the obligation of the injured patient to put forth quality, credible evidence of a defendant physician's existence of a duty to exercise reasonable care, and what that duty of care requires of the defendant physician. However, it is the right of the defendant physician to put forth quality, credible evidence to rebut the injured patient's claim. It is from this adversarial presentation of evidence that the liability in a medical malpractice lawsuit will be assigned.

See Also

Medical Malpractice – Medico-legal Perspectives: Negligence, Standard of Care; Negligence, Causation; Negligence Quantum

Further Reading

Conway v. *O'Brien*, 111 F.2d 611 (1947).
Dobbs D (2000) *The Law of Torts*. St. Paul, MN: West Group.
Furrow B, Greaney T, Johnson S, Jost T, Schwartz R (2001) *Health Law*, 4th edn. St. Paul, MN: West Group.
Morrison v. *McNamara*, 407 A.2d 555 (1979).
Pate v. *Threlkel*, 661 So.2d 278 (1997).
United States v. *Carroll Towing Co.*, 159 F.2d 169 (1947).
Zobel H, Rous S (1993) *Doctors and The Law*. New York: W.W. Norton.

Negligence, Causation

M Flynn, Nova Southeastern University, Fort Lauderdale, FL, USA

Introduction

Medical malpractice is the term commonly used to describe negligence on the part of a doctor, hospital, or other medical care provider. Although medical malpractice may also include the legal liability of medical care providers for intentional misconduct, medical malpractice usually refers to medical negligence. Negligence is the legal doctrine that imposes liability for failing to use adequate care. Therefore, medical negligence can be defined as the failure to exercise adequate care in the delivery of medical care and treatment. This article presents what might primarily be an American legal perspective on medical malpractice.

Negligence in General

Any discussion of medical malpractice, medical negligence, must begin with defining the tort of negligence. Tort, taken from the French word *tortum*, means a wrongful act. The tort of negligence refers to the type of wrongful act that falls below the standard of care required to protect others against an unreasonable risk of harm. There are four requirements to make out a legal claim for negligence against a potential defendant:

1. the potential defendant must possess a duty to exercise reasonable care
2. the potential defendant must breach the duty to exercise reasonable care
3. the potential defendant's breach of the duty to exercise reasonable care must be the proximate cause of injury to another – the potential plaintiff
4. the potential plaintiff must sustain a legally cognizable injury.

The potential plaintiff in a negligence claim has the burden of proving all four of these elements in any kind of negligence claim. The potential plaintiff's burden of proof requires that all four elements of negligence be proven by a preponderance of the evidence. The preponderance of the evidence burden requires that the potential plaintiff introduce enough proof to show that it is more likely than not that each of the four elements of a negligence claim is true. Failure to prove with a preponderance of the evidence each of the four elements of a negligence claim will be fatal to that negligence claim.

The four elements of a negligence claim and the burden of proof requirement for a negligence claim apply equally to a medical negligence claim.

The Application of Negligence to Medical Care and Treatment

The application of the legal elements of a negligence claim to medical care and treatment requires a specific application and analysis of the duty, breach of duty, proximate cause, and injury elements. This article will focus on the element of causation and proximate cause.

Causation as an Element of Medical Negligence Claim

The causation element of a medical malpractice, medical negligence, cause of action requires that the plaintiff prove by a preponderance of the evidence that the defendant medical care provider's breach of the duty to exercise reasonable care resulted in injury to the plaintiff. This causal connection between the medical care provider's breach of duty and the patient's injury is a crucial and often disputed element of medical negligence lawsuits. It is this causal connection that connects a medical care provider's fault to a patient's injury.

The element of causation in a medical negligence case – for that matter in any negligence case – breaks down into two separate requirements. First, a plaintiff must prove cause in fact. Cause in fact refers to the requirement that the plaintiff must prove that, more likely than not, the medical care provider's breach of duty actually caused injury to the plaintiff. This element is essentially the requirement to prove cause and effect. After sustaining the burden of proving cause in fact, the plaintiff must then prove proximate cause. Proximate cause refers to the requirement that the plaintiff must prove that, more likely than not, the medical care provider's breach of duty resulted in a foreseeable injury to a foreseeable plaintiff. This is essentially the requirement to prove that it is fair to hold the medical care provider liable for the plaintiff's injury. Whether you refer to the causation element of a medical negligence cause of action as the proximate cause or legal cause or some other similar requirement, every medical negligence case – for that matter every negligence case – requires proof of both cause in fact and proximate cause.

The Cause in Fact Requirement

The law of negligence subscribes to a number of tests that set out the framework within which the cause in fact requirement can be analyzed. This same set of tests applies to medical negligence cases. At its base is a set of questions used to isolate the proof required of a plaintiff to satisfy the cause in fact requirement in a number of different circumstances. There is a set of tests used to prove cause in fact when there is only one potential defendant. A second set of tests is used to prove cause in fact when there are multiple potential defendants. Finally, a third set of tests is used to prove cause in fact when the other sets of cause in fact tests cannot be applied. All of these tests (questions) are used to frame the proof requirements for cause in fact.

Single Defendant

In situations, when there is a single defendant, the plaintiff is attempting to prove that a single potential defendant is the cause in fact of the plaintiff's injury. In the context of a medical negligence case, this translates into a patient attempting to show that a single medical care provider is the cause in fact of the patient's injury. It is the simplest form of a medical negligence cause of action. For example, a patient who presents at a hospital to have his left leg amputated below the knee because of advanced diabetes but the surgeon amputates the patient's right leg below the knee instead would fit this category of cause in fact cases.

In this context, there are two different but equally applied tests for proof of cause in fact. The first test is often referred to as the "but for" test. This test asks the following question: Can you say, more likely than not, that but for the surgeon's breach of duty, that is cutting off the wrong leg, the patient would not have been injured? If the answer is yes, as it would be in this example, then the surgeon is the cause in fact of the patient's injury.

The second test is sometimes referred to as the "increased risk" or "multiply the risk" test. This test asks the following question: Can you say, more likely than not, that the surgeon's breach of duty, that is cutting off the wrong leg, increased the risk of the patient being injured? If the answer is yes, as it would be in this example, then the surgeon is the cause in fact of the patient's injury.

The difference between these two tests for cause in fact is a matter of closeness. The "but for" test requires proof of the closest connection between the surgeon's breach of duty and the patient's injury. In addition, the "increased the risk" test produces a more relaxed standard for proof of the connection between the surgeon's breach of duty and the patient's injury. The key is that proof that satisfies either test is sufficient to demonstrate that the surgeon's breach of duty is a substantial factor in producing the patient's injury.

Multiple Defendants

Not all medical negligence cases, just like other negligence cases, involve a single defendant. In fact, most medical negligence cases are much more complicated and may involve many potential defendants. In this situation, both the "but for" and "increased the risk" test do not effectively apply to this kind of situation. For example, what if a patient's injury can be traced to both the hospital's failure to maintain a heart–lung machine adequately and the surgeon's failure to make sure that the heart–lung machine was in working order before performing major heart surgery? In this instance, if you apply the "but for" test or the "increased the risk" test to each defendant, the hospital and the surgeon, then neither defendant alone can be said to be more likely than not the "but for" or "increased the risk" cause in fact of the patient's injury. Either is just as likely, by itself, to have caused the patient's injury. In the absence of some other cause in fact test, both potential defendants could escape liability.

In this case of potentially multiple defendants, cause in fact employs two other tests to satisfy the cause in fact requirement. The first test is referred to as "but for both" test. In this test, you ask the question: Can you say, more likely than not, but for both the hospital's failure to maintain the heart–lung machine and the surgeon's failure to check out the heart–lung machine, the patient would not have been injured? In this test, you are basically asking if it requires the breach of duty by both potential defendants, the hospital and the surgeon, for the patient's injury to occur. If the answer is yes, as it is in this example, then both defendants, the hospital and the surgeon, are the cause in fact of the patient's injury. In this kind of case, neither the hospital's failure to maintain the heart–lung machine nor the surgeon's failure to check out the heart–lung machine alone would be enough to injure the patient. If the hospital had properly maintained the heart–lung machine then the surgeon's failure to check out the heart–lung machine would not have resulted in injury to the patient. Further, even if the hospital had failed to maintain the heart–lung machine properly, if the surgeon had checked out the heart–lung machine before using it, the patient would not have been injured.

The second test for cause in fact with multiple defendants is referred to as the "both increase the risk" test. In this test, you ask the question: Can you say, more likely than not, that both the hospital's failure to maintain the heart–lung machine adequately and the surgeon's failure to check out the heart–lung machine before using it increased the risk of injury to the patient? In this test, you are asking whether, although either the hospital's or the surgeon's breach of duty may be enough to produce injury to the patient; both potential defendants contributed to the patient being injured. If the answer to this question is yes, as it is in this example, then both the hospital and the surgeon are the cause in fact of the patient's injury. Although either the hospital's failure to maintain the heart–lung machine or the surgeon's failure to check out the heart–lung machine may have been enough for the patient to be injured, both defendants increased the risk of injury to the patient.

The difference between these two tests is similar to the differences between the "but for" test and the "increased the risk" test as applied to single defendants. The "but for both" test requires a closer causal relationship of both defendants to the patient's injury than the "both increased the risk" test. It is important to note that these two tests apply to the situation of multiple defendants – two or more potential defendants. In addition, the application of either of these tests results in the defendants being concurrent causes in fact of the patient's injury. Further, either test applies equally to prove cause in fact. Finally, and most importantly, both tests sufficiently indicate that both defendants are substantial factors in bringing about the patient's injury.

Difficult Causation Problems

Some negligence cases just do not fit into the neat little boxes of the cause in fact tests. Most of these instances concern a negligence case in which the cause in fact appears to be indeterminate. In the context of medical negligence cases, one particular kind of factual scenario provides a good example. Using the noted cases of *Ybarra* v. *Spangard* (154 P.2d 687 (Ca. Supreme Court 1944)) and *Summers* v. *Tice* (199 P.2d 1 (Ca. Supreme Court 1948)) as guideposts, suppose that a patient enters the operating room for the surgical removal of his appendix. The operating room is staffed with a number of medical care providers, including the chief surgeon, but also anesthesiologists, nurses, radiologists, and others to assist in the surgical procedure. Suppose further that at the conclusion of the successful appendectomy, the patient awakes from the anesthesia only to find his left arm paralyzed.

In this kind of circumstance it may be very difficult to pinpoint which one of the people in the operating room was the cause in fact of the patient's paralysis. Every person in that operating room, from the chief surgeon to the anesthesiologist to the nurses to the radiologist and others, may have had some part in causing the paralysis of the patient. Yet, in fact, it only takes the act of any one of the people in that operating room to cause the patient's paralysis. None of the permutations of the "but for" or "increased the risk" tests for cause in fact can be successfully applied to satisfy the more likely than not burden of proof to one or all of the medical and other staff in that operating room. For example, can you say more likely than not, but for the anesthesiologist the paralysis to the patient would not have occurred? No, because it is just as likely that the chief surgeon or nurses placed the patient on the operating-room table in such a way as to damage the nerves in the patient's left arm. Can you say more likely than not that all of the staff and physicians in the operating room increased the risk of the patient suffering paralysis to his left arm? No, because it is just as likely that only one of the staff or the physicians' actions caused the patient's paralysis. In addition, in most of these kinds of cases, it is fairly safe to conclude that every person in that operating room is trying to blame any other person in the operating room for the patient's paralysis.

This example is a difficult cause in fact case because, from the patient's perspective, the cause in fact is essentially indeterminate.

In response to this particular kind of medical negligence case, the law of causation employs a modified cause in fact test. First, more likely than not, one or more of the staff or physicians in that operating room is the cause in fact of the paralysis of the patient who went into the surgery not exhibiting any symptoms or other predisposition to suffering paralysis. Second, the staff and physicians in that operating room are a team, an interdependent group of trained medical professionals who all contribute to the success or failure of any medical procedure. This interdependence of function and action on the part of the surgery team permits courts to rule that, in the absence of other testimony pinpointing the culpable staff person or physician, the patient will have satisfied his cause in fact burden by:

1. including all of the surgery team as defendants in the medical negligence lawsuit concerning his paralysis
2. describing the interdependence of function of all of the surgery team defendants
3. proving that pinpointing the particular member or members of the surgery team who were the cause in fact of the patient's paralysis is not possible
4. proving that the patient's preoperative condition and anything the patient may have done during surgery were not, more likely than not, the cause in fact of the patient's paralysis.

Upon satisfying each of these requirements, the courts shift the burden of cause in fact to each of the defendant members of the surgery team. This shift results in each member of the surgery team bearing the burden of proving more likely than not that the cause in fact of the patient's paralysis was some other member of the surgery team. The policy behind this shift in the burden of proving cause in fact is that the surgery team members are certainly in a much better position than the paralyzed patient, who was anesthetized during surgery, to know the cause in fact of the patient's paralysis. In the absence of such a shift in the burden of proof of cause in fact, the

paralyzed patient would be precluded from successfully presenting a medical negligence case against one or any group of the surgery team that caused his paralysis. The indeterminate cause in fact cases, like this particular example, provide the courts with an opportunity to seek a fair result by modifying the cause in fact tests.

The Proximate Cause Requirement

The burden of proving causation is only half satisfied upon proof of cause in fact. The second half of the burden of proving causation is proof of proximate cause. Many times the term "proximate cause" is also referred to as "legal cause" or "actual cause." By any name, the proof of proximate cause assumes proof of cause in fact first and then posits the question of whether or not it is fair for the particular defendant or defendants to be held liable for the injury to this particular plaintiff. In short, the issue of proximate cause is one of fairness based on the concept of foreseeability of injury to a specific person.

The Cardozo Test for Foreseeability

The American law of proximate cause owes its roots to the jurisprudence of the English courts in the In Re Arbitration Between Polemis and Furness, Withy & Co., Ltd (3 K.B. 560 (Court of Appeals 1921)) case and the Australian courts in the *Overseas Tankship (UK) Ltd.* v. *Morts Dock and Engineering Co., Ltd* cases. Relying on these judicial opinions, the American concept of proximate cause originate from the noted case of *Palsgraf* v. *Long Island R.R. Co.* (162 N.E. 99 (NY Court of Appeals 1928)). Chief Judge Cardozo of the New York Court of Appeals wrote the majority opinion in the Palsgraf case. Judge Cardozo's opinion sets out the classic framework within which the issue of proximate cause is analyzed – hence the name the Cardozo test for proximate cause.

The Cardozo test for proximate cause, that is to test the foreseeability of the injury to the particular plaintiff, begins with the view from the defendant's position. In other words, Judge Cardozo suggests that all proximate cause analysis needs to begin from the perspective of the defendant's alleged negligent act. Then, from this perspective, a jury must look forward to determine if the injury to specific people would be reasonably foreseeable from the defendant's negligent act. It is this "zone of danger" that is created by what is reasonably foreseeable from the defendant's alleged negligent act that limits the reach of proximate cause. Any injury to a person that does not fall within that zone of danger is not reasonably foreseeable and the alleged defendant would not be the proximate cause of the injury to that person. It is important to note that, although an alleged defendant may be the cause in fact of injury to a person, the defendant may not be the proximate cause of the injury to that person.

Perhaps the best way to understand how the Cardozo test for proximate cause works in the context of medical negligence is by way of example. Suppose that a patient presents to a physician with bladder cancer and the physician recommends surgery. The patient consents to the surgery, but the surgeon mistakenly damages healthy organs located next to the patient's bladder. Under the Cardozo test for proximate cause, the surgeon's mistake in damaging the healthy organs located next to the patient's bladder is foreseeable. From the surgeon/defendant's perspective, the organs next to the bladder fall within the zone of danger from the surgery because such organs are located so close to the bladder and any mistake in dissecting part of the patient's bladder could easily result in injury to other closely located organs. Therefore, it would be fair to adjudge the surgeon as the proximate cause of the patient's injury to organs located next to the bladder.

Alternatively, suppose that in the same example, in addition to claiming proximate cause for the damage to his organs located next to the bladder, the patient claims that his wife will no longer consent to sexual intercourse with him. In this example, the Cardozo test for proximate cause may preclude the patient from recovering for this type of loss. The argument against the patient in this instance would be that from the perspective of the surgeon/defendant, it is not foreseeable that the patient's wife would refuse sexual intercourse when the damage to the organs next to the bladder did not affect the patient's ability to have sexual intercourse. The wife's refusal does not fall within the zone of danger of a negligently performed bladder surgery and is therefore too speculative to be reasonably foreseeable by the surgeon/defendant. Under the Cardozo test for proximate cause, it would be unfair to adjudge the surgeon as the proximate cause of the patient's wife's refusal to engage in sexual intercourse with the patient.

The concept of proximate cause, as espoused by Judge Cardozo, limits the liability of potential defendants for negligence.

The Andrews Test for Foreseeability

The minority opinion in the Palsgraf case, authored by Judge Andrews, offers an alternative framework for the analysis of proximate cause, and hence the name the Andrews test for proximate cause.

The Andrews test for proximate cause, that is, the test to determine the foreseeability of injury to a specific plaintiff, begins with a view from the point in time of the plaintiff's injury. Unlike the Cardozo foresight test for proximate cause, the Andrews hindsight test looks back from the plaintiff's injury and tracks back to the defendant's alleged negligent act to see if there is a direct and unbroken chain of events that leads to the plaintiff's injury to determine foreseeability. Under the Andrews test, the jury examines whether any intervening act exists between the plaintiff's injury and the defendant's alleged negligent act. Further, the Andrews test evaluates the remoteness in time, space, and distance of the plaintiff's injury from the defendant's alleged negligent act. Finally, the Andrews test examines public policy to determine if there is any specific public policy that weighs in favor or against holding this particular defendant liable for the injury to the plaintiff. If the plaintiff's injury is the result of an unbroken chain of events that tracks back to the defendant's alleged negligent act and the injury to the plaintiff is not too remote in time, space, and distance, and there is no public policy that would preclude the defendant from being held liable for the plaintiff's injury, then the injury to the plaintiff is foreseeable and the defendant would be the proximate cause of the plaintiff's injury.

The same example of the patient who suffers damage to other organs located next to his bladder as a result of bladder surgery will illustrate the application of the Andrews test for proximate cause. In that example, there is a direct causal link between the plaintiff's injury to the organs located next to the bladder during bladder surgery – there is no other outside force that acts to cause the plaintiff's injury. Further, the timing of the injury to the plaintiff's other organs is contemporaneous with the bladder surgery. The space between the bladder and the other damaged organs is small because the organs are located next to the bladder. The spatial relationship between the bladder and the other damaged organs is also close because the organs are located next to each other with no other organs in between. Finally, there appears to be no public policy that would weigh against holding a surgeon responsible for his/her mistake in damaging other organs during bladder surgery. Consequently, just as in the analysis of the Cardozo test for proximate cause but based on a completely different analytical framework, the injury to the plaintiff's organs located next to his bladder during bladder surgery would be reasonably foreseeable and the surgeon would be the proximate cause of the patient's injury.

However, continuing to extend the application of the Andrews test to the same example, referring to the wife's refusal to have sexual intercourse with the patient after the surgeon's negligent performance of the bladder surgery, the result may be different. Under the Andrews test for proximate cause the plaintiff would argue that there is a direct causal link from the refusal of the wife to the surgeon's negligent bladder surgery; in fact, it is the direct result of the surgeon's alleged negligence. Further, the wife's refusal is not too remote in time, space, and distance because the refusal follows as a direct result after the surgeon's mistake in the bladder surgery. Finally, the plaintiff would argue that there is no public policy prohibition that would protect the surgeon from being held liable for such injury. Consequently, unlike in the application of the Cardozo test for proximate cause, the Andrews test for proximate cause might conclude that the loss suffered by the patient due to his wife's refusal of sexual intercourse is within the ambit of reasonably foreseeable injury.

Unlike the Cardozo test for proximate cause, the Andrews test for proximate cause does not create as much of a limitation on the liability of defendants for injury to plaintiffs.

Finally, it is important to note that, despite the majority and minority opinion status of the Cardozo and Andrews tests for proximate cause, both tests have been equally applied in modern American proximate cause jurisprudence.

Intervening Act Analysis

The final piece to the causation analysis in a negligence case concerns the concept of an intervening cause. An intervening cause is the act of some person or some force that intervenes or comes between the alleged negligent act of a defendant and the injury to a plaintiff. The character and foreseeability of that intervening act may make a difference. For example, an intervening intentional or criminal act may supersede and therefore remove liability from a negligent defendant. For example, a physician who negligently prescribes medication that is life-threatening to a patient would not be liable for the injury or death of that person from someone robbing the patient of the medication. In this example, the intervening act of the robber is an intentional, criminal act. This kind of intervening act, using the Cardozo or Andrews test for foreseeability, is not foreseeable and therefore eliminates the liability of the physician for negligence in prescribing the wrong medication.

In the context of medical negligence litigation, the most common application of the intervening act analysis occurs when the alleged medical negligence intervenes after a negligent act. For example, suppose a pedestrian is injured when a negligent driver of a car loses control and runs up on a sidewalk. Further suppose that the pedestrian is then taken to a local hospital where a physician negligently provides medical treatment for the pedestrian's injury. The medical negligence on the part of the physician is an intervening act. However, unless the intervening medical negligence on the part of the physician amounts to a reckless act, the intervening act of medical negligence will not supersede the liability of the car driver for the injury to the pedestrian. In other words, using either the Cardozo or Andrews test for foreseeability, the intervening act of medical negligence is foreseeable and will not negate the liability of the car driver for negligence. Although it may seem unusual ever to categorize medical negligence as foreseeable, in this instance, the injured pedestrian benefits from being able to sue both the original car driver and the physician in a negligence lawsuit.

Conclusion

In every medical negligence case, sooner or later the issue of causation will be presented and hotly contested. The issue of causation not only requires a complicated legal analysis but also is made doubly difficult because of the complexity of dealing with the science of medicine. It is the task of all involved, the lawyers, judges, and medical professionals, to try to simplify and make some sense out of the complexity that is the law of causation and the science of medicine.

See Also

Medical Malpractice – Medico-legal Perspectives: Negligence, Standard of Care; Negligence, Duty of Care; Negligence Quantum

Further Reading

Davies J, Levine L, Kionka E (1999) *A Torts Anthology*, 2nd edn. Anderson.

Dobbs D (2000) *The Law of Torts*. St. Paul, MN: West Group.

Keeton R (1978) *A Palsgraf Anecdote*. 56 Tex.L.Rev. 513.

Overseas Tankship (UK) Ltd. v. *Morts Dock & Engineering Co., Ltd.*, A.C. 388 (Privy Council 1961).

Overseas Tankship (UK) Ltd. v. *Miller Steamship Co.*, 1 A.C. 617 (Privy Council 1966).

Prosser W, Wade J, Schwartz V (2000) *Torts*, 10th edn. New York: Foundation Press.

Strachan (1930) *Scope and Application of the "But For" Causal Test*. 33 Mod.L.Rev. 386.

Wright (1985) *Causation in Tort Law*. 73 Cal.L.Rev. 1735.

Negligence Quantum

M Flynn, Nova Southeastern University, Fort Lauderdale, FL, USA

Introduction

Medical malpractice is the term commonly used to describe negligence on the part of a doctor, hospital, or other medical care-provider. Although medical malpractice may also include the legal liability of medical care-providers for intentional misconduct, medical malpractice usually refers to medical negligence. Negligence is the legal doctrine that imposes liability for failing to use adequate care. Therefore, medical negligence can be defined as the failure to exercise adequate care in the delivery of medical care and treatment.

Negligence in General

Any discussion of medical malpractice, medical negligence, must begin with defining the tort of negligence. Tort, taken from the French word *tortum*, means a wrongful act. The tort of negligence refers to the type of wrongful act that falls below the standard of care required to protect others against an unreasonable risk of harm. There are four requirements to make a legal claim for negligence against a potential defendant:

1. The potential defendant must possess a duty to exercise reasonable care.
2. The potential defendant must breach the duty to exercise reasonable care.
3. The potential defendant's breach of the duty to exercise reasonable care must be the proximate cause of injury to another – the potential plaintiff.
4. The potential plaintiff must sustain a legally cognizable injury.

The potential plaintiff in a negligence claim has the burden of proving all four of these elements in any kind of negligence claim. The potential plaintiff's burden of proof requires that all four elements of negligence be proven by a preponderance of the evidence. This is the quantum of proof required for a negligence claim. The preponderance of the evidence burden requires that the potential plaintiff introduce enough proof to show that it is more likely than not that each of the four elements of a negligence claim is true. Failure to prove with a preponderance of the evidence each of the four elements of a negligence claim will be fatal to that negligence claim.

The four elements of a negligence claim and the burden of proof requirement for a negligence claim apply equally to a medical negligence claim.

Application of the Negligence Burden of Proof to Damages

The application of the negligence burden of proof to the fourth element of a medical negligence claim, proof of a legally cognizable injury, involves at least two aspects. First, a potential plaintiff must show the existence of an actual physical or emotional or other injury. For example, proof of physical deformity caused by the negligence of a medical provider would satisfy this proof of injury requirement. Further, proof of psychological or emotional trauma caused by the negligence of a medical care-provider would also satisfy the proof of injury requirement.

The second aspect of proof of injury in a medical negligence claim concerns proof of money damages related to the physical and/or emotional injury suffered by a potential plaintiff. Although money damages will, in some cases, be inadequate to restore fully an injured patient to a life without the injury, money damages are primarily designed to compensate an injured patient for a life with the injury. In addition, money damages may be awarded against a medical care-provider to punish the wrongdoers and to act as a deterrent against future wrongdoings.

Proof of Money Damages – Economic Damages

One type of money damages available in a medical negligence case is damages for economic loss. A potential plaintiff is entitled to receive compensation for economic loss caused by the medical negligence of a medical care-provider. The potential plaintiff must prove to the satisfaction of the trier of fact in a medical negligence lawsuit by a preponderance of the evidence that the plaintiff is entitled to receive any money damage for economic loss. The amount and type of economic loss depend on the type of injury sustained by an injured patient and who the patient is. For example, a baby injured by the negligence of a medical provider presents very different economic damages considerations than perhaps an elderly person who is injured. Likewise, a patient who suffers a catastrophic injury resulting in death or a long-term disabling injury requires different money damages evaluation from a patient who suffers a temporary and treatable physical injury.

In any case of negligence, including medical negligence, there is a menu of potential economic loss claims that must be evaluated. Usually, these economic loss claims include claims for wage loss, including loss of earning capacity, medical expenses, including medical rehabilitation expenses, vocational rehabilitation and retraining, and other incidental expenses associated with the medical condition of the injured patient, like transportation expenses. Regarding wage loss, injured patients utilize the expert witness testimony of economists and other financial experts to calculate the amount of present and future wage loss caused by the negligence of a medical care-provider.

Concerning medical expenses as an element of economic damages, injured patients rely on the testimony of expert witnesses well versed in calculating the past, present, and future cost of medical treatment and care. In most medical negligence lawsuits, it is this portion of the money damages award that can be very substantial. For example, the cost of providing medical care and treatment, including additional surgical procedures, daily nursing care, and medications, for a severely brain-damaged baby for the remainder of the baby's life can sustain a multimillion-dollar award for economic damages.

Proof of vocational rehabilitation expenses involves the development of a comprehensive rehabilitation and retraining plan for the injured patient. Vocational rehabilitation experts testify as to the short-term and long-term disabilities of an injured patient and the cost of achieving and sustaining the maximum quality of life and work for the injured patient.

The defendant medical care-provider routinely challenges every aspect of an injured patient's claim for economic damages. The defendant medical provider will proffer expert testimony that counters the injured patient's entitlement to and the amount of money to be awarded for wage loss, medical expenses, and vocational rehabilitation. In the end, the decision as to the injured patient's entitlement to and the amount of any economic damages is left to the reasoned discretion of the trier of fact, namely, the judge or jury evaluating the evidence presented. In the case of a jury trial, the judge has the discretion to grant an additur or a remittitur after a jury has awarded economic damages. An additur is when the judge decides to increase the amount of economic damages awarded to an injured patient based on the evidence presented. A remittitur is when the judge decides to decrease the amount of economic damages awarded to an injured patient based on the evidence presented. An additur or a remittitur becomes the final amount of an award of economic damages absent a timely challenge by the affected party. In any case, the plaintiff patient has the burden of proving the entitlement and the amount of any economic damages by a preponderance of the evidence. The quantum of proof does not vary.

Finally, an injured patient's actual award of economic damages will in most states be reduced by the amount of collateral-source payments received by the injured patient. For example, if the injured patient collected workers' compensation benefits or other kinds of public benefits prior to the trial of the case or the injured patient's medical insurer paid some or all of the injured patient's medical expenses, then the injured patient's economic damages will be reduced by the amount of such payments. Based on a particular state statute, the providers of these benefits or payments may be entitled to receive reimbursement from the injured patient for those collateral source payments.

Proof of Money Damages – Noneconomic Damages

Besides economic damages, an injured patient may attempt to recover money damages for noneconomic losses. This type of damages award is more difficult to prove and to quantify. Essentially, noneconomic damages include money awards based on the physical pain, mental suffering, and other harm, including disfigurement and the loss of the capacity to enjoy life, sustained by an injured patient. The injured patient's burden is to prove an entitlement to such money damages and the amount of such damages by a preponderance of the evidence. The key is that any award of noneconomic damages must have a reasonable basis and not be based on speculation.

Proof of this kind of noneconomic loss is intensely personal to the injured patient. Although some expert witness testimony may be used to chronicle and categorize the level of physical pain or other emotional harm suffered by an injured patient, proof of noneconomic loss requires an indepth view of the injured patient's life before and after the medical negligence. For example, an injured patient who walks with a limp and is no longer able to stand for an extended period of time without back pain as a result of medical negligence can be found by trier of fact to experience physical pain. Likewise, a trier of fact could find that such an injured patient experiences mental suffering from the personal humiliation of walking with a limp.

The trickier proposition is to determine how much money physical pain and mental suffering are worth. This is not an exact calculation. However, there are various ways to transform and relate physical pain and mental suffering to money damages. For example, equating the cost of medications and other types of therapy for the relief of such pain can provide a reasoned basis for calculating what the physical pain and the mental suffering are worth. In addition, equating the cost of not being able to perform some kind of ordinary task can be a measuring stick for the value a particular injured patient may put on the physical pain and mental suffering. The goal of the injured patient is persuasively to present corollaries from that injured patient's life that are quantifiable in dollars and cents from which a rational award of damages can be measured. Though not an exact measurement of money damages, persuasive and creative examples can be enough proof to satisfy the preponderance of evidence burden of proof of noneconomic damages.

Likewise, proving the money loss of a permanent scar or the money value of the loss of the capacity to enjoy life requires the same kind of intimate portrayal of the life of the injured patient before and after suffering injury due to medical negligence. For example, take a concert pianist whose hands are injured due to medical negligence. Not only would the injured patient attempt to quantify the physical pain and the mental suffering of the pianist but also attempt to quantify any disfigurement to the pianist's hands and the void left in the pianist's life by being unable to play the piano at all. These losses could be translated into a money value that is based on the number of hours the pianist plays per day or some other measurement that enables a judge or jury to consider the real consequences of the medical negligence.

Just as in the proof of economic damages, the defendant's medical care-provider usually disputes the injured patient's claim for these "soft" damages. However, some states mandate that if medical expenses are awarded to an injured patient, then a judge or jury must award some amount of money for noneconomic damages.

Proof of Money Damages – Punitive Damages

Perhaps the most controversial of all of the categories of money damages awarded in any negligence case, including medical malpractice, is punitive damages. The entitlement to punitive damages is purely a question of state law. Some, but not all, states authorize by statute the right of an injured patient to claim punitive damages. Absent this kind of statutory authorization, punitive damages may not be awarded to an injured plaintiff. Further, most states that permit punitive damages awards require a threshold determination of whether the injured patient's case warrants consideration of a punitive damages award.

Simply stated, punitive damages, sometimes called exemplary damages, are designed to punish a liable defendant and to act as a deterrent to other potential defendants. Consequently, punitive damages are not routinely awarded, even in those states that permit such a recovery.

The US Supreme Court ruling in *State Farm Mutual Automobile Insurance Company* v. *Campbell*, 123 S. Ct 1513 (2003), citing numerous other Supreme Court decisions, reviews and analyzes the constitutional limitations of punitive damage awards. In this opinion, the Supreme Court comments on the application of a set of factors that a judge or jury must consider in deciding to award punitive damages and in deciding the amount of any punitive damages award. These factors include consideration of the nature of the defendant's wrongful conduct, the extent of the harm inflicted, the intent of the defendant committing the act, the financial wealth and standing of the defendant, and any mitigating factors that might operate to reduce the amount of any award, including the ratio between the amount of economic and noneconomic damages and the amount of a punitive damages award. In essence, the Supreme Court and the constitution require that there be some rational basis for the award and amount of punitive damages in any case.

Perhaps the most crucial threshold consideration involves an examination of the type of conduct engaged in by a defendant. Generally, some level of culpability above ordinary negligence is required to support a punitive damages claim. A defendant's conduct that rises to the level of an intentional act or a reckless act usually triggers consideration of a punitive damages award. An intentional act is conduct that amounts to a deliberate or purposeful act that results in injury to a person. This is the highest form of culpability. Fortunately, the instances of a medical care-provider purposefully and deliberately injuring a patient are rare.

In addition, and also unfortunately, there are several instances of medical care-providers acting recklessly in the treatment of patients. A reckless act is conduct that amounts to an egregious departure from the standard of care applicable to a defendant such that the defendant's actions amount to disregard for the person's well-being. This level of culpability is sometimes also referred to as gross negligence. For example, when a surgeon amputates a patient's right leg instead of the patient's left leg then an argument can be made that the medical care-provider's conduct was egregious and reckless. It is this kind of intentional or reckless conduct by a medical care-provider that may subject such a defendant to punitive damages.

Since the purpose of punitive damages is not only to punish the defendant, but also to deter other potential defendants from engaging in the same or similar conduct, the amount of punitive damages can be very high. In many cases, just like the State Farm case, the amount of economic and noneconomic damages may be relatively small while the amount of punitive damages is hundreds of times larger. The rationale for this unbalanced ratio is that effective punishment and deterrent for some wealthy defendants demand a high, punitive damages award. The key to these kinds of cases, as stated in the Supreme Court opinion in the State Farm case, is that the amount of a punitive damages award must be supported by some kind of rational basis. In any event, just as in the case of economic and noneconomic damages, a judge will have the opportunity to use additur and remittitur to control the amount of a punitive damages award.

Conclusion

There is no question that no matter how you analyze the entitlement to and award of money damages in a medical negligence case, the fundamental inadequacy of paying money to an injured patient remains. However, there is no alternative! Injured patients deserve first to be "uninjured", and then second, to be compensated by the liable medical care-provider. Negligent medical care-providers deserve first to be held liable for patient's injuries, and second, to pay for this liability. It is the injured patient's burden to prove this liability and entitlement to money damages by a preponderance of the evidence.

See Also

Medical Malpractice – Medico-legal Perspectives: Negligence, Standard of Care; Negligence, Duty of Care; Negligence, Causation

Further Reading

Bell PA, O'Connell J (1997) *Accidental Justice*. New Haven, Connecticut and London: Yale University Press.

Belli M (1951) *Demonstrative Evidence and the Adequate Award*. 22 Miss. L. J. 284.

BMW of North America, Inc. v. Gore, 116 S. Ct 1589 (1996).

Cooper Industries, Inc. v. Leatherman Tool Group, Inc., 121 S. Ct. 1678 (2001).

Dobbs D (2000) *The Law of Torts*. St. Paul, MN. West Publishing.

Fleming J (1996) *The Collateral Source Rule and Loss Allocation in Tort Law*. 54 Calif. L. Rev. 1478.

O'Connell J, Carpenter K (1983) *Payment for Pain and Suffering through History*. 50 Ins. Couns. J. 411.

O'Quinn (1997) *Common Elements of Recovery in Personal Injury Cases*. 18 S. Tex. L. J. 179.

Pacific Mutual Life Insurance Co. v. Haslip, 111 S. Ct. 1032 (1991).

Peck (1974) *Compensation for Pain: A Reappraisal in Light of New Medical Evidence*. 72 Mich. L. Rev. 1355.

TXO Production Corp. v. Alliance Resources Corp., 113 S. Ct. 2711 (1993).

Zabel (1985) *A Plain English Approach to Loss of Future Earning Capacity*. 24 Washburn L. J. 253.

MEDICAL MISADVENTURE

J J Buchino and J E Sullivan, University of Louisville, Louisville, KY, USA

Introduction

It is not uncommon for the forensic pathologist to be involved in the investigation of the unexpected death of a hospitalized patient. In such cases, medical misadventure must be a serious consideration as a cause of death. In order to have the best chance at elucidating the cause of death, the forensic pathologist must have access to a thorough scene investigation and familiarity with the various types of medical misadventures that can cause death. Therapeutic misadventures can be broadly divided into (1) medication errors and (2) those involving mechanical devices.

Medication Errors

The Institute of Medicine (USA) in 2000 gave a lengthy and detailed report of the types of medication errors that can result in the death of a patient. It is estimated that medication errors cause at least one death every day in the USA. The ten most common

Table 1 Ten most common lethal medication errors in hospitalized patients

Concentrated potassium chloride injections
Insulin errors
Intravenous calcium and magnesium
Inadvertently administered 50% dextrose
Known allergy to medication
Miscalculated digoxin (pediatric patients)
Confusing vincristine and vinblastine (look-alike names)
Concentrated sodium chloride injections
Intravenous narcotics
Aminophylline

Data from Argo AL, Cox KF, Kelly WN (2000) The ten most common lethel medication errors in hospital patients. *Hospital Pharmacy* 35: 470–474.

lethal medication errors are listed in **Table 1**. While the most likely cause of the error associated with these medications is the administration of the wrong dose, other possibilities must be considered. For example, in one case the correct amount of potassium chloride concentrate was added to D5W (Dextrose 5% water) but the contents were not mixed well and the patient died due to hyperkalemia. In the case of calcium administration, care must be taken to clearly identify the salt form being used. Calcium gluconate contains $4.65\,\text{mEq}\,\text{g}^{-1}$ of calcium, whereas calcium chloride contains $13.6\,\text{mEq}\,\text{g}^{-1}$. Some institutions have stored these two forms next to each other leading to a mistake by the pharmacist or nurse. Poor penmanship on the part of the ordering physician can result in the wrong drug being dispensed and administered. This is exemplified by the death of a 42-year-old man who received 20 mg of Plendil rather than Isordil because the illegibility of the prescription caused the pharmacist to dispense the wrong medication. It is imperative that the patient record be examined for both what was ordered and what was given to a patient who dies unexpectedly. Similarly, abbreviations can result in lethal medication errors. Another reported source of error is confusing patients with similar names. It is not unusual for a harried caregiver to have two patients with the same surname and inadvertently administer the correct drug to the wrong patient. Because they have a direct impact on the central nervous system, intrathecal medications can be particularly dangerous. There have been several reports of death due to intrathecal vincristine administration. Recently, a 49-year-old woman was reported to have died following an overdose of intrathecal tranexaneic acid.

Of particular concern is the susceptibility of children to medication errors. Key factors include the size of the patient, the need to compute small dosages, and the fact that a ten-fold error may appear deceivingly normal to the person administering the drug. In addition to dosage errors, some medications initially thought to be safe for use on children have resulted

in unexpected death, especially when used for other than the manufacturer's intended purpose. Newly approved drugs, although having passed Food and Drug Administration (FDA) testing, may result in death from side-effects undetected in the study population. Recent examples in adults include the weight reduction drug fen-fen. In pediatrics seemingly innocuous drugs can be catastrophic as in the vitamin E preparation eferol.

Another source of medical misadventure is laboratory testing. Perhaps the most common problem in this regard is patient or specimen misidentification. This in turn can lead to inappropriate and potentially life-threatening therapy. The area of greatest concern to the laboratory is the blood bank because administration of mismatched blood products can result in rapid death. The other main area of concern is electrolyte analysis. Errors in reporting abnormal values in potassium, calcium, or phosphorus can result in administration of these supplements and subsequently death.

Errors Involving Mechanical Devices

Medical care has been enhanced by an ever-increasing number of mechanical devices. Fortunately, most medical equipment has been thoroughly tested prior to approval for general use. Because of this, device failure is relatively rare. However, complications caused by user error or by device migration or displacement are a more common occurrence.

Endotracheal tubes and vascular catheters present the most frequent hazards. Respiratory arrest can result from displacement of endotracheal tubes and tracheostomy tubes. While these tubes are usually secured in place, patient movement may cause them to be dislodged. Furthermore, these tubes may be occluded by pulmonary secretions or other means. Resuscitation attempts are often thwarted by placement of the endotracheal tube in the esophagus. In 1986 Buchino and coworkers reported the unusual situation of two infants with tracheoesophageal fistula who died suddenly before surgery as the result of malpositioning of the endotracheal tube in the fistula.

Vascular catheters have also been a cause of medical misadventure and sudden death. We have seen unrecognized perforation of a large vessel during catheter insertion with subsequent hemorrhage into the abdominal or thoracic cavity causing exsanguination. Cardiac tamponade related to peripherally inserted central catheters has been reported. One review found 25 catheter-associated deaths over a five-year period reported from 83 newborn intensive care units. Pneumocardium has resulted from inadvertent injection of air into a central vascular catheter. In another instance, a 77-year-old woman, who received approximately

50 ml of enteral feed containing high-molecular-weight dextrin intravenously, died six hours later despite intensive emergency resuscitative attempts. Other tubing besides vascular catheters may be the source of error. Dramatic cases of inadvertent intracranial nasogastric tube placement have resulted in the death of patients. More recently, a fatal case of strangulation of an 11-month-old infant boy with intravenous tubing was reported.

A recent phenomenon has been patient deaths reported due to narcotic overinfusions resulting from the misprogramming of patient-controlled analgesic (PCA) infusion pumps. The incidents reported typically involve the entry of an erroneously low drug concentration when programming the pump for use, which causes the pump to deliver an excessive amount of the drug. Another cause for infusion pump error may be cellular technology. Hahn and coworkers reported the delivery of a toxic dose of adrenaline (epinephrine) because the rate setting of the intravenous pump was greatly accelerated by a nearby cell phone in the standby mode.

Investigation of Medical Misadventures

Adequate investigation of the death of a hospitalized patient due to suspected medical misadventure requires cooperation and coordination of hospital personnel, law enforcement officials, and forensic pathologists. A protocol, such as the example given in **Table 2**, is best followed to insure the highest yield of results. We suggest that forensic pathologists work with local law enforcement and hospital officials to proactively institute standard operating procedures in the event of a sudden, unexpected death of a hospitalized patient.

Following an unexpected death of a hospitalized patient, hospital personnel should secure the scene. This can be difficult because relatives and friends of the decedent may want to view the body. However, it should be explained to them that the best opportunity

Table 2 Protocol template

Control and limit access to body and room; institute time log of persons entering room
Secure all items in room
Notify coroner and law enforcement
Notify risk management personnel
Notify laboratory to retain all biologic samples pertaining to patient
Notify security to retain monitor videos
Perform complete forensic autopsy

Modified from Buchino JJ, Corey TS, Montgomery V (2002) Sudden unexpected death in hospitalized children. *Journal of Pediatrics* 140: 461–465. © 2002. With permission from Mosby.

to determine the cause of death is to allow a rapid investigation to take place without disturbance of the environment of the deceased. Similarly, hospital personnel will typically attempt to clean the room following a failed resuscitation. However, in the process, valuable clues and trace evidence may be discarded.

Most states require notification of the coroner or other legal authority in the case of any unexpected death, regardless of the length of hospital stay. Hospital personnel should be instructed that as a general rule it is always better to err on the side of notifying these officials and letting them have the opportunity to decide whether or not they wish to investigate the situation further.

While not essential to the investigation, most hospitals would prefer to have a representative from their risk management department present during the procedure. Involving risk management personnel from the outset usually helps facilitate cooperation between the hospital and law enforcement.

All medical devices such as monitors and intravenous pumps that were used in the patient's care should be secured. They should not be disconnected from their power supply until examined by biomedical engineers to determine whether or not memory loss will occur if disconnected.

All premortem specimens should be saved by the laboratory for possible analysis. Likewise, all intravenous fluids attached to the patient should be analyzed. Fluids contained in syringes discarded in the sharps container in the patient's room should also be analyzed.

Although a sudden, unexpected death of a patient is traumatic for caregivers, it is important that they be interviewed concerning the events surrounding the death. Experience has shown that the most accurate information obtained is in the period immediately after the death.

Security cameras are now commonly used to monitor many areas within hospitals. Therefore, videotape of the events leading up to the death may be available. The security department should be notified to save any such tape of the area pending review by the investigating authorities.

Given the information generated from the scene investigation and the results of a complete autopsy to rule out natural causes of death, the forensic pathologist is then in the best position to determine if a medical misadventure played a role in the cause of death.

Further Reading

Anonymous (2002) Medication safety: PCA pump programming errors continue to cause fatal overinfusion errors. *Health Devices* 31: 342–346.

Argo AL, Cox KF, Kelly WN (2000) The ten most common lethal medication errors in hospital patients. *Hospital Pharmacy* 35: 470–474.

Buchino JJ, Keenan WJ, Pietsch JB, *et al.* (1986) Malpositioning of the endotracheal tube in infants with tracheoesophageal fistula. *Journal of Pediatrics* 109: 524–525.

Buchino JJ, Corey TS, Montgomery V (2002) Sudden unexpected death in hospitalized children. *Journal of Pediatrics* 140: 461–465.

Byard RW, Cohle SD (1994) *Sudden Death in Infancy, Childhood and Adolescence.* Cambridge, UK: Cambridge University Press.

Kuhn LT, Corrigan JM, Donaldson MS (2000) *To Err is Human: Building a Safer Health System.* Committee on Quality Health Care in America, Institute of Medicine. Washington, DC: National Academy Press.

Nadroo AM, Lin J, Green RS, *et al.* (2001) Death as a complication of peripherally inserted central catheters in neonates. *Journal of Pediatrics* 138: 598–601.

MEDICAL RECORDS, ACCESS TO

G Morris, Nova Southeastern University, Fort Lauderdale, FL, USA

Introduction

The bedrock of the physician–patient relationship has always been mutual trust. Healthcare professionals must trust that their patients are being honest and forthright when they provide information, so that the proper medical judgment can be exercised. At the same time, patients must trust that their healthcare professionals will have the patient's interests at heart and will use professional judgment and skill on their behalf. In order for this trust to be present, all patients must know that whatever they tell their healthcare professionals, as well as the other information about them in the healthcare professional's records, will be held in strict confidence. Any distrust in this regard could lead to patients not fully cooperating in their medical care. If patients provide incomplete or inadequate information, it could result in misdiagnosis, mistreatment, and harm.

The fundamental duty of healthcare professionals to maintain patient confidentiality is reflected in various professional codes of ethics and in the law. As early as the fifth century BC, the Hippocratic oath required that "Whatever, in connection with my professional practice, or not in connection with it, I see or hear, in the life of men, which ought not to be spoken abroad, I will not divulge, as reckoning that all such should be kept secret."

The importance of this commitment remains undiminished to this day, although the practice of medicine has changed dramatically since Hippocrates' time. No longer do patients have a single physician who makes house calls, knows the entire family history, and can address all their medical needs. Modern healthcare by its nature involves the participation of a number of healthcare professionals and specialists in a variety of healthcare settings. This fragmentation of the modern healthcare delivery and payment systems requires the widespread sharing of patient information among healthcare professionals and third parties. Inherent in this is the risk of inadvertent or unauthorized disclosures.

As if these challenges to patient confidentiality were not enough, the expansion of modern technology and electronic communications into healthcare services also provides additional threats. Our increasing reliance upon telecommunication devices and computers offers unprecedented access, both authorized and unauthorized, to information of all sorts. Increasingly we use the internet for personalized healthcare information services and products. The expansion of "telemedicine," relating to the practice of medicine "at a distance," and the proliferation of "telehealth," which encompasses all of the other dimensions of healthcare services and activities, suggest that these risks will increase. Modern healthcare delivery and payment systems routinely utilize this growing technology to convey, use, and store confidential, sensitive, or potentially embarrassing medical information.

Accordingly, it is helpful to understand the rights, responsibilities, and limitations imposed on those who create or hold medical information, and on those others who seek to access, or use, this special category of information.

Medical Records – General

As discussed above, disclosure made by a patient to a healthcare professional within the framework of a physician–patient relationship is considered confidential. When those disclosures are memorialized in written form, these written records, as well as other information generated during the relationship, are also considered confidential.

Purpose of Medical Records

Patient medical records serve a number of important purposes. First and foremost, the medical record is an orderly collection of information about the patient and the care rendered to the patient. Medical records have become all the more important in our decentralized modern healthcare system with its heavy reliance on a primary care physician, specialists, diagnostic testing by third parties, and multiple providers. Complete and accurate medical records are essential to the decision-making by these participants and providers who may not know the patient or actually even see the patient.

Another important function of a patient medical record is to document the medical necessity for the care provided and the extent of the services rendered. For example, insurance companies and third-party payers generally require such written evidence before payment can be authorized. In the case of managed care, such documentation may be required even before the treatment is authorized. Patient medical records also serve as a basis for performing medical professional peer review, for quality improvement initiatives, and for verifying whether a healthcare provider's local, regional or national licensure requirements or accreditation standards have been met. Medical records are also an important source of information to governmental entities responsible for maintaining vital statistics, preventing or managing communicable diseases, and generally protecting the public health.

Content of Medical Records

Generally, patient medical records include three types of information. They are patient identification information, clinical information, and financial information. The patient identification information typically includes the patient's name, address, birth date, family or contact persons, and social security or other identification numbers. The clinical information may include a patient's medical and social history, the results of physical examinations, diagnostic tests, X-rays and other radiology reports, and any orders for medications. If hospitalization is involved, the medical records may also include admission notes, surgical reports, nursing notes, pharmacy records, laboratory test results, discharge planning, and a discharge summary. Medical records will typically also include information about advance directives and healthcare decision-making proxies

or surrogates. Also included in the medical record is financial information such as health insurance coverage, assignments of benefits, and the names of co-signing parties or guarantors for purpose of arranging payment.

Form and Content of Medical Records

Some important legal and practical distinctions must be noted on the form in which the medical records and their contents are kept. Historically medical records were only kept in paper form but increasingly they are now being maintained in an electronic form or a combination of paper and electronic form. Generally, the originator, creator, or holder of the medical record is considered its owner. At the same time, however, the person about whom the information pertains usually controls how the holder may make use of the information and therefore controls the disclosure of the medical information to third parties. As a result, when a patient changes physician, or seeks a second opinion, the patient is usually entitled to a copy of the medical record but not to the original medical records themselves.

Medical Records Access and Use

As a general rule, patient medical information may only be provided to those having a legal right to access it or to use it. Usually the patient is the primary recipient of the information and it is the patient who gives specific written consent to its use or to dissemination to third parties. However, it is important to note that there are times when public policy considerations and other important societal benefits may outweigh the patient's individual need for confidentiality. These may include investigations of communicable diseases or allegations regarding possible child or sexual abuse. In such cases access to what would otherwise be confidential information is permitted without patient knowledge or consent, or even over the patient's vehement objection. State or national laws and professional codes of conduct usually articulate these rights and the exceptions. For the most part, however, without the patient's specific consent or the presence of other compelling state interests that provide a justification, both access to and use of confidential patient medical information is improper and illegal. Specific instances that commonly arise are discussed below.

Patient/Authorized Representative Access

The patient or person about whom the medical information is collected is generally entitled to access to his/her information. The patient is also permitted to approve or restrict the further uses or dissemination of this medical information. Disclosures to third parties are usually accomplished by the use of a written medical record authorization form or release that the patient signs. In some cases, particularly if the form is signed elsewhere and merely presented to the holder of the records, it is appropriate to require that the patient's signature be notarized in order to authenticate that it is in fact the patient who has signed the form. At times the patient may wish to delegate to others this right to approve access or authority to approve disclosures. Patients may ordinarily do so through the use of legal documents such as power of attorney or perhaps pursuant to an advance directive naming a surrogate. The applicable law may also allow disclosure to legal guardians, surrogates, or proxies in cases where the patient is not mentally or physically competent.

Spouse/Immediate Family Members

As a general rule, even those persons who are closest to the patient are not permitted to have access to a patient's medical information unless the patient consents to the disclosure. This consent may be in writing or implied from the circumstances. Their legal status as a relative by blood or marriage, or close personal relationship, does not automatically grant status that permits access to medical record information. This can present difficulty when the healthcare provider is in need of medical treatment consent or in other situations where the provider is in possession of information about the patient's genetic condition that can be inherited, or perhaps about communicable diseases that may affect others but the patient may not wish to disclose.

Healthcare Providers – For Treatment

Generally, a physician may disclose a patient's confidential information to office personnel, other physicians, hospital personnel, and medical consultants in connection with the patient's care. This may be done even without specific approval or written consent by the patient. This is because the patient's approval for such disclosures is implied from the physician–patient relationship and from the fact that the patient has submitted to the physician's care. It is reasonable to assume that the patient's desire for treatment encompasses approval to make all disclosures reasonably necessary to obtain the appropriate medical care. Obviously, these other persons are in need of access to all relevant information necessary for them to fulfill their duties in connection with their shared undertaking.

In a similar vein, the office personnel and administrative staff of healthcare providers are also generally permitted to have access to confidential medical information. This is the case so long as the access is in connection with performance of their patient-related duties such as scheduling appointments, reporting results to patients, telephone orders, billing and collection, and communication with legal advisors in defense of malpractice claims.

Unless the patient directs otherwise, on the same basis, disclosure is also generally permitted to third parties providing related healthcare services such as those involved in discharge planning, pharmacies, durable medical equipment entities or short-term rehabilitation, or long-term custodial nursing care. However, abundance of caution suggests that written authorization be obtained.

Healthcare Providers – For Quality and Peer Review

Another important use of patient medical information is to evaluate the professional services of healthcare providers. Recent studies have focused attention on the prevention of medical mishaps and improved patient safety. Government entities that license healthcare providers, hospitals, and managed care entities have traditionally engaged in professional credentialing and peer review activities that require consideration of their patient care activities as gleaned from patient medical records.

Third-Party Payers

As modern healthcare has become more costly, reliance upon health insurance and government health benefit programs has also become increasingly important. Disclosure of patient medical information is frequently necessary in order to obtain payment by, or reimbursement from, these third-party payers. Generally patients will sign consents or give authorization at the outset of treatment or care to allow their providers to release medical information. Otherwise the patient risks denial of payment and will be personally responsible for payment.

Legal Obligations

There are times when patient medical information that is otherwise confidential must be disclosed without patient consent, or even over the patient's objection. There are a number of situations in which healthcare professionals or providers may have an affirmative duty to report such information, or a duty to respond when asked. In these situations the healthcare provider will not be liable to the patient for improper disclosure as immunity is usually provided under the following applicable laws.

Reporting mandated by law Many jurisdictions impose a requirement on healthcare providers to report suspected instances of child abuse, sexual abuse, elder abuse, or occasions where a patient may be a danger to him/herself or others. In these circumstances healthcare professionals may have virtually no discretion and must report even when aware of mitigating circumstances. In fact, these healthcare professionals can face possible civil liability, criminal prosecution, or professional licensure discipline if they fail to report so. As a result, patient medical information that may otherwise be confidential must be disclosed without the patient's consent or even over the patient's objection.

Public health Another instance when disclosure is frequently mandated involves the preservation of public health. Healthcare professionals are frequently under legal obligations to report cases of sexually transmissible diseases, as well as other contagious diseases such as hepatitis, tuberculosis, and human immunodeficiency virus/acquired immunodeficiency syndrome (HIV/AIDS). The worldwide threat of biological and chemical weapons of mass destruction may also impose duties on healthcare professionals to report under public health as well as national security requirements.

Discovery in legal proceedings Patient medical records are regularly the subject of discovery and used as evidence in connection with legal proceedings. Frequently, the health condition of the patient has been placed in issue by the patient as part of a civil lawsuit claiming personal injuries or professional negligence, or perhaps in cases seeking disability benefits. A person's mental or physical condition may also be an issue in child custody proceedings or guardianship proceedings. Medical information can also be relevant in criminal cases and administrative matters.

Generally, disclosure of patient medical information as part of pretrial discovery or as evidence in a judicial proceeding is compelled through use of a subpoena for production of records at a deposition or judicial proceeding or a subpoena seeking personal testimony. Sometimes specific court orders compelling production or testimony are also issued. With the exception of investigatory matters, the person about whom the records are sought usually has an opportunity to interpose an objection before disclosure occurs. In many jurisdictions, subpoenas for production of records in lieu of deposition may be issued in civil cases in which the opposing party is given a certain time within which to object. Failure to object timely constitutes an authorization for disclosure.

Refusal to honor a proper request for medical records can be punished by the court's contempt powers.

Disclosure in connection with searches and seizures There are times when law enforcement agencies or government entities may seek patient medical information in connection with investigations of the patient or of the healthcare providers. In the USA, the Fourth Amendment of the Constitution provides protection against unreasonable searches and seizures and provides an assurance that a basis exists for making this inquiry. Unless authorized by law or legal process, routine inquiries by law enforcement may be refused unless the patient's consent has been provided. Under these circumstances the healthcare professional is typically instructed not to alert the patient as to the receipt of the inquiry.

Employers

Another area where problems can sometimes arise is when access to patient medical records is sought by the patient's employer or even prospective employer. This situation may occur, for example, in the cases of preemployment health screenings and when employees seek compensation for work-related injuries, or other employer-provided benefits such as medical leave or disability. This can also become problematic in those places where employees receive their healthcare or benefits from their employers. In reaction to the rising costs of healthcare, many larger businesses operate self-funded plans under Employee Retirement Income Security Act (ERISA) and similar laws, which may give employers access to healthcare and claim data on their employees.

The concern is that the employer may use the medical information in connection with decisions about hiring, firing, promotion, and benefits coverage. Generally, unless the applicable law permits disclosure to employers without the patient's consent, the patient's authorization is required.

Scientific Research

Another instance where confidential medical information may be requested is in connection with clinical research. The evaluation of new medications, implantable devices, and treatments frequently involves testing on human subjects. The measurement of success over the long term also relies upon collection and evaluation of patient data. Ordinarily, if medical records are being reviewed for purposes of data collection and the information is aggregated and reported in a way that will not identify the patient to which the data pertain, then no specific patient authorization is required. However, if a person is participating in a clinical trial and his/her patient information is to be reported to the study sponsor in a way that is identifiable, then a consent for this will generally be included in the initial enrollment documentation presented to the patient.

Limitations and Liabilities

Limitations on Access

As expansive as the protections may already be to preserve confidentiality of patient medical records, there are a number of instances where additional limitations have been imposed, or special exceptions to the general rules are created in order to further various public policy considerations. Typically, these safeguards have been established to protect the needs of persons who are seen as the more vulnerable among us. Some examples are as follows.

Emancipated minors Generally the law provides that only persons who are considered adults are permitted to make decisions regarding access to their medical information or their medical care. Adult status is usually conferred when the person reaches the "age of majority," as defined in local law. However, in many jurisdictions the law allows those who are under the legal age of majority to be treated as adults if they have achieved emancipated status. Minors can demonstrate emancipation by serving in the military, upon becoming married, or by otherwise living independently and providing for their own support.

The law continues to struggle with the degree of respect to be shown to "mature minors" who do not meet the above criteria for adulthood, but who, by virtue of experience, education, acceptance of responsibility, and other circumstances, have demonstrated their ability to act as reasonably and appropriately as someone over the age of majority. In addition, in some jurisdictions unwed pregnant minors may also be granted legal status to make medical treatment decisions that may include decisions with respect to access to medical information.

"Superconfidential" medical information Special limitations on access are also provided to certain categories of medical information that are deemed "superconfidential." These special categories generally include medical records pertaining to sexually transmissible diseases or HIV/AIDs, drug or alcohol abuse, or mental health conditions. In these cases, the public policy benefits that result from encouraging early diagnosis and treatment, or the ability of the public health authorities to control spread of dangerous diseases, are seen as justifying a higher level of authorization to obtain such information or to compel disclosures without consent. Another public policy consideration favoring the imposition of these additional burdens is the desire to spare these patients from exposure to perceived or real discrimination that may result from disclosures that might occur in the usual course.

As a result, in the case of "superconfidential" medical records, a very specific form of consent from the patient is usually required to authorize disclosure. A general medical record release is not sufficient. In many instances subpoenas for medical records that are routinely issued in the course of litigation are also insufficient to reach these special types of medical records. Rather, in some jurisdictions an additional and very specific court order will be required to permit the disclosure and to delimit the circumstances under which any further dissemination or uses will be allowed.

Public figures In recent years the health conditions of celebrities, sports figures, political candidates, and government officials have become the subject of great public attention. More troublesome for these people and their family members is media interest in toxicology reports and autopsy photographs in cases of injury or death of the famous or celebrated. In order to avoid sensationalism or to ally unwarranted speculation, it is now commonplace for such figures to disclose health information voluntarily. As a rule, however, the status of the individual as a public figure does not change the character of the information or the rules governing access to it. Such medical or hospitalization information is confidential and may not be released to the media without the patient's family consent, court order, or as permitted by governing law.

Legal Duties and Causes of Action

In the event of a disclosure of confidential medical information where there is an obligation not to do so, the law provides several legal theories for legal redress.

Breach of confidentiality While patient medical information is generally considered "confidential" and the communications between a healthcare professional and patient are considered "privileged," it is helpful to understand the differences between them. This is the case because these differences can affect the legal duties, rights, and remedies in the event of an improper disclosure.

The special protection is based upon the concept that certain information, when shared with third parties under certain circumstances, should be kept private and confidential and that the obligation should be enforceable. Sometimes this duty is created by a special relationship of trust that exists between the parties such as physician and patient. Other times the duty is imposed by virtue of specific laws that apply to the relationship in question.

Generally, a physician who violates the confidentiality of the physician–patient relationship may be liable to the patient for damages. Likewise, any other holder of information that is by law considered confidential will be liable to the patient for any improper disclosures. Damages may include nominal damages for vindication of the legal right associated with the mere fact that the breach of duty happened and may also include compensatory damages for actual harm caused. If the breach is especially egregious, the law may also permit punitive or exemplary damages to be awarded. It is also likely that discipline by the applicable licensing authority will be imposed as well.

Privilege against disclosure   Another limitation on disclosure of medical information is associated with a privilege that attaches to the physician–patient relationship. Privileges are created by law and serve a special purpose. Privileges are used in legal proceedings to control the scope of information that can be discovered or introduced as evidence. Privilege may be seen as a right to withhold information. It is an affirmation by society about the value and importance assigned to the ability to speak and write freely about certain things in the knowledge that it will not be used later. Because privileges are legal in nature they are not absolute. There are instances, for example, in the case of a mentally incompetent patient, child custody, suspected abuse cases, or other compelling circumstances where the privilege may be overcome. But, for the most part, the privilege frequently does work to protect communication by a patient, or information about a patient, from being brought to light.

Among the privileges recognized by law, perhaps the most commonly recognized is the physician–patient privilege. It protects the patient's privacy, and therefore may be waived by the patient. The provider does not have an independent basis to refuse to disclose patient information if the patient has waived the privilege. Unless the patient waives the privilege, the provider is bound to maintain the confidentiality.

Invasion of privacy   A concept that is closely related to the above is privacy. This concept is not limited to the healthcare information and relationships. Some jurisdictions recognize a common law, statutory or even constitutional right to be "let alone." An invasion of an individual's right of privacy is considered a civil wrong. It involves an unwarranted making use of that individual's personality where the public has no legitimate interest, or a wrongful intrusion into his or her private activities. Under common law a claim for invasion of privacy could be made when there was an unjustified intrusion upon physical solitude or seclusion, the taking and use of a person's name or likeness for financial gain, for unreasonable disclosures of private facts, and for publicity that unreasonably placed the person in a false light before the public.

In the healthcare setting this issue has surfaced in connection with media demand for access to autopsy photographs or medical records of public figures, politicians, laboratory results of rock stars, and politicians. Healthcare professionals and providers must take care to take reasonable steps to protect the safety and confidentiality of patients and their records. In the USA the Health Insurance Portability and Accountability Act (HIPAA) privacy standards are applicable to protect broad categories of protected health information.

Other causes of action   Other possible causes of action for improper disclosures exist. For example, in the USA a cause of action may be made for violation of constitutional rights in those states that have enacted constitutional provisions that guarantee a right to privacy that may encompass health or medical information.

Alternatively, a claim could be made for breach of an implied contract to keep such things confidential based upon the circumstances, even though there is no agreement to do so. Another legal theory could be negligence for violation of a duty that is imposed by society or law. Still another possible claim could be for infliction of emotional distress stemming from the nature of the harm that might be suffered by a patient, if embarrassing or sensitive medical information were improperly shared.

Emerging Trends in Medical Records

There are several emerging trends that are reshaping the future of patient medical records, their retention, and their disclosure. The first is the ongoing effort internationally to encourage electronic medical records. The second is a direct result of the first. There are now widespread initiatives by patient advocates, industry, and government to provide enhanced protection against unwarranted disclosures of electronic records and to impose greater accountability by the holders of such confidential information.

Electronic Medical Records

Modern telecommunication and computer technology is contributing to rapid expansion of electronic medical informatics systems that will result in elimination of paper or handwritten medical records, which can be incomplete, illegible, or misplaced. The great promise of electronic health data is that it will permit creation of a comprehensive medical record that can overcome the difficulties of fragmented medical care, lack of ready access, and the frailties of paper records. Such electronic records will be readily accessible from even remote locations to meet emergent or ordinary medical needs. Electronic medical records will improve patient medical care by more efficiently coordinating the professional and support services required over the continuum of care, resulting in shortened hospitalizations and overall reduction of medical errors and costs.

Electronic medical records are vulnerable to the same threats that are already being faced by other sectors of business and government that rely heavily on telecommunications and computer support.

Additional Protections and Accountability

It is in response to the threats created by electronic medical records that many countries are imposing additional legal safeguards and requiring systemic accountability. For example, in the UK the Data Protection Act 1998 became effective on March 1, 2000. Among other things, this law requires that personal data shall be adequate, relevant, and not excessive in relation to the purpose(s) for which they are processed. Further, the law requires that appropriate technical and organizational measures shall be taken against unauthorized or unlawful processing of personal data and against accidental loss or destruction of, or damage to, personal data. In a requirement that perhaps reflects the increasing mobility of its populations and the reduction of geographic and political barriers, the Act also provides that personal data shall not be transferred to a country outside the EEA, unless that country or territory ensures an adequate level of protection for the rights and freedoms of the data subject in relation to the processing of personal data.

Similarly, in the USA privacy regulations became effective in April 2003, and have been adopted in connection with the 1996 HIPAA. Additional regulations imposing technical requirements on the holders or transmitters of electronic protected health information will be effective in 2005. These regulations require that healthcare providers give their patients written notices that describe their privacy practices and procedures. The regulations also require certain health providers to maintain logs about inquires made concerning their patients' personal health information (sometimes called PHI). The content of this log is available to patients for review. In addition, when responding to inquiries for PHI, the health provider must review the records and provide only the minimum PHI that is necessary to respond to the inquiry. A broad range of stringent penalties may be imposed for violation.

Caveat and Conclusion

It should be noted that this article reflects primarily on the law and principles found in North America and to some extent in the UK. Readers are cautioned that, although these broad principles apply globally, there will be local, regional, or national differences.

For example, a patient's right to access their own medical information may be more restricted in some nations such as Japan where cultural paternalism was historically present, or where religious traditions run deep. Similarly, while the European Council Convention on Human Rights and Biomedicine in 1997 embraced the principle of access to medical information, there remain great differences on what that truly means in a particular country. Even among the nations with shared English common-law traditions, no uniformity is necessarily present on the question of a patient's access to his or her own records. For instance, the Canadian Supreme Court has recognized a far-ranging right of access to medical information, but the Australian High Court has taken a narrower view.

Other disparities can be seen in the nature and extent of the privilege against disclosure. In France the privilege against disclosure is considered "general and absolute" such that even the patient may not relieve the physician of the obligation. In contrast, in Germany, under certain circumstances, the patient's consent to the disclosure automatically voids the physician's right to avoid making disclosure.

As illustrated above, every factual setting is unique and important differences and distinctions may be present when considering the legal implications. Consequently, this article is intended to provide general information and should not be construed as providing legal advice and it is not intended to be relied upon for that purpose.

See Also

Clinical Trials: Legal Aspects and Consent; **Consent:** Confidentiality and Disclosure; **Human Rights, Controls and Principles; Professional Bodies:** United Kingdom

Further Reading

American Medical Association. *Code of Medical Ethics, Current Opinions with Annotations, 2004–2005*. AMA Press.

Aspen Health Law and Comptiance Center (1996) *Hospital Law Manual*. Aspen Publishers, New York, USA.

British Medical Association (revised December 2002) *Access to Health Records by Patients* (discussing the Data Protection Act 1998). Available online at: http://web.bma.org.uk/ap.nsf/Content/accesshealthrecords? OpenDocument& Highlight. Accessed May 23, 2004.

Dunkel Y (2001) *Notes and Comments: Medical Privacy Rights in Anonymous Data: Discussion of Rights in the United Kingdom and the United States in Light of the Source Informatics Cases, 23 Loyola*. Law. A. Int'l & Comp. L. Rev. 41.

Gostin L, *et al.* (1995) Privacy and security of health information in the emerging health care system. *Health Matrix* 5: 1–36.

Harris R (1997) The need to know versus the right to know: privacy of patient medical data in an information-based society. *Suffolk University Law Review* 30: 1183.

Health Insurance Portability and Accountability Act of 1996 and the Standards for Privacy of Individually Identifiable Health Information, 45 C.F.R. Parts 160 and 164.

Joint Commission on Accreditation of Healthcare Organizations Comprehensive Accreditation Manual for Hospitals. Standard IM 7.1 et seq. (2004). Joint Commission Resources, Oak Brook, IL, USA.

Jost TS (2001) *Readings in Comparative Health Law and Bioethics*, pp. 189–226. Durham, NC: Carolina Academic Press.

Jurveic A (1998) When technology and health care collide: issues with electronic medical records and electronic mail. *University of Missouri – Kansas City Law Review* 66: 809.

The Geneva Declaration, 1 Declaration of Geneva (1949) *World Medicine Association Bulletin* 109–110.

Capron and Brrubaum (eds.) *Treatise on Health Care Law* (2003) Chapter 16. Patient Information and Confidentiality. Matthew Bender.

Win KT, Croll P, Cooper J, Alcock C (2002) Issues of privacy, confidentiality and access in electronic health record. *Journal of Law and Information Science* 12: 24–25.

MEDICAL RECORDS, DOCUMENTATION, CONFIDENTIALITY AND OBLIGATIONS

B A Liang, California Western School of Law, San Diego, CA, USA
L Ren, University of Houston Law Center, Houston, TX, USA

Introduction

Patient medical records represent a lifetime history that describes the healthcare experience of the patient. Generally, providers must be cognizant about potential invasion of privacy and breach of confidentiality suits for inappropriate use and/or disclosure of medical information. Also, providers should be aware of government regulations on medical privacy that may also result in significant penalties if their tenets are not adhered to. These issues and related concerns are reviewed below. In this article, we focus on the USA; however, the themes and concepts are similar in other western industrialized countries and we provide some information thereon when relevant.

General Considerations

It is important to note that medical record-keeping is not merely a legal construct to follow, but serves the purpose for allowing an adequate medical assessment and appropriate clinical intervention for use and interpretation by others involved in patient care. Comprehensive, quality medical records are a necessity for clear communications between healthcare professionals. Clinical documentation standards from medical organizations, accreditation groups, and provider entities thus emphasize the need to provide complete and accurate records to allow a reader other than the author to review the patient's history, care provided, and care plan to render the best care for the patient at hand. Indeed, facilities around the world have emphasized such a need in response to care that has been found suboptimal as a direct result of poor documentation in a wide and highly diverse array of clinical circumstances, such as psychiatric care in Singapore and Finland, nursing care in Taiwan, wound ostomy care in the USA, alcohol treatment in Canada, and critical care in Norway.

In most medical facilities, each test, procedure, provider visit, treatment consent, and medical impression is recorded in a patient's medical record. Further, sensitive information describing a patient's psychological state, personal beliefs, human immunodeficiency virus (HIV) status, financial status, and other important, but private, information is also collected in the medical record. As such, both private accrediting organizations and public law mandate patient record standards. For example, in the USA, the Joint Commission on Accreditation of Healthcare Organizations (JCAHO), a private accreditation entity, requires that the medical record be accurate; include information regarding physical exam, admitting diagnosis, results of all medical evaluations, complications, orders and notes as well as other reports, discharge summary without outcome and disposition of treatment, and final diagnosis; be documented in a timely manner with its information readily available and accessible for prompt retrieval; and be stored in a manner to maintain confidentiality and security. Substantively, JCAHO's standards are similar to those of federal regulations for hospitals serving the government Medicare and Medicaid programs and other sites for care. State requirements range from the very general to the very detailed and once again reiterate the need to assess local conditions to determine legal obligations. Generally, a complete record of the care provided and relevant supporting activities and discussions must be documented within the medical record. If care is not documented in the medical record, the provider and/or organization will often have to rebut the presumption that the specific event did not occur and may be held liable thereon. Indeed, this can extend to "criminal" liability if the omission from the medical record was committed to falsify business records or medical records to hide an event that should have been recorded.

Although there are standards relating to the form and substance of the medical record and information contained therein, the critical considerations for legal purposes are the confidentiality of medical information and when this confidentiality may be breached.

Confidentiality of Medical Records and Information

For the purposes of literal ownership, medical records are the property of the entity that created them, e.g., individual provider, hospital, managed-care organization, and group practice. However, the patient is generally considered to have some ownership interest in the information contained in these records. Physicians and other medical providers are under an affirmative duty to keep the information within these medical records confidential, as indicated by professional ethics

pronouncements, formal court decisions, as well as legislation. The policy is to encourage the patient to indicate all relevant information to the provider so that the provider can make a full clinical determination and then provide medically appropriate care. Without an assurance of confidentiality, the patient may not reveal such information and the therapeutic process could be hindered.

Under the common law, two general tort theories have been used for breach of medical record confidentiality. Under the first, the unauthorized disclosure of patient information by a provider constitutes an invasion of privacy. Such an invasion generally consists of an unauthorized release of medical records that constitutes an unwarranted appropriation or exploitation of the patient's personality, publicizing the patient's private affairs with which the public has no legitimate concern, or wrongful intrusion into the patient's private activities which would cause outrage or mental suffering, shame, or humiliation to a person of ordinary sensibilities.

The second theory by which courts hold providers liable for unauthorized release of medical records is through a common-law rule of confidentiality in the physician–patient relationship. If a medical provider discloses to a third party personal information learned about the patient during the course of treatment, the provider may be liable for breach of confidentiality between provider and patient, unless such disclosure is justified when there is a danger to the patient or another person. Thus, under this rule, all physicians have an obligation to keep confidential any information obtained during the physician–patient relationship and within the medical record; if they breach this rule, they may be liable for damages.

Other Issues Regarding Confidentiality of Medical Records

Altering, Appending, and Correcting Medical Records

Medical records can be altered and corrected for valid purposes, e.g., to correct transcribing errors or note new information relevant to the patient's care. These changes should be clearly indicated by making a single line through the portion of the record to be altered, corrected, or appended, with the date of the change and the person's signature or legible initials noted conspicuously. Further, an explanation as to why the record is being altered, corrected, or appended should be placed in the chart. The exact form by which these changes are made in the medical record is dictated by government regulation, medical bylaws, or both.

However, alterations that allow for view of previous notes will assist in avoiding any charges that the record was altered for self-serving purposes. Changes to a medical record that are made for purposes such as fraud or intent to deceive are, in some locations, subject to criminal and civil penalties (including punitive damages), and medical board or association sanctions for unprofessional conduct, and may result in loss of licensure and malpractice insurance.

Similarly, in England and Wales, the Data Protection Act of 1998 requires amendments to a record to be made in a way that clearly indicates why the alteration was made, to ensure the records are not tampered with for any underhand reason. The Act also authorizes patients either to petition the court to have inaccurate records amended, or to seek the assistance of the Information Commissioner.

Disclosure of Identity

The scope of the confidentiality is broad. The patient's identity, even to his or her own kin, is also within this right under the physician–patient relationship. Thus, a physician who delivered a patient's daughter was held to be answerable to the patient after the physician assisted the daughter in finding out her mother's identity after the child had been put up for adoption. Another concern is when patient information/likeness is used as materials in a book. This use is also within the scope of the confidentiality relationship and if a provider utilizes such materials without patient consent, the provider may once again be liable for damages in tort even if the patient's name is not disclosed.

Drug and Alcohol Information

There are strict requirements to maintain confidentiality of patient records regarding alcohol and drug treatment for patients who are participating in drug or alcohol rehabilitation programs. In the USA, government regulations for these facilities preempt any local laws that allow for purported disclosure of this information, although local government entities may pass valid laws that are more stringent than the national requirements. The consent for disclosure of this information will be valid only if the patient consents to disclosure to a particular party in writing; and the facility provides in writing to the patient-approved party: the facility's name or program name, the name/title of the person to receive the information, the patient's name, the purpose/need for the disclosure, the extent/nature of the information to be disclosed, a declaration that the consent may be revoked and the time when the consent will expire automatically, the patient's signature, and the date of the signature.

HIV Status

Generally, HIV status is strictly confidential. Many local governments have passed statutes that specifically apply to disclosure of medical information regarding HIV and impose both criminal and civil penalties (including punitive damages) against providers who violate these rules. Thus, whenever records or other information that includes any mention of a patient's HIV status is requested, the provider would be prudent to remove HIV information from the report unless specifically authorized in writing by the patient. Courts have stringently attempted to minimize identification of persons with HIV or acquired immunodeficiency syndrome (AIDS), although sometimes allowing for limited disclosure.

The law in the UK is even more strict. It prevents the disclosure of any identifying information about a patient examined or treated for a sexually transmitted disease beyond only HIV. However, like the USA, disclosure is allowed to a medical practitioner, or to a person employed under the direction of a medical practitioner, for valid diagnostic and treatment purposes.

Medical Malpractice

Breach of confidential information may also be brought as a malpractice claim in some jurisdictions. Because the provider has a duty to maintain appropriate confidences under a professional standard, a breach of that standard can be negligence and therefore malpractice.

Other Causes of Action

Beyond the standard tort causes of actions indicated above, patients have brought actions for breaches of medical record confidentiality under intentional infliction of emotional distress and breach of implied contract suits. Of importance is that the former requires extreme and outrageous conduct and the latter is amenable to the generally longer statute of limitations for breach of contract actions as opposed to general tort claims such as malpractice. However, as in the standard breach of confidentiality or privacy, the plaintiff must still show inappropriate disclosure of confidential information.

Physician–Patient Privilege

Some jurisdictions in the USA have laws that provide for a physician–patient privilege, which allows the provider not to disclose information in circumstances where the provider is compelled to testify, including testimony at trial, depositions, or administrative hearings. These statutes apply where the patient may not be suing and/or has not placed his or her condition at issue. This privilege is held by the patient, and therefore only he/she may waive it to allow the provider to testify. Note, however, that this privilege does not apply when the patient is putting his/her medical condition at issue or has waived his/her right in some other manner.

Localities without such statutes generally do not have a physician–patient privilege because the common law does not generally recognize this form of privilege, and thus the provider must testify in these circumstances. However, some of these jurisdictions are adopting a psychiatrist–patient privilege and a psychologist–patient privilege due to the sensitive nature of mental health therapy and communications. The privilege extends only to circumstances where there is a true provider–patient relationship and only to communications between the parties; hence, there is some question as to whether third parties, such as nurses, are included within it. This latter concern requires careful assessment of the laws to determine if and when the privilege applies.

Other common-law jurisdictions also have a tendency to reject the physician–patient privilege. For example, an early English case, Duchess of Kingston's Trial in 1776, rejected such privilege. The court reasoned that "even absent a privilege, a patient's self-interest would ensure that he/she would reveal all necessary information to his or her physician" and held that "while a physician must generally protect a patient's confidences, to reveal such information in court was not a breach of duty to the patient." England and its former colonies, such as Singapore and Australia, still follow this common-law rule and reject the physician–patient privilege.

Allowable Disclosures

Certain situations exist where the medical provider can disclose potentially embarrassing or private information without the patient's consent. However, these disclosures are very circumscribed and thus quite limited in scope.

Waiver

The first method by which a provider may validly disclose medical record information is through patient waiver. Waiver generally relates to providers giving their opinion about the patient in a dispute that directly relates to the condition of the patient, i.e., the patient is putting his or her very medical status in question in the dispute. Under these circumstances, when the focus of the conflict is upon the patient's medical status, generally the provider who discloses such information is not liable for invasion of privacy or breach of confidentiality.

Public Duty

The second basis for allowed disclosure stems from some official public duty. Generally, if providers are asked to give an official opinion for a court or provide information pursuant to an official government requirement or law, reporting the relevant information therein to the appropriate authority is not a violation of the patient's right to privacy or confidentiality.

Public Welfare

Disclosure without the patient's permission is also permitted when the disclosure is necessary to protect the public interest. Public interest in this context generally includes warning of a foreseeable danger or circumstances of possible death.

Beyond simply addressing acute dangers, Denmark and England allow disclosure of patient information for broader general welfare and public interest. Both have governmental registries of birth parents and adoptees, as well as records of patients (and their names) who have genetic disorders. Government possession of such information is presumed to be beneficial for the citizens' healthcare and social services and thus is presumptively disclosed to the relevant government databases.

Other Issues Regarding Allowable Disclosures

Disclosure of Information to Employer

Generally, it has been held that information disclosure by a provider to an employer is not in violation of a patient's right to confidentiality or privacy if that information is of direct and legitimate interest to the employer. These circumstances are akin to workers' compensation cases; courts will often hold that employers have a right to this information and thus providers who supply the information are not liable. However, it is important to note that, once again, the information that can be legitimately disclosed is limited to that directly relevant to the employer with respect to the employee; other information disclosure, even if relevant to the present work-related injury or circumstance (such as a previous history of a similar injury), may be a violation of the patient's confidentiality and privacy if disclosed without authorization. Further, if providers obtain information regarding HIV-positive status that is not directly relevant to the patient's workers' compensation claim, it has been held that liability may attach to the provider if this information is disclosed to employers, since the disclosure by the provider in these circumstances is not privileged.

Duty to Warn in the Public Interest – Variations

Information on foreseeable harm obtained through the special relationship between providers and patients usually creates some duty to warn. While some courts require that a specific individual be identified, others impose a more general duty. Providers may also be liable if they merely warn instead of implementing other precautions, including confinement. This liability may extend to providers not warning their patients of potential risks and harms of their medical conditions, including a duty to warn children regarding ramifications of their genetic disease transmissibility. In addition, this requirement to warn may be applicable to warning family members of a contagious or sexually transmissible disease including, in some localities, HIV. Of course, if the warning is provided under appropriate circumstances, there will be no liability of the provider for such disclosures.

Other duties to warn are also extant. For example, in Australia, Brazil, Denmark, Italy, and Norway, disclosure of a Huntington's disease diagnosis is routine and permitted. Australia, Brazil, and Denmark also permit disclosure of a hemophilia A diagnosis. In England, the Abortion Regulations of 1991 require that medical practitioners, who carry out termination of pregnancy, notify the Chief Medical Officer and provide detailed information about the patient. The Chief Medical Officer may then disclose that information under provisions of the Regulations.

HIV Status

Prohibitions against reporting do not apply to circumstances when the provider is required by law to report information regarding AIDS incidence (as compared with HIV infection) and other epidemiological factors to specific authorities "as specifically delineated by law." Sexual partners, spouses, and/ or needle partners in some jurisdictions may also be allowed knowledge of the HIV status of a patient and, under specific circumstances, are allowed access to that information regardless of patient authorization.

Disclosure may also be allowed to other specified third parties, including coroners and funeral directors, epidemiologists, facilities which procure transplant organs, semen for artificial insemination, or blood products, quality assurance and accreditation committees, parents of minors who have been diagnosed with HIV infection, researchers, and victims of sexual offenses. Further, disclosure of a physician's HIV status by hospitals to individuals who may have been treated by the physician has been allowed. However, beyond these narrow circumstances, providers should not release HIV information to any entity without the express consent of the patient or before checking with legal counsel. Finally, many laws either require or rely on voluntary reporting and disclosure of providers who are HIV-positive.

Other countries, however, have very different approaches to the HIV disclosure problem. France requires mandatory reporting, which was used to develop epidemiological information within the context of a universal healthcare system that provides 100% coverage for AIDS patients and their healthcare needs. Japan imposes no legal restriction or requirement concerning disclosure, and scholars have criticized the Japanese society for not recognizing patients' rights. However, a recent court ruling found the dismissal of an HIV-infected worker based upon his HIV status illegal and an infringement on the worker's human rights. In addition, the court found the disclosure of the worker's HIV status by his employer to third parties to be an infringement upon his right to privacy. For Japanese society, that has traditionally viewed employers and physicians as paternal guardians, this ruling signifies deviation from this traditional value. Australia takes an intermediate position on this issue. Legislation in New South Wales, Victoria, South Australia, and Queensland imposes duties of nondisclosure of HIV status and other medical information acquired during the course of employment of health professionals employed in public hospitals and other government-funded facilities. However, statutory restrictions are not applicable to private clinics and hospitals.

Other Public Policy Exceptions

In addition to circumstances of a foreseeable harm to others, additional circumstances have been held to be within the purview of allowable disclosures. Two major circumstances include when formal legal authorities such as the police pursuant to a valid court order request the information; and when another's life is being threatened. Note again, however, that it is important to limit the disclosure to that requested and directly relevant to the circumstance; additional information that is beyond this scope may subject the provider to liability under a breach of privacy or confidentiality.

Other Legal Disclosures

Practical disclosures are also generally allowed. For example, medical records may be released when transferring the patient to another facility or when requested by medical or forensic examiners. Other areas of permitted disclosure include suspected child abuse, wounds that are inflicted by sharp instruments that could cause death and all gunshot wounds, or simply all wounds that were a result of a criminal act. These laws are consistent with protection of the public welfare.

Patient Consent and Minors/Incompetents

If a patient consents to have his/her records released to a particular party, then the provider must release the specific records to that party, and no liability should result for such disclosure. What this implies in law is that patients have a right of access to their records. With regard to minor patients, parents generally have the right of access to a minor child's medical records, but in specific circumstances the parent may not have complete access if a provider determines that access is detrimental to the child.

Similarly, guardians of mentally incompetent patients generally have access to medical records, but again, there may be a limit on the disclosure if the information sought contains sensitive family information or if full disclosure would be detrimental to the patient's well-being. Disclosure of psychologically sensitive information that may harm the patient has been decided differently in different countries. For example, physicians in Switzerland favor the disclosure of Down syndrome carrier status, while physicians in Japan are generally against such disclosure as it may threaten marriages and other social institutions.

International Comparative Perspectives on Patient Record Access

Privacy appears to be a concept often seen native to the USA. For example, the Danish Council of Ethics began a study of medical privacy only in 1992. In other countries, the general focus of medical records is generally the access to one's own records. Physicians are given wide discretion in handling medical information and patients' access may be restricted for reasons such as lack of medical knowledge to understand their content. While Canada, the Netherlands, China, and Norway recognize patients' right specifically to medical records, Germany and Austria have only recognized such right of access through the individual citizen's right to self-determination.

In the UK, access has been a hotly contested issue. Under the universal healthcare system, physicians maintain a lifelong medical record for each patient. If the patient applies for life insurance, it is the physician who supplies the patient's medical information to the insurer. In a well-publicized High Court decision, a patient was denied access to her own records held by her plastic surgeon, which she sought for the purpose of legal action against a breast implants manufacturer. The Royal College of Physicians

forbade its members to provide any such information to lay persons. Addressing this issue, under the Data Protection Act of 1998, competent patients in England and Wales may now apply for access to their own records; Scotland is now implementing access to immediate discharge of documents under the 1998 Act. Authorized third parties, such as attorneys and parents, may also gain access under the 1998 Act. However, disclosure of any third-party identities is prohibited, unless the third party consents, or it is reasonable to dispense with that third party's consent. In addition, the 1998 Act also requires important explanations: the Act mandates the patient's record to be accompanied by an explanation of any terms that are or may be unintelligible. It should be noted that the law still requires the decisions about disclosure be made by the appropriate health professional, who is usually the patient's primary care physician. Courts under the law are authorized to order disclosure or nondisclosure, especially regarding information as to the physical or mental health condition of the patient. However, the 1998 Act specifically restricts the disclosure about the keeping or use of gametes or embryos, but genetic information is not covered by the Act.

In Australia, where the English common-law tradition is often followed, patients have very limited access to their own records, especially those held by private clinics. The Commonwealth Freedom of Information Act of Australia only enforces access to records in the public sector, and hence only these patients are afforded access rights. The six judges of the High Court unanimously rejected the notion that patients should have a right of access to medical records held by private physicians. Only the Australian Capital Territory and New South Wales have legislated for patients to access records in private healthcare facilities. The New Zealand legislature enacted the Health Information Privacy Code in 1993 to ensure patients' access to records, which generally grants broad access by patients for medical records and information.

The US Health Insurance Portability and Accountability Act (HIPAA)

In response to possible inappropriate use of private medical information, attention has resulted in national US laws to address the growing concern. HIPAA rules in this area cover all identifiable patient healthcare information in any form – oral, written, or electronic – maintained or transmitted by a wide array of "covered entities," including providers, healthcare clearinghouses, contractors, subcontractors, and health plans.

This extensive rule requires significant administrative policies, physical safeguards, technical security services, and mechanisms to be put into place by the covered entities. These entities must designate a privacy official or contact person to address complaints and provide privacy information, develop employee privacy training programs, implement "appropriate" systems against unauthorized access and mistaken misuse, create a mechanism of complaint for the entity's privacy practices, and develop employee sanctions for violations of the rule and the covered entity's privacy policies.

In addition, business associates of all of these entities are subject to the privacy regulations, including those who provide legal, actuarial, accounting, consulting, management, accreditation, and data aggregation, and financial services and any other entity that receives protected health information from or performs a function or activity for the covered entity. Contracts between the parties must limit business associate use and disclosure of patient information to parties specified and must require particular security, inspection, and reporting mechanisms by the business associates, and their subcontractors; internal records must be made available to the US Secretary of the Department of Health and Human Services, and all protected information must be returned or destroyed at the end of the contract period if practicable. The healthcare entity may be held responsible for rule violations of its business associates if it has knowledge thereof.

Patients have the right to inspect their healthcare information, copy and amend it, authorize (or not authorize) its use, and receive formal accounting of how their information is used. When patients request access, copying, inspection, and amendments to their medical records, covered entities have time limits to respond to these requests.

When disclosure and use of medical information are allowed, disclosure is limited to that "minimum necessary," with limited exception for treatment-related disclosures to providers. This standard requires that only the information necessary to accomplish the purpose for which the information is used or disclosed be released. The rule provides significant incentives for providers to err on the side of too little information use or disclosure: criminal and civil sanctions. Civil monetary penalties of up to $25 000 and criminal penalties of imprisonment of up to 10 years and a fine of up to $250 000 for each standard violation may be imposed, with providers subject to both for the same violation. The law represents a floor of protection for privacy; stricter local laws are not preempted. The rule also encourages providers to make a good-faith effort to obtain patients' written acknowledgment that they have received notice of their privacy rights and the entity's privacy practices.

There are exceptions to the patient authorization requirements. Authorization exceptions include information use for health oversight activities, public health activities, and research; in addition, law enforcement, legal proceedings, marketing, public safety and welfare circumstances, and listing in facility patient directories require no or limited patient approval.

See Also

Consent: Confidentiality and Disclosure; **Medical Malpractice:** General Practice

Further Reading

Aronsen T, Rekkedal LM, Hole A, Aadahl P (2003) Medical records of critically ill patients. *Tidsskrift for Den Norske Laegeforening* 123: 2257–2259.

Bishop RH (2003) The final patient privacy regulations under the health insurance portability and accountability Act – promoting patient privacy or public confusion? *Georgia Law Review* 37: 723–754.

Care First – Blue Cross Blue Shield (2003) *Medical Record Documentation Standards*. Available at: http://www.carefirst.com/providers/html/MedicalRecord.html.

Feldman EA (ed.) (2000) *The Ritual of Rights in Japan*. Cambridge, UK: Cambridge University Press.

Fletcher JC, Wertz DC (1990) Ethics, law, and medical genetics. *Emory Law Journal* 29: 747–789.

Frankel M (2001) Do doctors have a constitutional right to violate their patients' privacy? Ohio's physician disclosure tort and the first amendment. *Villanova Law Review* 46: 141–169.

Greenfield EL (1997) Maintaining employees' privacy of HIV and AIDS information in the workplace. *Hofstra Labor and Employment Law Journal* 15: 277–316.

Huefner DS, Daggett LM (1997) FERPA update: balancing access to and privacy of student records. *West's Education Law Reporter* 152: 469–491.

Laurila JV, Pitkala KH, Strandberg TE, Tilvis RS (2004) Detection and documentation of dementia and delirium in acute geriatric wards. *General Hospital Psychiatry* 26: 31–35.

Lee TT, Change PC (2004) Standardized care plans: experiences of nurses in Taiwan. *Journal of Clinical Nursing* 13: 33–40.

Liang BA (2001) The adverse event of unaddressed medical error: identifying and filling the holes in the healthcare and legal systems. *Journal of Law, Medicine and Ethics* 29: 346–356.

Lu M, Ma CT (2002) Consistency in performance evaluation reports and medical records. *Journal of Mental Health Policy and Economics* 5: 141–152.

Mamun K, Goh-Tan CY, Ng LL (2003) Prescribing psychoactive medications in nursing homes: current practice in Singapore. *Singapore Medical Journal* 44: 625–629.

Piorkowski JD (1987) Between a rock and a hard place: AIDS and the conflicting physicians' duties of preventing disease transmission and safeguarding confidentiality. *Georgetown Law Journal* 76: 169–198.

Rosenman H (1998) Patients' rights to access their medical records: an argument for uniform recognition of right of access in the United States and Australia. *Fordham International Law Journal* 21: 1500–1556.

Spong SG (1988) AIDS and the health care provider: burgeoning legal issues. *Michigan Bar Journal* 67: 610–618.

Strong JW (1992) The privacy for confidential information secured in the course of the physician–patient relationship. *McCormick on Evidence*, 4th edn., vol. 1, pp. 368–372. St. Paul, MN: West.

Wertz DC (1993) International perspectives on ethics and human genetics. *Suffolk University Law Review* 27: 1411–1443.

Winn PA (2002) Confidentiality in cyberspace: the HIPAA privacy rules and the common law. *Rutgers Law Journal* 33: 617–670.

Zeleznik J, Agard-Henriques B, Schnebel B, Smith DL (2003) Terminology used by different health care providers to document skin ulcers: the blind men and the elephant. *Journal of Wound Ostomy Continence and Nursing* 30: 324–333.

MUNCHAUSEN-SYNDROME-BY-PROXY

R Meadow, University of Leeds, Leeds, UK

Introduction

The term "Munchausen syndrome by proxy" (MSbP) was first used in 1977 to describe two children who had incurred severe abuse as a result of their mothers' persistently fabricating illness over a long period of time. One of the children died as a result of salt poisoning; the other suffered greatly as a result of the mother's false story and her fabricating the child's hematuria. Both children had many hospital admissions and had incurred many needless, unpleasant investigations, procedures, and treatment because of their mother's false story and creation of factitious signs, in much the same way as adults who have Munchausen syndrome incur needless investigations and treatment. For these two children the falsification was not by the children, but by another person acting on their behalf (a proxy). Therefore, the term "Munchausen syndrome by proxy" was used to describe the abuse which the two children had incurred.

Deliberate poisoning and other forms of child abuse had been reported before, but the originality of the 1977 report was, as its title implied, in drawing attention to parents who seemed to abuse children in order to gain the benefits of the child's illness for themselves. In both the initial cases, the mothers themselves had a degree of somatoform behavior and they extended their own behavior to the children, causing death in one case and severe harm in the other.

MSbP is an uncommon, but not rare, form of child abuse throughout the world; similar abuse may occur to elderly or other dependent relatives for whom an adult fabricates illness, and also to pets whose owners may fabricate illness. Nevertheless, the term is used primarily to describe the type of abuse incurred by children who have illness persistently fabricated by an adult.

In most countries MSbP describes a particular form of child abuse, though some psychologists and psychiatrists use the term to describe the behavior of the adult perpetrating the abuse, rather than the abuse itself. There has been considerable debate about the use of MSbP and many synonyms have been proposed or used, including factitious illness by proxy, fabricated disorder by proxy, illness induction syndrome, induced illness syndrome, and fabricated or induced illness. In this review, the term "Munchausen syndrome by proxy" (MSbP) will be used to describe a particular type of child abuse, rather than as a psychological/psychiatric diagnosis applicable to the perpetrator.

The criteria for MSbP abuse are as follows.

1. Illness fabricated (faked or induced) by the parent or someone *in loco parentis*.
2. The child is presented to doctors, usually persistently; the perpetrator (initially) denies causing the child's illness.
3. The illness disappears or diminishes when the child is separated from the perpetrator.
4. The perpetrator is considered to be acting out of a need to assume the sick role by proxy, or as another form of attention-seeking behavior.

It should be noted that this definition stresses the persistent presentation of the child to doctors, who are unwittingly part of the abusive process. The fourth criteria, identifying the motive of the perpetrator, is necessarily somewhat subjective, but helps to distinguish MSbP from other forms of harm that come to children as a result of misunderstandings and mismatches between parental expectations and anxieties, and medical beliefs and practices.

Features

A child incurring MSbP abuse will always have had a false story of illness provided by the carer. Sometimes the parent will also fabricate signs or induce illness in the child. There may be escalation from the first stage to the third, but each on its own can be very harmful to the child.

False-Illness Story

Even if a parent is not directly harming the child, a false medical history given to a doctor results in needless investigations, treatments, and admissions, and may result in advice limiting the child's life, education, or opportunities.

Fabricated Illness Story and Falsification of Signs and/or Samples

The perpetrator fabricates signs, alters samples from the child, or interferes with charts and records.

Induced Illness

In addition to the false-illness history, the parent (usually the mother) harms the child with drugs/poisons, or by smothering and other physical injuries so that she can present the child to doctors with the features of serious illness. This third stage is less common than the other two, but tends to feature in court cases because of the strength of evidence, which may include detailed toxicology, video recordings, or other robust forensic evidence.

Epidemiology

Boys and girls are equally affected. Most are young preschool children, for whom the doctor relies on the story of illness from the carer, and who are not under the regular observation of teachers or persons other than their parents. The abuse is most common in the first 2 years of life, and usually starts within a few months of birth. It is often many months, or even years, before the false nature of the child's illness is discovered. MSbP is identified much less often in children of school age. In such older children sometimes the child is complicit in the deception,

having been taught by the parent to give a false-illness story to others, and to feign illness by deception. In some cases the older child appears to have been "brainwashed" into adopting an illness role, and in others to have been taught to deceive so that the young adult presents him/herself to doctors with the features of Munchausen syndrome.

Although most case reports and series have come from Europe or North America, there have been reports from all parts of the world, and it is clear that MSbP occurs in countries that have very different social and medical systems, and that it is not confined to affluent societies or to those in which healthcare for children is free.

The only large-scale epidemiological survey is the 2-year prospective study, 1992–1994, of the British Pediatric Surveillance Unit concerning the incidence of MSbP, nonaccidental poisoning, and nonaccidental suffocation in the UK and the Republic of Ireland. For children under the age of 1 year, the combined annual incidence was found to be at least 2.8 per 100 000 children. A follow-up study 2 years later did not identify any child, originally diagnosed as MSbP, who had subsequently been found to have a genuine illness; thus there were no clear false-positive diagnoses of MSbP, suggesting a clinical tendency to underdiagnose such abuse. In fact, because doctors are such an integral part of MSbP (i.e., criterion 2), the pressures from both professional pride and litigation can be a forceful barrier to the identification of abuse and the safeguarding of children. It is less easy for doctors to identify abuse when they know that they are implicated actively or passively in that abuse.

As with most child abuse, there is a high incidence of abuse in the siblings of the index child; at least 50% are likely to have incurred, or be at risk of, similar abuse or other forms of child abuse.

Presentation

Particularly common presentations are seizures and apnea, partly because the doctor rarely sees such periodic events, and relies mainly on the story of the child's carer as the basis for investigation and treatment of the child. Alleged bleeding, diarrhea, vomiting, fever, and rashes are common presentations. Although some children present with apparent multisystem disorder, it is more usual for them to be presented with symptoms and signs suggesting a single-system disorder, thus after initial assessment they tend to be referred to one of the pediatric specialties, such as pediatric neurology, nephrology, or gastroenterology. Others will be referred to ear, nose, and throat, ophthalmic, orthopedic, or to system specialists who may have much less familiarity with disorders of young children than of adults. There are certain services and groups of children who are more likely to include children with MSbP, for instance those with intractable or unusual epilepsy, infants presenting with recurrent severe apnea or near-miss sudden infant death, older infants referred for Nissen fundoplication, or for sleep studies, and children receiving long-term parenteral nutrition, or who have had gastrostomies created because of unusual feeding problems (both groups of children provide easy access for insertion of drugs or foreign material directly into the body).

The commoner presentations of MSbP in relation to the different systems are shown in **Table 1; Table 2** shows some of the ways in which signs have been fabricated or induced by a parent.

Diagnosis

Child abuse is sufficiently common for it to be a necessary part of the differential diagnostic list for many childhood illnesses and accidents. The diagnosis of abuse depends on assessing carefully the clinical story and background to seek a genuine natural reason for the child's illness or injuries, and at the same time seeking positive evidence of falsification or induction of illness.

In the first instance the clinician is likely to have become suspicious because of a child's illness being unusual, unexplained, and prolonged, with symptoms and signs that are incongruous or apparent only when the mother is present, or because of standard treatments being either ineffective or not tolerated. Study of the family may reveal other unusual

Table 1 Clinical presentations of Munchausen syndrome by proxy

Nervous system	Seizures, apnea, drowsiness, ataxia
Gastrointestinal	Vomiting, diarrhea, failure to thrive, bleeding
Respiratory	Apnea, breathlessness, hemoptysis
Renal	Hematuria, biochemical chaos
Endocrine	Glycosuria, hypernatremia, biochemical abnormality
Allergy	Rashes, diarrhea, vomiting, fever
Otorhinolaryngological	Chronic otitis, foreign bodies
Educational	Dyslexia, disability, special needs
Skin	Dermatitis artefacta, abscesses, burns
Orthopedic	Locked joints, arthritis
Hematological	Anemia, bleeding
Cardiovascular	Sick sinus syndrome, hypertension
Child abuse	False allegations of sexual or physical abuse
Immune system	Immunodeficiency, fevers, osteomyelitis

Table 2 Fabricated signs

Bleeding	Hematemesis, hemoptysis, hematuria, and bleeding from other sites are fabricated, usually by the mother adding blood to a sample obtained from the child, or alternatively smearing blood around the perineum, nose, or other orifice. Generally she obtains the blood by pricking herself, or using a vaginal tampon during menstruation. Occasionally raw meat is used. Alternatively she causes bleeding by injuring the child
Seizures/apnea	Anoxia caused by smothering or drugs, usually one that has been prescribed for the child or another member of the family
Failure to thrive	Withholding or diluting food, sucking back food from the stomach via a nasogastric tube
Diarrhea	Laxatives
Fevers	Feigned, by falsifying temperature charts or heating the thermometer. Genuine, by injecting contaminated solutions into intravenous lines, or intramuscular injections of foreign bodies
Diabetes and endocrine abnormalities	Addition of sugar, salt, cooking ingredients, or other additives to the child's urine or to a blood sample whilst it is waiting to be sent to the laboratory. Poisoning of child. Deprivation of water
Hypertension	Altering entries on blood pressure charts or instructions concerning size of cuff to be used for measurement. Poisoning
Feculent vomitus	Vomiting is induced by salt administration or pushing fingers down the child's throat and then feces are stirred into the bowl of vomit
Dermatitis	By applying caustic solutions (e.g., oven cleaner or bleach) or repetitively scratching, burning, or rubbing the child's skin
Chronic discharge	From ears, vagina, anus, or other orifice by repetitively poking the orifice with a nail or other small object
Anemia	By disconnecting intravenous lines to drain blood from the child, or by venepuncture
Renal stone	Addition of gravel to the child's urine. Child may be given a stone to eat in food, and then taken with a falsely blood-stained sample of urine to the accident department where X-ray reveals the radiopaque stone

happenings to children, including abuse, unexplained death, a parent who seems deliberately to prevent her partner becoming involved in the child's illness, or a parent who has somatoform disorder.

The clinician has to review all the medical records very carefully and check the history for temporal associations between parental presence and childhood illness, consistency of reported illness episodes, and verification of episodes that are said to have occurred in the presence of another person. The hospital-based specialist needs to liaise with the primary care doctors and nurses, and vice versa, as well as with other family members. Sometimes it will be possible to secure direct forensic proof of induced illness by toxicological analysis of the urine, blood, or vomit, or by DNA or blood group testing of other samples. Polygraphic recordings and, particularly, covert video surveillance of infants being cared for by their parents in hospital have, at times, yielded indisputable evidence of poisoning, induction of vomiting, injection of foreign material into intravenous lines, and smothering by obstruction of the child's airways with the parent's hand, body, or a pillow.

Separation of the child from the parent can be an important diagnostic stratagem, and may be a valuable way of avoiding dangerous invasive procedures. It necessitates very careful assessment before and after separation from the parents, and the need to recognize that, in some cases, the child will have a genuine medical condition, usually mild, which is being magnified and distorted by the parent to create a major life-threatening illness.

Consequences

A false-illness story causes a child to have the multiple assessments, hospital admissions, investigations, and treatments that would be appropriate for a genuine illness. Young children are frightened, hurt, and, at times, put in danger by investigational procedures, treatments, and needless operations. Many have had prolonged therapy with steroids, cytotoxic drugs, and psychotropic drugs.

When the mother induces signs of illness, direct physical harm is involved, for instance, by scarifying, or burning the skin with caustics, obstructing the child's airways to cause anoxia and seizures, by injecting contaminated solutions to cause polymicrobial septicemia, and by the administration of drugs.

A third consequence is that, if the deception is undetected and continues for many years, the child may grow up believing him/herself to be disabled, and to be unsuitable for normal activities and opportunities. In some extreme cases children seem to have been programmed into taking on the role of an adult

with Munchausen syndrome, so that by their late teens they are presenting themselves to hospitals with false-illness stories, independent of their parents.

The biggest factor influencing morbidity is the speed with which the deception is uncovered. Most of the worst outcomes, such as blindness, deafness, organ transplant, lengthy parenteral nutrition, and death, have been in children who have incurred false illness for several years. There are many reports of MSbP resulting in the death of one or more children, but mortality rates are difficult to interpret and have been reported variously in the range of 5–30%.

Even with prompt intervention, the long-term outcome may not be as good as was hoped. Studies suggest that risk of recurrence of abuse is significant, and that MSbP abuse, which in the UK is categorized as physical abuse, usually has a much stronger core of emotional abuse and reflects a very abnormal parent–child relationship.

Perpetrator

In well over 90% of cases the child's mother is identified as the perpetrator. Usually her partner is unaware and disbelieving of the abuse. However, the striking noninvolvement of some partners in the care of their children, at times, implies an element of passive complicity. Fathers are the perpetrators in less than 5% of cases. It is even rarer for both parents to be working together to create a false illness in a child.

Systemic study of perpetrators of MSbP show that over half have personal abnormal-illness behavior in the form of factitious or somatoform disorder. Often the parental illness alternates with that of the child: the self-injurious behavior of the parent may wax and wane as the factitious illness of the child wanes and waxes. The limited information concerning male perpetrators suggests that parenteral abnormal-illness behavior is even more prevalent, with overt Munchausen syndrome (a very rare disorder) being unusually frequent.

Most perpetrators, when assessed by psychiatrists, are found not to have an identifiable mental illness. By virtue of their behavior they are considered to have a personality disorder.

Intervention

Procedures for assessing child abuse and for intervention vary from country to country. In most developed countries there are local guidelines, based upon national guidelines and national laws relating to children and families, which direct the lead clinician. In the UK the lead clinician is likely to be a pediatrician who at an early stage liaises with other medical colleagues, and with social services. Local authority social services then take the lead in organizing a full multidisciplinary assessment and, if necessary, intervention to protect the child. In the UK the safety of the children is organized through the procedures of the Children Act 1989, whose proceedings are heard in family courts. Although family courts have an adversarial nature, in that the local authority, the parents, and the children all have separate legal representation, the court also has a limited inquisitional role, which is best demonstrated at the highest level in the Family Division of the High Court where very experienced judges adjudicate on the most serious cases of MSbP and unusual childhood death. In these courts it is uncommon to hear the term "Munchausen syndrome by proxy," used, or one of its synonyms, because the task for the court is to decide whether a child has been abused, the detail of it, and whether that child is at risk of significant harm. The motivation of the parent, or the term MSbP, is irrelevant to those decisions. Once the facts and degree of abuse have been established, it becomes more relevant to establish why a parent behaved in a particular way, and such understanding may influence how best to help the family. Such assessment of the perpetrator's personality, motivation, and behavior is an important second stage.

In the UK the Crown Prosecution Service has instigated separate criminal proceedings in only a small proportion of cases, presumably depending on their perception of the public interest and the robustness of the evidence.

MSbP Interrelationships

Since its first description there has been a tendency to overuse the term. Worldwide recognition of MSbP drew attention to many previously unrecognized ways in which young children were being seriously abused. The extent of that abuse was beyond the imagination of most people, and still causes skepticism. Recognition of MSbP led to much wider recognition of nonaccidental poisoning and of repetitive smothering of infants, and to the realization that some dead infants previously categorized as sudden infant death syndrome had been smothered by their parents. In turn this led some people to use the term MSbP for any child who had been covertly killed. That is inappropriate. The British Pediatric Surveillance Unit's survey indicated that, although about half of the cases of nonaccidental poisoning or smothering occurred in the context of MSbP abuse (repetitive episodes causing them to be presented recurrently to doctors), nevertheless just under half of the cases were isolated events more akin to a sudden outburst of physical violence by a parent against a child. Study of MSbP has also led to a better recognition of the many different ways in which the parents' perception of the children's illness and inappropriate health-seeking behavior may combine with overrigid medical practice to cause immense harm to children. The links with somatoform behavior, doctor shopping, unusual health beliefs, delusional disorder, overanxiety, and hysteria are apparent, as well as the harm that may come to children because of combinations of inappropriate actions by parents and doctors. The link between unusual types of parental behavior and discrepant patient–doctor interactions needs to be remembered within the complexity of child–family–doctor consultations.

See Also

Children: Physical Abuse; **Forensic Psychiatry and Forensic Psychology:** Multiple Personality Disorder; **Head Trauma:** Pediatric and Adult, Clinical Aspects; **Imaging:** Radiology, Pediatric, Scintigraphy and Child Abuse; **Injury, Fatal and Nonfatal:** Blunt Injury; Burns and Scalds

Further Reading

Eminson M, Postlethwaite RJ (2001) *Münchausen Syndrome by Proxy Abuse: A Practical Approach.* London: Arnold.

Levin AV, Sheridan MS (1995) *Münchausen Syndrome by Proxy. Issues in Diagnosis and Treatment.* New York: Lexington Books.

McClure RJ, Davis PM, Meadow SR, Sibert JR (1996) Epidemiology of Münchausen syndrome by proxy, non-accidental poisoning and non-accidental suffocation. *Archives of Disease in Childhood* 75: 57–61.

Meadow R (1977) Munchausen syndrome by proxy: the hinterland of child abuse. *Lancet* 2: 343–345.

Meadow R (1999) Unnatural sudden infant deaths. *Archives of Disease in Childhood* 80: 7–14.

Parnell TF, Day DO (1998) *Münchausen by Proxy Syndrome.* London: Sage.

Reece RM, Ludwig S (2001) *Child Abuse, Medical Diagnosis and Management,* 2nd edn. Philadelphia, PA: Lippincott/Williams & Wilkins.

Rosenberg DA (1987) Web of deceit: a literature review of Münchausen syndrome by proxy. *Child Abuse and Neglect* 11: 547–563.

Royal College of Paediatrics and Child Health (2002) *Fabricated or Induced Illness by Carers.* London: Royal College of Paediatrics and Child Health.

Schreier HA, Libow JA (1993) *Hurting for Love: Münchausen by Proxy Syndrome.* New York: Guilford Press.

Southall DP, Plunkett ML, Banks MW, Falkov AF, Samuels MP (1997) Covert video recordings of life threatening child abuse. Lessons for child protection. *Pediatrics* 100: 735–760.

MURDER–SUICIDE

C M Milroy, University of Sheffield, Sheffield, UK

Introduction

Murder-suicide, more correctly termed homicide-suicide, is the phenomenon of an unlawful killing or killings together with the suicide of the assailant. These episodes are also referred to as dyadic death, from the Greek meaning paired. These deaths show features that are different from homicides in which the assailant does not kill himself or herself. Although sometimes called murder-suicide, they are more correctly referred to as homicide-suicide, as murder has a specific legal definition, depending on the legal jurisdiction, and requires a full criminal trial for final determination. Killings that are followed by the suicide of the assailant will not come to trial and though in some legal systems an inquest may be held, the killer is not able to put a defense, which might have resulted in a manslaughter verdict on the basis of mental illness, provocation, or similar grounds that allow partial or complete defenses to murder.

Definition of Homicide-Suicide

Marzuk and coworkers classified murder-suicides as a homicide followed by the suicide of the assailant within a week. However, there are a number of patterns of homicide followed by suicide that include:

1. Typical cases where the victim(s) and assailant are known and the suicide of the assailant rapidly follows the killing of the victim or victim(s).
2. Where the assailant commits suicide after arrest. In these cases, factors that influenced the reason for killing may have changed and the suicide might be for different reasons.
3. Pseudo-commando pattern. In these cases, the killer will go on a destructive mission with the intent to kill as many people as possible before destroying himself/herself. The victims are typically strangers.
4. Political/religious motivation where there is a specific group of victims targeted and the assailant dies as an intentional part of the act.
5. Culturally based homicide-suicide episodes such as "amok," originally described in young Malaysian men, and "windigo," a pattern of homicide-suicide seen amongst the Ojibwa tribe in sub-Arctic Canada.

Homicide-Suicide Studies

West published his seminal work *Murder Followed by Suicide* in 1965. This study examined episodes of killing followed by suicide in London, England between 1948 and 1962. The study was based on inquest findings that recorded verdicts of murder and suicide. Until 1977, English coroner's courts could return verdicts of murder, rather than unlawful killing. Based on these data, West concluded that one-third of all murderers in England committed suicide. This figure has often been quoted to state that England has a high suicide rate of its killers. These data did not include those cases where there was a verdict of manslaughter and overstated the overall rate of suicide by England's killers. However, West's study was important as a large study of such episodes and pointed to important differences from other patterns of homicide. In particular, he found that women formed a large cohort of killers, and that their victims were their own children. In his study 40% of killers were women. Of the male killers, most killed their wife or girlfriend. Other early studies of homicide also included data on suicide rates. A high percentage of homicide followed by suicide was seen in Denmark, Israel, and Australia, but with lower percentages in the USA. Subsequent studies have shown both similarities and differences in patterns of homicide-suicide.

Assailants and Victims

In 1992, Marzuk and colleagues proposed a classification for homicide-suicide episodes (**Table 1**). Their classification has been used as the basis of other classification systems, notably that of Hanslick and Kopenon. The principal relationships can be divided into spousal, familial, and extrafamilial. The most common patterns are spousal and familial. In the study of West, it was suggested that women may form a large group of assailants in homicide-suicide episodes, but studies over the last three decades from a number of different countries have indicated that men are the principal perpetrators of homicide-suicide, with most survey's revealing the male perpetrator rate above 90%. The principal victim is the man's spouse or partner. The man may also kill his children. When women kill, the victims are most commonly their own young children. Extrafamilial killings are rare, but include work colleagues, random victims of mass shooting episodes, religious cults, and victims of terrorism.

Table 1 Classification of homicide-suicide

1 Spousal or consortial
Perpetrator
(a) Spouse
(b) Consort
Type of homicide
(a) Uroxicidal (spouse-killing)
(b) Consortial (killing of lover)
2 Familial
(a) Mother
(b) Father
(c) Child (under 16 years)
(d) Other family member
Type of homicide
(a) Neonaticide (child <24 h old)
(b) Infanticide (child >1 day <1 year)
(c) Pedicide (child >1 year <16 years)
(d) Adult family member
3 Extrafamilial
Class
(a) Amorous jealousy
(b) Mercy killing
(c) Altruistic or extended suicide
(d) Family, financial, or social stressors
(e) Retaliation
(f) Other
(g) Unspecified

Reproduced with permission from Marzuk P, Tardiff K, Hirsch CS (1992) The epidemiology of murder-suicide. *Journal of the American Medical Association* 267(23): 3179–3183. Copyright © 1992 American Medical Association.

Methods of Killing and Suicide

In West's study of homicide followed by suicide, the most common method of killing and suicide was carbon monoxide poisoning. During the period of his study (1948–62), domestic gas in the UK was produced from coal (known as "town gas") and contained a high concentration of carbon monoxide. It was therefore relatively easy to kill young children and commit suicide at the same time using domestic gas. This raised the interesting question of whether a change in availability of method of killing would alter the pattern of killing. In the 1960s, the supply of domestic gas in the UK was changed to natural gas, which contains no carbon monoxide. This resulted in a significant drop in female suicide rates. A subsequent study of homicide-suicide in the UK examining deaths between 1975 and 1992 showed a low rate of female killers in the UK and revealed lower rates of carbon monoxide poisoning, with car exhaust fumes the source. Women formed a small proportion of the killers and used passive methods of killing, poisoning with medication or chemicals being the chosen method of the killing and suicide. The studies by West and Milroy identified a high rate of use of firearms in a country that has very restrictive firearms legislation. In the later study by Milroy, firearms accounted for nearly 40% of these killings, although fewer than 10% of all homicides involve the use of firearms. However, in a study from Hong Kong, firearms use in homicide-suicide was unusual.

In countries that have higher firearm ownership rates and where firearms are the principal weapon in homicides, such as the USA, there is a very high rate of use of firearms homicide-suicide episodes. In Victoria, Australia, where there is a higher rate of firearms-related homicide than the UK, this rate was found to be 70% whilst in studies from the USA rates of over 90% have been found. Thus availability of firearms does appear to have a significant effect on the pattern of killings as well as possibly the rate of these episodes. Even in low-ownership countries, firearms are an important factor in homicide-suicide episodes.

Epidemiology

An analysis of the studies of homicide-suicide reveals varying rates of homicide-suicide episodes between countries. In studying homicide-suicides some authors have looked at the percentage of homicide-suicides compared with total number of homicides. This however, does not always allow easy comparison between different jurisdictions. Examining the rate, that is the number of episodes per 100 000 people, allows more accurate comparison between countries and with time.

In 1983 Coid examined published data on homicide-suicide episodes and proposed three laws. They are:

> The higher the rate of homicide in a population, the lower the percentage of offenders who were found, (a) to be mentally abnormal and, (b) to have committed suicide.
> The rate of mentally abnormal offenders and those who commit suicide appears to be the same in different countries, despite considerable differences in the overall rates of homicide.
> There is some indication that the rate of mentally abnormal offenders, and those who commit suicide, remains the same, despite a fluctuation in the overall rate over time.

The rate of homicide-suicide episodes from published studies is shown in **Table 2**. It can be seen that the percentage of homicides to homicide-suicide episodes can vary quite significantly between countries, but an analysis of the rate of these episodes shows there is actually less variation in homicide-suicide episodes between different countries than overall homicide rates. The countries with the higher rates of homicide-suicide tend to have

Table 2 Epidemiology of homicide-suicide

Country/region	Years of study	Homicide rate (per 100 000)	Homicide-suicide (%)	Homicide-suicide rate (per 100 000)
Australia	1989–91	2.00	8.0	0.16
Australia (Victoria)	1985–89	1.87	9.0	0.19
Bermuda	1920–79	2.35	5.5	0.13
Canada	1968	1.50	18.0	0.27
Canada	1961–66	1.36	15.6	0.21
Denmark	1968–83	0.99	8.0	0.08
Denmark	1946–70	0.79	30.0	0.20
England and Wales	1980–90	1.11	7.2	0.07
England (Yorkshire)	1975–92	1.50	4.6	0.07
Finland	1955–70	2.20	8.0	0.18
Hong Kong	1961–71	1.57	5.0	0.07
Hong Kong	1989–98	1.50	13.0	0.09
Iceland	1900–79	0.72	8.5	0.06
Israel (Oriental Jews)	1950–64	1.07	25.6	0.27
Israel (Western Jews)	1950–64	0.59	67.8	0.40
New Zealand	1976–89	1.5	3.4	0.05
Scotland	1986–90	1.7	3.0	0.05
Sweden	1970–81	0.7	15.6	0.09
USA (Albuquerque)	1978–87	12.0	4.0	0.25
USA (Atlanta)	1988–91	38.8	1.4	0.46
USA (Houston)	1969	23.3	1.8	0.42
USA (Kentucky)	1985–90	5.0	6.0	0.30
USA (Los Angeles)	1970–79	17.1	2.1	0.36
USA (Miami)	1977–85	27.1	2.27	0.55
USA (New Hampshire)	1995–2000	1.7	14.7	0.26
USA (North Carolina)	1972–77	16.1	1–2	0.19
USA (Philadelphia)	1948–52	6.1	3.6	0.21
USA (Virginia)	1980–84	12.7	2.6	0.34
USA (Virginia)	1990–94	14.6	2.6	0.38
USA (Washington)	1974–75	29.3	1.5	0.43

a higher rate of overall homicide, with a greater availability of firearms. There is therefore some evidence to support Coid's contentions formulated above. In addition an examination of homicide data from England and Wales since 1945 reveals evidence to support the assertion that over time the rate of homicide-suicide episodes remains relatively unchanged, despite a significant increase in the overall homicide rates.

Reasons for Homicide-Suicide

Motives behind homicide-suicide episodes have been less studied than other episodes of homicide because of the non-survival of the assailant. However, suicide notes are left (in 27% of the cases in the series of Milroy), and other surrounding evidence allows elucidation of these events. Spousal/consortial killings account for greatest proportion of cases. In the study of Milroy they accounted for 50% of all episodes. The main reason for spousal killings is a breakdown in the relationship. In most cases the woman is about to leave, although in some cases the

man returns to kill his partner. A depressive mood may be present. Often a degree of jealousy is present. These killings are motivated by anger and revenge and not remorse. In older couples, however, often stress factors are often present. Studies of homicide-suicide in Australia and England found ill health and financial stress to be important factors in elderly couples. In Hong Kong economic factors were also important. Cohen has also pointed to the importance of homicide-suicide in elderly couples. When these episodes are studied in the elderly, they show resemblance to suicide pacts. Mental illness is the principal factor in a small percentage, and avoidance of criminal responsibility is an unusual reason for committing suicide. These episodes appear to involve the intention of destruction of both victim and assailant *ab initio*, rather than as an afterthought by the assailant.

With female killers, where the victims are their children, the motive is typically a misplaced altruism founded on mental disorder in the mother. These cases have been called altruistic suicide or extended suicide.

Generally, the killers have a higher socioeconomic status than other killers, though in Hong Kong homicide-suicide episodes were seen in more deprived couples. Alcohol is well recognized as a factor in homicidal violence and this also applies to homicide-suicides; Milroy found that one in five assailants had a blood alcohol above $100\,\mathrm{mg\,dl^{-1}}$. Felthous and colleagues found high concentrations of blood alcohol in assailants in cases in their study from Texas.

The Investigation of Homicide-Suicide

The investigation of a homicide-suicide episode should not be undertaken with the preconceived view that no assailant need be found as he or she is lying dead at the scene of the crime. A number of episodes have been recorded where an assailant has made one of his victims appear as though they have committed suicide (e.g., the English case of *R* v. *Bamber*). In approaching any homicide-suicide episode the pathologist and the investigating authorities should start from the basis that there is a homicide and then consider carefully whether the injuries seen in the apparent suicide are definitely self-inflicted. It is also important to exclude the deaths as being part of a suicide pact. Occasional cases of double natural deaths may occur as do accidental deaths from carbon monoxide poisoning. All these scenarios should be considered before a determination of the causes and manner of death is made.

Conclusion

Homicide-suicide forms a distinct subgroup of homicide that has been reported from many different societies. The assailants are predominantly men who kill family members, most commonly their wives. Firearms are the most common method of killing. Spousal breakdown is the most common triggering factor. The rate of occurrence of homicide-suicide is relatively uninfluenced by overall rates of homicide.

Further Reading

Barraclough B, Harris C (2002) Suicide preceded by murder: the epidemiology of homicide-suicide in England and Wales 1988–92. *Psychological Medicine* 135: 577–584.

Chan CY, Beh SL, Broadhurst RG (2003) Homicide-suicide in Hong Kong, 1989–98. *Forensic Science International* 137: 165–171.

Cohen D, Llorente M, Eisdorfer C (1998) Homicide-suicide in older persons. *American Journal of Psychiatry* 155: 390–396.

Coid J (1983) The epidemiology of abnormal homicide and murder following by suicide. *Psychological Medicine* 13: 855–860.

Felthous AR, Hempel AG, Heredia A, et al. (2001) Combined homicide-suicide in Galveston County. *Journal of Forensic Sciences* 46: 586–592.

Hanslick R, Koponen M (1994) Murder-suicide, Georgia 1988–91: comparison with a recent report and proposed typology. *American Journal of Forensic Medicine and Pathology* 15: 168–173.

Lecomte P, Fornes P (1998) Homicide followed by suicide: Paris and its suburbs, 1991–96. *Journal of Forensic Medicine and Pathology* 43: 760–764.

Marzuk P, Tardiff K, Hirsch CS (1992) The epidemiology of murder-suicide. *Journal of the American Medical Association* 267: 3179–3183.

Milroy CM (1993) Homicide followed by suicide (dyadic death) in Yorkshire and Humberside. *Medicine Science and the Law* 33: 167–171.

Milroy CM (1995) The epidemiology of homicide-suicide (dyadic death). *Forensic Science International* 71: 117–122.

Milroy CM (1995) Reasons for homicide and suicide in episodes of dyadic death in Yorkshire and Humberside. *Medicine Science and the Law* 35: 213–217.

Milroy CM (1998) Homicide followed by suicide: remorse or revenge? *Journal of Clinical Forensic Medicine* 5: 61–64.

West DJ (1965) *Murder Followed by Suicide*. London: Heinemann.

N

NEONATICIDE

R W Byard, Forensic Science Centre,
Adelaide, SA, Australia

Introduction

Generally, infanticide refers to the killing of a young child under the age of 12 months, with the term neonaticide being reserved for murders where the victims are under 1 month of age. The boundaries are blurred however, with variable cut-off points for neonaticide being reported at 24 h, 28 and 30 days. The majority of neonaticides occur within several hours of birth and are a response to unwanted pregnancies and deliveries. The assessment of such cases is often difficult as the bodies of the victims are usually hidden and injuries may not be found on autopsy examination. Due to the unique situation of a newborn child, simple omission of adequate care may result in rapid death. Even determining whether an infant was alive at the time of delivery may not be possible from the scene and autopsy investigations. Further methods for determining whether live birth had occurred or whether the infant was born dead are also inexact and may not be able to be applied with any precision. For these reasons extreme caution must be taken in the assessment of these cases. Generally, this article will deal with deaths occurring at or soon after birth.

Historical Background

Both neonaticide and infanticide have been practiced in most communities since earliest recorded times. Unwanted infants were sometimes drowned or smothered if they were perceived to be a financial burden for the family or community, and female infants were particularly vulnerable. In groups as diverse as the Spartans, Inuit, and Bedouin, unwanted infants would be left in the open to die from exposure, dehydration, animal attack, or hypo/hyperthermia. The Vikings and Celts sacrificed newborns to various gods as part of complex pagan rituals. In Europe during the reformation, church leaders advocated the drowning of infants with intellectual impairments. Such infants were sometimes allowed to starve to death and a separate category for "overlaid and starved at nurse" can be found in the Bills of Mortality for the City of London in the seventeenth century. Decline in the numbers of cases of neonaticide has been reported in more recent times in communities where there have been alterations in social attitudes to pregnancies outside marriage, improvements in contraception and sex education programs, and better social welfare programs for single mothers.

Case Characteristics

Mothers who kill their newborn infants are typically young and single, with a low level of formal education. They usually do not have a criminal record and have not attempted to seek an abortion. The pregnancy may have been denied by the mother, or she may simply not have been aware of it. When the delivery occurs it is often a solitary and secretive act with subsequent concealment of the infant. Death may have been actively induced by a variety of methods including suffocation by smothering or strangulation, drowning, or head trauma from blunt-object impact. Alternatively death may have occurred from hemorrhage due to failure to tie off the umbilical cord, or from suffocation from being wrapped in a plastic bag for disposal (**Figure 1**). Failure to provide nutrition may result in fatal dehydration or starvation, and lack of appropriate clothing may lead to death from hypothermia.

The secretive nature of the delivery means that there will have been no provision of medical care. Thus, mothers may present to emergency departments shocked from blood loss with continued hemorrhage, or with retained products of conception. In spite of the presence of a retained cord and placenta, the pregnancy and recent delivery may still be forcefully denied.

The motivations for such an act are ill understood; however despite assertions that the mothers show no

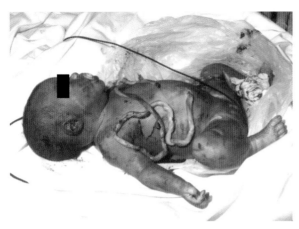

Figure 1 A term infant who was found wrapped in a plastic bag in a garbage bin following a concealed pregnancy and delivery. The end of the cord had been cut but not tied. A Guedel airway and monitoring lead were left with the body following unsuccessful attempts at resuscitation.

evidence of psychiatric illness, cases have occurred where there have been dissociative hallucinations and depersonalization. Mothers have described being removed from the event and of "watching" themselves during the delivery. The pregnancy and delivery may be denied and this may be a manifestation of underlying florid psychosis, possibly triggered by the event. Legislation in the UK acknowledged the possibility of puerperal psychiatric disturbance or depression, stating that a mother may have "the balance of her mind … disturbed by reason of her not having fully recovered from the effect of giving birth to the child or by reasons of the effect of lactation consequent on the birth of the child." There may be long-standing psychiatric disturbance with occasional reports documenting mothers who have committed multiple neonaticides/infanticides over a number of years.

In other cases, however, the motivations may be more obvious, with neonaticide committed to hide the birth from family members because of feelings of shame and concern that there may be rejection or punishment. Contraception may have failed or a mother may have delayed too long to enable an abortion, or may have been prevented from obtaining one by societal, family, or religious restrictions. Delivery may be hidden from a spouse if the pregnancy was the result of an extramarital affair. Other motives include financial anxieties about raising a child, not wanting the responsibility of parenthood, or concerns that parenthood may interfere with employment. In these cases there may have been quite elaborate lengths taken to ensure a private delivery and successful disposal of the body. These features mitigate against underlying mental impairment or incapacitating mental illness.

Scene Examination

Infant bodies may be disposed of in a variety of ways. In cases where mothers are suffering from psychosis, there may be minimal attempts to disguise the birth. In these situations the infant may be found at the site of delivery. Alternatively, young mothers may attempt to hide bodies around the house in a box in the attic, in the back of a cupboard, or they may bury the body in the garden or in an under-floor space (**Figure 2**). In other instances the body may be taken away from the place of birth and hidden in isolated woodland, a rubbish dumpster, or a public washroom. The method of disposal reflects access to locations and varies among countries. For example, a favored method of disposing of infants and/or their bodies in Japan has been to leave them in coin-operated lockers in railway stations. This method has declined in recent years with increased surveillance of stations.

In cases where the body of a recently delivered infant has been found in a house with limited access there is often minimal difficulty in determining who the likely mother was. When a body has been found in a public area with unrestricted access, for example a rubbish bin at a university campus, the list of possible mothers may be extensive.

Materials that are found with the body, such as blankets, sheets, or household rubbish, should be retained for formal examination as these may provide significant clues to the origin of the infant and possible places of delivery.

Pathological Findings

Examination of the infant should be undertaken in a standard fashion with careful external examination of the body for evidence of inflicted injury. Cases of asphyxia or drowning will not usually have any unusual findings. Blood-staining and vernix caseosa (white material that is normally adherent to the skin of a fetus) may be present, indicating recent delivery. Conversely, their absence may merely mean that the body was washed before disposal. The finding of injuries such as stab wounds or skull fractures and cerebral lacerations from blunt trauma suggest that the infant was live-born.

Evidence of dysmorphism should be documented and photographed as this may indicate significant underlying associated diseases or conditions that may have been responsible for death. Growth parameters such as crown–heel and crown–rump lengths, head and chest circumference should be measured, as well as weight and foot length.

Internal examination may reveal conditions that are incompatible with survival, such as severe

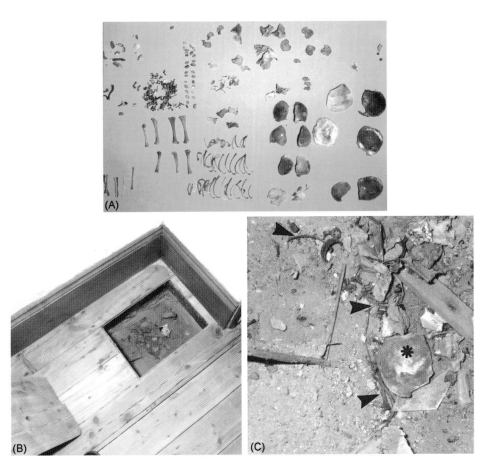

Figure 2 (A) The skeletonized remains of three near-term infants were found beneath the floor of a 70-year-old house. No bony injuries were found and the causes of death remained undetermined. Given the likely age and nature of the remains it was not surprising that police investigators were unable to shed any light on the discovery. (B) A trapdoor in a floor that had been concealed by a carpet. (C) A close-up of debris beneath the trapdoor, including infant long bones (arrowheads) and skull fragments (asterisk).

pulmonary hypoplasia from congenital diaphragmatic hernia (**Figure 3**). Microbiological samples, including blood cultures and swabs in nonputrefactive cases, are important in identifying or excluding significant infectious conditions.

Major difficulties often arise in the pathological assessment of these cases as injuries may be very subtle, and proving live birth may not be possible. The legal definition of live birth may also not be particularly clear and may differ from jurisdiction to jurisdiction. Requirements for "independent existence" also vary and may include complete expulsion from the birth canal, a detectable heartbeat, and/or respiratory efforts.

Cases of intrapartum death of normally formed term infants may occur during deliveries in hospital. Autopsies in such cases may be noncontributory, revealing no abnormalities, demonstrating clearly that mechanisms of death may be far from clear even under highly controlled conditions.

The goals for the pathologist faced with a case of possible neonaticide are to estimate the gestational age of the infant, to check for underlying diseases or conditions that may have caused death, to document injuries, to make an assessment of whether live birth occurred, to help establish the identity of the mother, and to determine the cause, mechanism, and manner of death. None of these goals may be achievable in certain cases, for example when all that is left are skeletal remains.

The gestational age can be determined from an examination of both the placenta and the infant. Maturation of chorionic villi may provide an approximate guide to gestational age while growth parameters such as foot length can be plotted against standard charts found in texts and on internet sites. Radiological examination is mandatory, as ossification centers will provide a more accurate determination of infant age than pathological assessment. Standard charts listing the time of appearance of ossification centers are widely available. In addition, radiographs may pick up significant underlying conditions such as skeletal dysplasias that will not be found by routine autopsy examination.

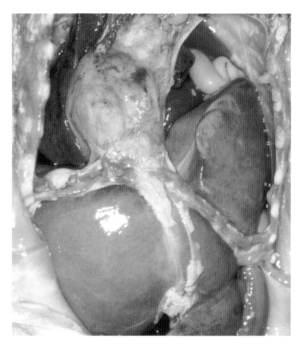

Figure 3 A diaphragmatic hernia responsible for death in a term infant showing herniation of the stomach, small intestine, and part of the liver through a defect in the left dome of the diaphragm, with pulmonary hypoplasia and displacement of the heart and mediastinum to the right.

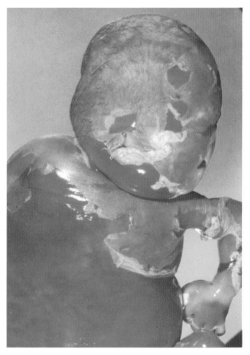

Figure 4 Marked maceration indicating *in utero* death in an infant with dysmorphic facial features, suggesting the possibility of an underlying chromosomal abnormality.

The chance of fetal survival increases with gestational age, with otherwise well infants born at 28 weeks now expected to live. Even less mature infants may survive, although often requiring medical support. In different jurisdictions an infant of 24 or 28 weeks' gestation or more is considered viable and capable of independent existence.

Determination of live birth is often difficult as there may be no way to prove that an infant had independent existence, with a heartbeat and complete expulsion from the birth canal. It is far easier to suggest that an infant was not born alive if there are signs of intrauterine death. A maternal history of cessation of fetal movements may be obtained. In addition, when a dead infant has remained *in utero* for some time sterile tissue breakdown occurs, producing characteristic changes of maceration (**Figure 4**). It can be confidently stated that a macerated infant has not been alive outside the uterus. Typical changes include reddening of the skin with peeling and slippage occurring approximately 12 h after death, with purple mottling and blister formation after 24 h, and the accumulation of reddish autolytic effusion fluid in the peritoneal, pleural, and pericardial spaces after 48 h. The body loses tone and joints become hyperextensible. After several days the brain softens and the skull begins to collapse with overriding of cranial bones. This may be picked up on radiographs and is known as Spalding's sign.

Although it has been proposed that shed fetal skin (squames), and/or meconium within the alveoli indicates stillbirth, this is incorrect. Meconium staining of the body (**Figure 5**) or under the nails merely indicates that fetal distress has occurred before or during delivery and suggests that the infant may have been compromised before labor was initiated. While there are certainly increased amounts of intraalveolar squames when there has been fetal stress, they are not an uncommon finding in the lungs and may be detected for some time after an apparently normal delivery. Frothy pulmonary edema fluid within the airways may be an indication of survival. While pulmonary interstitial emphysema has been proposed as a marker for live birth, its reliability is yet to be determined.

The usefulness of the so-called "birth line" in teeth is arguable. This finding results from disturbance of ameloblast activity at birth and may be detected at about 3 weeks of age. Although scanning electron microscopy may detect changes as early as the first 1–2 days of life, this is of limited use as the majority of neonaticides occur immediately after delivery.

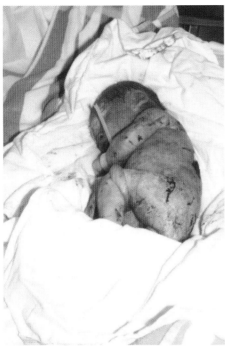

Figure 5 Meconium staining of a term infant indicating intrapartum stress. Delivery had occurred into a toilet bowl following a concealed pregnancy.

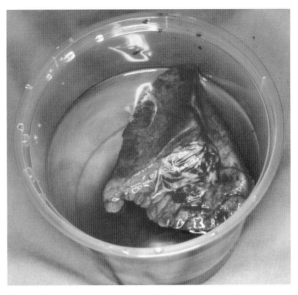

Figure 6 Well-aerated lungs floating in water in a case of alleged stillbirth without attempted resuscitation. The infant was not putrefactive.

Flotation Test

This test, known initially as "docimasy" or "hydrostasy," was first proposed by Swammerdam in 1667 to differentiate stillborn lungs from those of infants who had breathed. It involves placing the lungs in water to see if they float. Although variations have been proposed in which the heart and lungs are placed in water *en bloc*, in an attempt to increase the sensitivity and specificity of the test, it remains controversial.

The basis of the test is an assumption that the lungs from an infant who has breathed will be inflated, with expansion of the distal airways, and will therefore float in water (**Figure 6**). Their spongy texture and salmon-pink color contrast with the dense texture and dark-red appearance of lungs (**Figure 7**) from a stillborn infant that will sink when "hydrostasy" is attempted.

Significant problems exist, however, as lungs from stillborn infants may float if there is putrefaction with gas generation by bacteria, or if there has been attempted resuscitation with inflation of the airways by positive pressure. Infants who are born alive may breathe only very weakly, or may exhibit agonal gasping that may not be of sufficient force to open alveoli. There may be only patchy and partial inflation with an admixture of collapsed and inflated alveoli producing a mottled appearance. These lungs

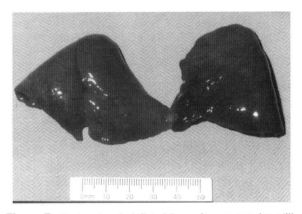

Figure 7 Dark-red underinflated lungs from a genuine stillbirth contrast with the salmon-pink lungs from the previous case (**Figure 6**) that showed obvious inflation. They failed to float in water.

may not float. Liver has been used as a control tissue on the basis that normal liver will sink, whereas putrefied liver with gas cysts will float.

Alternatives to the flotation test such as the test of Ploucquet have also been discredited. This relied upon comparisons of the absolute weight of the lungs to the body weight to determine whether respiration had taken place, i.e., inflated lungs that are perfused with blood will be heavier than lungs where respiration has not occurred. This has also been shown to be highly inaccurate.

Radiographs may be used to assess whether air is present uniformly throughout the lung fields and/or

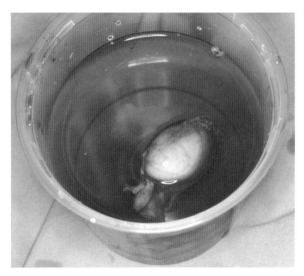

Figure 8 An air-filled stomach from an alleged stillbirth floating in water. There had been no attempts at resuscitation.

in the stomach. Again, the presence of air in the stomach (**Figure 8**) and small intestine may indicate that the infant has survived long enough to swallow air. However, the possibility of air being forced into the stomach during attempted resuscitation or being generated by bacteria during postmortem putrefaction must be considered. Putrefactive gas formation may be confirmed if abdominal radiographs show gas within the vessels of the liver. Air within the middle ears has been used as an indicator of live birth but is subject to the above caveats.

Another feature of live birth that may be present is milk within the stomach indicating that an infant had been fed prior to death. Histological examination of the umbilical cord may also reveal a vital reaction. Reports from the mother or independent observers of an infant crying or moving may confirm live birth.

Cause of Death

Failure to provide adequate care to a newborn infant may result in death from exsanguination if the cord is not clamped, from upper-airway obstruction if the airways are not cleared, or from hypothermia if an infant is not kept warm or is left exposed to a cold environment. Other common methods of neonaticide are asphyxia due to smothering or strangulation, or blunt-head trauma. Drowning may occur if an infant is delivered into a toilet bowl or is held underwater in a bath. Stabbing is less common and poisoning is rare. In the past it was alleged that midwives caused deaths of unwanted infants by pushing needles through fontanels or under eyelids. Deaths in these cases would

result from intracranial hemorrhage if venous sinuses were torn, or from sepsis.

As previously noted, the autopsy findings in cases of smothering or drowning are usually nonspecific, and unless the event has been witnessed or the perpetrator confesses, the cause of death may not be established. Delay in finding the body may also result in putrefactive changes with insect infestation that may alter, disguise, or simulate injuries. Smothering may result from a hand being placed over the mouth and choking may occur if cloth is forced into the mouth. Circumferential marks around the neck may be left from ligature strangulation, although it is important not to confuse these with normal skin creases or impressions from the umbilical cord if it has been wrapped around the neck during delivery or postmortem. Facial petechiae are usually not present in cases of infant smothering or strangulation. Although a cloth ligature around the neck suggests ligature strangulation, even this must be viewed circumspectly, as it has been reported that cloth may be tied around the neck by a mother to assist with traction in cases of obstructed self-delivery. Fingertip bruising or fingernail scratches may be found on the neck in cases of manual strangulation. Again, it is important not to mistake these for marks caused by the mother attempting to deliver the infant by herself.

If injuries are detected they must be differentiated from birth trauma that is most likely to occur with malpresentation of the infant and/or from prolonged labor. Comparing the pattern of injury to that of inflicted injury reveals differences which are explainable when the history of the labor and presentation of the infant are ascertained. For example, difficult breech deliveries may be associated with fractures or separation of parts of the occipital bone, so-called occipital osteodiastasis. When this occurs there may be tearing of venous sinuses in the posterior part of the cranial cavity with extensive subdural hemorrhage and cerebellar lacerations. Unfortunately, due to the nature of many of these cases, specific information about the labor and delivery will not be available.

Common birth-related injuries include caput succedaneum (bleeding and edema within the soft tissues of the scalp) and cephalhematoma (bleeding under the periosteum). The amount of hemorrhage associated with these injuries is not life-threatening. Skull fractures are not common and are usually linear fractures of the parietal bones occurring during difficult forceps deliveries. There may be associated extra- and subdural hemorrhages.

Other birth-related injuries include spinal injuries, fractures of the clavicles and long bones, and trauma to internal organs such as the spleen and liver.

Obstructed labor from cephalopelvic disproportion or shoulder dystocia may result in infant death from asphyxia. This may also occur in smaller infants if there has been rapid delivery. If a mother was standing or crouching during a precipitate delivery head injuries may result from the infant striking the floor. Obviously the cord has to be of sufficient length for this to happen. Measurements of the cord length should, therefore, be compared to measurements of the height of the mother's perineum from the ground.

Evidence of lethal natural diseases should also be carefully sought. These may be reasonably obvious, with conditions such as congenital diaphragmatic hernias with pulmonary hypoplasia, anencephaly, or chromosomal disorders providing acceptable causes of death. Subtle but serious cardiovascular anomalies, metabolic conditions, or sepsis may, however, be harder to identify. If death has occurred during delivery there may be evidence of previous intrauterine stress with reduced subcutaneous fat, poor growth, and meconium staining of the skin and under the fingernails. Findings at autopsy to support death due to an acute asphyxial event during delivery may include epicardial, pleural, and thymic petechiae with histologic findings in the lungs of intraalveolar hemorrhage, aggregates of meconium, and squames.

If a mother is located there are certain maternal conditions that can be checked for that are associated with poor fetal growth and the possibility of intrapartum asphyxia. These include diabetes mellitus, preeclampsia, hypertension, anemia, and heart or kidney diseases. Prolonged gestation (>42 weeks) and a high number of previous pregnancies may also be associated with poor infant outcome.

Maternal Identification

DNA comparisons between an alleged mother and an infant can be undertaken to assist in maternal identification. For this reason tissue and blood sampling at autopsy should be performed.

Placental Examination

As placental abnormalities may be responsible for the demise of an infant it is important to conduct a careful examination of the placenta if possible. Unfortunately the body of an infant may have been disposed of separately from the placenta and so the placenta may not be available for examination.

Conditions that may be responsible for infant death include premature separation of the placenta, abruptio placentae with extensive retroplacental hemorrhage (**Figure 9**) and compromise of cord blood supply. A large blood clot may still be present

adherent to the maternal surface of the placenta, or if it has been dislodged there may be an indentation indicating its position. Marked hemorrhage may also occur with placenta or vasa previa when the placenta or cord is overlying the entrance to the birth canal. Vessels and tissues become traumatized at the initiation of labor. Similarly, vessels may be damaged when there is velamentous insertion of the cord into the membranes rather than the body of the placenta, again with substantial and potentially life-threatening hemorrhage. Although infant mortality with such an occurrence is 60–70%, autopsy examination of an affected infant in isolation may not reveal any abnormalities.

Other problems leading to intrauterine or peripartum death include marked placental infarction (**Figure 10**) or sepsis. Cultures of the placenta may reveal the causative organism and histological examination of the cord and the placenta may show funisitis, villitis, or chorioamnionitis. Immunohistochemical staining has been used to delineate pathogenic infectious agents within placental tissue.

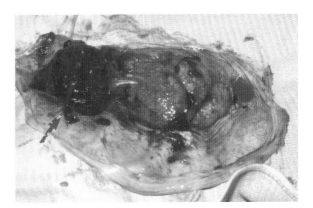

Figure 9 Significant amounts of retroplacental clot (arrow) in a case of abruptio placentae causing infant demise in an out-of-hospital delivery.

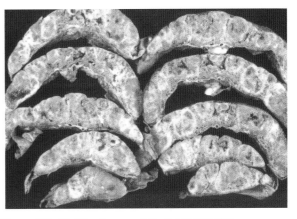

Figure 10 Multifocal areas of placental infarction.

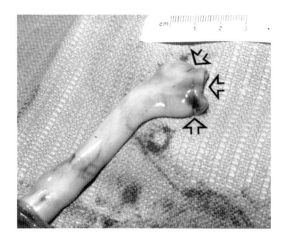

Figure 11 Three irregular incisions at the end of an umbilical cord (arrows) in a case of home delivery of an alleged stillborn term infant. No vital reaction was seen on microscopy.

The length of the umbilical cord should be measured as it may have a direct bearing on the reasons for infant demise. Asphyxia has been reported during labor from traction on excessively short cords (<30 cm), whereas long cords (>100 cm) have been associated with torsion, prolapse, knotting, and wrapping around the neck. The average cord length is 54–61 cm. The cord should also be examined for the presence of knots that may have interfered with the infant's blood supply. Loose knotting is not uncommon and is not significant; however, a tightly knotted cord will have narrowed vessels with congestions and edema on one side and pallor on the other. Histologically, there may be thrombi within cord vessels. The significance of twisting of the cord may be even more difficult to ascertain. Cords that have wrapped around the neck may also be important if there has been compromise of the infant's cerebral blood supply or airway. The severed ends of the cord should be examined and photographed to document whether the cord was cut (**Figure 11**) or torn, possibly during a precipitate delivery.

Dessication and separation of the umbilical stump begin after 24–48 h. An earlier change seen microscopically may be the presence of a vital reaction at the severed ends, indicating that there had been survival for some time after delivery. There may also be thrombosis of umbilical cord vessels with early organization. If death occurred immediately after delivery none of these changes will be present.

Conclusion

The investigation of possible neonaticide and concealment of birth is difficult as pathological findings may be subtle or nondiagnostic. For these reasons it is important to realize that in certain cases it may simply not be possible to determine whether live birth occurred, or to arrive at the cause of death with any certainty. In these cases it is appropriate to assume that an infant was stillborn until evidence to the contrary can be produced, with death being classified as "unascertained" or "undetermined."

See Also

Children: Sudden Natural Infant and Childhood Death; Non-inflicted Causes of Death; **Sudden Infant Death Syndrome, Etiology and Epidemiology**

Further Reading

Bove KE and the Autopsy Committee of the College of American Pathologists (1997) Practical guidelines for autopsy pathology. The perinatal and pediatric autopsy. *Archives of Pathology and Laboratory Medicine* 121: 368–376.
Bowen DAL (1989) Concealment of birth, child destruction and infanticide. In: Mason JK (ed.) *Paediatric Forensic Medicine and Pathology*, pp. 178–190. London: Chapman and Hall Medical.
Byard RW, Cohle SD (2003) Homicide and suicide. In: Byard RW *Sudden Death In Infancy, Childhood and Adolescence*, 2nd edn., pp. 125–135. Cambridge, UK: Cambridge University Press.
Keeling J (1987) *Fetal and Neonatal Pathology*. London: Springer-Verlag.
Kellett RJ (1992) Infanticide and child destruction – the historical, legal and pathological aspects. *Forensic Science International* 53: 1–28.
Knight B (1996) *Forensic Pathology*, 2nd edn. London: Arnold Press.
Schwartz-Kenney BM, McCauley M, Epstein MA (2001) *Child Abuse-A Global View*. Westport, CT: Greenwood Press.

Nuclear Terrorism *See* **Terrorism:** Nuclear and Biological

OCCUPATIONAL HEALTH

Contents
Police
Autopsy

Police

D McLay, Formerly Strathclyde Police, Glasgow, UK
C Shuttleworth, FGI, Ontario, Canada

Introduction

This article emphasizes the occupational health needs of police officers and the (nonsworn) staff employed to support their activities from a predominantly UK point of view. Despite that perspective, the broad principles apply widely although the organization, extent, and resourcing of police functions vary throughout the world. In the UK, nearly all duties not requiring police powers – in general, the authority to pursue, arrest, charge, and detain suspects – are devolved to civilian or support staff. Examples include the search of scenes of crime and the desk officers or station assistants who are often the first contact for members of the public. In addition, police forces have many clerical and administrative employees.

The distinction between police officers and support staff has become blurred. Specialists in computer crime and forensic science, for instance, are integral to investigations requiring their skills. Some police officers find it difficult to concede high status to these experts. Such cultural attitudes contribute to the organizational stress prevalent within police forces. Unless this problem is firmly addressed, the aim of achieving and maintaining a healthier police service will not succeed. There is no reason to think this is solely a UK problem.

In the UK, doctors are subject to standards contained in the General Medical Council's *Good Medical Practice*. These standards apply in an occupational health setting, in which a careful balance has to be struck between the interests of management and those of the work force. An occupational health service for the police should be led (or overseen) by a physician whose ethical standards apply to all staff, whether clinical or administrative. Management must also acknowledge the obligations owed by the occupational health service to individuals, despite any expectation that force objectives will have priority. To add to their difficulties, occupational health professionals have a role as employer advisers.

For simplicity, the acronym OHU (occupational health unit) will be used both for the unit itself and for occupational health staff who, depending on contractual arrangements, may be employed by the police force or by an external provider.

Do Police Officers have Different Occupational Health Needs from Other Employees?

Police officers are expected always to be "on duty," to maintain a standard of behavior during leisure time that is quite at odds with the norms of society. Self-control exercised at work spills over into personal lives, often to the detriment of family relationships. It is easy to forget that the sudden deaths, injuries, and fatalities in road traffic accidents, deaths of young children, as well as criminal acts, are far beyond normal experience. There are psychological consequences for police and other emergency-service personnel. If the response of supervisors is that this is the job they were employed to do, such lack of understanding merely adds to the stress of these experiences. Similar attitudes are found in other enforcement agencies (prisons, customs and excise, and military) in which there is a hierarchical, regimented structure.

The prevalence of marital, addiction, and post-traumatic stress issues in police forces and similar organizations is far higher than in other occupations. There is also a higher incidence of injury sustained on duty, and longer-term poor physical health is more common.

How Should Occupational Health Services be Supplied?

Nurses with occupational health qualifications fulfill the bulk of the day-to-day work, but an integrated OHU could usefully employ physiotherapy staff (physical therapists) and occupational therapists to provide treatment and speed return to work. Clinical psychologists, dentists, and dependency counselors are valuable resources. Circumspect referral of personnel to specialists such as psychiatrists, orthopedic surgeons, experts in physical medicine, or physicians is cost-effective. The work of welfare officers or of an employee-assistance program (EAP) is discussed later.

Economic and logistic factors determine the provision of services. A cost/benefit analysis should establish a total budget and how it is managed. In-house staff have the benefit of close cultural identification with police officers but may suffer greater management interference. A fully or partially contracted-out service at a fixed price assists overall budgeting.

Chemical, thermal, radiation, biological, or infective hazards concern occupational health in a conventional industrial context, but when police officers encounter these, they are more likely to do so unexpectedly or inadvertently rather than as part of their working environment. Police forces in the UK employ health and safety officers, who provide current guidance on hazards, but exposure to body fluids spilt in the course of assault or accident causes great anxiety. Questions are likely to devolve to the OHU. Bloodborne virus diseases are considered later. There is a need to maintain close liaison with external health providers because only the largest police organizations have the resources to cope in-house with the active management of emergencies.

A central issue for professional and administrative staff is confidentiality. Without reassurance of confidentiality, patients or clients will not avail themselves willingly of whatever services are provided. It is crucial that these services are not seen to be linked to management departments dealing with human resources or personnel. Whenever OHU believes there is a need to breach confidentiality in the interest of the individual, to comply with some legal obligation or (particularly in a police context) because of a criminal inquiry, the problem should be shared with colleagues. In any case, the desirability of disclosure will normally have been discussed with the patient/client.

Staff of an external EAP provider, being neither fellow employees nor agents of the police organization, have independence that increases their credibility with officers using their services. A disadvantage is that external providers sometimes do not have a good understanding of the police culture. This can lead to clients feeling misunderstood or that the counselor does not appreciate their working environment. A counselor may create an unrealistic expectation, for example, by suggesting that the client request a job where he or she never has to deal with death in any form! Subject to agreement with the client, direct liaison between the counselor and manager is to be preferred.

Working Conditions of Police Officers

The need for the police to provide 24-h service, ready to react to whatever incident presents, has become intensified within cities as entertainment and the consumption of alcohol continue well into the night. Wherever crowds gather, there is a duty (for reasons of public safety) to ensure an adequate police presence. To cope, officers must work a shift pattern to match patterns in both crime and public activity. Although some police officers relish the comparative freedom to pursue other interests, most find a rotating shift enervating due to both the adverse physiological effects and the spillover into family life and relationships. Prevalent working conditions make it difficult to maintain a fitness regime and to eat regular, balanced meals. Police premises should have at all reasonable times: sports or gymnasium facilities for use on or off duty; well-appointed changing rooms and hygienic bathrooms; facilities for the preparation of meals; and (in larger buildings) cafeterias that serve a range of nutritious food. The benefits for both staff and management need repetition and reinforcement.

The requirement to be on duty at hours outside the core working day results in: an increased risk to officers' health; a likelihood of disturbed sleep patterns; increased fatigue and impaired judgment; greater risk of accidents; an adverse effect on enjoyment of life. The manifestations of impaired sleep resulting from rotating shift patterns are well documented. The variation in tolerance to night work arises from a complex of commitment to the job, physical and psychological fitness, and daily habits.

From a physical standpoint, much of the work of a police officer is sedentary (at a desk or in a car), whatever the assigned duties. The demands for speed or stamina come without warning: there is no opportunity to warm up in preparation. A satisfactory level of athletic fitness is a requirement for officers working in an operational post.

Safety obligations come with the everyday activity of driving, but particular responsibilities fall on professional drivers, who include police officers, and their supervisors. Sleep-related vehicular accidents (SRVAs) account for up to one-fifth of road traffic accidents, with peaks occurring in early morning (mainly affecting young male drivers) and mid-afternoon (older males). Sleep deprivation due to rotating shifts puts police officers at increased risk during the clusters of SRVAs; in addition, many have to drive home after their shift, when their attention span is reduced. The problem of excessive daytime sleepiness is compounded if the officer is attending court during the day, has family commitments keeping him or her from adequate rest, or has a second occupation.

Confrontation leading to a physical struggle puts an officer at risk of injury, as does involvement in crowd disorder. Instruction and training emphasize techniques designed to help the officer defuse a situation and preserve "personal space." Even with the use of protective equipment such as batons, CS, or pepper sprays, conflict cannot always be avoided. Neither Tasers (Taser International Inc.) designed to deliver a disabling electric charge, nor firearms guarantee safety. The protective, armored vests commonly worn may impede movement. During a struggle, all types of injury may be sustained, blood is likely to be spilt, and some of those resisting arrest will attempt to intimidate officers by spitting into their eyes or mouth potentially infected sputum.

At incidents, or following an arrest, officers may be required to move vehicles or equipment or to lift and carry those they have arrested or injured people. In the heat of the moment, it is easy to forget the danger of suffering a handling injury.

Recruitment

The traditional aim in assessing candidates has been to exclude those who are "unfit" and those, such as diabetics, thought to be at increased risk of becoming unfit in the future. The question is, "fitness for what?" The physical and mental attributes demanded of officers have changed radically: medical advice must be pragmatic. OHU should help promote programs encouraging recruits to maintain, or even improve, the standard of physical fitness they possess on entry. Again, positive cultural influences (especially support from immediate supervisors and older colleagues) are important.

Standards

An effective recruiting department will state clearly in its literature the standards demanded, with a list of potentially disqualifying disorders. These standards

require medical guidance. Some candidates may challenge published exclusions, but it is fair to intimate that the job requires some fixed level of fitness (mental, physical, and emotional) as well as educational achievement. The evidential basis for standards has proved difficult to establish. Both male and female officers are expected to engage in the same level of physical activity, but most females are slighter and shorter than their male counterparts. The effort not to discriminate unfairly between males and females has resulted in the acceptable height for male recruits being reduced. Similarly, many more males than females have impaired color vision: to reject on the basis of defective color vision would adversely affect more males than females (unless it can be shown that perfect color vision is essential to accomplish police duties). In essence, these considerations are societal, not medical, but doctors are likely to have to manage them on behalf of the police force.

For these reasons, the standards set out in **Table 1** are merely advisory. With age and seniority, athleticism is required less because fewer operational demands are made on officers in promoted posts.

Disability Discrimination Legislation

The UK Disability Discrimination Act of 1995 exempted police recruitment procedures, but this protection is coming to an end. The Department of Work and Pensions calculates that the disability level in the working population is approximately 9% and assumes the comparable figure for the police to be 7% (there are about 166 000 police officers). The recruitment of disabled police officers is likely to increase that figure to 8%. Of course, during their career, some police officers will develop disability but be retained in office due to their skill and experience. A more general recruitment of the disabled may result in unfairness to other officers because blocks on redeployment seem inevitable.

Special Categories

The ability to drive a car is an almost universal requirement. Police officers are "professional" drivers for whom the UK authorities prescribe medical screening to exclude a wide variety of potentially disabling conditions.

Additional standards apply when officers take specialist posts, for instance, as divers, aircrew, and in mounted detachments.

Physical Health

Force management, representative organizations (police trade unions), and OHU have roles to play

Table 1 Standards for recruits[a]

System	Reject	Consider carefully	Comments
Eyes	Squint	Latent squint	Laser surgery under review
	History of detached retina	Lens implant	
	History of glaucoma	Corneal graft with good uncorrected visual acuity	
	Radial keratoplasty		
	Laser corneal correction		
Visual acuity (unaided)	Worse than 8/18 in either eye (binocular worse than 6/6 requires correction)	Consider effects of age on acuity	An independent specialist's eye opinion may be helpful, especially when higher standards are demanded
Color vision	Failure on City University Test	Failure on Ishihara Test	City University Test: 7 of 10 correct within normal limits
Ears	Hearing aid	Any chronic ear, nose, and throat condition	
	Active chronic suppurative otitis media		
	Current perforation		
Hearing	>average of 20 db loss over range 500–4000 Hz	Consider effects of age on acuity	Audiometry routine at preemployment assessment, using a soundproof booth
Cardiovascular	Hypertension requiring treatment	Hypertension >140/90	
	Severe varicose veins	Minor varicose veins	Defer until treated
	Uncorrected congenital heart disease	Hemorrhoids	Defer until treated
	History of coronary artery disease	Cardiac surgery in childhood	Routine ECG not required
	Cardiac surgery, adult		
Neurological	Any proven epileptic seizure after 5 years of age	Any episode of altered consciousness after 5 years of age	
		History of migraine	
	Degenerative neurological disease	History of brain surgery	
		Any significant head injury	
Metabolic	Diabetes mellitus	History of thyroid or any other metabolic disorder	Well-controlled diabetic may merit consideration
		BMI between 25 and 30	
		BMI <19	
Weight	BMI >30	BMI between 25 and 30	
		BMI <19	
Body fat		Percentage greater than Male, 21 Female, 30	
Gastrointestinal	Peptic ulcer	Occasional dyspepsia	
	Hiatus hernia	Hernia	Defer until treated
	Crohn's disease		
	Ulcerative colitis		
	Irritable bowel syndrome		
Respiratory	Nonasthmatic chronic respiratory disorders	Sinusitis, chronic URTI, hay fever	Routine chest X-ray not required
	Asthma currently on treatment (including inhalers)	Past history of asthma	Routine spirometry required

Continued

Table 1 Continued

System	Reject	Consider carefully	Comments
	Spontaneous pneumothorax on two or more occasions	Spontaneous pneumothorax on one occasion	
	FEV_1 or FVC >2 SD below predicted norm	FEV_1 <75%	
Musculoskeletal	History of back disorder requiring hospital treatment	History of minor back disorder	
	History of laminectomy	History of arthroscopy, including partial meniscectomy	
	History of major knee surgery, including open meniscectomy	Isolated dislocation of any joint	
	Recurrent dislocation of major joint	History of knee injuries not requiring surgery; significant fracture	
	Major foot deformities	Major soft tissue injury	
	Muscle wasting, effects of cerebral palsy	Chondromalacia patellae	
	Chronic orthopedic condition		
Psychiatric	Psychotic illness	History of isolated reactive depression	
	Most neurotic or stress-related psychiatric disorder		
	History of drug abuse		
	History of alcoholism		
	History of eating disorder		
	History of sociopathic behavior		
Genitourinary	Chronic genitourinary disorders	Any significant disorder of reproductive system	
Skin		Severe eczema, psoriasis, pustular acne	
Reticuloendothelial	All reticuloendothelial disorders		

[a]Adapted from McLay WDS (ed.) *Clinical Forensic Medicine*, 2nd edn. London: Greenwich Medical Media. Data published courtesy of FGI World.

in maintaining officers' physical fitness. The first need is to imbue staff with enthusiasm. Exhortation, example, publicity, and competitive sport all help, but so do facilities. The force may provide these, but the representative organizations often operate sports clubs. Good working relationships between officers' representatives and the OHU are worth all the effort expended to achieve them. Sports carry the probability of injury. The force must endure the consequent absences from duty. Certainly, in the UK and Canada, community services cannot cope with sporting injuries effectively, but there are many excellent sports-injury clinics that offer immediate treatment. Concession rates can often be negotiated for police officers or even provided as part of a benefits package.

Similarly, the delay in health service care for minor and chronic injuries suggests that police forces should consider the legitimacy of spending public money on private provision, either on a case-by-case basis or as part of overall medical and dental care.

Training in Techniques

The medical implications of such training are of interest to OHU. Instruction in combat and self-defense has the potential for injury during training as well in operational use. Two examples are self-injury during the deployment of CS spray (when particles strike the officer's face or contaminate clothing) and when attempting awkward lifts (e.g., when arresting a drunk). For the latter, direct input by a physical therapist on posture and back care is likely to be appreciated.

Injury

Recording of injuries that officers sustain on duty is essential. The financial consequences to the officer and to the force are major if the injuries are, or become, disabling. The UK Police Pensions Regulations 1987 defines a qualifying injury as one received in the execution of that person's duty as a constable;

while on duty; or while on a journey necessary in order to report for duty or return home after duty; or received because he or she was known to be a constable. These simple words are a rich source of litigation. Is an officer injured on duty if he/she twists his/her knee when rising from a chair? What about a defective chair? At the end of the day, these are legal, not medical, decisions.

Mental Health

The force must put in place a mechanism that is easily accessible to officers who face welfare problems, including debt, marital disharmony, discrimination, and anxiety about duties. The remit will vary, but welfare officers are usually employed directly. They will be less effective (and less trusted) if they report to central management. Many forces have contracted out the work to an EAP. **Table 2** provides information on the economics of using such a provider in Ontario, Canada, based on average utilization of 7%; in 2002, police utilization was 9.4%.

Critical Incident Stress Management

It is common for forces to have peer support programs to help officers deal with distress or emotional "highs" provoked by traumatic events. In some forces, debriefings are carried out by a mental health professional together with one of the peers as part of critical incident stress management (CISM). Such an arrangement allows the mental health professional to help in training and assessment of peer facilitators. Some explanation of the concepts underlying these procedures is necessary because they have become controversial.

Trauma can be provoked by a wide range of events, from child death to all sorts of catastrophe and brutality. The core feature of the officers' reaction is that some may begin to question their own security and the safety of family and friends. Actual bodily injury does not need to have been sustained: the essence is an existential doubt. Anyone who believes life has been in danger, who has seen death and destruction, is likely to be distressed, irritable, and perhaps irrational, but these feelings subside in hours or days. The purpose of debriefing or defusing is to demonstrate to members of a team that such feelings are expected, that they are "normal," and will probably diminish rapidly. An opportunity is given within a safe environment for members of the team to question themselves and their colleagues about what happened and why, about the outcome, and about what other steps they might have taken together. (This is not to be confused with operational debriefing, in which blame may fall on individuals.) The process allows

them to appreciate their own vulnerability, to put it into a context with which they can come to terms. Such a session may become quite heated but needs to be led by properly trained facilitators. Their role includes the responsibility to provide information on further services available and to be sensitive to those participants exhibiting warning signs of distress beyond the level anticipated. Promises of help must be given only where skilled support is in place.

Controversy arises over claims that these procedures cause harm rather than benefit. Readers are referred to the extensive literature on the topic but should bear in mind that the studies reviewed frequently do not relate to emergency personnel in their role as helpers and are often conducted by a single counselor (not a trained colleague) with individual patients who have suffered injury. CISM is a supportive technique, not a treatment. Adequate records and any follow-up should allow audit of the process to ensure that no harm results. The mechanism for ensuring assessment by a mental health professional when signs of distress are exhibited, or when participants request it, must be watertight. Voluntary follow-up also helps to ensure that individuals do not fall through the cracks.

Organizational Stress

Psychological distress does not result predominantly from traumatic incidents. OHU has a duty to bring resolutely to the attention of senior management patterns of behavior giving rise to organizational sources of stress, such as conflict, bullying, and discrimination. It is the duty of representative bodies, not OHU, to act as an officer's advocate. The doctor or nurse cannot undertake the inquiries necessary to establish facts. Nevertheless, good liaison with all levels of management allows beneficial input, supporting officers in achieving reasonable hours, family time, manageable workloads, some control over one's career, and a sense of security at work as well as being valued by management. Extensive studies throughout the world confirm that the lack of such factors influences the psychological ill-health contribution to sickness absence.

The force will have a policy toward sickness absence, probably involving some form of return-to-work interview by supervisors. It is crucial that the supportive purpose of such an interview is understood, otherwise it will fail. Training requires regular reinforcement. The interview gives a valuable opportunity for supervisors to assess colleagues, to understand undercurrents, and to refer for skilled assistance. Such skilled assistance may require counseling techniques but often no more than a listening ear or the institution of practical supportive measures.

Table 2 Economics of using an employee assistance program[a]

Estimated return on productivity

Assumes: 10% workforce distressed
       20% productivity loss for distressed staff
       65% success through EAP counseling

Costs without EAP

A. Number of employees in the plan	1000
B. Number of troubled employees (A × 0.10)	100
C. Average annual wage/benefits to troubled employees	$40 000
D. Wages to troubled employees (B × C)	$4 000 000
E. Cost of reduced productivity without EAP (D × 0.20)	$800 000

Costs with EAP

F. Number of troubled employees contacting EAP (B × 0.08)	80
G. Number of troubled employees who contact EAP and reach goal (assume 65% success) (F × 0.65)	52
H. Number of employees who contact EAP and do not reach goal as well as those who are assumed to be distressed and do not contact EAP (B − G)	48
I. Cost of reduced productivity for employees "H" (H × C × 0.20)	$384 000
J. Cost of reduced productivity for employees "G" (assumes that even those who are successful in EAP require time to return to productivity) (G × C × 0.20 × 0.167)	$69 500
K. Cost of EAP	$45 000
L. Cost of reduced productivity with EAP (I + J + K)	$498 500

Savings with EAP

M. (E − L)	$301 500

Return on investment

N. (M ÷ K)	6.7:1

Estimated return on supervisory time

Assumes: 10% workforce distressed
       9 h of additional supervisory time, beyond that typically provided, is required to manage the troubled employee (reduced productivity, impact on other employees, etc.)
       6.88% EAP utilization rates
       65% success through EAP counseling

Cost of supervisory time without EAP

A. Number of employees in the plan	3300
B. Number of troubled employees (assumes 10% of workforce is distressed) (A × 0.10)	330
C. Number of supervisory hours per troubled employee per year above normal supervision	9
D. Cost of supervisory time per troubled employee without EAP (assume supervisory rate of $25/h) (B × C × $25)	$74 250

Cost of supervisory time with EAP

E. Number of EAP users (A × 0.685)	226
F. Number of EAP users who reach successful goal (E × 0.65)	147
G. Number of EAP users who do not reach successful goal (E − F)	79
H. Cost of supervisory time for employees who did not use EAP and those who did but were unsuccessful [(B − E + G) × C × $25]	$41 175
I. Cost of supervisory time for those employees in "F" (assume that employees in EAP require at least 3 h of supervisory time until issues are resolved and return to productivity) (F × 3 × $25)	$11 025
J. Cost of supervisory time with EAP (H + I)	$52 200

Savings on supervisory time with EAP

L. (D − J)	$11 700

Employee turnover

Assumes: 6.88% usage rate
       5% of users are at "high risk" to leave job
       $60 000 in replacement costs (assumes $40 000 wage/benefits × 1.5 replacement costs; Conference Board of Canada, 1994)
       65% success rate through EAP counseling

A. Number of employees in plan	3300
B. Number of EAP users (A × 0.07)	226
C. High-risk (5% of EAP users at high risk for turnover (B × 0.05)	11
D. Success rate in EAP (i.e., number of high-risk employees who do not leave) (C × 0.65)	7
E. EAP users who do leave (C − D)	4

Continued

Table 2   Continued

Savings on employee turnover with EAP	
F. (D × $60 000)	$420 000
Cost of employee turnover with EAP	
G. (E × $60 000)	$120 000
Net savings	
H. (F − G)	$180 000

Estimated savings on short-term disability costs
Assumes: 3% of employee population will go on STD leave
        6.88% usage rate in EAP
        65% success in counseling
        $8400 average cost of STD case (assumes $200 per day × 28 day absence × 1.5 salary for replacement
costs)

A. Number of employees	3300
B. Number of employees at risk of STD (A × 0.03)	99
C. Number of employees at risk of STD who use EAP (B × 0.07)	7
D. Number of high-risk employees who reach goal and do not utilize STD benefit (C × 0.65)	4
E. (D × $8400)	$33 600

Summary

Estimated return on productivity	$821 688
Estimated return on supervisory time	$22 050
Employee turnover	$180 000
Estimated saving on STD costs	$33 600
Total cost savings for EAP	$1 057 338

[a]Data published courtesy of FGI World.
Abbreviations used: EAP, employee assistance plan; STD, short-term disability.

Vulnerable Groups

Among officers requiring routine psychological support are: those working on major criminal enquiries undercover; those dealing with vice, pornography, and sex offenders; liaison officers with families during lengthy murder enquiries; and officers using deadly weapons.

Chemical Dependency

Substance abuse (the nontherapeutic use of alcohol, prescription drugs, over-the-counter drugs, illicit drugs, and solvents/inhalants) may affect as many as one in five persons in a work force, with one-fourth of these addicted to alcohol. A police officer's job demands the exercise of judgment but is performed very much under public scrutiny. Violent crime is often alcohol-related, petty crime supports a drug habit, and drug trafficking is the root cause of much major crime. Officers with a "habit" are therefore in an especially invidious position. Their vulnerability to loss of position increases their need for concealment of the problem and the difficulty in seeking help.

Awareness of an officer's chemical dependency presents OHU with a dilemma because the rules of confidentiality are liable to put them at odds with management where strict disciplinary rules apply to officers who have consumed alcohol. Before any form of remedial action is taken, an unambiguous contract with the officer must make clear what is demanded of both sides. The force policy on alcohol and drug abuse must be well publicized to all personnel. It should warn of the consequences of alcohol and its effects on work, but it must also make clear how help is accessed. The response of colleagues is often to collude with the drinker, a course likely to prolong and worsen the problem.

Rehabilitation and Return to Work

One purpose of any management return-to-work interview is the detection and assessment of underlying problems, particularly if a pattern indicative of excessive drinking, family problems, disaffection, or malingering is established. The danger for both participants is that the interview can become confrontational rather than supportive. OHU may be able to resolve some of these problems and also facilitate negotiations for a program of, for example, parttime or light duties or reassignment to another department.

An arrangement of this kind is often necessary as an officer recovers from childbirth, bereavement, or some psychological crisis; it may be employed in association with continuing therapy. It is easier for managers to accept the need for a program following injury, particularly when physical or occupational therapy is in progress. Acceptance is particularly difficult when the need arises due to dependency on alcohol or drugs. If a timetable is not applied, these arrangements become open-ended, causing dissatisfaction for management, loss of OHU credibility, and ultimately, a disservice to the client. Regular monitoring is essential.

Infectious Disease

Wherever there is intravenous drug abuse and sexual promiscuity, there will be a pool of bloodborne viruses in the community. Operational officers need to be protected against hepatitis B by adequate immunization. There is a much greater fear of human immunodeficiency/acquired immunodeficiency syndrome (HIV/AIDS), and a lesser fear of hepatitis C, although these attitudes do not reflect actual risk. Priorities include:

- awareness of the dangers officers face
- sound hygienic practice
- use of rubber gloves
- covering broken skin
- use of heavy-duty gloves when handling broken glass at a road accident
- use of a device to perform mouth-to-mouth resuscitation
- thorough washing after the incident
- reporting any possible contamination via a wound.

Postexposure harm can be mitigated by antiviral therapy, following a proper protocol. Such treatment carries its own risks, and officers must be made aware of these.

Discharge from Service

Discharge is likely when an officer is unable, due to infirmity of body or mind, to perform the ordinary duties of a member of the force. To be "permanent," there must be no reasonable prospect of recovery in the foreseeable future. The UK regulations further define an injury on duty as one received without the officer's default in the execution of duty. Doctors have been left to perform a financial assessment, for the regulations link degree of disability with loss of earnings, not with medical loss of capacity. The inequities of the system have been widely accepted for many years, but governments have failed to implement necessary reforms.

See Also

Professional Bodies: United Kingdom; Rest of the World; **Professional Bodies, France – Forensic, Medical and Scientific Training**

Further Reading

Arnott J, Emmerson K (2001) *Managing Medical Retirement in the Police Service.* Briefing note 3/01. London: Home Office, Policing and Reducing Crime Unit (also available at www.homeoffice.gov.uk).

Arnott J, Emmerson K (2001) *In Sickness and in Health: Reducing Sickness Absence in the Police Service.* Police Research Series paper 143. London: Home Office, Policing and Reducing Crime Unit (also available at www.homeoffice.gov.uk).

Brown J, Cooper C, Kirkcaldy B (1994) Impact of work pressures on senior managers in the United Kingdom. *Policing and Society* 4: 341–352.

Collins PA, Gibbs ACC (2003) Stress in police officers; a study of the origins, prevalence and severity of stress-related symptoms within a county police force. *Occupational Medicine* 53: 256–264.

Connor J, Norton R, Ameratunga S, et al. (2002) Driver sleepiness and risk of serious injury to car occupants: population based control study. *British Medical Journal* 324: 1125–1128.

Costa G (2003) Shift work and occupational medicine: an overview. *Occupational Medicine* 53: 83–88.

DVLA (2003) At a glance guide to the current medical standards of fitness to drive. For medical practitioners. www.dvla.gov.uk/at_a_glance/content.htm.

General Medical Council (2001) *Good Medical Practice*, 3rd edn. London: General Medical Council.

Michie S, Williams S (2003) Reducing work related psychological ill health and sickness absence: a systematic literature review. *Occupational and Environmental Medicine* 60: 3–9.

Mitchell JT (1983) When disaster strikes – the critical incident stress debriefing. *Journal of Emergency Medicine Services* 8: 36–39.

Strategy for a healthy police service (2002) http://www.policereform.gov.uk/docs/healthypolice/strategy_healthy_police.

Autopsy

M B Nashelsky, University of Iowa Carver College of Medicine, Iowa City, IA, USA

Introduction

The Occupational Safety and Health Act in the USA (1970) and the Safety at Work Act in the UK (1974) are legal codes with broad influence throughout the industrialized world. They mandate employer recognition of work hazards with the goal of ensuring a safe work environment for employees. Each act has been followed by relevant codes that address safety issues in numerous work settings, including healthcare. In the USA, such codes include the well-known Bloodborne Pathogens Standard. In the UK, a guide has been published entitled *Safe Working and the Prevention of Infection in the Clinical Laboratories*, among many others.

These laws and regulations recognize that healthcare professionals at all levels are vulnerable to diverse work-related hazards. These include exposure to microorganisms in fluids or air, exposure to radiation or toxic materials, performance of ergonomically incorrect manual tasks, and psychological effects of the healthcare work environment. Although autopsy workers perform only one medical procedure, they are confronted by a similar constellation of occupational health issues.

The Autopsy as a Medical Procedure

An autopsy consists of a detailed external and internal examination of a dead body. Aside from the comprehensive visual examination, there are common additional studies including histology (microscopic examination of body tissues), microbiology (laboratory cultures of fluids and/or tissues for microorganisms), and toxicology examinations (analysis of fluids and/or tissues for drugs). The objectives of an autopsy are to: (1) confirm all features of the body that are structurally within normal limits and (2) describe and characterize all developmental, disease, and injury-related abnormalities. Synthesis of autopsy observations allows one to offer an opinion on cause of death, and will often facilitate interpretation of circumstances of death.

Autopsies are performed by physicians who have specialized in anatomic pathology (and often forensic pathology). Others present at an autopsy may include autopsy assistants, attending and resident physicians in pathology and other specialties, medical students, and law enforcement officers. Autopsies usually require long periods (hours) of uninterrupted standing and concentration on the part of pathologists and assistants. Most autopsies are performed in dedicated space in a hospital, a medical examiner's office, or a coroner's office. Fewer autopsies are performed in funeral homes. Autopsy tools include the spectrum of common surgical instruments: scalpels, scissors, forceps, and oscillating saws. Large knives and rib shears are other instruments more specific to the autopsy procedure.

The Autopsy and Occupational Health Issues

The occupational health challenges of the autopsy procedure may be subdivided into:

- exposure to infectious, toxic, radioactive, and other external agents
- facilities' design effects on autopsy workers
- ergonomics
- psychological effects of autopsy work.

While these areas will be discussed separately, they should be considered in aggregate as the dominant issues of autopsy safety. In the healthcare setting, employers must recognize and remedy a vast array of potential hazards, including those most pertinent to an institution's autopsy service. These employer obligations extend beyond reactive problem-solving and include proactive strategies such as availability of occupational health medical specialists.

Potential Transmission of Infectious and Other External Agents

The internal portion of an autopsy consists of examination of contents of the head, neck, chest, abdomen, and pelvis. Opening body cavities, cutting blood vessels, and subsequent direct examination of dissected organs release a large volume of blood and other body fluids. Contemporary autopsy techniques are essentially unchanged from those employed by the great anatomists of the eighteenth century (Morgagni) and nineteenth century (Rokitansky and Virchow). Sharp instruments (scalpels, scissors, and knives) and blunt dissection were and are low-tech mainstays of the dissection procedure. The orthopedic oscillating saw has replaced the traditional handsaw for removal of the skullcap. The oscillating saw may also be used to remove the chest plate. Needles and syringes are used to collect fluids from the eyes, heart, urinary bladder, and femoral area. Running water is used to rinse organs during dissection.

Percutaneous transmission   Scalpels, scissors, knives, and needles carry an obvious risk of percutaneous injury. There is near-continuous handling of or proximity to sharp instruments during an autopsy, as well as potential exposure to fractured or cut ends of bone, broken glass, and other sharp objects. Virtually all internal areas of the body and eviscerated organs are bathed in body fluids, especially blood.

A bloodborne pathogen is a disease-causing organism that may be transmitted from one person (or body) to another person via exposure to infected blood. While the list of bloodborne pathogens covers the spectrum of bacteria, viruses, fungi, spirochetes, and prions, a few viral diseases are common (especially in the forensic autopsy population) and may be transmitted via skin injury. These are the hepatitis B and C viruses (HBV and HCV) and the human immunodeficiency virus (HIV).

Worldwide, an estimated 350 million people have chronic HBV infection. Chronic HCV infection affects 170 million individuals worldwide. HIV infection is an expanding global epidemic, with an estimated 42 million affected individuals. In most cases transmission is via body fluids. Chronic HBV and HCV infections may evolve to hepatic cirrhosis and cancer of the liver. HIV infection may progress to the acquired immunodeficiency syndrome (AIDS), an often fatal compromise of the immune system.

There is an effective HBV vaccine. Postexposure therapy in the unvaccinated consists of the dual strategy of hepatitis B immunoglobulin and initiation of the vaccination series. This regimen is effective in the large majority of cases. HCV and HIV vaccines are not yet available. For HIV, postexposure antiretroviral drug regimens are used. Although probably effective in most cases, this has not been adequately studied. Effective treatment of a percutaneous HCV exposure is not yet available.

These viral infections are fairly common but the prevalences underestimate the exposure risk for autopsy workers. Autopsies are infrequently performed in the contemporary western world except for cases that are in the jurisdiction of a medical examiner or coroner (ME/C). ME/C cases have higher prevalences of HCV, HBV, and HIV than in the general population. In some areas, 90% of intravenous drug abusers may have chronic HCV infection (and people in this group are likely to be examined by the ME/C in case of death). A study of the medical examiner autopsy population of Baltimore, Maryland, revealed seroprevalence of HBV at 23.2%, HCV at 19.1%, and HIV at 5.6%. Due to the frequency of sharp injuries at autopsy, these high prevalences are a significant safety issue.

Studies have shown that: (1) pathologists and pathology resident physicians sustained a sharp injury in 1 of 55 and 1 of 11 autopsies, respectively, and that (2) 8% of gloves are punctured during an autopsy without underlying incision or puncture of skin. In the first study, cutting injuries such as from a scalpel blade outnumbered needle puncture injuries. In the second study, one-third of glove punctures were undetected by the autopsy pathologist at the time of injury, resulting in prolonged bathing of skin in blood from another individual. Most pathologists would agree that both studies likely underreport the true prevalence of skin and glove injuries. The risk of sharp injury during an autopsy, even when performed by experienced hands, is ever present.

Given that infected individuals are commonly autopsied and that sharp injuries in autopsy workers are not uncommon, it is fortunate that most percutaneous occupational exposures to these viruses do not result in transmission. Among these three viruses, HBV transmission is most likely, at a rate of 30% per exposure in the unvaccinated. Previous HBV vaccination effectively eliminates transmission of infection. HCV transmission occurs in 1.8% of exposures. Transmission of HIV is even less common at 0.3% of exposures. Although percutaneous transmission is infrequent, it does occur in healthcare and autopsy workers.

Airborne transmission   An airborne pathogen may be transmitted from both living and dead patients via aerosols or droplets. With a living infected patient, coughing and sneezing transfer infectious material to air around the patient. Another person in nearby space may inhale the suspended infectious material. In the case of a deceased patient, manipulation of infected organs (especially the lungs) and use of an oscillating saw aerosolize potentially infectious material. This phenomenon is an ever-present specter for autopsy workers, and is amply demonstrated by examination of one's face shield after an autopsy. Even gentle application of water to organs from a hose creates aerosols and droplets. Manual manipulation of organs may also produce aerosols and droplets. Oscillating saws produce an extraordinary concentration of aerosolized particles. HIV has been identified in aerosolized blood.

Tuberculosis (caused by *Mycobacterium tuberculosis*) is a disease that illustrates the principles of airborne transmission. Lung disease is most common. Transmission is airborne via coughing or sneezing by infected individuals (transmission is rarely percutaneous). The suspended infectious material may be inhaled by nearby individuals, thereby initiating a new cycle of lung disease in a previously uninfected person. A healthy individual usually does not develop active tuberculosis, although latent bacteria may persist in the lungs for many years or a lifetime. Onset of active disease in the previously infected person is usually associated with a compromised immune system. HIV co-infection – in which there is suppressed cellular immunity – is the classical setting that allows activation of latent tuberculosis bacteria.

Tuberculosis is the most common severe infectious disease in the world. Approximately one-third of the global population harbors the infection. Millions die annually of tuberculosis. The disease is far more prevalent in developing countries of Asia, Africa, the Middle East, and Latin America. Tuberculosis is usually treatable with medicines but there are drug-resistant tuberculosis bacteria. Tuberculosis vaccine is derived from a bacterial strain closely related to *M. tuberculosis*. It is variably effective and used predominantly in areas of high tuberculosis prevalence (usually developing countries).

Contemporary healthcare workers, especially autopsy workers, are at high risk for tuberculosis infection. Sobering research indicates that tuberculosis infection in pathologists (10%) exceeds the infection rate in pulmonologists (4%) and other clinicians (1%).

The recently recognized severe acute respiratory syndrome (SARS) is a viral disease of the lungs. Severity ranges from mild respiratory illness to death. Like tuberculosis, the coronavirus that causes SARS demonstrates classical airborne transmission. Coughing and sneezing by infected individuals produce infectious airborne particles that may be inhaled by close contacts. Neither a vaccine nor specific medical therapies are available for SARS.

ARS amply demonstrates the efficiency of airborne transmission of an infectious disease. SARS was first recognized in Asia in February 2003. The disease spread rapidly worldwide and infection was documented in 8000 individuals through July and August 2003, at which time SARS was considered contained. The mortality rate of the 2003 outbreak was 10%. Most deaths occurred in China, Taiwan, Singapore, and Canada. Healthcare workers were affected and there were fatalities in this group.

Risk management for percutaneous and airborne transmission Risk management in autopsy pathology consists of:

- assessing the risk of transmission of a known or unrecognized infectious disease from a dead body to an autopsy worker
- recognizing inherent hazards of the autopsy procedure
- modification or elimination of known hazards.

As noted, potentially transmissible infectious diseases are common and frequently undiagnosed at the time of death. One should approach each autopsy case as if it presents a potential threat. Preautopsy risk assessment strategies include careful review of medical records and other provided behavioral history (if known), external examination of the body for possible indicators of an underlying infectious disease or risk factors, and rapid HIV and hepatitis serological testing. These procedures are generally inadequate to assess risk due to possible incomplete medical records, occult disease without external stigmata, and technical limitations of serology testing of postmortem blood. Risk assessment is therefore somewhat moot (one should consider all bodies infected). Instead, one must recognize

and modify hazards inherent to every autopsy procedure.

Strategies to reduce autopsy hazards relative to infectious disease transmission may be grouped into:

- personal protective equipment (PPE) and vaccinations
- techniques and procedures
- facility design.

Personal protection is barrier protection, including use of airway "barriers." Barrier protection to protect skin, eyes, and mucous membranes consists of surgical scrub shirt and pants, a fluid-impervious gown with full coverage of the arms and legs, a surgical cap, eye protection (preferably a face shield that provides more coverage than eyeglasses), a face mask, and shoe covers. Barrier protection may be enhanced by waterproof rubber boots that cover at least the ankle and mid-calf. The fluid-impervious gown should descend below the top of the rubber boots (**Figure 1**).

Barrier protection of the hands consists of two latex gloves with an interposed cut-resistant synthetic mesh glove (**Figure 2**). This strategy should be used on both hands. Both the dominant and nondominant hands are vulnerable to sharp injury from bone or bullet fragments and cutting instruments. Cut-resistant gloves will not protect against needle

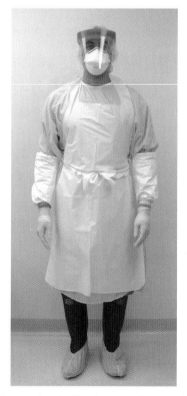

Figure 1 Personal protection for autopsies, consisting of skin and airway barriers.

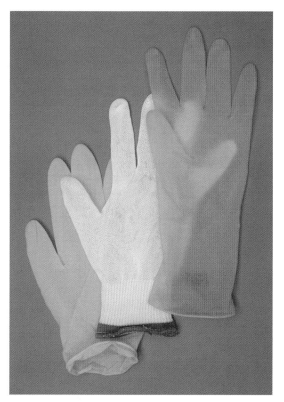

Figure 2 Three-layer barrier protection for the hands, including cut-resistant gloves.

punctures. With experience, triple gloving does not impair sensation or dexterity.

Aerosolized pathogens present additional challenges. Use of the N-95 respirator mask is the least intrusive method to reduce inhalation of airborne pathogens substantially, including the bacterium that causes tuberculosis. Airborne transmission of viral particles may require further filtration of inhaled air via a powered air-purifying respirator (PAPR) equipped with a high-efficiency particulate air (HEPA) filter. This device is cumbersome and consists of a battery-powered respirator attached to the waist. Through a tube, the respirator provides positive-pressure filtered air in a hood covering at least the head and shoulders.

There is an effective vaccine directed against HBV. Due to extensive fluid exposure by autopsy workers, HBV immunization should be a mandatory condition of employment. A tuberculosis vaccine (bacille Calmette-Guérin, BCG) is widely used in the UK, although it is rarely used in the USA. Vaccines specific for HIV and HCV are not currently available.

Techniques and procedures to reduce surface and inhalation exposure to pathogens encompass a wide range of work practices. In general terms, all autopsy workers must have training that sufficiently emphasizes the hazards of the autopsy procedure and the

autopsy suite environment. It is assumed that autopsy pathologists and physicians-in-training understand the transmission and biology of infectious diseases. It is equally important for the autopsy assistant to possess a broad science background appropriate to the task of daily autopsy work. This is particularly important as it pertains to his/her consistent recognition of and response to the varied hazards of the autopsy suite.

Every autopsy contaminates surfaces and air in the autopsy suite. All autopsy workers and visitors must be diligent in maintaining separation of contaminated and "clean" areas of an autopsy facility. There should be a high level of confidence that surfaces and air in "clean" areas are relatively uncontaminated by biological materials produced by an autopsy.

Any maneuver related to handling a body and eviscerated organs may contaminate the autopsy area. The goal is to minimize exposure to pathogens. All contaminated objects must be handled with care, anticipating splash and/or aerosol generation as two or more objects or surfaces impact each other. These activities are as diverse as movement of a bloody body surface from a gurney to the autopsy table, handling of individual moist organs during dissection on a wet dissection surface, and placement of autopsy instruments on a wet/bloody surface at the edge of the dissection area. Each of these activities, if performed carelessly, may cause a significant splash. As noted, application of running water on dissected organs has high splash and aerosol generation potential. Management of aerosols generated by an oscillating saw is a significant challenge. A plastic bag may be applied to enclose the head during use of the saw. The head of the oscillating saw may be modified to accept a vacuum attachment. The autopsy table may be equipped with downdraft ventilation. Gloves or other surfaces of PPE should be considered "dirty" even if not visibly contaminated. A PPE item in use should never touch areas of an autopsy suite that are considered "clean." These "clean" areas include a dry work surface used for writing notes, a telephone, and a door handle.

All autopsy instruments and work surfaces must be thoroughly cleaned and disinfected between autopsies. While there is great emphasis on safe work practices during an autopsy, adequate cleaning of all areas after an autopsy is no less important to minimize exposure. Additionally, autopsy workers must correctly dispose of sharp tools (needles, scalpels, and disposable knife blades). Housekeeping and biosafety disposal staff depend on autopsy personnel to dispose safely of any potentially sharp materials used during the autopsy.

Proper facility design is essential for safe performance of autopsies. There must be clear designation of clean (administrative) and contaminated (autopsy) areas of an autopsy facility. Movement of personnel between the two areas should be through a passageway or anteroom that, by nature of the physical design, establishes a definite transition between clean space and administrative space. An anteroom (not a changing room) between the clean and contaminated areas provides space for dressing in PPE and shedding of PPE when moving between clean and contaminated areas. Within the autopsy room itself, locations of door(s), autopsy table(s), dissection area(s), counters, storage areas, and photographic equipment should facilitate movement and flow of autopsy workers, bodies, and biological materials.

Strategies have been previously discussed to control dissemination of aerosols produced by the autopsy procedure and minimize inhalation of aerosolized pathogens. On a larger scale, rooms in which autopsies are performed should adhere to a standard of at least 12 air exchanges per hour. Optimally, air is drawn from clean to contaminated areas of an autopsy room, then directly vented outside the facility. Negative pressure in the autopsy rooms is essential in order to eliminate dissemination of aerosols from the autopsy area to the administrative area, and potentially beyond. Inadequate facility ventilation has resulted in well-publicized outbreaks of tuberculosis infection among administrative staff in a few medical examiner offices.

The size of the autopsy and administrative space must satisfy both employee and workload needs of the facility. Crowding, from too little space per person or too much work for a given amount of space, has an impact on morale, productivity, and safety. The autopsy is a complex procedure requiring numerous sequential technical and medical decisions. To this end, an autopsy facility in which there is a high density of workers, visitors, bodies, and equipment will be prone to inefficiency, accidents, and errors in judgment. While individual personalities and style may compensate for some measure of crowding, the overall mission of an autopsy service (hospital-based or medicolegal) can be compromised in the setting of a facility with inadequate space.

Exposure to Toxic and Radioactive Materials, Defibrillators, and Foreign Bodies

Poisonings from cyanide and other chemicals are widely popularized in the nonmedical media, but one poison is truly ubiquitous in the practice of autopsy pathology: formaldehyde. Formaldehyde (called formalin in the dilute form) is a clear liquid used in large volumes to preserve tissues. The funeral industry also uses formaldehyde as a tissue preservative. It is a volatile compound that irritates skin,

mucous membranes, and the eyes through direct exposure to body surfaces and inhalation. An increased risk of cancer is associated with long-term inhalation exposure. Periodic monitoring of 15-min and 8-h cumulative exposure to formalin allows early detection of potentially dangerous exposure.

Other poisons intentionally or unknowingly ingested by humans include cyanide (metal industries), metallic phosphides (rodenticides), and organophosphates (pesticides). With each material, the primary danger to autopsy workers is exposure to gastric contents. Each compound reacts with gastric acid to produce poisonous gas. A well-ventilated autopsy suite is essential but the autopsy facility must be further equipped with a chemical fume hood in which the stomach can be opened.

Some diagnostic and therapeutic procedures rely on localization of injected radioactive material in specific organs or areas of the body. These nuclear medicine procedures create a radioactive depot in the body of a patient. Technetium-99m is commonly used because of its short half-life (6 h) and versatility in combining with a variety of carrier molecules. A related procedure in nuclear medicine – brachytherapy – consists of implantation of a sealed radioactive source in or near a tumor. The therapeutic design dictates the duration of implantation and the type of radiation.

These materials present a potential radiation exposure hazard to autopsy workers. One must notify the institution's radiation safety department if there is a history of brachytherapy or injected radioactive material. In consultation with radiation safety experts, autopsy workers must use strategies for personal protection against radiation and appropriate techniques for the recovery and disposal of brachytherapy devices.

The implantable cardioverter defibrillator (ICD) detects potentially fatal heart rhythms and immediately delivers a shock intended to return the heart to normal rhythm. An ICD may discharge in a dead body. The electrical discharge ranges from 25 to 40 J, 1 million times more than a pacemaker's electrical discharge. Discharge of an ICD in a dead body may be precipitated by handling or cutting of the detection lead during the autopsy. Autopsy workers must stop the procedure upon detection of an ICD. Manufacturers' representatives are generally willing promptly to assist autopsy staff in inactivation of an ICD. Further, interrogation of the device may provide invaluable information about the decedent's perimortem cardiac function.

Foreign bodies or sharp internal structures may be encountered during an autopsy. These include bullets, broken knife ends, metal filters, fractured or cut rib ends, and irregular calcification of the aorta or cardiac valves. Advance knowledge of one or more of these items is often not available, hence preautopsy radiographs are prudent in selected cases that may harbor a dangerous foreign body. There is no specific technique to eliminate these hazards. As is usual when considering a possible percutaneous injury, risk is markedly reduced by appropriate personal protection and careful manual technique.

Ergonomics

Ergonomics is a multidisciplinary area that studies the physical interactions between humans and work. It exists in large part to recognize and study how work practices and tools may injure workers, and to provide solutions. Routine autopsy suite functions include activities that are well-recognized ergonomic challenges. These consist of pushing and pulling heavy loads and prolonged standing.

Although procedures will vary somewhat between hospitals and medical examiner/coroner (ME/C) offices based on how an autopsy suite is equipped, there will be at least two (and possibly more) transfers of a dead body between carts and a separate dedicated autopsy table or customized autopsy cart. Sometimes, the transfer is further complicated because the two surfaces are of unequal height. These transfers are physically demanding maneuvers that include sudden loading and significant static exertion over a long distance between the spine and hands. Performed once or repetitively over time, an autopsy worker may sustain injuries of the hands, arms, neck, shoulders, or back. Pushing a heavy load, as when moving a loaded cart, is a similarly demanding procedure.

Performance of a routine autopsy requires prolonged standing adjacent to a body as the evisceration is performed and subsequent prolonged standing adjacent to the dissection surface as the individual organs are examined. The posture assumed by autopsy workers is very similar to that seen in surgeons and other surgical personnel: prolonged static standing with slight flexion of the neck and back. This position increases the likelihood of a chronic musculoskeletal injury, especially low-back pain.

Simple solutions to these ergonomic issues are elusive. Regarding body transfers, there are mobile lifts designed to move bodies from surface to surface. They are expensive and cumbersome. They require additional floor space and, often, customized carts. There are much simpler devices that somewhat reduce the resistance of a body sliding between a cart and an autopsy surface. Although somewhat reducing muscular work effort, these devices have seen little acceptance.

Body posture of autopsy workers, especially pathologists, may be partially addressed by use of chairs. Sitting is possible during much of the individual organ dissection if the dissection area is appropriately designed, somewhat like an elevated desktop.

Psychological Effects

Physical health and mental health are intimately linked areas of occupational health. Physical workplace challenges (i.e., risk of an inadvertent needle puncture) lend themselves to quantitative evaluations and similarly structured solutions. Psychological workplace challenges are much less amenable to discrete, packaged descriptions yet are ever present and perhaps more pervasive than the physical aspects of occupational health.

Stress is a body's adaptive response to stressors. Stressors are those poorly characterized demands of life and work that motivate individuals to care for self and family and to interact productively with others in the course of personal and professional lives. Low stress is associated with inertia and low productivity. Moderate stress is normal and stimulates people to engage in the usual activities of life and profession, which are inherently productive. High stress yields high production in the short term but prolonged high stress precipitates exhaustion and low productivity (burnout).

A major genesis of stress among healthcare workers is the recurring direct or indirect interaction with patients (and their families) who are ill, vulnerable, and potentially very demanding. This occurs in the setting of significant competing stressors from the highly structured bureaucracy and hierarchy of the modern western healthcare complex. Stressors more specific to autopsy workers include: (1) daily exposure to death as the healthcare and/or behavioral outcome; (2) regular interactions with bereaved family members; and (3) intense involvement in institutional quality assurance and quality improvement efforts through evaluation of autopsy findings. An individual's response to these diverse stressors is evident through measurable work product and less tangible behavioral and physical manifestations.

There are no simple solutions to the psychological challenges of autopsy and general healthcare work. Institutional acknowledgment of stress and its potential adverse effects must form the foundation of realistic, sensitive, and confidential procedures that emphasize employee mental health as a high priority. Prevention, recognition, and treatment of stress-related illnesses should be a core function of the occupational health clinic in every healthcare system.

Conclusion

The autopsy procedure and the autopsy suite are inherently hazardous. Infectious diseases such as AIDS, viral hepatitis, and tuberculosis are present in many decedents coming to autopsy. Foreign bodies, radiation, electrical devices, and toxins may be present. Foreknowledge of these details of an individual case may not be available to autopsy workers. The physical maneuvers of body handling and autopsy performance are ergonomically unsatisfactory. In the setting of sharp autopsy instruments, a very large amount of liberated body fluids, and an oscillating saw that aerosolizes biological materials, there must be strict adherence to strategies of personal protection, procedures that minimize risk of injury or contamination, and thoughtful facility design that further reduces the likelihood of injury or exposure. Lastly, healthcare work, including autopsy work, is inherently stressful. Daily interactions with death, families of decedents, and objective quality of care issues associated with each patient's death are significant stressors for all autopsy workers.

See Also

Autopsy: Medico-legal Considerations; Pediatric; Adult

Further Reading

Al-Wali W (2001) Biological safety. In: Burton J, Rutty G (eds.) *The Hospital Autopsy,* 2nd edn., pp. 25–36. London: Arnold.

Antony SJ, Stratton CS, Decker MD (1999) Prevention of occupationally acquired infections in posthospital healthcare workers. In: Mayhall CG (ed.) *Hospital Epidemiology and Infection Control,* 2nd edn., pp. 1141–1158. Philadelphia, PA: Lippincott, Williams & Wilkins.

Buerger R (1999) Surgery and ergonomics. *Archives of Surgery* 134: 1011–1016.

Burton JL (2003) Health and safety at necropsy. *Journal of Clinical Pathology* 56: 254–260.

Hasselhorn H-M, Toomingas A, Lagerstrom M (eds.) (1999) *Occupational Health for Health Care Workers. A Practical Guide.* Amsterdam: Elsevier.

McCullough NV (2000) Personal respiratory protection. In: Fleming DO, Hunt DL (eds.) *Biological Safety. Principles and Practices,* 3rd edn., pp. 339–353. Washington, DC: ASM Press.

McCunney RJ, Barbanel CS (eds.) (1999) *Medical Center Occupational Health and Safety.* Philadelphia, PA: Lippincott, Williams and Wilkins.

Murphy TM (2001) The effects of a crowded workplace on morale and productivity. *Journal of Histotechnology* 24: 9–15.

Nolte KB, Taylor DG, Richmond JY (2002) Biosafety considerations for autopsy. *American Journal of Forensic Medicine and Pathology* 23: 107–122.

ODONTOLOGY

Contents
Overview
Bite Mark Analysis

Overview

J G Clement and A J Hill, Victorian Institute of Forensic Medicine, Southbank, VIC, Australia

Examination of the Mouth to Corroborate Identity

Starting from the premise that all forensic odontologists have a degree in dentistry, an examination of the oral cavity of deceased persons might be looked upon as a straightforward procedure. This is far from the case in many instances. Bodies requiring identification by odontological means are by their very nature often unrecognizable in a conventional way. This may be due to the effects of trauma, incineration, or putrefaction singly or in combination.

In extreme circumstances where a body or bodies have been badly burned, the first problem may be even to locate the head and the oral structures that remain. Large-format radiography, preferably realtime fluoroscopy, often has to be used to locate structures of interest (**Figure 1**). This problem obviously does not confront the dentist treating living patients.

Generally, oral structures that are useful in the corroboration of identity are preferentially preserved

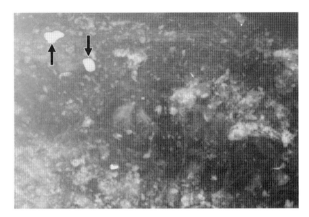

Figure 1 Large-format X-ray photograph (radiograph) of debris from a house fire in which some human remains were discovered. The two silhouettes (arrowed) are human teeth displaced from the corpse. Without this simple radiographic screening technique it may be impossible to find such small remains. Fortunately their very high density gives good X-ray contrast.

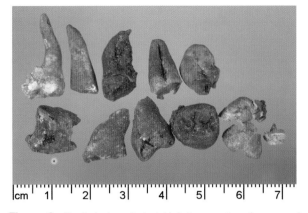

Figure 3 Teeth incinerated at high temperature for several hours. There has been some fragmentation of the teeth with enamel tooth caps lost from some of them. The bulk of the tooth is composed of dentine which has a similar composition to bone but is more highly mineralized.

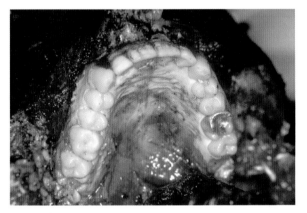

Figure 2 Badly burned body. All superficial soft tissues have been destroyed. Simple dissection reveals preserved teeth, dental restorations (a metal crown), and ridges in the soft tissue of the palate (rugae) which may indicate a racial affiliation or population of origin.

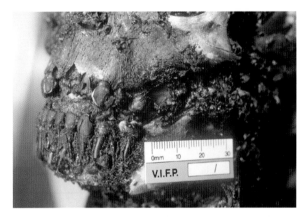

Figure 4 Badly burned jaws with the bone, that once covered the roots of the teeth, now destroyed.

during the destruction of a body by fire, hence the value of forensic odontology. The teeth are initially protected by the overlying soft tissues until they succumb to combustion. The heating of soft tissues often causes the tongue to protrude from the oral cavity (perhaps due to shrinkage of strap muscles in the neck) and for a time this too confers additional protection to the anterior teeth as the tissues of the tongue become fixed by heat covering the tooth crowns. The soft-tissue structures of the palate may also be useful features for identification (**Figure 2**). As the incineration progresses further, the soft tissues of the face and the protruding tongue are lost and then the facial surfaces of the teeth bear the brunt of the fire. Individual dental hard tissues are extremely resistant to heat, but the tooth crowns, comprising

two different tissues, each of which responds to heating differently, quickly become friable as enamel cleaves from underlying dentine (**Figure 3**). Ideally, these fragments need to be located and collected at the scene of the fire so that the dentition may later be reconstructed as far as possible.

Eventually, as the bones of the jaws become exposed, they too begin to burn. As the outer plate of bone from the maxilla and mandible are lost the roots of the teeth are exposed and they too begin to be destroyed (**Figure 4**).

It is therefore important that body recovery teams have ready access to an odontologist who can identify orodental structures and stabilize them by wrapping so that fragile evidence is not lost at the scene or later dislodged, only to become lost or further reduced in size amongst the other contents of the body bag. If this precaution is not taken then a potentially positive identification can easily be thwarted. Crumbling tooth crowns can be stabilized with low-viscosity, quick-setting resins such as LocTite® or the more expensive dental fissure sealant. Burned heads should be bubble-wrapped and sealed with packing tape and bagged prior to any moving of the body. This will greatly enhance the value and efficiency of the dental examination, which will take place later in the mortuary. A further option to be considered is the *in situ* examination of the remains by the odontologist, but this does require adequate lighting and access to adequate dental instruments if the examination is to be conducted to the standard normally achieved in the mortuary setting.

At the mortuary, for a meticulous dental examination to be possible, it is very important to have access to high-quality illumination similar to that used in a dental surgery. Many materials used to restore tooth crowns are specifically designed to match the existing color and translucency of natural teeth and so can be very difficult to detect even under optimal conditions. Dental instruments used in a mortuary for autopsy work need to be more robust than those commonly used in clinical dentistry. In living subjects a great deal of interaction takes place between the dentist and the patient to optimize compliance and minimize discomfort for mutual benefit. In the postmortem setting not only is there no compliance, but also the tissues are often rigidly fixed due to the temporary effects of rigor mortis or the permanent effects of heat fixation of tissues. (Similarly, overenthusiastic cooling of the corpse to below freezing by mortuary staff also makes access to oral structures a practical impossibility for many hours, sometimes days.)

After discussion with the pathologist (who will probably wish to examine the body first) and the coroner, and with the feelings of the next of kin firmly in mind, a decision about the removal of facial tissues to gain access to the mouth needs to be taken. This decision should never be taken lightly. The final decision is often determined by the degree of disfigurement of the remains prior to autopsy. Obviously, incisions that would mutilate the face of undamaged bodies cannot be condoned. However, if a detailed, direct examination of the orofacial skeleton is mandated in such a case there are methods whereby the soft tissues of the face can be removed and replaced in a virtually undetectable manner. Such procedures require skill and take time – and time is a commodity that is often in short supply in the forensic context. The decision to dissect the face rather than remove damaged tissues to gain access needs to be carefully balanced between additional costs in time, any potential loss of trust by the community in the forensic practitioners involved, and the value of any benefits gained in additional forensic information.

If a body is very badly disfigured it has often been advocated that the jaws be removed to facilitate their more careful examination in a cleaner and more tranquil setting away from the distracting influences of bad odors and noise in the mortuary. Excision of jaws is simple and rapid, but cannot be achieved without destroying the maxillary sinuses. If the saw cut is too close to the crowns of the teeth the roots will be damaged and, if far enough away to avoid this problem in the maxilla, the paranasal structures have to be disrupted (**Figure 5**). So, whilst the narrow requirements of the dental examination may be made easier, features such as radiographic outlines of paranasal sinuses, which can be just as important for an identification, can be rendered completely useless. For this reason, provided that mortuary facilities in terms of lighting, ventilation, and adequacy of hand instruments can be relied upon, resection of the jaws should be avoided wherever possible. An additional argument against initial resection of the jaws is that at the time of the dental autopsy not all the antemortem records which may be available will have always been identified and located. This means that the best approach in the beginning should always be the most conservative and the least destructive.

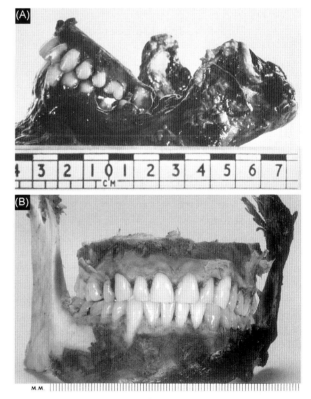

Figure 5 Resected jaws. The example shown in (A) was sawn too close to the teeth and the roots will have been damaged. Example (B) may have spared the tooth roots but has now destroyed paranasal sinus outlines which could have been useful for identification.

Should any organs be removed for examination elsewhere, an auditable continuity of evidence trail needs to be in place so that all organs removed for coronial purposes can be replaced in the body prior to its release for burial or cremation. Failure to observe this important point is highly likely to lead to the inadvertent retention of body parts, which then cannot be returned to the next of kin without causing additional distress and giving rise to more complications relating to the final disposal of tissues and organs.

As dental identification is essentially a comparative process, the form of the dental autopsy closely follows the conventions of a typical dental examination in a living person. This is because treatments or clinical findings recorded antemortem by the treating dentist are being verified or contradicted during the postmortem dental examination by the odontologist. In adults the dental autopsy records any teeth present together with any dental restorations or evidence, such as prepared cavities, that such restorations existed. It is common to find bodies in which restorative materials have either burned or melted from where they had been placed in the teeth. Nevertheless, the fine machining marks of the dental drill and the shape of prepared cavities can enable a reasonably comprehensive dental record still to be reconstructed, often sufficient for the remains to be identified.

With a temporal gap in the antemortem dental records prior to death it is quite possible that some additional restorations may have been placed in teeth, other existing ones enlarged, and some teeth extracted. If retrieval of all antemortem records is unsuccessful then these later modifications to the dentition will not be available for comparison. None of the unrecorded changes mentioned present an incompatible inconsistency when antemortem and postmortem records are compared. Furthermore, certain specific anatomical features or particular treatments like a single root canal filling or a fixed dental bridge may remain which, on their own, can provide ample evidence for individualization and matching (**Figure 6**). At the same time, teeth previously recorded as extracted cannot reappear during the postmortem examination. However, care has to be taken and clinical judgment exercised because not all dental charting is perfect and some teeth are often misidentified by the dentist when other teeth in that particular series of teeth are missing, thereby precluding comparison. This is a good example of where differences can arise between a specialist dental practitioner's opinion and that of an anthropologist who may have little knowledge of dentistry when looking at the same evidence. For a comprehensive interpretation the examiner must possess both the

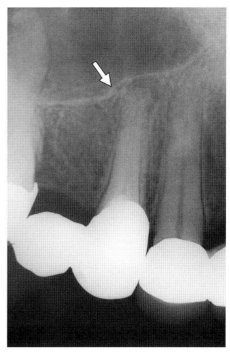

Figure 6 Radiograph of a fixed metal bridge (white). The shape of the roots present within the bone is seen. One has some pathology associated with the root apex. The floor of the maxillary sinus is seen as a thin white line (arrow) running just above the apices of the tooth roots.

anatomical and anthropological knowledge of human tooth morphology and have an expert knowledge of dentistry and dental materials commonly employed in the treatment and repair of teeth.

Radiology

Dentists frequently take X-ray images of their patients' jaws and teeth and usually keep such radiographs as part of the clinical records. Additional larger radiographs requiring larger and more specialized X-ray equipment may have been taken elsewhere for the assessment of cranial anatomy in the context of an orthodontic assessment, or to assess the position of unerupted teeth such as third molars in young adults. These radiographs may be retained by the orthodontist or oral surgeon but may also have been given to the patient or his/her parents for safekeeping. As radiographs are so valuable to the identification process, it is important that agencies such as the police, who are frequently required to collect dental records on behalf of the coroner or other investigating authority, appreciate the need for early expert interpretation of any records obtained from any practitioner. Hidden in the clinical shorthand of the busy practitioner there is often a reference to other sources of

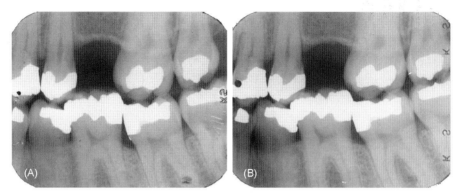

Figure 7 Intraoral radiographs (A) antemortem; (B) postmortem. There is an excellent match between the two images no matter which characteristics are compared. This is very good evidence to corroborate identity. Courtesy of Dr Richard Bassed, Victorian Institute of Forensic Pathology.

records but again, it may take a person with dental experience to appreciate this fully.

The most common dental radiographs are intraoral (**Figure** 7). These images are recorded on small packaged films which protect the contents from the oral fluids because the films are placed in the oral cavity inside the dental arches and the X-rays then directed at them from outside the mouth. These films, and their more modern digital equivalents, conveniently record the condition of tooth crowns and the periodontal tissues. Images, recorded at the quite high resolution needed to detect leakage of dental restorations and small carious lesions, contain a myriad of features which may be used for comparison (**Figure** 7). Unfortunately, the antemortem records may not match the quality of the radiographs recorded postmortem but the forensic scientist, like the archeologist or the paleontologist, has to work with whatever evidence is available. Some defects of poor or degraded antemortem images can be partially corrected by the careful application of image processing. Any improvements must be accompanied by the necessary audit trail so that others may reproduce the same transformations.

Extraoral films are larger and while being positioned prior to exposure are protected from the fogging effects of light by cassettes, many of which contain intensifying screens to optimize the performance of the film for the minimum radiation dose needed to record the image. It is these extraoral films that are commonly taken in specialist radiological centers. Lateral cephalometric films taken for orthodontic assessment and orthopantomograms taken more as a summary of the condition of the jaws and the position of the teeth within them (**Figure** 8) can be invaluable for comparative purposes. The lateral cephalometric radiograph often records the midline soft-tissue profile of the face. These features may be

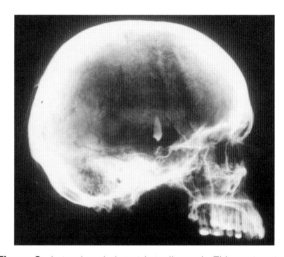

Figure 8 Lateral cephalometric radiograph. This postmortem specimen is unusual because it appears to shows a tooth inside the cranial cavity. This is due to postmortem displacement of teeth (the tooth is under the skull in the body bag) but images like this are sometimes seen when teeth have been displaced due to gunshot injury. Such radiographs reveal much about the anatomy and dimensions of the skull and these features can be compared with any similar preexisting antemortem images of a known person.

used as an aid to reconstructive anatomy and facial approximation methods used in forensic art which attempts to reproduce a likeness of someone in life from remnant skull evidence (**Figure** 9).

The use of dental implants to replace natural tooth roots to carry either a fixed or removable prosthetic superstructure like a bridge or denture is becoming a more popular, if still expensive, treatment option for some people in more prosperous societies. Implants are usually metallic and are therefore completely radiopaque, giving excellent silhouettes on radiographs. Postmortem images of implants within the jaws can be excellent for comparison with corresponding images taken at the time of surgery

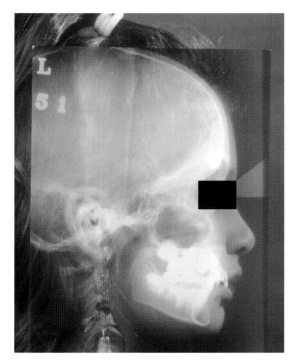

Figure 9 Lateral cephalometric radiograph superimposed over a lateral view of a child's face. The relationship between the face and the underlying facial skeleton is revealed. An appreciation of these relationships is essential for reconstructive sculpting of faces upon remnant skull evidence.

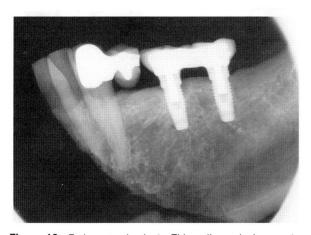

Figure 10 Endosseous implants. This radiograph shows natural teeth at the front of the mouth and metallic implants used to replace missing posterior teeth. There are many different designs of implant, each with its own silhouette. Images like this are unique.

or during healing to verify that osseointegration has occurred (**Figure 10**). The individualization and identification of remains where a putative identity has to be corroborated is aided by the wide range of implant systems which have found use to date. The durability of implants and their resistance to fire further add to their value as an aid to forensic identifications.

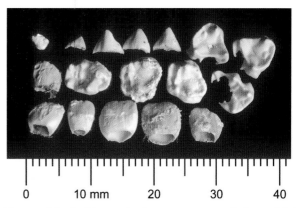

Figure 11 Deciduous tooth caps recovered from fetal remains. Gestational age can be estimated from the stage of tooth development.

Aging using Morphological Criteria

The determination of age from the dentition relies upon a balanced consideration of a number of factors, some related to the chronology of development, and some to physiological age changes which are much more susceptible to modification by customs, habits, and diet and which must therefore be given much less weight when all the available evidence is being considered together.

Prenatal Period

Aging of human remains in the prenatal period often cannot be separated from the corroboration of a human origin for skeletal remains. If the remains have been wrapped or enclosed in some way it is possible to recover most or all of the developing tooth caps which are easy to identify but which tend to become dislodged from the jaws after burial and later disinterment (**Figure 11**). As teeth develop in a known pattern and sequence, the chronology of tooth development can accurately age human remains in the prenatal period. Of course, osteological indicators of maturity should be cross-checked against the dental evidence but where there is a discrepancy, dental development, so vital to survival in times past, should be given more weight. The possibility of commingled remains or twins should always be borne in mind and the checks of number and symmetry always carried out.

The First Few Months of Postnatal Life

This period of human dental development still remains the one which least is recorded in the literature. For this reason it is illustrated here (**Figure 12**). The independent human is growing at its fastest

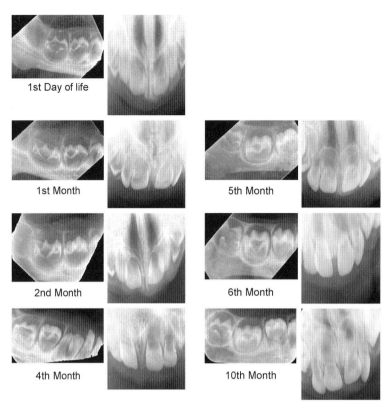

Figure 12 Radiographs of the stages of tooth development in the first 10 months of postnatal life. This period of tooth development has not previously been extensively studied and recorded. Each stage is illustrated by a radiograph of anterior teeth in the upper jaw and a corresponding radiograph of the posterior teeth for one quadrant of the mouth.

during this period. The jaws, so essential for nutrition and communication, develop rapidly but still amount to little more than a thin veil of bone enclosing the growing tooth germs of developing teeth. This period comes to an end about 6 months after birth when the first deciduous teeth emerge into the oral cavity. These are usually the mandibular central incisors.

Later Development of the Deciduous Dentition

The period of emergence of deciduous teeth into the mouth spans a period of about 2 years usually (but not invariably) beginning with the front teeth in the lower jaw. Since the third month *in utero*, some of the deciduous teeth have been forming within the jaws in bony crypts, yet tooth emergence does not begin until 6 months after birth. Similarly, root formation will continue in the last teeth to erupt for a period of another year or 18 months. This means that reliable criteria for age determination using the deciduous dentition alone may be available for examination for a period roughly twice as long as it takes for all the crowns of the teeth to emerge. The deciduous dentition should be considered as a transitional structure. The young child needs teeth during early childhood

but those teeth would be inadequate for the demands placed upon them by the adult musculature.

The deciduous teeth emerge sequentially and in a pattern which approximates to the order in which their formation commenced, front teeth first with lower (mandibular) teeth often emerging just prior to their upper (maxillary) counterparts. Symmetry in tooth development within the jaws means that contralateral pairs of teeth emerge at similar times. Even the discovery of a few forming tooth caps allows the developmental status of the entire dentition to be reconstructed and hence an age at death inferred. Once all the deciduous teeth have formed completely it is much less reliable to estimate age using these features alone.

It is highly likely that the whole deciduous dentition never exists in its entirety at any one time. Just as the tips of the last deciduous molars are forming at the back of the mouth, the roots of the incisors, which formed much earlier, are beginning to resorb. Resorption of the deciduous dentition is an internal cell-mediated process whereby the hard tissues of the tooth roots and even some of the enamel of the crown of the tooth are degraded and solubilized. The process is phasic with periods of resorption being interposed with periods of hard-tissue repair. This occurs by the reformation of cementum, a bone-like tissue that normally covers the outer surface of tooth roots providing anchorage for the fibers of the periodontal ligament, the structure by which teeth are attached to the tooth socket. In living children who are shedding their deciduous teeth it is common to see teeth loosen as resorption shortens the tooth roots and then retighten as one period of resorption ceases and is followed briefly by cementum repair and temporary reattachment of the periodontal ligament. Each period of resorption erodes progressively more and more of the tooth roots until the tooth crown is eventually lost. This provides space in the jaw for the permanent successor. If the successional tooth is absent or displaced, deciduous teeth may be retained long into adulthood, but this is quite uncommon and would provide a characteristic which in itself would be individualizing.

When deciduous teeth are found with incomplete roots it is important to be able to distinguish between those teeth which are incomplete because their initial formation was interrupted and those teeth whose later resorption had begun because the two events occur at quite different periods in the life history of the tooth. It is also worth noting that teeth are often found which may simply have been fractured either antemortem or postmortem (even during recovery of the remains) and this can provide yet another example of teeth with incomplete roots. Generally good lighting and some modest magnification, either using dental surgical loupes or a dissecting microscope, are enough to be able to distinguish clearly between forming, resorbing, and fractured teeth (**Figure 13**).

Mixed Dentition

At the age of 6 years all the crowns of the 20 teeth of the deciduous dentition remain in the oral cavity despite resorption of roots occurring within the jaws. Growth of the facial skeleton makes space for the first permanent molar to erupt at the back of the dental arch in each quadrant of the mouth, thereby enlarging the dentition. For the ensuing 5 or 6 years there is then a progressive complete replacement of deciduous teeth by their permanent successors (**Figure 14**). This process ends around 12 years of age when the permanent maxillary canines emerge. However, there is some slight variation in the pattern of replacement, often influenced by local factors such as tooth crowding, and so it may be the replacement of some deciduous molars which occurs last. Once the last deciduous tooth has been replaced the period of the mixed dentition comes to an end. Many studies of dental maturity have studied this period of human life, often using data obtained from radiographs. In

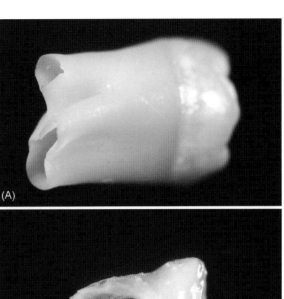
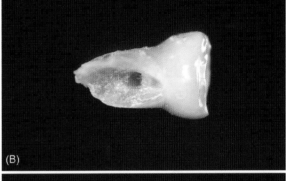
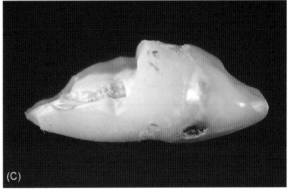

Figure 13 Teeth in three stages (A) forming permanent tooth root indicating that tooth formation was not complete at the time of death; (B) a resorbing deciduous tooth root prior to exfoliation or shedding; (C) a fractured tooth root. Such fractures can occur in life, perimortem, or postmortem during recovery of remains. Photos courtesy of Dennis Rowler School of Dental Science, University of Melbourne.

some studies tooth development is divided into an arbitrary number of identifiable stages, whilst in others indirect measurement of tooth size from the radiograph is used as the growth parameter plotted against known age to obtain the necessary regression equations then used for the aging of unknown remains thought to come from the same population at the same period in history. Many of these studies are based upon concerns that data from one population may not apply to others but, in fact, interpopulation variation is quite small, perhaps another

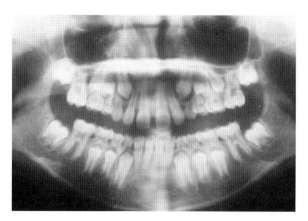

Figure 14 A panoramic radiograph of the jaws (orthopantomograph or OPG) taken during the period of the mixed dentition. Some of the erupted teeth are deciduous and some are permanent. Within the jaws, under their remaining deciduous predecessors, several developing permanent teeth can be seen. These will still have incomplete roots for about 18 months after they have emerged into the oral cavity.

reflection of the imperative in past times for all humans to develop a functional dentition rapidly in order to survive.

Permanent Dentition

At the age of 12 or 13 years all the teeth present in the mouth are now permanent. It is around this age that the second permanent molars are added to the dental arches, bringing the number of teeth present to 28. Only the third molars or wisdom teeth remain to erupt between 17 and 25 years of age. These teeth are frequently congenitally absent or restrained from entering the dental arches due to lack of available space when they become jammed (impacted) against other teeth.

By the third decade of life most of the minor adjustments of the position of teeth within the dental arches to optimize alignment and fit of the teeth with one another are complete. After this period it becomes much harder to estimate age because the features which have to be used for this purpose are much more susceptible to modification due to environmental factors, some of which cannot be known or inferred when postmortem remains are being examined.

The consolidation of known progressive changes such as tooth wear, recession of soft-tissue attachment (i.e., "getting long in the tooth"), infilling of the pulp chambers with more hard-tissue deposition, continued accretion of cementum (an attachment tissue) around the apices of tooth roots, and increasing translucency of dentine (due to infilling of dentinal tubules with mineral) has been used to construct regression formulae from which age at death can be

estimated. Such efforts were partially successful in Scandinavia in the mid twentieth century, probably due to the fact that Sweden still had a very ethnically homogeneous population at that time. Almost everyone enjoyed a similar high standard of living and education and probably ate a similar diet including constituents all prepared in a similar way. In essence the ethnic, cultural, and environmental influences that may affect the rate of change of structure in the teeth and jaws were largely controlled. Unfortunately, with greater mobility of peoples around the world in the late twentieth and early twenty-first centuries, such methods are of little use today.

Several later workers have striven to refine these early methods, but as might be anticipated, have had only partial success. However, of all the known changes with age, the increasing translucency of dentine is probably the least influenced by environmental effects and is likely to be the most physiologically regulated. Changes in the color of tooth roots with age have been studied and this color change may be related to the same changes in the optical properties of the dental tissues, which also give rise to translucency. Age estimation techniques based on color change alone have never found widespread application. The problem remains as to how to quantify the amount of translucent dentine deposited. Traditionally, teeth have been sawn lengthways to produce a longitudinal section which is then lapped down to a standard thickness (100 μm) when the proportion of the root length occupied by translucent dentine can be measured under a light microscope and plotted against known age. This method, whilst quite accurate, is subject to sampling errors. Once a section has been cut in one plane the tooth cannot be sectioned in another. Yet once the section has been cut the length of translucent dentine on one side of the root is frequently observed to be quite different from that on the other. Similarly, the acquisition of translucency may occur irregularly in zones which do not extend through the full thickness of the dentine and so are difficult to measure or estimate in terms of length. Hopefully modern technology will soon be able to provide a solution to this dilemma. High-resolution microcomputed tomography scanning is now becoming more available and is capable of quantifying mineral density in three dimensions throughout the entire domain of the dentine of the tooth. This will remove the sampling problems implicit in any two-dimensional method and should improve correlations between a progressive structural change in teeth and known age at death by permitting volumetric measurements of changes to dentine mineralization to be compared with the residual volume of still unaltered tissue.

Concluding Remarks

Despite advances in DNA technology, forensic odontology remains a very cost-effective and rapid means of confirming identity of deceased persons when teeth remain and antemortem records exist. This position is not likely to alter in the foreseeable future. These advantages come to have special importance in cases of mass disaster or in the investigation of mass graves after massacres following periods of civil unrest or warfare.

Similarly, dental examinations of living persons can be used to corroborate identity in cases where identity is disputed, such as in cases involving immigration authorities and questioned documents.

See Also

Anthropology: Bone Pathology and Antemortem Trauma; Morphological Age Estimation; **Crime-scene Investigation and Examination:** Recovery of Human Remains; **Fire Investigation, Evidence Recovery**; **Mass Disasters:** Principles of Identification; **Odontology:** Bite Mark Analysis; **War Crimes:** Site Investigation; Pathological Investigation

Further Reading

Aboshi H, Takahashi T, Tamura M, Komuro T (2000) Age estimation based on the morphometric analysis of dental root pulp using ortho cubic super high resolution CT (ortho-CT). In: Willems G (ed.) *Forensic Odontology: Proceedings of the European IOFOS Millennium Meeting, Leuven (Belgium)*, p. 199 (abstract). Belgium: Leuven University Press.

Burgman G (1992) Examination of the unidentified body: mortuary procedures. In: Clark DH (ed.) *Practical Forensic Odontology*, pp. 53–66. UK: Wright.

Ciapparelli L (1992) The chronology of dental development and age assessment. In: Clark DH (ed.) *Practical Forensic Odontology*, pp. 22–42. UK: Wright.

Clement JG (1998) Dental identification. In: Clement JG, Ranson DL (eds.) *Craniofacial Identification in Forensic Medicine*, pp. 63–81. UK: Arnold.

Clement JG, Kosa F (1992) The fetal skeleton. In: Clark DH (ed.) *Practical Forensic Odontology*, pp. 43–52. UK: Wright.

Clement JG, Olsson C, Phakey PP (1992) Heat induced changes in human skeletal tissues. In: York LK, Hicks JW (eds.) *Proceedings of an International Symposium on the Forensic Aspects of Mass Disasters and Crime Scene Reconstruction*, pp. 212–213. FBI Academy Quantico 1990, Laboratory Division of the FBI. Washington DC: US Government Printing Office.

Demirjian A, Goldstein H (1976) New systems for dental maturity based on seven and four teeth. *Annals of Human Biology* 3: 411–421.

Fasekas I, Kosa F (1978) *Forensic Fetal Osteology*. Budapest: Akademiai Kiado.

Gustafson G (1950) Age determination on teeth. *Journal of the American Dental Association* 41: 45–54.

Kraus BS, Jordan RE (1965) *The Human Dentition Before Birth*. Philadelphia, PA: Lea and Febiger.

Kvall SI (1995) *Age Related Changes in Teeth. A Microscopic and Radiographic Investigation of the Human Permanent Dentition*. PhD thesis. Oslo, Norway: University of Oslo.

Liversidge HM, Lyons F, Hector MP (2003) The accuracy of three methods of age estimation using radiographic measurements of developing teeth. *Forensic Science International* 131: 22–29.

Logan WHG, Kronfeld R (1933) Development of the human jaws and surrounding structures from birth until the age of fifteen years. *Journal of the American Dental Association* 20: 379–427.

Maples WR, Rice PM (1979) Some difficulties in the Gustafson dental age estimation. *Journal of Forensic Science* 24: 168–172.

Mornstad H, Staaf V, Welander U (1994) Age estimation with the aid of tooth development: a new method based on objective measurements. *Scandinavian Journal of Dental Research* 102: 137–143.

Nkhumeleni FS, Raubenheimer EJ, Monteith BD (1989) Gustafson's method for age determination revisited. *Journal of Forensic Odontostomatology* 7: 13–16.

Ranson DL (1998) Craniofacial dissection. In: Clement JG, Ranson DL (eds.) *Craniofacial Identification in Forensic Medicine*, pp. 95–104. London: Arnold.

Schour I, Massler M (1941) The development of the human dentition. *Journal of the American Dental Association* 28: 1153–1160.

Solheim T (1993) *Dental Age-Related Regressive Changes and A New Method for Calculating the Age of An Individual*. PhD thesis. Oslo, Norway: University of Oslo.

Ten Cate AR, Thompson GW, Dickinson JB, Hunter HA (1977) The estimation of age of skeletal remains from the colour of roots of teeth. *Journal of the Canadian Dental Association* 43: 83–86.

Bite Mark Analysis

J G Clement, Victorian Institute of Forensic Medicine, Southbank, VIC, Australia
S A Blackwell, The University of Melbourne, Melbourne, NSW, and the Victorian Institute of Forensic Medicine, Southbank, VIC, Australia

Introduction

Bite mark analysis is currently an extremely contentious topic. For a subject with such potentially serious outcomes for both suspect and victim, little research in analyzing methods and evaluating outcomes is reaching peer-reviewed journals. Although admissibility of bite mark evidence has been explicitly established and routinely accepted in the USA and other legal systems for a long time, some odontologists argue that bite mark methodology has never really undergone critical examination and legitimately passed the "Frye" test for admissibility. Other legal observers are rightly concerned that forensic odontologists are giving insufficient critical attention to the quality of bite mark evidence presented to the courts.

In Australia, there are many uncertainties surrounding bite mark evidence. The natural tendency to see what one wants to see, thereby tempting examiners to overinterpret bite marks, has led to serious difficulties when bringing such evidence before the courts. Two pivotal Australian cases have seen bite mark evidence rejected as "unsafe" and convictions overturned on appeal. Perhaps for such reasons this area of forensic science is currently undergoing review and reevaluation. Generally, courts now look for quantitative rather than simply descriptive analysis before accepting scientific evidence and it can be anticipated that future developments in bite mark analysis will have to comply if convictions are going to be made with confidence.

Current Techniques

Collection of evidence from suspects may include obtaining impressions of their dentition, and their bite is analyzed from the resulting stone cast. This is a process where features of the suspect's dentition are compared with impressions or marks left by the teeth on a variety of substrates, usually parts of the human body. A wide variety of techniques for bite mark analysis have been described in the literature, including computer axial tomography (CAT), scanning electron microscopy (SEM), video imaging, radiography, and the use of fingerprint powder to dust the impression. However, the predominant technique for comparison of exemplars is transparent overlays – analysis of the bite made using a 1:1 transparent overlay of the biting surface of the suspect's dentition placed over a 1:1 photo of the bite (**Figure 1**). The five following commonly used overlay techniques are relatively cheap and the equipment and materials are easily obtainable:

1. computer-based (**Figure 2**)
2. radiopaque wax
3. hand-traced from wax
4. hand-traced from study casts; used in the Carroll and Lewis cases (see below)
5. xerographic.

With an abundance of methods and no standard agreed tests of their effectiveness, the analysis of bite

marks and the consequences of presenting questionable bite mark testimony to the courts will continue to promote skepticism. The following two Australian

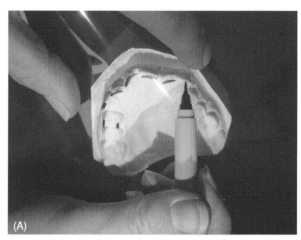

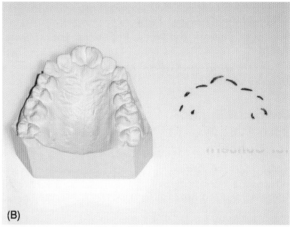

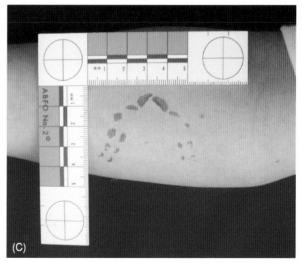

Figure 1   Historical method of bite mark analysis, hand-traced from study casts on to acetate sheet to provide overlay to be used for comparison with either photographs of injury at life size or directly with the wound: (A) highlighting of incisal edges and cusps with pen on to acetate; (B) tracing and model of suspect compared; (C) photograph of bite mark simulated using inked model shown in (A) and (B).

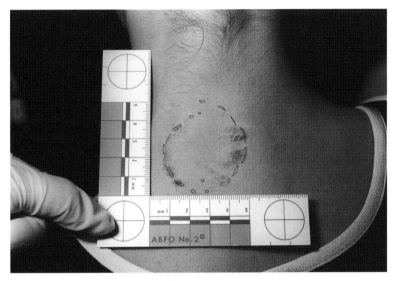

Figure 2 New method of bite mark analysis, computer-based overlays. In such cases the characteristics of the biting edges of the teeth have been highlighted from models scanned on a flat bed scanner using simple image processing techniques (i.e., lasso tool in Adobe® Photoshop®. Refer to Digital Analysis of Bite Mark Evidence using Adobe Photoshop by RJ Johansen and CM Bowers.).

cases remain controversial, and illustrate the issues at hand.

Two Australian Cases – Grounds for Concern

Raymond John Carroll v. The Queen

In 1973 a 17-month-old girl, Deidre Kennedy, was abducted, raped, and strangled and her body, dressed in women's undergarments, was discovered on top of a toilet block in Ipswich, Queensland. A bruise was found on her inner thigh just above the knee. This mark was identified by a forensic odontologist as being inflicted by human teeth. The odontologist went on to say that it would be "impossible to establish the identity of the biter."

Just under 9 years later another offense was committed in Ipswich at the women's quarters of the Royal Australian Air Force (RAAF) base. Items of ladies' underwear had been stolen and found vandalized along with pictures of scantily dressed women. Suspicion fell on Raymond Carroll, who was stationed at the RAAF base at the time. As both cases involved deviant behavior with women's clothing, Carroll became a suspect in the earlier murder of Deidre Kennedy.

In October 1983, 10 years after the Kennedy murder, casts of Carroll's dentition were made. The casts were then altered by an odontologist, based on dental records, in an attempt to recreate features obscured or altered by dental treatment in the 10 years since the child's murder. Comparisons were then made

between a hand-traced overlay of Carroll's altered dentition and a photograph of the bruise on the child's leg. The bite mark evidence was examined by three odontologists who testified at the 1985 trial "that the bite-mark was made by the accused Carroll and no other." Subsequently the jury found Carroll guilty, largely on the unanimous conclusions of the three odontologists.

Carroll appealed, and in November 1985 the appeal was upheld and Carroll acquitted. The determination was based on the grounds that the judges of the Court of Criminal Appeal considered the evidence given by the three odontologists, although coming to the same conclusion, contained too many inconsistencies in methodology. Two odontologists associated the upper bruise pattern with all four upper central teeth, while the third associated the bruise with three of the four central teeth. Further, two odontologists associated the upper bruise pattern with the incisal edges while another with the palatal edges. One odontologist associated the lower bruise pattern with all four lower central teeth while the other associated it with only three of the lower central teeth. The judges concluded that a verdict based on this evidence would be unsafe, and because the original bite mark evidence had been pivotal to the case there was, therefore, no need for a retrial.

Twenty-seven years after the murder of Deidre Kennedy, police revisited the case in 2000 and reexamined the bite mark evidence. In highly unusual circumstances, Carroll was charged with perjury in relation to his 1983 murder trial. This reexamination of the bite mark evidence employed a new technique that involved three-dimensional imaging of a cast of Carroll's dentition. A computer model of Carroll's dentition was created by superimposing sequentially photographed layers of the cast as it had been gradually immersed in opaque ink. During biting, the teeth impinge on the skin at nonperpendicular angles, so the investigators estimated this angle. The immersion was then performed with the cast on this angle, generating a contour map that would reproduce the different contributions of individual teeth to the bite pattern. Numerous odontologists were consulted who testified to the reproducibility of this new scientific method and its acceptance by their discipline. The Supreme Court in Queensland deemed the evidence admissible and Carroll was convicted of perjury. However, at a later appeal the court concluded that to have brought a perjury charge before a criminal court in this case had been in conflict with the double-jeopardy principle of the common law and was an abuse of the process of the court. This decision, made almost 20 years after Carroll first became a suspect in the child's murder, gave him freedom and guaranteed his liberty.

Lewis v. The Queen

In 1986, whilst a young woman was walking home from a disco in Darwin, Northern Territory, a man approached her and offered to walk her home. She claimed that after she had refused his advances many times, he raped her. After the attack, the woman and the assailant were intercepted by the woman's boyfriend, who confronted the assailant. It was also alleged that the boyfriend was then bitten on the chest by the same assailant during a scuffle. Lewis, the suspect for these attacks, had been a regular patron at the disco and was arrested in connection with these offenses. This occurred despite alibis placing him elsewhere at the time of the alleged offense. He willingly supplied body samples and underwent a dental examination that included taking an impression of his teeth. It is important to note that Lewis had undergone dental treatment as a result of an injury to his teeth that occurred between the time of the alleged attack and the taking of the impression. Police investigations at the scene yielded no evidence to link Lewis to the location, and clothing seized from the accused was not contaminated with any blood, hair, or other evidence to link him to the rape or later attack on the boyfriend. Notwithstanding the fact that both the woman and her boyfriend were highly intoxicated on the night of the rape, which may have affected their recall of the attacker's identity, and that a taxi driver present during the later attack on the

boyfriend had clearly stated that it was not the accused who had sat in the front seat of his taxi, Lewis was identified as the biter by two odontologists and convicted. This conclusion was reached by reference to a single black-and-white photograph of the bruise left on the victim's chest. This photo was compared with an acetate overlay that had been constructed by hand-tracing around the biting edges of the cast made of Lewis' dentition. The odontologists claimed with confidence, one with "100% certainty," that it was the incisal edges of five teeth from Lewis' lower jaw that had made the mark on the victim's chest. On appeal the following year, like Carroll, Lewis was acquitted, the basis being that the judges did not believe that the evidence of the odontologists was sufficiently sound for Lewis' conviction to stand, using the Carroll case as a precedent.

Problems with Bite Mark Analysis in the Carroll and Lewis Cases

Identification of Lewis was made using a black-and-white photograph of a bruise pattern of five teeth on a man's chest. Carroll was identified by a bruise pattern that was said to identify three or four of his upper anterior teeth. Bowers, a forensic odontologist in the USA unconnected to either case, wrote that the ability to attain a positive match has more to do with the number of tooth marks seen in the bite and not the uniqueness of each individual characteristic of either the defendant's dentition or the bite mark injury. Applying this criterion, there were probably not enough tooth marks present in either of the Carroll or Lewis cases for a detailed comparison to be made and definite conclusions to be reached about the origin of source of the injuries.

Each stage in the analysis of bite marks provides the opportunity for the incorporation of additional errors. The hand-tracing on to acetate of features from the study casts in both the Lewis and Carroll examinations is a method that has been shown to be one of the least accurate in terms of production of two-dimensional overlays. The validity of alterations made to the study cast of Carroll's dentition must also be questioned; the accuracy of the resulting replicas is difficult to quantify or validate.

Marks made by teeth on the human body are often left on curved surfaces such as the breast, arms, and buttocks. These bite marks may appear in the form of a bruise, or as indentations in the skin. When there are indentations, a replica of the bitten surface may be made and morphometric analysis carried out. However, when only a bruise is left, the exact origin of source of the mark is less easily determined. The bite mark evidence may only be good enough to exclude certain suspects whose dentition bears no resemblance to the pattern of injuries. Bruises heal, migrate, and smudge. The blood of the bruise may drain away from the site of initial injury and these factors can further hinder an accurate comparative analysis.

Forensic odontologists confidently testified in both the Carroll and Lewis cases that the poorly defined bruises seen on the surface of skin were made by the accused men and no other person. This was surprising because one odontologist who gave evidence at both trials agreed that "there was a body of opinion, held by experts whom he would not rate as being inferior in skill to himself," who believed that identification of teeth by comparing them to bruises was not reliable.

Consequences of the Carroll and Lewis Cases

Outcomes of the Carroll and Lewis cases have reduced the credibility of bite mark analysis, and future cases involving bite mark testimony will be forced to face the precedent set by these cases. Following these trials a Victorian report by Coldrey into the taking of body samples and examinations of suspects in custody concluded that the taking of bite mark evidence was of little value in criminal cases. This view was reached because bite mark evidence had been ruled inadmissible on a number of occasions and because the committee believed that bite mark evidence was subjective and rarely secure enough to support a conviction. However, the Coldrey report overlooked the potentially important exculpatory significance of even poor bite marks to an investigation.

Bite Mark Evidence Later Contradicted by DNA

The criminal justice system is not perfect and can be subject to error. The possibility of obtaining a false-positive conviction always exists. This is when an innocent person is imprisoned in error whilst the perpetrator is free and has the opportunity to reoffend. Although the number of false positives may be quite small compared to the number of true-positive convictions, wrongly "doing time" in prison or being executed cannot be reversed by monetary compensation for the accused or his/her family.

In February 2003, the annual meeting of the American Judicature Society focused on the conviction of innocent persons. Six causes of injustice were identified, including confirmatory bias in police investigations and false scientific evidence. The chance of obtaining false positives via erroneous scientific evidence (e.g., inaccurate bite mark analysis) is one issue that is currently under investigation in the American criminal justice system.

DNA Exoneration – Correcting the False Positives

In the USA, there has been a major shift in the criminal justice system over the past decade due predominantly to the impact of exonerations based on later DNA analysis. Currently, 30 states have enacted statutes addressing postconviction DNA testing.

In 1992, a nonprofit legal clinic was established at the Benjamin N. Cardozo School of Law in New York to assist convicted people who claim innocence. Over a period of 14 years, a total of 131 convictions have been overturned. In the following case, a man was wrongly convicted on the basis of bite mark evidence.

An American Case – *State* v. *Krone*

On December 29, 1991, the stabbed body of a 36-year-old woman was found in the men's toilets of the bar where she worked. Little physical evidence was found; however there were bite marks on the breast and neck of the victim's body. She had apparently told a friend that a regular customer named Ray Krone was to help her close the bar on the night she was killed. Krone was arrested and charged with murder and kidnapping. An odontologist took Styrofoam impressions of Krone's teeth for comparison with the bite marks on the woman's body. At the trial, dental experts for the prosecution testified that these bite marks matched the impression that Krone had made in the Styrofoam, and he was convicted and sentenced to death for the murder and received a consecutive 21-year term of imprisonment for the kidnapping. Krone appealed in 1996, but was again convicted, mainly on testimony relating to the bite mark evidence. This time he received a reduced sentence, life imprisonment. In 2002, DNA testing was conducted on the saliva and blood found on the victim. The samples matched a man named Kenneth Phillips, who had worked nearby but had never been questioned. After the unfortunate Krone had served more than 10 years in prison, all charges against him were dismissed, and he was exonerated and released.

Bite mark evidence in this case was incorrectly interpreted and this emphasizes the need to question current standards of bite mark analysis to prevent similar situations arising in the future.

Admissibility of Bite Mark Evidence

Currently, two tests exist for the admissibility of new scientific techniques in courts of law, implemented to protect the accused from being persecuted by methods that have not been proven or established. The "Frye" test, established in 1923 as an outcome of *Frye* v. *United States*, specifies minimum requirements that a new scientific procedure must undergo before being deemed admissible in a court of law: it must be "demonstrable," sufficiently "established," and have gained the "general acceptance of experts" working in the field/s to which the evidence belongs.

In 1993 the US Supreme Court abandoned Frye and adopted a more flexible validation standard resulting from the case *Daubert* v. *Merrell Dow Pharmaceuticals*. Daubert states that the reasoning or methodology underlying testimony must be "scientifically valid," determined by examining testability, error rate, peer review and publication, and general acceptance.

The problem with Daubert is that the responsibility is placed on judges to screen evidence for reliability and relevance, but many judges would agree that they are not sufficiently founded in science to be able to determine if expert testimony is reliable and risk admitting inappropriate testimony. Widespread concern is expressed that judges will become amateur scientists. Judges themselves express disquiet, one stating that "federal judges ruling on admissibility of expert scientific testimony face a far more complex and daunting task in the post-Daubert world" and that "we judges are largely untrained in science and certainly no match for any of the witnesses whose testimony we are reviewing." In 1994, Jonakait wrote that "if Daubert was taken seriously, then much of forensic science is in serious trouble." This statement is particularly relevant for the analysis of bite marks. However, because the Court decided Daubert on statutory rather than constitutional grounds, it remains the decision of individual states in the USA to determine the method by which scientific evidence is admitted. In 1995, 22 states apparently remained committed to Frye. Perhaps understandably, there has also been some reluctance to introduce Daubert into the Australian legal system.

In Carroll's original murder trial, the techniques used in the examination of the bite marks were deemed admissible by the court in accord with the Frye test; however, the conviction was overturned on appeal due to inconsistencies in methodology. It seems that existing methods for bite mark analysis are not robust enough to withstand courtroom challenges and the reputation of all bite mark analysis has been marred as a result. The scientific basis for bite mark analysis is yet to be established, and until this happens, it will be a difficult task to restore the credibility of bite mark analysis as a science.

Factors Affecting Our Ability to Analyze Bite Marks and Identify the Biter

Uniqueness of the Dentition May Not Translate into a Unique Bite Mark

The evidential value of bite mark analysis is predicated on an assumption of uniqueness in both the dentition of the biter and the corresponding injury left after biting. Although uniqueness of the dentition is well established in the identification of a person's remains by his/her teeth and uniqueness of a bite mark, the transfer of features of the same dentition to another surface is much more problematic. Taroni suggested that a perfectly sharp broken tooth could be viewed as unique. However, the same feature transferred to another surface by pressure can look blurred and merge into other adjacent patterns in the substrate.

In 1982, Sognnaes loosely examined individuality of the human dentition in a small study of five sets of identical male twins. This paper is often quoted as proof for the uniqueness of a bite mark in skin. The authors pressed stone dental casts of the dentitions of 10 twins into various substances such as wet plaster of Paris, wax, polyether, and silicone to record the mark left. These indentations were then filled with radiopaque material, radiographed, digitized, and computerized. The resultant bite patterns of each pair of twins were then superimposed and analyzed with respect to each other. From these superimpositions, Sognnaes concluded that the "illustrations of these computerized comparisons show the uniqueness of the human dentition" and that "in terms of occlusal arch form and individual tooth positions, even so-called identical twins are in fact not dentally identical."

Whilst Sognnaes' conclusions may well have been correct for plaster of Paris, wax, silicone, and polyether materials, these conclusions probably could not have been made if human skin had been used as the recording material. In addition, despite a careful approach, the researchers had no control over the depth of penetration of the dentition into the recording medium. In 2001, Pretty and Sweet considered this point and showed that variations in a bite mark pattern can be produced using the same dentition by only changing the pressure when it is forced into dental wax.

Other Factors to be Considered

Skin and underlying tissue are highly deformable substrates and there are many variables that affect the representation of the transfer of the biting surface of the teeth to human skin. A mechanism is required that accounts for these variables:

- amplitude and direction of biting forces
- sucking action (which may cause additional bruising)
- depth of penetration of the skin (if any)
- three-dimensional (curved) morphology of the substrate
- movement of assailant and/or victim during bite
- capacity of wounds to change during healing.

To illustrate some of these problems, DeVore conducted a simple experiment using an inked rubber stamp of a concentric circle which he pressed on to the arm of an individual. The stamp was then photographed with the individual flexing, extending, and rotating the arm in different directions. Included in the photograph was a ruler used to make accurate comparisons from the prints. DeVore concluded that there was up to 60% linear distortion of the stamp on the skin depending on the position of the body. Therefore, photographic images of bite marks to be used in comparative analysis should perhaps only be used if the position of the body at the time of the infliction of the injury can be replicated. This is a difficult requirement when it is understood that most bites are made during an attack, some of which are fatal for the victim (**Figure 3**).

Overlays still being the most common form of bite mark analysis, in 1986 the American Board of Forensic Odontology (ABFO) recommended guidelines for the collection of bite mark data and their analysis sufficient to inculpate or exculpate suspects, but, despite these recommendations, problems still exist that require resolution.

Admirably, much effort has been devoted to developing a reproducible method of overlay production using the medium of Adobe® PhotoShop®, but although this method corrects for certain types of distortion, it cannot completely compensate for the three-dimensional nature of the dentition and the surface that has been bitten. In photography, extremities of curved surfaces are distorted with respect to features seen at the center of the field of view. It will therefore be necessary to produce a set of rules that can make provision not only for the

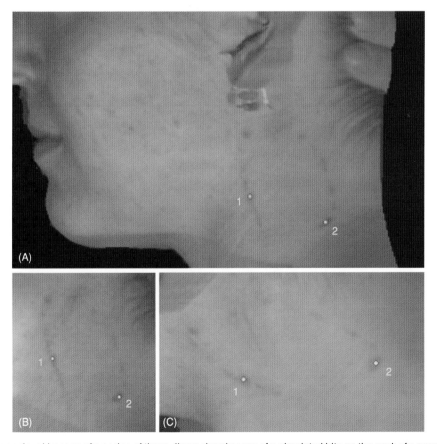

Figure 3 Two-dimensional images of a series of three-dimensional scans of a simulated bite on the neck of a person showing effects of simple postural distortion: (A) head erect 35.2 mm between points labeled 1 and 2; (B) head tilted away from bite 38.7 mm between points 1 and 2; (C) head rotated 49.7 mm between points 1 and 2. Distances measured in three-dimensional space, not simply in the plane of the two-dimensional image.

three-dimensional morphology of the skin but also the dynamics of biting and the distortion caused.

The issue of unconscious bias should not be ignored. The odontologist may work closely with police and prosecution lawyers. They are often requested to make a dental cast from a suspect's dentition and then asked to match the bite marks found on the victim with the dentition of the person in custody. This introduces confirmatory bias into the identification from the outset. Rothwell suggested using a line-up of dental casts that may or may not include the suspect's dentition, thus eliminating any bias the forensic odontologist might feel to "match" the mark with the suspect's dentition. In the Lewis case, an attempt was made by a third odontologist to demonstrate that the cast of another person's teeth (a person completely unrelated to the case) exhibited some similarities when compared with the photo of the bite on the boyfriend's chest, but this evidence was disallowed by the court. This makes it even more surprising that the opinion of the odontologists inculpating Lewis as the only possible biter could be held with such firm conviction.

The Future Direction of Morphometric Analysis in Bite Mark Identification

Bite mark, fingerprint, and DNA analyses, and more recently morphological facial identification, are similar in that a certain minimum number of points of concordance between two objects must be observed for a positive match to be concluded. Scientists have composed databases whereby fingerprint and DNA analyses can be expressed quantitatively as a numerical probability in the population. Although the individuality of the human dentition is commonly observed by dentists in practice, there is presently no database to express the uniqueness of the human dentition quantitatively.

It is not enough to believe that each dentition is unique. Where bite marks are being considered, what is important is the ability to discriminate between different individuals using morphometric criteria. The differences between some individuals may be so slight that, when they are masked by the degraded nature of the information contained in the wound, differences that could be measured between the dentitions of two or more potential suspects cannot be detected in the bite mark. Hence it becomes impossible to attribute the bite to any particular individual with certainty. The present lack of statistics relating the characteristics of the biter to the bite mark injury continues to spark controversy, prompting the need for further research efforts.

Three-Dimensional Imaging and Quantification of Bite Marks and Dentitions

Research on three-dimensional imaging and quantification of bite marks is progressing. It is only when the bite of the offender and the bite mark arising from the action of biting (both three-dimensional structures) can be compared in three dimensions that progress can be made toward scientifically valid quantification in bite mark analysis. Even when this has been achieved, the dynamic nature of the interaction between the teeth and the skin needs to be modeled. This will require an understanding of the behavior of tissues during the process of being bitten. This has yet to be achieved and, furthermore, it will require input from disciplines outside dentistry.

In research by the authors, dental stone models and simulated bite marks in an imperfect impression

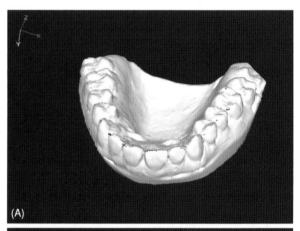

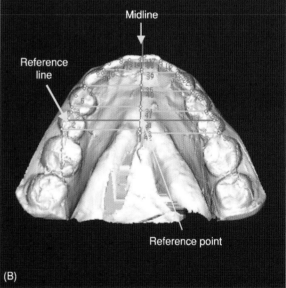

Figure 4 (A) and (B) Three-dimensional laser scans of stone dental models with some landmarks identified, which could be used for comparisons with potentially corresponding three-dimensional scans of wounds or bite mark injuries.

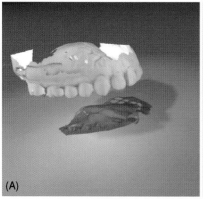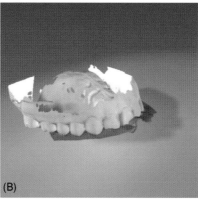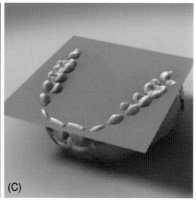

(A)   (B)   (C)

Figure 5 Stills taken from three-dimensional animations of comparisons between impressions in wax (red) and model of biter (white) (Website 5: www.dent.unimelb.edu.au/3dbitemarks): (A) Approaching contact; (B) In contact showing near perfect registration; (C) Use of a cutting plane to illustrate topography of biting surfaces of teeth. With three-dimensional scans of the body such simple cutting planes could be replaced by curved surfaces that are descriptive of the undeformed surface of the skin at sites of bite mark injuries. This could then be used to predict depth of bite in resulting injury patterns.

medium (dental wax) have been laser-scanned and a series of two- and three-dimensional measurement categories quantified (**Figure 4**). A numerical matrix has been developed to try to determine the proportion of dentitions that match a particular bite mark exactly within the tolerances introduced by the use of wax as a recording medium, the number that could possibly match, and the number that do not match at all. We strive to calculate the probability of predicting matches, possible matches, and definite nonmatches for a particular cohort. Animation of matching and nonmatching dentitions and bites has also been explored, and may prove to be of use in the future in assisting juries in a courtroom situation (**Figure 5**).

It is just such statistics that need to be presented to the courts in order to give the appropriate weighting to the opinion of the expert. At the end of the day, the process of coming to a conclusion may be less important than the performance of the expert in tests of competence, these coming in the form of correct answers in bite mark analysis simulations.

Summary

Pretty and Sweet's extensive critical review of bite mark literature confirmed that the scientific basis of bite mark analysis is currently very weak. Their research exhorts us to increase the rigor of our analyses. To address these deficiencies, we need to utilize experts in other fields, such as dermatology, mechanical engineering, and motor vehicle crash simulation, to gain a better understanding of the interactions of human skin with three-dimensional objects capable of inflicting injuries which leave a signature in the wound pattern.

See Also

Odontology: Overview

Further Reading

Bowers CM, Johansen RJ (2001) Digital analysis of bite marks and human identification. In: Fixott RH (ed.) *The Dental Clinics of North America*, vol. 45(2), pp. 327–342. USA: WB Saunders.

Carroll (1985) 19 A Crim R 410 at 417 (Court of Criminal Appeal, Queensland, Australia).

Clement J (2000) Odontology: bitemarks, bruising and other injuries to skin. In: Siegal JA, Saukko PJ, Knupfer GC (eds.) *Encyclopedia of Forensic Sciences*. San Diego, CA: Academic Press. Available online at: http://dx.doi.org/10.1006/rwfs.2000.0000.

DeVore DT (1971) Bite marks for identification? A preliminary report. *Medicine, Science and the Law* 11: 144–145.

Forrest AS, Davies I (2001) Bite marks on trial – the Carroll case. *Australian Society of Forensic Dentistry* 18: 6–8.

Gundelach A (1989) Lawyers' reasoning and scientific proof: a cautionary tale in forensic odontology. *Journal of Forensic Odonto-Stomatology* 7: 11–16.

Jonakait RN (1994) The meaning of Daubert and what that means for forensic science. *Cardozo Law Review* 15: 2103–2117.

Lasser AJ, Warnick AJ, Berman GM (2002) A unique way to analyse bite marks using 3D laser scanners and comparative software. *Proceedings for the American Academy of Forensic Sciences 54th Annual Meeting*. Atlanta, GA, USA, February 2002.

Lewis v. *The Queen* (1987) *Federal Law Reports, Court of the Appeal of the Northern Territory* 88: 104.

Pretty IA, Sweet D (2001) The scientific basis for human bitemark analyses – a critical review. *Science and Justice* 41: 85–92.

Rothwell BR (1995) Bite marks in forensic dentistry: a review of legal, scientific issues. *Journal of the American Dental Association* 126: 223–232.

Sognnaes RF, Rawson RD, Gratt BM, Nguyen NB (1982) Computer comparison of bitemark patterns in identical twins. *Journal of the American Dental Association* 105: 449–451.

State v. *Krone* (1995) 182 Ariz. 319 (Supreme Court of Arizona, USA).

Sweet D, Bowers CM (1998) Accuracy of bite mark overlays: a comparison of five common methods to produce exemplars from a suspect's dentition. *Journal of Forensic Sciences* 43: 362–367.

Taylor RV, Blackwell SA, Yoshino M, *et al.* (2002) *Proceedings for the American Academy of Forensic Sciences 54th Annual Meeting*. Atlanta, GA, USA.

ORGAN AND TISSUE TRANSPLANTATION, ETHICAL AND PRACTICAL ISSUES

S Cordner and H McKelvie, Victorian Institute of Forensic Medicine, Southbank, VIC, Australia

Introduction

That transplantation of human organs and tissues is a desirable activity is no longer seriously debated, if ever it was. Furthermore, given the availability of a sufficient number of organs and tissues, there seem to be no moral reasons why the practice of transplantation should not increase, although there may well be discussion about the ethics of some forms of transplants; for example, the recently reported possibility of face transplants for cosmetic purposes. This increase, however, has been slower than it might have been because of a shortage of organs and, to a lesser extent, tissues. For example, in the late 1990s in the USA, "only about 5500 deaths of an estimated 8000–15 000 deaths of suitable donor candidates each year led to organ donation." At the same time, the number waiting for organs was estimated to be over 63 000, with 4000 dying annually while they wait. Thus, it is issues of procurement that have preoccupied the minds of policy-makers more than other aspects of transplantation. It is in this realm that current debates also take place – for example, debates about xenotransplantation, living donors, and commerce are all issues related to increasing the supply of organs or tissues.

The important distinctions that encompass the critical issues in human tissue or organ supply and usage relate to:

1. the provider; whether:
   a. a living human being
   b. a beating heart (systolic, brain-dead) cadaver
   c. a nonbeating heart (asystolic) cadaver or
   d. a fetus or embryo

2. the nature of the tissue or organ; whether:
   a. regenerative or nonregenerative
   b. single or paired
   c. if single, whether vital
   d. used immediately, or stored
   e. gametes
   f. excretions, byproducts, or wastes (e.g., urine, feces, tears)
   g. sui generis (e.g., hair, teeth, fingernails) or
   h. altered or developed by human agency

3. the use to which the tissue or organ will be put; whether:
   a. diagnosis
   b. transplantation (with or without banking)
   c. research, e.g., epidemiological nonidentifying use; results of possible consequence to the provider
   d. education
   e. commercial development and exploitation (e.g., cell lines) or
   f. other uses such as public display, cannibalism, cosmetics, information-gathering (e.g., DNA from hair roots).

A large range of issues arises from these distinctions and it is difficult to imagine a comprehensive regulatory or ethical schema that would deal comprehensively with them, let alone cope with the dynamic nature of the issues around their supply and demand. Such a task is beyond the scope of this article, which will focus on ethical and practical issues relevant to transplantation of organs and tissues from the systolic or asystolic cadaver into another human being. These are:

1. organs
   a. heart, lung, liver, kidneys, pancreas, and others
2. other transplantable tissues
   a. cardiovascular tissue (heart valves, blood vessels)

b. ocular tissue (corneas, sclera)
c. skeletal and related tissue (bone, ligaments, tendons, cartilage, fascia)
d. skin.

The article is therefore not concerned with xeno-transplantation, living donors, or with fetal or embryonic donors/sources of tissue, as clearly they invoke quite distinct considerations. Neither are issues related to the banking of blood, gametes, or bone marrow canvassed, nor are those related to manipulating or propagating tissues. Other usage of organs and tissues, such as research, education, diagnosis, commercial development, and exploitation, are not considered. (Listing these exclusions serves to remind one of the contextual ranges, or depending upon one's point of view, complexity, of practical and ethical considerations in this and related areas of medicine and science.)

Organs and Tissues

Much effort has been expended trying to demarcate precisely the boundary between organs and tissues. An organ can be defined as "a distinct part of an animal or plant adapted for a particular function." In the same *Oxford Dictionary*, tissue is "any of the distinct types of material of which animal or plants are made, consisting of specialized cells and their products." On this basis, a heart valve is probably better regarded as an organ, although it is retrieved, prepared, and stored in "tissue banks" worldwide. Ultimately, laboring over the boundary between organs and tissues is a futile exercise, because it is only one of a number of distinctions that can be made that are important for ethical, policy, and regulatory purposes.

Developments in tissue banking and transplantation have generally paralleled but been overshadowed by those in organ transplantation. Organ donation has a close association with changing notions of death, and solid organ transplantation the mystique of a highly developed and complex medical science that saves lives. One effect of this has been that the separate and distinct issues associated with the removal, processing, storage, and transplantation of tissues removed from asystolic (nonbeating) heart donors have received less attention. This is despite the number of people whose health and quality of life are improved by tissue transplantation far outnumbering those who receive organ transplants. For example, in recent years in Australia, with a population of around 19.7 million, approximately 200 organs per year were transplanted, compared with over 5000 allografts per year (including heart valves,

bone, skin, and corneas). Whatever the difference in numbers and public profile of organ and tissue transplantation, they share the characteristic of being procedures for which there is an ongoing demand that exceeds supply.

Developing an Understanding of the Body

Such perceptions are highly culturally dependent. This discussion will be limited to mainstream western perceptions, whilst acknowledging the range of philosophical and religious positions informing perceptions of the body around the world. Given the increasingly multicultural nature of the societies one lives in, there is a growing need for greater cross-cultural knowledge of these matters, to ensure all beliefs are respected, especially in the context of procuring organs and tissue for transplantation. Unfortunately, it is beyond the scope of this article to explore them all here.

The scarcity of human tissue to meet medical demand has precedence, starting with early anatomical investigation of human corpses. In 1504, the town council of Edinburgh granted a charter to the Guild of Surgeons and Barbers allowing them to claim the body of one executed criminal a year for dissection. Similarly, in England in 1540, Henry VIII granted to the United Company of Barbers and Surgeons the corpses of four executed felons "yearly for anatomies." Elizabeth I gave an equivalent grant to the College of Physicians in 1564, leading occasionally to unseemly squabbles between the physicians and barber surgeons over possession of the body. The activities of resurrectionists (or grave-robbers) were well known in the eighteenth century to meet the needs of the medical schools for bodies for anatomy classes. The tale of Burke and Hare is now infamous: they became multiple murderers in order to supply corpses for a fee.

These investigative activities added tangible knowledge to the development of medical practice and to the modern western medical model of the body. Various philosophical traditions also contributed to understandings of the human body and the emergence of scientific thought and method. For example, the ancient Greeks developed a dualistic view of the spirit as separate from the body. In the seventeenth century, Francis Bacon argued the notion of the body as morally neutral ground, related to the idea of nature being secular and separate from the spiritual realm – the body and nature therefore being subject to study and control. René Descartes saw the body as a machine and disease as an attempt to repair the parts of the machine. The mind/spirit he saw as morally superior to, and distinct from, the body. John Locke was also influential. He wrote about property rights, and argued that if any individual "invests labour in raw material to produce a product" he acquires property rights over the product. Locke did not discuss the body as such, but his views on property and ownership have influenced expectations of modern medical research.

The western medical view emerging from these major philosophical positions is of human beings as fragmented – mind and spirit separate from mechanistic bodies, requiring outside intervention for repair and healing. This model of the body has been dominant, as modern medicine and biotechnology have developed, although since the 1980s there has been a recovery of the Judeo-Christian holistic understanding of the mind/body/spirit. In this tradition the physical body is seen as integrated with mind and spirit, a vehicle through which they find expression. Contemporaneously, there has been an exponential increase of interest in alternative, holistic healthcare models and spiritual practices such as prayer and meditation, in which the link between body, mind, and spirit is seen as central to healing and personal growth. These understandings place emphasis on the power of the individual's role in healing and healthcare, undermining the position occupied by western healthcare with its reliance on professional disease cure.

This holistic view of the human person also undermines claims that body parts after death are merely matter, with their only real value being linked to medical scientific uses. The significance accorded to the body and its parts by many, whether symbolic, moral, or spiritual, can be difficult to articulate, compared with the "factual" language and demonstrable benefits arising from medical science's use of human tissue. However, in recent years this difficulty was overcome with a significant outpouring of feeling and public outcry when it was revealed that public institutions in the UK (and elsewhere) had retained organs and other body parts from autopsies without the knowledge or consent of parents and family members. (The fact that in Australia the retention was, broadly speaking, lawful offered no protection to the pathologists involved in the court of public opinion.) This situation clearly demonstrated a gap between the general community's expectations of respectful treatment of human body parts and the approach of the medical community to human tissue as a (disembodied) resource. It may be that the response was partly a reaction – fueled by the influence of the consumer movement of the last few decades – against the paternalism inherent in taking without asking. Many of the family members indicated that it was the fact that they had not been consulted that concerned them

the most. The distress of others was clearly linked with their views about the moral and spiritual significance of their children's bodies being disposed of "whole." In general, the experience of the "organ retention scandal" highlighted a tension between the western medical model and other more holistic understandings of human beings and the significance of bodies and their parts.

This tension creates a difficult position for organ and tissue transplantation. As stated at the outset, the desirability of transplantation as an activity is not seriously debated. But thinking about the symbolic, moral, spiritual, and physical reality of making one's own or a loved one's organs and tissue available for this purpose is a more daunting proposition for many, as it involves contemplation of one's own mortality. Arguably, the reluctance to confront these issues is in part a consequence of the success of medical technologies such as those that make transplantation possible. Whatever ambiguity exists around attitudes to bodies and their parts, there is a generalized expectation of the medical profession (often unarticulated until personally relevant and urgent) to provide ways of prolonging life in circumstances where, before the advent of the relevant medical technologies, suffering and death were more easily accepted as "normal outcomes." This expectation of longevity (and fear of confronting death) has evolved alongside advancements in medicine, untempered by the reality of limited resources – in this particular context, the disparity between available organs for transplantation and those in need of them. It will be interesting to see what, if any, influence the emerging interest in holistic healing and spirituality has on this pressurized situation. Perhaps we will see more acceptance and less desperation around prolonging life by means of major medical intervention such as organ transplantation, which after all is not always successful – a point which is often lost in what has become an increasingly politicized debate about boosting organ donation rates. It may also be that the medical community will play a part in modifying unrealistic expectations: Richard Smith, former editor of the *British Medical Journal,* has suggested a new covenant for the twenty-first century between the public, the profession, and politicians, one which would include recognition that "death, sickness, and pain are part of life; medicine has limited power particularly to solve social problems and is risky; patients cannot leave [all] problems to doctors; doctors should be open about their limitations and politicians should refrain from making extravagant promises and concentrate on reality."

Brain Death

Brain death is another concept relevant to organ transplantation that is well accepted amongst the medical and related professions, but which may not be well understood or accepted by the lay community. Traditionally, the physical death of an individual equated with the cessation of heartbeat and the absence of respiration. However, technologies developed during the twentieth century for resuscitating patients whose heartbeat and respiration have stopped made the traditional criterion indeterminate in many cases. A person whose heart had stopped beating could be restored to life by means of medical intervention. The concept of brain death was based on international acceptance that a patient cannot recover once there has been irreversible cessation of all brain functions.

The other practical reason to define death by reference to brain function was to provide certainty in the context of medical procedures around the removal of organs and tissues for transplantation. The diagnosis of brain death in many, if not most, countries of the world means that the patient is dead, just as if the patient had died because of irreversible cessation of his/her circulation. When the clinical and legal criteria for the diagnosis of brain death have been satisfied, the patient is dead, even if the cardiovascular and respiratory systems are functioning with artificial support – circumstances which provide the optimum conditions for "harvesting" organs for transplantation use.

However, there is evidence that as many as 20% of families in some settings retain doubts that their family member was indeed dead at the time their organs were removed. Although called brain death, the diagnostic criteria are essentially assessments of brainstem death. It is well recognized that brainstem death is compatible with aspects of "brain life." For example, neurological regulation of hormonal secretion and electroencephalographic (EEG) activity possibly representing cortical function commonly exist even when the formal criteria for diagnosing brain death are satisfied. This discordance, while neither understood nor articulated well in the public mind, may contribute to some of the disinclination in some communities to donate organs and tissues for transplantation.

Measures Taken to Improve the Supply of Organs and Tissues

With an ever-increasing number of people around the world needing organ or tissue transplants to save, or vastly improve the quality of, their lives, the issue of improving the supply of available organs and tissues is one that continues to occupy governments, and policy-makers, and those who would seek to profit from this situation. Many of the measures that can be considered to improve the supply of human tissues for transplantation, within the constraints of this article, fall under three headings:

1. presuming consent/opting out
2. improving the efficiency of the existing system
3. commercialization.

Presuming Consent or "Opt-Out" Systems

Presuming consent or opting out are terms used to describe a system where all body parts of a deceased person are available for use, unless the person has registered an objection in his/her lifetime. If no objection is registered, a person is presumed to consent to his/her organs and other tissues being donated on death. This system places the onus on individuals to be proactive and think about the issue of organ donation and to act to register their objection. Assuming there are the personnel and facilities available, it can have the effect of making organ donation a more "routine" event, and eliminates the necessity for next of kin to make decisions at a difficult time.

Opt-out systems are operating in several European countries following the 1978 adoption by the Committee of Ministers of the Council of Europe of Resolution 78(29), a model legal code concerning the removal, grafting, and transplantation of human organs and tissues. The code, as well as prohibiting commerce in body materials, allowed "presumed consent" (for the procurement of cadaveric organs and tissues) provided there was no recorded objection by the deceased (so-called "opting out"). No inquiry of the relatives was needed.

The Council was persuaded in coming to a conclusion favoring "presumed consent" by:

- the invaluable importance of organs and tissues for transplantation
- their shortage
- the interests of sick people.

The Council of Europe affirmed its position in 1987, but noted: "The practice in most countries shows that relatives are consulted and though in most cases its opinion is not overriding, none would go against the expressed refusal of the family." Quite apart from anything else, pragmatic concerns mean that the families have to be consulted. They are the repository of vital information about the deceased's lifestyle, and such information is critical to decisions about the transplantability of the organs and tissues.

If during this consultation families disagree with the decision to donate, it is difficult to see how the donation can proceed. Consequences associated with bad publicity initiated by the family could affect the whole organ donation program and the attitude of the family may affect the confidence one could have in the lifestyle information provided. If families are heeded at this stage, then essentially the presumed consent regime has been defeated. At this stage, the only remaining value attaching to a presumed consent regime for organ and tissue donation would be as a statement of the importance attached to the value of organs and tissues and their availability for sick people.

Underpinning arguments about presumed consent is that it actually works to increase the availability of organs and tissues for transplantation. The answer is not as clear-cut as might be supposed, especially in relation to organs. For example, some countries with a high organ donation rate together with a presumed consent regime also have high road death rates. It is not simply a matter of comparing rates of donations in countries with and without presumed consent laws. Simply the awareness generated by public debate prior to the introduction of presumed consent laws may be responsible for some of the increase that might be claimed to be due to the new laws. There is, however, evidence in the USA about the positive effect of presumed consent laws in relation to the availability of corneas. States such as Florida, Michigan, Texas, and Ohio followed the 1975 lead of Maryland in authorizing procurement of eye tissue when:

- a body is in the jurisdiction of a coroner or medical examiner for forensic autopsy purposes;
- there is no known objection to corneal tissue procurement; and
- procurement would result in neither disfigurement of the body not interference with the autopsy.

Such laws (Law Reform Commission of Canada, Procurement and Transfer of Human Tissues 1992) led to increases in corneal transplantation in Florida from 500 to 3000. The desirability of this, however, is still subject to some of the concerns expressed above, in particular, notwithstanding the availability of testing, the need to obtain reliable information about lifestyle from the family.

Some commentators regard presumed consent as a contradiction in terms, or a fiction. Consent is the active exercise by a person of an aspect of his/her autonomy. It can never be presumed. One might develop criteria for when consent is not necessary because of some overriding consideration (e.g., the desperate shortage of organs and tissues), but this is not presuming consent. Rather, it is not being

concerned with the wishes of the deceased or his/her family (unless the deceased took steps in life to register his/her objection to donation) to meet what society has determined is an overriding need. In using the language of consent, one might be accused of disguising what one is actually doing, however well motivated that might be, by appealing to our respect for individual autonomy. The option of registering an objection during life, of course, does not mitigate this; the realities of civic life are such that a very small proportion of the population will engage with the issue, and even smaller numbers will take the option even if it represented their wish. As with brain death, at some level this type of labeling of public policy probably contributes to the disinclination of some communities to respond to pleas to support organ and tissue donation.

Improving the Efficiency of Existing Systems

Other measures taken to increase supply of organs and tissues do not rely on altering the principle of positive consent to donation on which many countries' systems are based. In the USA, an attempt has been made to enhance the effectiveness of the system by introducing "required request." This policy presumes that the problem lies not with engendering altruism but with helping people to act on their good intentions and overcoming any reluctance of health professionals to approach families. Although there are some variations from state to state, generally the system requires hospital staff to assess and document the suitability for organ and tissue donation of every patient who dies in hospital. This information is passed to designated organ procurement organizations (OPOs) who are responsible for ensuring that approaches are made to the deceased's family. In general, exceptions are made where:

- the wishes of the deceased were already known
- healthcare staff could not locate the family in time
- it seemed that the inquiry or request would add to the relatives' mental distress.

There is evidence to suggest that this approach has generally failed to increase the rate of organ donation, primarily because of continued objections by next of kin. By contrast, the rate of tissue donation has risen. This may be because the circumstances in which solid organ donation can occur are very limited, but many more of the notifications to the OPOs would have potential for tissue donation. The required request system has increased awareness of the possibility of tissue donation and the rate at which families are approached. It could also be that family members are more comfortable with the idea of donating musculoskeletal tissue rather than whole organs for reasons relating to their beliefs about the human body, as canvassed above.

A further way of promoting donations of organs and tissue is known as "mandated choice." This entails indicating willingness or refusal to donate (in the event of the required circumstances arising at the time of demise) when performing some task mandated by the state, e.g., obtaining a driver's license or filling in a tax return. Some see this as having an ethical advantage over opt-out systems, as it encourages individual autonomy. It also provides family members with an expression of the deceased's choice, making it easier for them to agree to retrieval of organs or tissue at a very stressful time. However, there are some major limitations on the effectiveness of this system:

- Not everyone obtains a driver's license or files a tax return.
- Coordination of an electronic register of individuals' choices is necessary to allow access at the time of a potential donation. This is not easy to achieve, especially on a national or regional basis.
- If the mandated choice is not backed by legislation allowing hospitals to act on the choice registered, the choice may be vetoed by family members. Also individuals may have changed their minds about donation since the time of registering their choice. Reliance is therefore placed on family members to confirm the choice, in any event.

Further initiatives for improving donation rates focus on coordination of relevant services and active education of health professionals and the community. Reviews of donation systems have identified as critical the attitudes of clinicians at the donating end: emergency and intensive care physicians, and, for tissue, hospital staff responsible for care before death and pathologists undertaking autopsies. Education programs have been implemented for medical practitioners to cultivate a positive outlook about donation, and promote awareness of the requirements for organ and tissue donation, including how families should be approached with information and support. However (and this may also be true of what has occurred in the USA with the required request system), these have a limited effect on actual donation rates where they are not backed with the necessary resources. For example, having sufficient intensive care beds to accommodate a brain-dead patient and sustain respiration and circulation while the necessary tests are performed can be a major issue. Having transplant coordinators who can work with clinicians and who are trained and experienced in approaching families is also important. Similarly, staff and resources are required for emergency room doctors to have the time to identify and deal with potential donors and liaise with intensive care units and transplant coordinators, otherwise their primary role – saving lives in the emergency room – will always come first.

Commercialization as an Alternative or Additional Means of Supplying Organs or Tissue

There are already significant elements of commercialization in organ and tissue transplantation wherever it exists. Surgeons, operating theater staff, and the staff of tissue banks earn their livelihood; goods and services at commercial rates are consumed in obtaining, processing, storing, and distributing organs and tissues which contribute to the profits of those providing them. Therefore, not only commercialization, but profit-making by some is inherent in organ and tissue transplantation. However, amidst all of this, most regard the tissue itself as privileged and to be protected at all costs from the mammon-virus. The organ or tissue is not to be thought of as a commodity; it is a priceless gift of life or health which cannot be bought or sold but only donated.

As a matter of ethics, how are we to regard a donor (now a provider) receiving valuable consideration in return for tissue to be used for transplantation? This is more than a theoretical problem. Liver4you.org makes the claim that for specified fees it will arrange transplant surgery with either cadaver or live organs in the Philippines. Kidney transplants cost from $US35 000 to $US85 000 and liver transplants from $US150 000 to $US250 000. That arrangements associated with this service may be ethically dubious is obviously something to be considered.

For the purpose of understanding something of the ethics, it is easiest to consider a live kidney donor. The following arguments are usually advanced against paying a person to provide a kidney:

1. The whole idea is abhorrent and unthinkable. Some things are so obvious that there is no need to contemplate otherwise. For example, so the argument goes, views purporting to show that the Holocaust did not happen are so offensive and patently wrong that the principles of free speech do not apply. Human tissue is so linked with personhood that to allow it to be equated with money is to undermine that for which our respect (save in exceptional circumstances) should be absolute and unconditional: the human person.
2. The ability of poor people to sell one of their kidneys will lead to exploitation of the poor. The

poor and indigent have yet another indignity heaped on top of a pile of misfortune: undergoing an operation (with associated risks) which, by force of circumstances of hunger and deprivation, they have no real choice to refuse. Such exploitation should not be allowed.

3. The voluntary donation of a kidney is a noble act, and altruism is a community good which should be encouraged and supported. Paying for kidneys will undermine this because:

   a. Potential donors may now not donate. They might dislike the commercialized environment. If the going rate for a person selling a kidney was $1000, a potential donor might well think s/he is giving $1000, not life, and hence not donate.

   b. Many or most volunteers might now sell.

In the first case, the actual number of kidneys from the living for donation may actually decrease (leaving aside drives for organs from the developing world). In the second case, the community may not lose supply but would have lost the altruism surrounding it.

Consequentialist arguments against allowing the purchase of kidneys from living providers can also be made. These are based on conclusions reached by Titmuss in relation to a private market in blood. Kidneys purchased as opposed to donated:

- entail much greater risks to the recipient of disease, chronic disability, and death because the providers, keen to obtain the money, will lie about their health
- are potentially more dangerous to the health of the suppliers who will be induced to take greater than acceptable risks
- may, in the long run, because of the above two factors produce greater shortages of kidneys.

The level of abuse of commercialization has proved difficult to quantify, although the number of horror stories is accumulating.

The website for Organ Watch: Social Justice, Human Rights, and Organ Transplantation is http://sunsite.berkeley.edu/biotech/organswatch/index.html. This is a small university-based attempt to monitor organ trafficking globally. The website includes a compilation of news and journal articles about a range of abuses that have occurred in recent years around the world, many involving the active participation of members of the medical profession.

Let us move to the argument in favor of paying providers. Kidney donation is a laudable practice but there is a great shortage of organs. Paying people for kidneys will not stop altruistic donation; in any event we pay for many other things and services which could otherwise be regarded as altruistic, e.g., medical care itself, foster care, and care for the elderly. Individuals can voluntarily sell their labor and be paid to take risks (e.g., professional boxing, being an airforce pilot) without it necessarily being said that they are being used as a means, so why should people not be able to sell a kidney? If, in my informed judgment, I will be better off for having done so, not to allow this infringes my personal autonomy, a right that extends to the taking of risks and which underscores human dignity and the respect owed to me by others. It is acceptable that there is the potential to exploit the poor, but regulation will prevent abuses. Furthermore, regulation will extend to the distribution of kidneys, which will be governed by need and medical efficacy and not by purchasing power.

The European Parliament is in no doubt about its position. It has recently strengthened its position against the purchasing of organs. The measures proposed will render patients liable for criminal penalties if they go abroad and pay for organs. These will be extremely difficult offenses to prove, so it is questionable whether this will have any impact on trafficking in relation to European patients. That is not to be critical of the proposals, which embody important values, but they bring to mind the difficulties of dealing with trafficking whatever position one adopts on commercialization.

Some jurisdictions have moved to an intermediate position in relation to commercialization. In 1999, the US state of Pennsylvania, having already improved its donation rate by introducing various measures, proposed the payment of $US300 of funeral expenses to donor families. This was not regarded in any way as a payment for the tissues, but was a recognition of society's appreciation for the donor family. The initiative was never implemented because of a conflict with federal law. It did however stimulate heated debate, with many ethicists viewing it as an incentive to donate that should properly be characterized as providing a monetary benefit to donor families and, therefore, a step down the path to paying for organs.

Conclusion

There are many issues not covered here, even in this narrow field of cadaveric organ and tissue donation and transplantation. For example, confidentiality issues (e.g., test results with consequences for donor families; confidentiality as between donor and recipient) have not been dealt with; the safety and quality of the organs and tissues including the potential for disease transmission (e.g., human immunodeficiency virus (HIV), hepatitis B and C, rabies, bacteria, fungi, malignant disease); the particular issue of the use of organs and tissues provided from executed prisoners; whether or not there is any commercial element associated. Neither has the fascinating issue of property rights in human tissues been explored. Finally, nothing has been said about the allocation of organs and tissues, the paradigm of a scarce resource.

In conclusion, a note of caution is appropriate. Enthusiasm for tissue transplantation must be tempered by knowledge of the known and respect for the unknown. Scott waxes lyrical about the success of the Australian National Pituitary program which prevented over 600 children who would otherwise have been dwarfs from being so and which enabled over 1400 previously infertile women to have children. As with similar programs around the world, a number of these patients subsequently developed Creutzfeldt–Jakob disease, and more will probably do so as time passes. As with the disastrous infiltration of hepatitis C and HIV into the blood supply everywhere in the 1980s and 1990s, this serves as a warning, if one was needed, about the caution and humility with which tissue banking and transplantation should proceed. The situation is different for organ transplantation. Unless serious international action is developed to arrest and stop organ trafficking, public revulsion at

the practice may well impact upon domestic attitudes to organ donation.

See Also

Consent: Treatment Without Consent; Confidentiality and Disclosure; **Religious Attitudes to Death**

Further Reading

Erin CA, Harris J (1999) Presumed consent or contracting out. *Journal of Medical Ethics* 25: 365–366.

Hakim NS, Papalois VE (eds.) (2003) *History of Organ and Cell Transplantation.* London: Imperial College Press.

Kerridge IH (1999) *Death, Dying and Donation: Organ Transplantation and the Diagnosis of Death.* Victoria, Australia: Australian Institute of Health, Law and Ethics.

Price D (2000) *Legal and Ethical Aspects of Organ Transplantation.* Cambridge, UK: Cambridge University Press.

Shelton W (2001) *The Ethics of Organ Transplantation.* Amsterdam, Netherlands: Jai Press/Elsevier Science.

ten Have HAMJ, Welie JVM (eds.) (1998) *Ownership of the Human Body: Philosophical Considerations on the Use of the Human Body and its Parts in Healthcare.* Dordrecht: Kluwer Academic.

Titmuss RM (1970) *The Gift Relationship: From Human Blood to Social Policy*, p. 157. London, UK: George Allen and Unwin.

P

PARENTAGE TESTING

G S Williams, Northern Illinois University, DeKalb, IL, USA

Introduction

Parentage testing before 1986 involved only the use of serology to determine red blood cell (RBC) surface antigens, human leukocyte antigens (HLA), serum proteins, and RBC enzymes for identifying family members. Serology is literally defined as the study of serum (blood serum). However, forensic serology also included immunological study of biological tissues, body fluids, and biological stains.

Forensic serology has been changed to forensic biology as analysts now also perform deoxyribonucleic acid (DNA) testing on cells other than from blood. In 1986, nucleic acid testing (NAT) became legally acceptable to establish DNA markers, thus increasing the power to identify or exclude individuals as biologically related. The expanded definition is the natural outgrowth from the increase in knowledge of polymorphic genes from 1980 to 2003. The human genome has been sequenced and it is estimated that 0.1% or 3 million basepairs are polymorphic; one in every 1000 bases has more than one allele. These polymorphic sites are either true coding regions and transcribed into proteins or are in noncoding regions. Most DNA-based testing is on the highly polymorphic noncoding DNA regions due to the increased ability to exclude a wrongfully accused person. The most recent addition to DNA parentage testing is single nucleotide polymorphism (SNP) analysis which is automated.

The bulk of this article will focus on paternity testing of the typical trio of mother (Mo), child (Ch), and one alleged father (AF). In addition to the typical trio, parentage testing and identity testing within families include maternity confirmation, determination of identical versus fraternal twins, identification of recovered kidnapped children, matching grandparents to grandchildren, analysis of paternity without maternal specimens, settling immigration and inheritance disputes, and sibling confirmation.

History

Landsteiner discovered the ABO blood groups between 1900 and 1901. In 1926, the first use of the ABO system to exclude (rule out) an AF occurred in Vienna. The following year, M and N antigens were discovered. Ten years later, ABO and MN were first used in parentage testing in the USA. In 1939, RBCs were shown to have rhesus (Rh) system antigens also. Four Rh system antigens, C, c, D, and E, are used by most labs that do RBC antigen typing for parentage testing. Other RBC systems or antigens that have added more power to the exclusion rate include K in the Kell system in 1946, S in the MN system in 1947, Cellano (k) in the Kell system in 1949, the Duffy system in 1950, the Kidd system in 1951, and the addition of s to the MNS system, also in 1951.

The ability to rule out a wrongfully accused man (exclusion power) using RBC antigens was good but not good enough for many cases. In 1955, polymorphism of haptoglobin (Hp) was described and subsequently, other RBC enzymes and serum proteins were found to be polymorphic and useful for identity testing. The recognition that polymorphisms occur in serum proteins and RBC enzymes added more markers to help improve exclusion and inclusion percentages.

Prior to DNA testing, HLA testing was the best method to exclude and improve inclusion (possible biological father) probabilities of an AF. In 1972, HLA became available as a highly polymorphic system for use in paternity testing. By 1976, most laboratories used six RBC antigen systems of the more than 400 RBC surface antigens now known and HLA for parentage testing, and a few laboratories performed enzyme and protein testing.

DNA testing is now the norm throughout the world for determining genetic relatedness. In 1976, restriction fragment length polymorphism (RFLP) analysis was first described and it was used in 1980 to show a highly polymorphic region of DNA. By 1986, RFLP was used for paternity testing. RFLP analysis requires large amounts of good-quality intact DNA and the procedure takes several days to perform. Newer testing methods for DNA are highly automated, do not require intact DNA, and are completed in a few hours.

When the polymerase chain reaction (PCR) became automated, new markers were amplified and used for identity testing. Variable number of tandem repeats (VNTR) genetic loci were identified as powerful markers for forensics and were soon used in parentage disputes. Both long tandem repeats (LTR) and short tandem repeats (STR) frequencies for most populations are established. These markers are now used more frequently than the traditional serological markers. By 1995, STR testing became practical and also replaced RFLP analysis for forensic identity testing and parentage studies. The most recent addition to parentage testing, SNP analysis, was approved for parentage testing by the American Association of Blood Banks (AABB) in 2003.

Current Practice

Most laboratories now use DNA analysis for parentage testing, some continue doing serological analysis of HLA, and fewer continue to offer the less expensive RBC antigen methods. Blood protein analysis has only been offered by specialized laboratories since 1976. **Table 1** lists most markers currently used in parentage testing.

Specimen Collection

The specimens used for parentage testing vary depending upon the methods that will be used to analyze the sample. RBC antigen tests may be performed on clotted blood or anticoagulated blood in ethylenediaminetetraacetic acid (EDTA), or acid citrate dextrose (ACD). For HLA testing, ACD is

Table 1 Markers used in parentage testing[a]

Serology			DNA			
Red blood cell antigen systems	Red blood cell enzymes and serum proteins	Human leukocyte antigens (HLA)	Restriction fragment length polymorphism	PCR SSP	PCR LTR	PCR STR
ABO	PGM1	HLA-A	D1S339	HLA-DQA1	D1S80	FGA
Rh	ACP	HLA-B	D2S44	LDLR		HUMTHO1
MNSs	ESD		D4S139	GYPA		HUMTPOX
Kell	Hp		D4S163	HBGG		HUMCSF1PO
Kidd	GC		D5S110	D7S8		HUMF13AO1
Duffy	Gm		D6S132	GC		HUMVWA13/A
Lutheran	Am		D7S467			HUMFESFPS
Xg	Km		D10S28			HUMLIPOL
	AK		D12S11			D6S818
	ADA		D14S13			D9S302
	6-PGD		D17S26			D22S683
	TF		D17S79			D18S535
	BF					D7S1804
	M					D7S820
	C3					D3S2387
	GLO					D4S2366
	GPT					D5S1719
	UMPK					D3S1358
	PGP					D8S1179
						D13S317
						D16S538
						D18S51
						D21S11

[a]Tables 2, 3, and 6 have expanded listings of markers for HLA, and DNA analysis.
ACP, acid phosphatase; ADA, adenosine deaminase; AK, adenylate kinase; Am, immunoglobulin A polymorphic alleles; BF, Properdin factor B; C3, third component of complement; DNA, deoxyribonucleic acid; ESD, esterase D; GC, group-specific component; GLO, glyoxalase; Gm, immunoglobulin G polymorphic alleles; GPT, glutamate pyruvate transaminase; HBGG, hemoglobin G; Hp, haptoglobin; Km, light-chain polymorphic alleles; LDLR, low-density lipoprotein receptor; LTR, long tandem repeat; M, M subtyping of alpha$_1$-antitrypsin; PCR, polymerase chain reaction; 6-PGD, 6-phosphogluconate dehydrogenase; PGM, phosphoglucomutase; PGP, phosphoglycolate phosphatase; Rh, rhesus; SSP, sequence-specific primer or probe; STR, short tandem repeat; TF, transferrin; UMPK, uridine monophosphate kinase; GYPA, glycophorin A.

preferred for preservation of viability of white cells. ACD or Alsever's solution is also best for RBC enzyme studies to preserve the enzymes. Serum protein analysis is best done with serum from clotted blood.

For DNA tests, a wide variety of samples will do. If blood is drawn, 2–5 ml EDTA blood provides the best results because it preserves DNA by inhibiting DNase activity. FTA® paper also preserves DNA and samples can be stored for extended periods at room temperature. Alternative DNA samples include buccal cells or other tissue cells. When buccal samples are collected, different-colored swabs designated for each person help to avoid mix-up. For instance, a laboratory could have yellow, red, green, and blue swabs and always use yellow for a Ch, blue for AF 1, green for AF 2, and red for the mother.

After informed consent is obtained from each adult in the case, the collection of specimens must be performed by someone with no vested interest in the outcome and witnessed by another disinterested party. Each specimen must be properly labeled and processed.

Selection of Genetic Loci

Not all genetic loci are created equal. Even those with multiple alleles may have drawbacks. Establishing Hardy–Weinberg equilibrium for the locus increases the reliability of the data analysis. Several assumptions are made in using the Hardy–Weinberg approach: (1) random mating; (2) large population; and (3) migration unlikely. The frequency of a given allele at a polymorphic (at least two alleles) locus is established for each population.

Polymorphisms in the human genome occur in coding and noncoding regions. Polymorphisms of proteins, lipids, and sugars are differences in the structure that do not change their function significantly. The mutations in coding regions can lead to a functional gene product that will subsequently be passed on as an allele at that locus. Other mutations lead to changes incompatible with normal function resulting in a miscarriage or shortened life span. In parentage testing, normal alleles, resulting in expression of carbohydrates, lipids, and proteins on the RBC surface, inside the RBC, and in serum are useful markers. These traditional systems have been well evaluated, and exceptions to the normal expected outcomes of inheritance and testing have been well described. All of these parentage markers are genetically stable with rare mutations of less than one in a million individuals.

As opposed to the low mutation rate of RBC antigens, HLA, or serum proteins by classical serological methods, mutations are a significant issue when using DNA-based methods. Noncoding DNA mutations do not have a selective disadvantage or advantage whereas mutations in the coding region often lead to a dysfunctional protein.

Co-dominant alleles inherited by classic Mendelian rules are best (segregation and independent assortment). Segregation refers to the mode of inheritance of alleles; two alleles at the same site (locus) are never found in the same gamete (ova or sperm). For instance in the MNS system, when a parent is genetically *MS/Ns*, only *Ns* or *Ms* will be in any one gamete. Independent assortment refers to the way genes for different traits are inherited. For instance, the inheritance of *O* is independent of the inheritance of *MS* because these genes are on different chromosomes. Other genes, like *D*, are far apart from *Fy* on chromosome 1. This is also referred to as linkage. *O* and *MS*, *D* and *Fy* are not linked to each other. Some genes are so closely linked that they are inherited together, like *MN* with *SsU*. Phenotypes that lead to probable genotypes are most useful. For instance, someone who phenotypes D+C+ c+e+ and is white is most likely *DCe/ce*. Silent alleles make the analytical process more complicated, as illustrated in a later section.

Genetic markers or loci should have databases established for all potentially tested races or ethnic groups. The distribution of the selected alleles should be effective in excluding an unrelated person (e.g., an AF who is not the biological father). In calculating probability of parentage or relatedness, the laboratory must take into account all loci that have linkage disequilibrium or are linked genetically. One common example of linkage disequilibrium occurs in the HLA system. HLA-A1 and HLA-B8 are found together more frequently than would be expected by their independent gene frequencies. In addition, HLA-DQA1 DNA testing results are not independent of HLA-A and HLA-B serological results because they are all closely linked on chromosome 6.

By contrast, although DNA testing for RFLP, PCR-VNTR, PCR-short tandem repeat (STR), PCR-SNP, or sequencing (SQ) is extremely powerful in including a possible father as perhaps the only person on the planet who could have contributed the sperm, it is also more likely to have confusing results from mutations in the noncoding regions that are most widely used for these tests. Some of the markers have a mutation rate of 0.03. Refer to **Tables 2** and **3** for lists of mutation rates for DNA markers. DNA markers must also be stable under different host conditions and testing methods. This high rate of mutation could result in a male being excluded when he really is the father. An AF may have a very high inclusion rate of 99.9% and have one STR locus that appears to

Table 2 Mutation rates summarized for genetic markers analyzed by RFLP mapping[a]

System	Maternal[b] (%)	Paternal[b] (%)	Null[c] (%)	Multi-banded
D1S7	9/580 (1.55)	11/721 (1.52)	1/560 (0.17)	2/461 (<0.43)
D1S339	206/87600 (0.24)	388/104432 (0.37)	77/91846 (0.081)	143/69999 (0.20)
D2S44	335/203411 (0.17)	239/225733 (0.17)	465/233293 (0.20)	361/224260 (0.16)
D4S139	35/76809 (0.05)	951/100806 (0.94)	18/78545 (0.02)	778/83024 (0.94)
D4S163	4/21669 (0.02)	42/41635 (0.10)	32/46065 (0.07)	16/29731 (0.05)
D5S110	135/24567 (0.55)	412/23684 (1.74)	10/25879 (0.04)	502/30372 (1.65)
D5S43	0/525 (<0.191)	0/536 (<0.187)	UNK	UNK
D6S132	11/56265 (0.02)	67/84917 (0.08)	2/98399 (<0.01)	39/132922 (0.03)
D7S21	20/979 (2.04)	41/1317 (3.10)	UNK	1/1235 (0.081)
D7S22	15/2734 (0.55)	91/3187 (2.86)	UNK	UNK
D7S467	18/91022 (0.02)	156/140441 (0.11)	15/165771 (<0.01)	46/145815 (0.03)
D10S28	337/183546 (0.18)	180/188480 (0.10)	60/165265 (0.04)	144/167649 (0.09)
D12S11	5/15054 (0.03)	14/19043 (0.07)	3/19022 (0.02)	5/16199 (0.03)
D14S13	19/30596 (0.06)	108/33085 (0.33)	3/21391 (0.01)	119/26343 (0.45)
D16S309	0/176 (<0.06)	2/2129 (0.09)	UNK	UNK
D16S85	0/518 (<0.19)	2/542 (0.55)	0/676 (<0.148)	0/676 (<0.148)
D17S26	60/63059 (0.10)	157/65205 (0.24)	3/21165 (0.01)	32/55997 (0.06)
D17S79	7/15329 (0.05)	21/21222 (0.10)	12/10345 (0.12)	14/17582 (0.08)

[a]The mutation rates include data from the 2000 AABB Annual Report Summary.
[b]The data under these column headings refers to the number of inconsistencies/number of total meioses expressed as a percentage within the parentheses.
[c]Null alleles are assumed to exist in cases of paternal or maternal exclusion due to nonmatching homozygous banding patterns when there is otherwise overwhelming evidence in favor of paternity or maternity.
Reprinted from American Association of Blood Banks (2002) *Guidance for Standards for Parentage Testing Laboratories*, 5th edn., p. 140. Bethesda, MD: American Association of Blood Banks with permission.

exclude him because of a common mutation. Refer to the AABB *Guidance for Standards for Parentage Testing Laboratories* for examples.

Methodology

The methodology chosen for testing must comply with standards set by each country. In general, all samples should be assessed by two independent analysts using a different set of reagents from different sources. Quality assurance of testing personnel and procedures is essential. In order to trust data from different laboratories, the same procedures should be used by multiple laboratories for comparison by proficiency testing.

Serological RBC antigen testing, RBC enzymes, serum proteins, and HLA testing have been standardized for many decades and frequency tables have been established. NAT by STR or SNP databases on the other hand have discrepancies in nomenclature. For example, one group describes the repeat for HUMTH01 in the STR analysis as AATG and GenBank (a public database) uses the other strand of DNA and calls it TCAT. All investigators working on establishing these databases must agree upon nomenclature and frequencies to ensure accuracy.

RBC Typing

The six most common families of cell-surface proteins tested are ABO, MNS, Rh, Duffy, Kell, and Kidd. In the USA, the combined exclusion power for RBC antigens is 65.5%. The following is a list of the exclusion power of different systems of RBC antigens: (1) ABO: 20%, (2) MNS: 31%, (3) Rh: 25%, (4) Duffy: 7%, (5) Kell: 4%, (6) Kidd: 6%. In addition, Lutheran (3.5%) and Xg (varies) are tested by some laboratories. **Table 4** lists RBC antigens, nomenclature, and where their genes are located. These are stable markers on intact RBCs usually available for most parentage testing. **Table 5** lists the RBC phenotype frequencies for various ethnic groups in the USA.

Typing samples for RBC surface antigens involves the use of antisera from human or monoclonal sources. For tests using antihuman globulin, special controls of the individual's RBCs without reagent antibody must be included to ensure that they are not already coated with antibody. These Coombs-positive cells would test positive for every marker requiring antihuman globulin as part of the procedure.

ABO, Rh, and MNS systems are the most powerful RBC antigen systems to use for exclusions. The common phenotypes of the ABO system are O, A_1, A_2, B, A_1B, and A_2B. Several rare subgroups of

Table 3 Apparent mutations summarized for genetic systems analyzed by PCR[a]

System	Maternal[b] (%)	Maternal null (%)	Paternal[b] (%)	Paternal null[c] (%)
D1S80	4/14052 (0.03)	UNK	75/199543 (0.04)	2/60372 (<0.01)
D1S2131	0/1212 (<0.08)	UNK	3/1240 (0.24)	UNK
D1S533	UNK	UNK	6/3830 (0.16)	UNK
D2S1338	UNK	UNK	9/45170 (0.02)	0/605 (<0.20)
D2S548	1/1212 (0.08)	UNK	0/1240 (<0.08)	UNK
D3S1358	5/18182 (0.03)	2/13293 (0.02)	77/52153 (0.15)	5/18094 (0.03)
D3S1744	16/10131 (0.16)	0/5697 (<0.02)	83/19555 (0.42)	0/8462 (<0.02)
D3S2386	0/1212 (<0.08)	UNK	1/1240 (0.08)	UNK
D5S818	29/127601 (0.02)	3/51327 (<0.01)	300/213999 (0.14)	18/67046 (0.03)
D7S820	19/120930 (0.02)	1/46032 (<0.01)	281/220861 (0.13)	5/73184 (<0.01)
D8S306	1/1212 (0.08)	UNK	3/1240 (0.24)	UNK
D8S1179	9/26510 (0.03)	3/14451 (0.02)	105/53114 (0.20)	4/22417 (0.02)
D9S302	19/8332 (0.22)	0/5669 (<0.02)	49/11179 (0.44)	0/8568 (<0.02)
D10S1214	28/2903 (0.97)	UNK	114/2938 (3.88)	UNK
D12S1090	9/4894 (0.18)	UNK	108/11957 (0.90)	0/5865 (<0.02)
D13S317	65/128422 (0.05)	112/68583 (0.16)	242/159361 (0.15)	131/134466 (0.10)
D13S764	0/1212 (<0.08)	UNK	0/1240 (<0.08)	UNK
D14S297	0/1212 (<0.08)	UNK	0/1240 (<0.08)	UNK
D16S539	19/97307 (0.02)	4/54649 (<0.01)	118/112872 (0.11)	14/58079 (0.02)
D17S5	0/228 (<0.44)	UNK	7/6568 (0.11)	UNK
D17S1185	0/1212 (<0.08)	UNK	0/1240 (<0.08)	UNK
D18S51	17/26804 (0.06)	2/12363 (0.02)	113/55362 (0.20)	3/20396 (0.02)
D18S535	1/2676 (0.04)	UNK	2/2624 (0.08)	0/5300 (<0.02)
D18S849	0/4281 (<0.03)	UNK	15/9594 (0.16)	0/5904 (<0.02)
D19S253	8/2997 (0.27)	1/1785 (0.06)	17/3247 (0.52)	7/2007 (0.35)
D21S11	31/28305 (0.11)	1/16244 (<0.01)	79/51202 (0.15)	2/18790 (0.01)
D21S1437	0/1212 (<0.08)	UNK	1/1240 (0.08)	UNK
D22S445	2/1212 (0.17)	UNK	1/1240 (0.08)	UNK
D22S683	2/2670 (0.08)	UNK	9/2625 (0.34)	0/5295 (<0.02)
ACTBP2	0/330 (<0.30)	UNK	330/51610 (0.64)	UNK
CYP19	6/343 (1.75)	UNK	205/177210 (0.12)	321/47259 (0.68)
CYAR04	2/3539 (0.06)	UNK	UNK	UNK
FGA	14/26123 (0.05)	0/15175 (<0.01)	690/236659 (0.29)	6/24689 (0.02)
HUMCSF1P0	21/109907 (0.02)	1/60275 (<0.01)	451/314702 (0.14)	5/68573 (<0.01)
HUMFESFPS	3/16264 (0.02)	1/7606 (0.01)	78/143297 (0.05)	0/11761 (<0.01)
HUMF13A01	0/8152 (<0.01)	0/283 (<0.40)	35/62820 (0.06)	0/2724 (<0.04)
HUMF13B	1/9857 (0.01)	0/4435 (0.02)	8/24314 (0.03)	0/7675 (<0.01)
HUMLIPOL	0/6200 (<0.02)	0/2311 (<0.05)	6/8918 (0.07)	0/2961 (<0.04)
HUMTHO1	10/100219 (0.01)	2/56371 (<0.01)	21/154685 (0.01)	2/74346 (<0.01)
HUMTPOX	2/79616 (<0.01)	0/50850 (<0.01)	21/112758 (0.02)	2/66052 (<0.01)
HUMvWA31	44/135789 (0.03)	1/66959 (<0.01)	1130/351664 (0.32)	22/120230 (0.02)
Penta E	1/6248 (0.02)	0/6248 (<0.02)	10/8315 (0.12)	0/8315 (<0.01)

[a]The mutation rates include data from the 2000 AABB Annual Report Summary.
[b]The data under these column headings refer to the number of inconsistencies/number of total meioses expressed as a percentage within the parentheses.
[c]Null alleles are assumed when cases of paternal or maternal exclusion occur due to nonmatching homozygous banding patterns in cases in which there is overwhelming evidence in favor of paternity or maternity.
Reprinted from American Association of Blood Banks (2002) *Guidance for Standards for Parentage Testing Laboratories*, 5th edn., p. 141. Bethesda, MD: American Association of Blood Banks with permission.

A and a few subgroups of B also exist. Rh typing for parentage testing is usually limited to testing for D, C, c, and E antigens. Antisera are not always monospecific and care must be taken when dual specificity is found, such as anti-Ce, for a person who is e-negative would not react well with this antiserum. It is so rare to be e-negative in most populations that anti-e is not used routinely. Exceptions include Mexicans, Native Americans, and Asians (**Table 5**). Testing for MNS system antigens is complicated by anti-N that cross-reacts with M. Careful controls must be run to ensure monospecificity. *MS, Ms, NS*, and *Ns* are the four haplotypes for MNSs and another antigen, U, may be useful to type in blacks who are S−s−. The combined exclusion power in the USA is 59%.

Table 4 Parentage markers and their chromosomal location

System/marker	ISBT symbol	Gene (ISGN)	Chromosome
ABO	ABO	ABO	9
MNS	MNS	GYPA, GYPB, GYPE	4
Rh	RH	RHD, RHCE	1
Kell	KEL	KEL	7
Duffy	FY	DARC	1
Kidd	JK	SLC14A1	18
Lutheran	LU	LU	19
Xg	XG	XG	X
HLA			6

ISBT, International Society of Blood Transfusion; ISGN, International System for Human Gene Nomenclature.

Duffy, Kidd, and Kell system antigens are all detected by the antihuman globulin test. Common Duffy system genes include Fy (a silent allele found primarily in blacks), Fyᵃ, and Fyᵇ. Common Kidd antigens are Jkᵃ and Jkᵇ); however, anti-Jkᵇ is very rare. In the Kell system, the common antigens are K and k. The addition of Lutheran to the set increases the combined rate to 67% but antiserum is very rare.

Enzymes and Proteins

Although testing for polymorphisms of enzymes and proteins is rare in current practice, a discussion is included for historical completeness. The polymorphic RBC enzymes and serum proteins are listed in **Table 1**. Immunoglobulin polymorphisms can only be tested on someone over 6 months old because maternal immunoglobulin remains in the infant until then. In addition, rare variants exist for each enzyme and protein and these must be cataloged.

The procedure to determine different alleles involves electrophoresis of serum proteins and subsequent staining to reveal multiple bands of human proteins. Most proteins have alleles that migrate to sufficiently different distances in the gel. When electrophoresis is insufficient to resolve alleles, isoelectric focusing (IEF) can be used; PGM1i would designate the use of IEF rather than standard electrophoresis. The least used are Gm, Am, and Km due to lack of reagents and difficulty interpreting the results. NAT for PGM and GC now substitutes for protein electrophoresis.

HLA

Compared to the RBC antigen system, the HLA system is highly complex. Its power to exclude is much higher but the technical expertise to do the testing and

Table 5 Frequencies for red blood cell phenotypes in the USA

Phenotype	Blacksᵃ	Whitesᵇ	Asiansᶜ	Native Americanᵈ	Mexican
ABO					
O	49	45	43		56
A	27	41	27		28
B	19	10	25		13
AB	4	4	5		4
Rh/DCE					
DCe	17	42	70	44	
DCE	<1	<1	1	6	
DcE	11	14	21	34	
Dce	44	4	3	2	
dCe	2	2	2	2	
dCE	<1	<1	<1	<1	
dce	<1	1	<1	6	
dcE	26	37	3	11	
MNS					
M+N+	44	50			
M+N−	26	28			
M−N+	30	22			
S+s+	28	44			
S+s−	3	11			
S−s+	69	45			
S−s− U−	<1	0			
Duffy					
Fy(a+b+)	1	49	8.9ᵉ		
Fy(a+b−)	9	17	90.8ᵉ		
Fy(a−b+)	22	34	0.3ᵉ		
Fy(a−b−)	<1	68	0		
Kell					
K−k+	96.5	91			
K+k+	3.5	8.8			
K+k−	<0.1	0.2			
Kidd					
Jk(a+b+)	34	49	50		
Jk(a+b−)	57	28	23		
Jk(a−b+)	9	23	27		
Jk(a−b−)	<1	<1	<1		

ᵃBlack refers to origins from any of the African Negro racial groups who indicate their race as "black" or African-American.
ᵇWhite refers to people of original Caucasian (before massive immigration) European, Middle East, or North African origin who indicate their race as "white". This includes hispanic, unless otherwise indicated.
ᶜAsian refers to those with origins in the Far East (Asian Indian, Chinese, Filipino, Korean, Japanese, Pakistani, Vietnamese, etc.) unless specifically indicated.
ᵈNative American refers to those with origins from tribes in North or South America considered "first people" and who indicate their race as "Native American" or "Alaskan Native" or from a particular tribe.
ᵉChinese.

analysis is also much greater. The microlymphocytotoxicity test takes much more time and is also very costly to perform. Antisera are derived primarily from multiparous women (women who have had many babies, preferably with the same father) and monoclonal preparations. Different sets of antiserum are used for different ethnic groups. Every part of the

Table 6 Complete listing of WHO-Recognized HLA-A, -B serologic specificities[a]

1980		2000		
HLA-A	HLA-B	HLA-A		
HLA-A1	HLA-B5	HLA-B		
HLA-A2	HLA-B7	A1	B5	B51(5)
HLA-A3	HLA-B8	A2	B7	B5102
HLA-A9	HLA-B12	A203	B703	B5103
HLA-A10	HLA-B13	A210	B8	B52(5)
HLA-A11	HLA-B14	A3	B12	B53
HLA-Aw19	HLA-B15	A9	B13	B54(22)
HLA-Aw23(9)	HLA-Bw16	A10	B14	B55(22)
HLA-Aw24(9)	HLA-B17	A11	B15	B56(22)
HLA-A25(10)	HLA-B18	A19	B16	B57(17)
HLA-A26(10)	HLA-Bw21	A23(9)	B17	B58(17)
HLA-A28	HLA-Bw22	A24(9)	B18	B59
HLA-A29	HLA-B27	A2403	B21	B60(40)
HLA-Aw30	HLA-Bw35	A25(10)	B22	B61(40)
HLA-Aw31	HLA-B37	A26(10)	B27	B62(15)
HLA-Aw32	HLA-Bw38(w16)	A28	B2708	B63(15)
HLA-Aw33	HLA-Bw39(w16)	A29(19)	B35	B64(14)
HLA-Aw34	HLA-B40	A30(19)	B37	B65(14)
HLA-Aw36	HLA-Bw41	A31(19)	B38(16)	B67
HLA-Aw43	HLA-Bw42	A32(19)	B39(16)	B70
	HLA-Bw44(12)	A33(19)	B3901	B71(70)
	HLA-Bw45(12)	A34(10)	B3902	B72(70)
	HLA-Bw46	A36	B40	B73
	HLA-Bw47	A43	B4005	B75(15)
	HLA-Bw48	A66(10)	B41	B76(15)
	HLA-Bw49(w21)	A68(28)	B42	B77(15)
	HLA-Bw50(w21)	A69(28)	B44(12)	B78
	HLA-Bw51(5)	A74(19)	B45(12)	B81
	HLA-Bw52(5)	A80	B46	Bw4
	HLA-Bw53		B47	Bw6
	HLA-Bw54(w22)		B48	
	HLA-Bw55(w22)		B49(21)	
	HLA-Bw56(w22)		B50(21)	
	HLA-Bw57(17)			
	HLA-Bw58(17)			
	HLA-Bw59			
	HLA-Bw60(40)			
	HLA-Bw61(40)			
	HLA-Bw62(15)			
	HLA-B63(15)			
	HLA-Bw4			
	HLA-Bw6			

[a]1980 "WHO-Recognized Specificities" are those *without* "w" designations.
Reprinted from American Association of Blood Banks (2002) *Guidance for Standards for Parentage Testing Laboratories*, 5th edn., p. 109. Bethesda, MD: American Association of Blood Banks with permission.

procedure must be done in duplicate by two different analysts. The complexity of interpretation, which includes cross-reactivity, antigen splits, and linkage disequilibrium, requires highly skilled analysts to evaluate results. World Health Organization-specified HLA-A and HLA-B alleles are listed in **Table 6**.

DNA Testing

Most laboratories use DNA-based procedures to establish parentage or relatedness. RFLP was the first method used and it is still used to exclude or include siblings, fathers, and mothers. Only four or five RFLPs are required to have a high power of inclusion. Discrimination between individuals can also be achieved by detecting VNTR (STR and long tandem repeat (LTR)), SNP, and SQ. When using STR loci, 9–10 loci must be tested to have the same power of inclusion as LTR/RFLP analysis. When only two alleles are at one locus, as with SNP testing, 50 loci must be tested to have strong inclusion likelihoods. SQ is not yet widely used for parentage studies due to cumbersome procedures. New rapid sequencers are becoming available and SQ may be more widely used in the future. Mitochondrial DNA testing is extremely challenging and not routinely done for parentage studies. Mitochondrial DNA is used to identify decomposed or badly damaged remains of military personnel and other samples that are badly damaged, as in the World Trade Center attack on September 11, 2001. It requires special facilities and equipment so only special laboratories perform these tests. It is the only way to match grandmothers to grandchildren when the parents are missing.

VNTR may be LTR or STR. LTR are sequences of DNA that contain 9–80 bases as a core sequence that is repeated consecutively a few to hundreds of times. STRs are sequences of 2–5 bases repeated 4–40 times. LTRs are detected by either Southern blot for RFLPs or by PCR. STRs are detected by PCR procedures. STRs of four repeats are the most widely used in identity testing.

RFLP RFLP refers to the variable sizes of DNA fragments resulting from the cutting with a restriction endonuclease (also called restriction enzyme: RE). The Southern blot procedure is used for RFLP and is illustrated in **Figure 1**. Most regions of use in parentage testing are listed in **Table 1**. Sample cases are shown in **Figure 2**.

Restriction endonucleases are isolated from bacteria and named to indicate the source. Hae III and Pst I are two commonly used REs used for parentage testing in the USA. Hinf I is used in Europe. Hae III is the third RE to be isolated from *Haemophilus aegyptius*. Pst I is the first RE to be isolated from *Providencia stuartii*. REs recognize double-stranded DNA in 4, 6, 8, or 10 basepair sequences and cut at particular sites within that sequence. Hae III recognizes 5'-GG^CC/3'-CC^GG and cuts between the C and G. Pst I recognizes 5'-CTGCA^G/3'-G^ACGTC and cuts between G and A. Hae III cuts

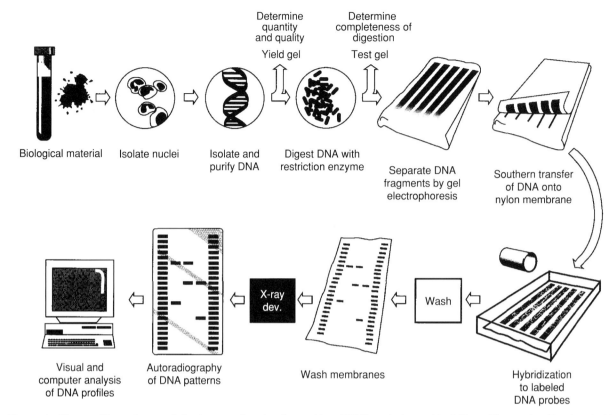

Determine quantity and quality
Yield gel

Determine completeness of digestion
Test gel

Biological material   Isolate nuclei   Isolate and purify DNA   Digest DNA with restriction enzyme   Separate DNA fragments by gel electrophoresis   Southern transfer of DNA onto nylon membrane

Visual and computer analysis of DNA profiles   Autoradiography of DNA patterns   X-ray dev.   Wash membranes   Wash   Hybridization to labeled DNA probes

Figure 1   Diagram illustrating restriction fragment length polymorphism (RFLP) analysis used for DNA profiling testing. Reprinted with permission from Baird ML (1993) Quality control in DNA profiling tests. In: Farkas DH (ed.) *Molecular Biology and Pathology: A Guidebook for Quality Control,* p. 203. San Diego, CA: Elsevier.

so frequently that sometimes small fragments run right off the end of the gel. Hinf I is from *Haemophilus influenzae* and recognizes G^ANTC/CTNA^G and cleaves between A and G. REs can exhibit star activity (cut at inappropriate sites) if the conditions of the digestion vary from the optimal, as indicated by the manufacturer.

Each fragment will be assigned a size in kilobases by comparing the fragment to a known sizing ladder. The ladder is loaded into several wells of the gel about five lanes apart so that it is easier to identify the correct size. In **Figure 2**, one can see that some fragments migrate to nearly the same place on the gel and to be sure that the bands are identical in paternity testing, the AF and Ch's DNA will be combined and run in one lane. When the bands of the AF and Ch appear as one, they are the same. When an indentation occurs between them at the edge of the bands, they are different. Band sizes will vary depending on the RE used and variability in electrophoresis procedures and conditions. A band that is 2.0 kb at one lab using Hae III may be the same allele as one at 1.97 or 2.03 on a different day or a different lab. Therefore, the range of sizes (often 10% of average) that a laboratory decides is not separable is classified as one band and called a

bin. In parentage testing, bins and running two samples of DNA together help cover for errors.

PCR   Beginning in 1994, PCR testing for parentage markers has increased the speed and inclusion power of molecular testing. The markers used include D1S80, a VNTR that is an LTR, and numerous STRs. Like all DNA testing of noncoding regions, the mutation rate must be included in deciding which alleles to test and what conclusions may be made from the results. Sequence-specific primers under special conditions of high stringency (the primers bind only exactly matched complementary sequences) allow for the amplification of specific alleles without transferring and hybridizing probes. The amplicons (amplified DNA target sequence) are analyzed by electrophoresis and gels stained with fluorescent stains to visualize by eye and/or machine. Newer methods use fluorescent tags on the primers so that the fluorescing amplicons can be directly evaluated by an optical scanner or charge coupled device camera. These results may be analyzed by human eye or machine and calculated for paternity index (PI) by hand or computer. An alternative method for coding alleles involves the amplification of the gene region

Paternity   PSTI   Lumigraph
Chemiluminescent-labeled D12S11 + D17S79
18-hr exposure

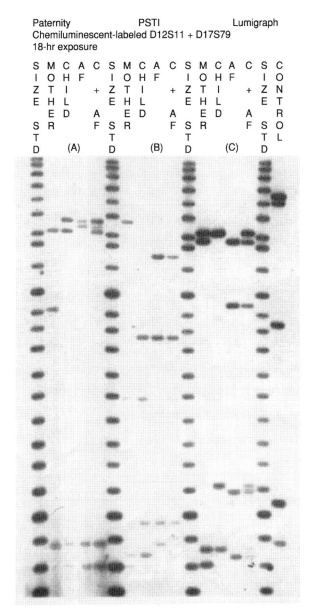

Figure 2 Photograph of a lumigraph from the analysis of three paternity trios A, B, and C. DNA was isolated from blood samples from the mother, child, and alleged father in each trio, digested with *PstI*, size-separated by electrophoresis, transferred to a nylon membrane, and hybridized with alkaline phosphatase-labeled, chemiluminescent probes which recognize the D12S11 (top) and D17S79 (bottom) loci. The size standard (STD) lanes contain fragments of known size used to measure the fragment lengths of the bands in the sample lanes. The control lane contains human DNA from cell line K562 digested with *PstI*. The alleged fathers in trios A and B are included while the alleged father in trio C is excluded as the biological father. C, child; AF, alleged father. Reprinted with permission from Baird ML (1993) Quality control in DNA profiling tests. In: Farkas DH (ed.) *Molecular Biology and Pathology: A Guidebook for Quality Control*, pp. 208–209. San Diego, CA: Elsevier.

using generic flanking primers and then reverse dot blots with allele-specific probes to determine phenotypes. These are usually read colorimetrically by hand by two independent observers. These markers

include HLA-DQA1, low-density lipoprotein receptor (LDLR), glycophorin A (GYPA), hemoglobin G (HBGG), D7S8, and GC. GYPA will show the same data as for the classical serological testing of MNS system antigens, and thus should not be considered an independent marker. In addition, HLA-DQA1 is closely linked to HLA-A and HLA-B and must be figured separately when using both types of data.

Amplified fragment length polymorphisms from LTR: D1S80 or STRs have become the most widely used platforms for paternity testing up to 2003. Multilocus chips have been created that detect dozens of different alleles at once; therefore, the throughput has increased dramatically.

In May 2003, the AABB approved the used of SNP analysis called SNP-IT tag array (formerly called APEX). It is highly automated and fast in analyzing cases and has increased the number of cases that may be analyzed per day tremendously. SNP analysis has the potential to supplant STRs as the preferred multilocus testing procedure.

SNPs occur about every 100 bases in the human genome and many occur at a frequency of 0.5. There are only two alleles at each locus and the required number of tested loci must be large to equal the power of inclusion of five RFLPs or 10 LTRs or STRs. Suggested platforms use 30 as the starting number of loci and additional ones when the first 30 do not result in an adequate inclusion of paternity value. Automated testing for SNPs is now approved for use in parentage testing. Microchips with multiple SNP allele detection systems can determine parentage in a couple of hours. **Figure 3** shows the results from a paternity test using APEX (now SNP-IT technology).

SQ is finding the exact spelling of the AGCT nucleotides in a piece of DNA. With the completion of the Human Genome Project, polymorphisms are being discovered rapidly. These can be used for all sorts of identity testing. New small rapid sequencers are now available, making this method of parentage testing practical.

Mitochondrial DNA Mitochondrial DNA is passed from the maternal ovum to children. When parents are unavailable and family matching to grandparents is possible, mitochondrial DNA from the grandmothers can be used to determine family linkage. A segment of noncoding DNA is amplified and sequenced. This has been used in South America where children were stolen from parents who were killed for political reasons, and to verify the remains of the family of Tsar Nicholas' family. The South American children were returned to their grandparents by matching not only chromosomal but mitochondrial DNA.

Multiplex PCR for APEX reaction

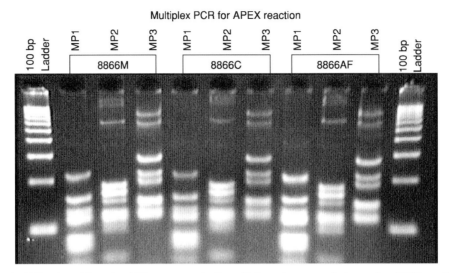

Figure 3 Image of ethidium bromide-stained 4% agarose gel with multiplex polymerase chain reaction (PCR) amplicons from a single case (#8866 TRIO). Three multiplex reactions were performed on genomic DNA from each individual in the case. MPI, multiplex 1 (ADH3, ARSB, LDLR, METH, PROS1, PRP, HSD3B, LPL, IGF2, BCL2); MP2, multiplex 2 (WI-1417, D3S2344, D2S1301, D7S1760, FUT1, DUF-1, TCRVB17); MP3, multiplex 3 (TCRVB12, DNASE1, CETP-1, CPT1, APOC3, CA2, COL2A1). 8866M, mother; 8866C, child; 8866AF, alleged father. Reprinted with permission from White LD, Shumaker JM, Tollett JJ, Staub RW (1998) *Human Identification by Genotyping Single Nucleotide Polymorphism (SNPs) Using an APEX Microarray.* Genetic Identity Conference Proceedings: Nineth International Symposium on Human Identification. Available at: http://www.promega.com.

Potential Errors

Many opportunities for errors occur in parentage testing. Several safeguards are built into specimen collection and analysis to catch most of these errors. The errors before and during testing include: (1) interchange of samples at collection accidentally or on purpose (fraud); (2) interchange of samples at the lab; (3) typing errors; (4) deficient test sera or technique; (5) deteriorated samples; (6) clerical errors; and (7) rare variants commonly missed by routine testing. During the interpretation phase, an analyst may disregard linkage disequilibrium, unbalanced gene frequencies, and silent alleles in the calculations, resulting in skewed calculations. Many of these problems are alleviated by automation; some are not. Prevention measures for errors at collection must be in place, including having a witness by a disinterested party, two independent specimen collections, photos, fingerprints, and signatures at collection. In the laboratory, errors may be prevented by using controls for antisera and other reagents, independent double testing using antisera from different sources, independent checking of results, and testing of duplicate samples. During analysis, errors may be prevented by consideration of the possibility of rare variants (**Table 7**) in the testing and analysis. For interpretation of the results, understanding the relationships between the people sampled including consanguinity, incest, and the ethnicities of all

Table 7 Rare variants of red blood cell (RBC) antigens

RBC system	Examples of variants
ABO	*cis*-AB, A_3, A_x, A_{el}, B_x
Duffy	Fy3, Fy4, Fy5, Fy6, Fy_x
Kell	Ko, Kx, KL
Kidd	Jk, Jk^3
MNS	M^g, M^k
Rh	C^w, hr^B, C^G

parties is important in selecting gene frequency databases. Correct evaluation of phenotypes and usage of more than one system to achieve an outcome are also essential. Evaluation of the probability of paternity of nonexcluding systems is also an important step. Further testing may be indicated and estimating the error risk is also required as a part of the final report.

Analysis

For analysis of markers of expressed proteins on RBCs, white cells, or plasma, a single nonmaternal marker carried by the Ch that an AF does not carry is classified as an exclusion. Direct and indirect exclusions are terms used in classic protein-based testing. The markers used in these studies have well-established inheritance patterns. Using DNA technology, the mutation rate is too high to say that one nonmaternal band not shared by the AF is enough to exclude; therefore, the term is mismatch and two mismatches are required to exclude an AF or declare nonmaternity. Several online databases exist, such as GenBank and ALFRED (allele frequency database for diverse populations and DNA polymorphisms) containing allelic frequencies for DNA markers for different populations.

The terms used for all paternity testing include PI, probability of paternity (PP) and probability of exclusion (PE), and random man not excluded (RMNE). Other terms sometimes used are cumulative paternity index (CPI) and cumulative probability of paternity (CPP). The PI refers to the ratio of the chance that the AF passed the gene to the chance that a random man could have passed it to the child. The cumulative PI is found by multiplying the PI for each locus. The PP includes the nongenetic evidence (prior chance) into the equation. It compares the AF chance to pass a gene to that of an untested man of the same race. PE is based exclusively on the maternal and child allelic frequencies. PE shows the chance that a falsely accused man would be excluded and is calculated as 1 − RMNE.

Direct Exclusion

There are two ways to have a direct exclusion: (1) when a Ch has a marker that neither the Mo nor AF carries; (2) the AF has two markers and the Ch has neither of them. An example of the first situation includes a Ch that is D-positive, the Mo is D-negative, and the AF is D-negative. The D must be contributed by one of the two parents of the Ch, therefore the AF is excluded. An example of the second situation includes an AF with Fy^a and Fy^b and a Ch who is Fy(a−b−) for the Duffy antigens on RBCs. The Ch would carry at least one of these markers if the AF was the biological father. Nonpaternity is established by one of these direct exclusions.

Indirect Exclusions

When a Ch has a single marker and the AF has a different single marker, homozygosity or a silent allele may be present at that locus. For an indirect exclusion the assumption is that both Ch and AF are homozygous. If there is a silent allele, the AF may indeed be the biological father and the test system cannot detect the marker. Suppose the Ch is Jk(a+b−) and assumed homozygous for Jk^a. The AF is Jk(a−b+) and assumed homozygous for Jk^b. There is a rare null allele *Jk* that is found in some parts of the Pacific Islands, Brazil, and in a few white families. The AF could be *Jk Jk^b* and the Ch *Jk Jk^a*. Thus the AF could be the true father. This allele is rare, thus, unless special circumstances are present in the racial

profile or AF origin, an indirect exclusion would be accepted.

False Exclusions

When one of the tested parties has a chimera, dispermy, an unlinked suppressor gene, no precursor for another gene to act upon, or a significant mutation, an apparent direct exclusion may be false. In the ABO system, H substance is required for the expression of glycosyl transferase genes that modify H substance to become A or B or AB. Although very rare, some individuals do not have H substance. They are genetically *hh*. They can pass A or B genes to offspring that they do not express. Thus the mother may be O, the Ch B, and the father types as an O (genotype *hh, BB*) by both forward and reverse typing. The mother would provide an H for the Ch to be able to express the B gene product. This situation requires an additional testing with O cells in the reverse typing (not routinely used). The father and all others with Bombay phenotypes would have strong anti-H activity that would agglutinate H+ O cells, whereas a typical group O serum would not agglutinate group O cells.

For the Rh system it is important to type for all typical antigens to help rule out the possibility of a null phenotype. Someone could type D-negative and really be D-positive. The person may carry a suppressor gene located on an unlinked locus. The D gene may be passed without the suppressor gene so that the Ch successfully expressed the gene. Full typing of the DCcEe reveals the suppressor gene. The person would appear not just D-negative but C−c−E−e− as well.

False indirect exclusions occur because of weak, untyped, or silent alleles. **Table 7** lists unusual variants of the typical alleles typed for parentage testing. Silent or weak or unusual variants occur in most RBC antigen systems. A single indirect exclusion is not adequate to establish nonparentage. Not all typing sera detect all variations of expression of weak alleles and most parentage testing does not test for rare variants like Ko, Fy4, or Fy5.

Ethnicity must be taken into consideration for antigen systems that are expressed in extremely different frequencies depending on the racial background. Blacks express a silent allele on RBCs, *Fy*, at a very high frequency of 82%. Middle Eastern populations and hispanics also express this silent allele due to natural selection in populations where malaria is endemic; Fy(a−b−) RBCs are not infected by *Plasmodium vivax*, the most common cause of malaria worldwide. The silent *Fy* is extremely rare in whites. Therefore, an indirect exclusion in a white trio with a

Ch who is Fy(a−b+) and an AF typing Fy(a+b−) would have a high level of confidence while the same phenotype in a black trio would not lead to the same conclusion. The AF is likely to be genetically Fy^aFy, the Ch Fy^bFy, and true paternity is highly possible.

The MNS system also has peculiarities based on linkage, linkage disequilibrium, and ethnic frequencies. M and N are antigens on glycophorin A, and S, s, and U are on glycophorin B. They are closely linked and only extremely rare recombinants or mutations have been described. Therefore, these linked loci are passed on as haplotypes of *MS*, *Ms*, *NS*, or *Ns* to our offspring. An illustration of linkage disequilibrium in the MNS system occurs because the frequency of *NS* (7%) is much less frequent than *Ns* (38%). The frequencies of the other two haplotypes are similar, *MS* (25%) and *Ms* (30%). Although rare phenotypes occur in other ethnic populations, the U− phenotype is present in 1% of blacks. Someone typing S−s− may also be U−.

A sample case using the MNS system follows. The Mo phenotypes MNSs and the undisputed biological father of the first three children is MSs. The Mo claims he is also the father of the fourth child. The children's phenotypes are as follows: Ch1 is MNS, Ch2 is MNS, Ch3 is MSs, Ch4 is MNs. The haplotypes passed by the mother must be *NS* and *MS* by the father for the first two. *Ms* is passed by the Mo for the third child and *MS* by the father. The fourth child received *Ms* from the mother so the biological father would have to pass *Ns* to Ch4. The biological father of the other three children is excluded as the father of the fourth child in this example.

Inclusion of Paternity

The Hardy–Weinberg formula and assumptions are used to calculate the chance of true paternity. There is a predictable relationship between observed allele frequencies and gene frequencies at any locus. This allows for the estimate of genotype frequency using the formula by multiplying the individual allele frequencies from one person's observed phenotype as follows:

$$p^2 + 2pq + q^2 = 1$$

where p = frequency of allele 1; q = frequency of allele 2; $2pq$ = frequency of heterozygotes (allele 1, allele 2); p^2 = homozygote for allele 1; and q^2 = homozygote for allele 2.

Linkage equilibrium is also assumed for these loci. Linkage equilibrium is established when haplotype frequencies match the expected frequency for each independent gene frequency multiplied. One key

assumption is that the frequency of a phenotype with many alleles is the product of the individual allelic frequencies. The Hardy–Weinberg assumptions and linkage equilibrium do not always apply. Certain ethnic groups in a large population of multiple ethnic groups are more likely to mate within their group. However, in practice the formulas have been shown to be valid.

Paternity Index

Inclusion criteria for an AF (X) involves multiplying allele frequencies for each of the loci by each other and dividing by the chance these could be from a random man (Y) to arrive at a PI or system index. Table 8 shows the formulas to determine PI for various combinations of maternal phenotypes, child phenotypes, and AF phenotypes. The result gives an idea of the likelihood that the AF is the biological father.

The following is a sample case calculating the PI. Suppose, for a white trio, that the mother is type MS

Table 8 Formulas used to calculate paternity indices in biallelic SNP systems

Combination	M	C	AF	PI
1	X	X	X	$1/x$
2	X	X	XY	$0.5/x$
3	X	XY	XY	$0.5/y$
4	XY	XY	XY	$1/(x+y) = 1$
5	XY	X	X	$1/x$
6	XY	XY	X	$1/(x+y) = 1$
7	XY	X	XY	$0.5/x$
8	X	XY	Y	$1/y$
9	Not tested	X	X	$1/x$
10	Not tested	XY	X	$0.5/x$
11	Not tested	XY	XY	$0.25(x+y)/xy = 0.25/xy$
12	Not tested	X	XY	$0.5/x$

PI formulae for the eight possible combinations of SNP phenotypes in paternity trios and four possible combinations of SNP phenotypes where the mother is not tested. Homozygosity is assumed when individuals only display a signal for one nucleotide at any SNP locus. X and Y represent the nucleotide signals obtained while x and y are the gene frequencies for the respective SNP alleles. It should be noted that the calculations for combinations 10 and 11 assume that the mother and the alleged father are of the same race (as they are in all cases presented here). If they differ in race, the PI formula for Combination 10 becomes $PI = x_M/x_{AF}y_M + x_My_{AF})$ where x_M = freq(X) from mother's racial database, x_{AF} = freq(X) from AF's racial database, y_M = freq(Y) from mother's racial database and y_{AF} = freq(Y) from AF's racial database. Likewise, the PI formula for combination 11 becomes $PI = (x_M + y_M/[2(x_{AF}y_M + x_My_{AF})]$. Formulae derived according to Brenner in *Transfusion* (1993) 33:51–54. Reprinted with permission from White LD, Shumaker JM, Tollett JJ, Staub RW (1998) *Human Identification by Genotyping Single Nucleotide Polymorphisms (SNPs) Using an APEX Microarray*. Genetic Identity Conference Proceedings: Nineth International Symposium on Human Identification. http://www.promega.com.

Table 9   Genotypes of individuals scored from 24 loci on identity chip

SNP locus	Polym	%	Trio			8875 PI calc.	8875 PI	MNT		8879 PI calc.	8879 PI
			8875M	8875C	8875AF			8879C	8879AF		
ADH3	A-G	56	AA	AA	AA	1/0.56	1.79	AA	AG	0.5/0.56	0.89
ARSB	A-G	67	GG	GG	FF	1/0.33	3.03	AG	AG	1/(4*0.67*0.33)	1.13
LDLR	T-C	45	TC	TC	TC	1	1.00	TC	TC	1/(4*0.45*0.55)	1.01
METH	T-C	58	TC	TC	TT	1	1.00	CC	CC	1/0.42	2.38
PROS1	T-C	58	TT	TT	TC	0.5/0.58	0.86	TC	TC	1/(4* 0.58* 0.42)	1.03
PRP	A-G	66	AG	AG	AA	1	1.00	AG	AG	1/(4* 0.66* 0.34)	1.11
HSD3B	A-C	77	CC	CC	AC	0.5/0.23	2.17	AC	AC	1/(4*0.77*0.23)	1.41
LPL	A-G	52	AG	AG	GG	1	1.00	GG	GG	1/0.48	2.08
IGF2	A-G	20	AA	AA	AG	0.5/0.2	2.50	AG	AG	1/(4*0.2*0.8)	1.56
BCL2	A-G	56	AA	AA	AA	1/0.56	1.79	AG	AA	0.5/0.56	0.89
W1-1417	C-T	48	TC	TC	TT	1	1.00	TT	TC	0.5/0.52	0.96
D3S2344	G-C	48	GC	GC	GG	1	1.00	CG	CG	1/(4*0.48*0.52)	1.00
D2S1301	G-A	55	AG	AG	GG	1	1.00	AG	AA	0.5/0.45	1.11
D7S1760	T-C	50	TT	TC	CC	1/0.5	2.00	TT	TC	0.5/0.5	1.00
DNASE1	A-G	56	AA	AA	AG	0.5/0.56	0.89	GG	GG	1/0.44	2.27
CETP-1	C-A	53	CC	CC	CC	1/0.53	1.89	CC	CC	1/0.53	1.89
FUT1	A-T	50	AA	AA	AA	1/0.5	2.00	AA	AA	1/0.5	2.00
DUF-1	A-G	41	AG	AA	AA	1/0.41	2.44	AA	AG	0.5/0.41	1.22
TRCVB17	C-T	48	TC	TC	TT	1	1.00	TT	TT	1/0.52	1.92
TCRVB12	C-T	53	TT	TT	TT	1/0.47	2.13	TT	TT	1/0.47	2.13
CPT1	G-A	49	AG	GG	AG	0.5/0.49	1.02	AG	AG	1/(4*0.49*0.51)	1.00
APOC3	T-C	58	TT	TT	TC	0.5/0.58	0.86	TT	TT	1/0.58	1.72
CA2	T-C	50	CC	CC	TC	0.5/0.5	1.00	CC	CC	1/0.5	2.00
COL2A1	C-T	48	TC	CC	CC	1/0.48	2.08	TC	TC	1/(4*0.48*0.52)	1.00
Cumulative PI							2901.30				1802.14

Reprinted with permission from Toll White LD, *et al.* (1998) *Human identification by genotyping single nucleotide polymorphism (SNPs) Using an APEX microarray.* Genetic Identity Conference Proceedings: Nineth International Symposium on Human Identification. Available at: http://www.promega.com.

for the RBC antigen system, the Ch is group MSs, and the father is group Ms. Since these are inherited as haplotypes, the mother contributed *MS* so the father contributed *Ms* and the chance for AF is 1 for contributing the *Ms* haplotype. A random man with this haplotype occurs at a frequency of 0.291. Therefore the PI (*X/Y*) is $1/0.291 = 3.43$. In the same trio for D1S80, the mother is 24, 33, the Ch is 15, 24, and the AF is 15, 18. The AF has a 0.5 chance of passing either the 15 or the 18 to a Ch. The population frequency of the LTR D1S80 allele 15 is 0.0015. Therefore $X/Y = 0.5/0.0015 = 333.33$. In this same trio for HUMFESFPS the mother is 10, 11, the Ch is 10, 11, and the AF is 10, 12. The mother could contribute the 10 to the Ch and then the chance for the AF for contributing the 10 allele is 0, the chance for a random man to contribute the 10 allele is 0.225. If the mother contributed the 11 allele then the chance for the AF contributing the 10 is 0.5 and a random man's chance is 0.284. Therefore, $X = 0.5 \times 0.5 + 0.5 \times 0 = 0.25$. $Y = 0.5 \times 0.225 + 0.5 \times 0.284 = 0.2545$. $X/Y = 0.25/0.2545 = 0.982$. Since these are not linked loci, the PI is the product of these systems. $3.43 \times 333.33 \times 0.982 = 1122.7$. The AF is 1122.7 times more likely to have contributed these

Table 10a   A sample, no mother case: phenotypes

System	Child	Alleged father
DIS80	17, 18	18, 21
YNZ	4, 5	4
FGA	3	2, 3
P450	2, 6	2, 6
THO1	6	6
VWA	3, 4	4, 5
FES	1, 3	3, 4
CSF	4, 6	4, 7

alleles to the Ch than a random man. **Table 9** has examples using SNP analysis to determine PI in a case with a maternal sample available and without. **Table 10** illustrates the calculations used when no maternal sample is available, the race of the father is either black or white, and LTR and STR loci are used.

Probability of Paternity

A statistical theory created by Bayes uses an estimate of previous probability to come up with a percentage of paternity probability. This is based on social

Table 10b A sample, no mother case: allele frequencies[a]

System	Allele	White	Black	System	Allele	White	Black
DIS80	17	0.004	0.044	THO1	6	0.224	0.135
	18	0.248	0.075				
				VWA	3	0.115	0.257
YNZ	4	0.293	0.105		4	0.197	0.282
	5	0.043	0.102				
				FES	1	0.008	0.099
FGA	3	0.323	0.319		3	0.320	0.221
P450	2	0.131	0.477	CSF	4	0.037	0.133
	6	0.379	0.101		6	0.328	0.271

[a]Allele frequencies modified from data supplied by Laboratory Corporation of America.

Table 10c A sample, no mother case: results. There are three calculations: the first is for the case in which mother and alleged father are both White; in the second case they are both Black; in the third case the mother is Black and the alleged father White

System	X	Y	PI
Mother White, alleged father White, alternative father White			
DIS80	0.002000	0.001984	1.01
YNZ	0.043000	0.025198	1.71
FGA	0.161500	0.104329	1.55
P450	0.255000	0.099298	2.57
THO1	0.224000	0.050176	4.46
VWA	0.057500	0.045310	1.27
FES	0.004000	0.005120	0.78
CSF	0.164000	0.024272	6.76
Combined PI			205
Mother Black, alleged father Black, alternative father Black			
DIS80	0.022000	0.006600	3.33
YNZ	0.102000	0.021420	4.76
FGA	0.159500	0.101761	1.57
P450	0.289000	0.096354	3.00
THO1	0.135000	0.018225	7.41
VWA	0.128500	0.144948	0.89
FES	0.049500	0.043758	1.13
CSF	0.135500	0.072086	1.88
Combined PI			1042
Mother Black, alleged father White, alternative father White			
DIS80	0.022000	0.011212	1.96
YNZ	0.102000	0.034401	2.97
FGA	0.159500	0.103037	1.55
P450	0.289000	0.194014	1.49
THO1	0.135000	0.030240	4.46
VWA	0.128500	0.083059	1.55
FES	0.049500	0.033448	1.48
CSF	0.135500	0.053651	2.53
Combined PI			346

Reprinted from American Association of Blood Banks (2002) *Guidance for Standards for Parentage Testing Laboratories*, 5th edn., pp. 128–129. Bethesda, MD: American Association of Blood Banks with permission.

evidence such as fertility of the AF, possible access to the mother at the time of conception, whether other male family members might have had the opportunity, and other factors. Testing laboratories do not have access to these data and assign 0.5, assuming the AF being tested and any other man would have an equal chance of being the father. The PI is used for the calculation as well. The final $PP = PI/(PI + 1)$. For the previous example, $PP = 1122.7/(1122.7 + 1) = 1122.7/1123.7 = 99.9\%$. In the USA, the range of required PI and PP in different states is from "20 to 1 and 95%" to "1000 to 1 and 99.9%," respectively. In our test case, the AF would be held liable for child support in any state.

Probability of Exclusion

The probability of exclusion is determined to put a value on the chances of excluding a man based on the phenotypes of the Mo and Ch. Calculate the number of men who would not be excluded (RMNE) and subtract that number from 1. The exclusion formula excludes all males who do not have the paternal allele on either chromosome and this equals $(1 - (\text{frequency of paternal allele}))^2$. RMNE $= 1 - \text{exclusion value}$. In the sample case for Ms, the probability of exclusion is 0.7054. For D1S80, the exclusion value is $(1 - 0.0015)^2$, thus the RMNE is $1 - 0.997 = 0.003$. For HUMFESFPS, the exclusion value is $(1 - 0.284)^2$, the RMNE is $1 - 0.513 = 0.487$. The cumulative RMNE is $0.705 \times 0.003 \times 0.487 = 0.001$. The cumulative power of exclusion is $1 - \text{RMNE} = 0.999$ or 99.9%.

Calculating a PI is more challenging when there are homozygous alleles or silent alleles that are possible in the population in question. When only one of two potential co-dominant alleles is expressed or found, the possible options include homozygosity, a silent allele, or the system does not pick up some rare allele. The report of the case should indicate the possible errors due to these factors.

Other issues that must be addressed when setting up a parentage testing service and the analysis of samples include the complexity of testing procedure, amount and type of sample required, the complexity of calculations, and the fragility of marker tested. RBC enzyme procedures, protein electrophoresis, HLA microlymphocytotoxicity testing, and RFLP analysis require many days to perform and highly skilled personnel such as a credentialed clinical laboratory scientist. While RBC antigens are easier to test for and less expensive in most cases, the analysis of the data can be quite challenging. Knowledge of rare alleles and variation in quality of antisera and antigens on the cell surface is important to a successful analysis. The background for these esoteric facts comes with a specialty in transfusion medicine also known as blood banking. For HLA testing, knowledge of cross-reactive groups and linkage disequilibrium is required to analyze a case correctly. HLA genes are all linked, but certain haplotypes (all tested genes close to each other on the same chromosome) are more frequent than would be expected if gene frequencies of each gene were multiplied. These situations must be carefully addressed for each case. In addition, HLA proteins show cross-reactivity with each other in serological systems. Cross-reactive groups have been established and the analysis must include each of these potential gene frequencies. Ethnicity must be factored in when known.

See Also

Anthropology: Role of DNA; **Blood Grouping**; **Children:** Legal Protection and Rights of Children; **Crime-scene Investigation and Examination:** Collection and Chain of Evidence; **DNA:** Basic Principles; Risk of Contamination; Mitochondrial; Postmortem Analysis for Heritable Channelopathies and Selected Cardiomyopathies; Hair Analysis; **Evidence, Rules of**; **Identification:** Prints, Finger and Palm; **Immunoassays, Forensic Applications**; **Mass Disasters:** Principles of Identification; **Serology:** Overview; Blood Identification

Further Reading

American Association of Blood Banks (2001) *Standards for Parentage Testing Laboratories,* 5th edn. Bethesda, MD: American Association of Blood Banks.
American Association of Blood Banks (2002) *Guidance for Standards for Parentage Testing Laboratories,* 5th edn. Bethesda, MD: American Association of Blood Banks.
Baird ML (1993) Quality control in DNA profiling tests. In: Farkas DH (ed.) *Molecular Biology and Pathology: A Guidebook for Quality Control,* pp. 201–215. San Diego, CA: Academic Press.
Brecher ME (ed.) (2002) *AABB Technical Manual,* 14th edn. Bethesda, MD: American Association of Blood Banks.
Gaensslen RE (1983) *Sourcebook in Forensic Serology, Immunology, and Biochemistry.* Washington, DC: US Government Printing Office.
Harrison CR (1999) Parentage testing. In: Harmening DM (ed.) *Modern Blood Banking and Transfusion Practices,* 4th edn., pp. 507–519. Philadelphia, PA: FA Davis.
Inman K, Rudin N (1997) *An Introduction to Forensic DNA Analysis.* Boca Raton, FL: CRC Press.
Issitt PD, Anstee DJ (1998) *Applied Blood Group Serology,* 4th edn. Durham, NC: Montgomery Scientific.
Mollison PL, Engelfriet CP, Contreras M (1997) *Blood Transfusion in Clinical Medicine,* 10th edn. Oxford, UK: Blackwell Scientific.
Parker PP, Snow AA, Schug MD, Booton GC, Fuerst PA (1998) What molecules can tell us about populations: choosing and using molecular markers. *Ecology* 79: 361–382.
Race RR, Sanger R (1975) *Blood Groups in Man,* 6th edn. London: Blackwell Scientific.
Strachan T, Read AP (1996) *Human Molecular Genetics.* New York: BIOS Scientific/John Wiley.
Sussman LN (1976) *Paternity Testing by Blood Grouping,* 2nd edn. Springfield, IL: Charles C Thomas.
Walker RH (1983) *Inclusion Probabilities in Parentage Testing.* Arlington, VA: American Association of Blood Banks.

PATTERN EVIDENCE

D W Davis, Hennepin County Medical Examiner's Office, Minneapolis, MN, USA

Introduction

In the usual course of performing an autopsy examination, the pathologist will make descriptions of gunshot wounds, sharp-force and blunt-force injuries. Any of these broad causes of injury can produce a pattern on the skin (or occasionally bone) that reflects the shape of the inflicting instrument. An effort to identify the type of instrument, and possibly the specific instrument, can be of paramount importance in solving a homicide. It is the responsibility of the pathologist to recognize and document patterned injuries, and then in appropriate cases offer opinions as to the likelihood that a particular weapon or instrument was involved in their creation. Beyond appreciating that a particular injury demonstrates a pattern, certain steps must be taken to allow for a valid injury–instrument comparison that can be supported in a court of law.

Patterned Injury Definition

Broadly speaking, it is any injury (abrasion, contusion, laceration, and sometimes even a knife or gunshot wound) that suggests an inflicting instrument or unique means of its creation. Some patterned injuries are instantly recognizable as to causation based on the type of injury, location, and the circumstances of the incident and a search for the inflicting instrument may be unnecessary. For example, a large, uniform abrasion on the upper neck of a car accident victim is likely an airbag injury (**Figure 1**). The cause of some patterned injuries is intuitively obvious without circumstantial information and the identification of the specific instrument (and therefore assailant) would be extremely helpful. An example might be a slap contusion on the buttock of a child that leaves a clearly recognizable handprint as evidence of child abuse (**Figure 2**). Although the handprint is clearly recognizable, it is very unlikely that we would be able to identify the specific hand that caused the injury as most people have a hand of average size with five fingers. Patterned injuries having characteristics that reflect manufactured objects provide the best opportunity for accurate instrument identification. For example, the horizontal patterned abrasion on the neck of a hanging victim faithfully reflects the width and texture of the ligature used (**Figure 3**). Associating the injury with an instrument in suicides is usually not an issue as the ligature, gun, or knife is almost always there with the body. Occasionally, family members will alter a suicide scene and remove the instrument, creating some difficulty.

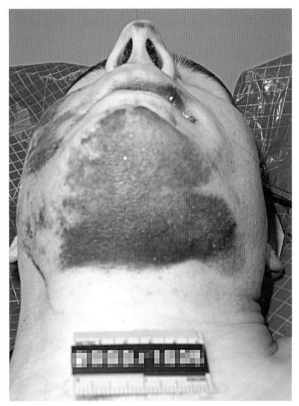

Figure 1 Airbag abrasion on the upper neck and undersurface of the chin in a motor vehicle accident victim.

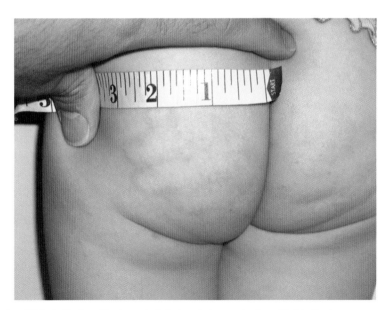

Figure 2 Photograph of a child's buttocks with characteristic hand slap contusion of left buttock.

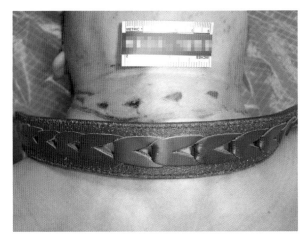

Figure 3 Hanging victim with patterned abrasion injury around neck identical with the ligature (belt).

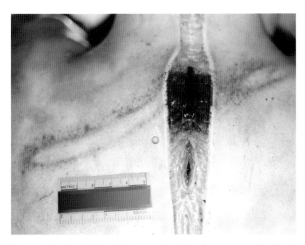

Figure 4 Homicide victim struck with pipe across the back, leaving "tram track" parallel contusions on skin surface. (The vertical incision was made by the pathologist.)

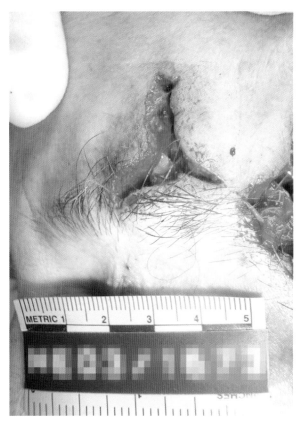

Figure 5 Homicide victim with pistol-whip laceration to forehead. A corner of a roughly cube-shaped pistol grip makes a three-pointed laceration.

Mechanism of Patterned Injury Creation

Most contusions created by forceful impact with an object will leave a blanched area on the skin that was in actual contact with the object. Blood will rupture from rapidly compressed capillaries under the object into surrounding tissue, outlining the object. For example, a heavy pipe struck across the back will leave the characteristic "tram track" appearance of bruising from ruptured blood vessels to the sides and deep to the impact (**Figure 4**).

Abrasions are the result of the offending object scraping across the skin. If the scrape is discrete, a very accurate reproduction of the object may be left behind. Bite marks frequently allow for easy suspect identification if the bite is abraded.

Incised or lacerated wounds divide the skin and subcutaneous tissue. The major difference between the two is that lacerations generally maintain so-called tissue bridges across the wound gap composed of small blood vessels, connective tissue, and nerves. Incised wounds do not. Most incised wounds leave little additional useful information beyond their length and depth. Lacerations, on the other hand, are the result of impact forces that crush the skin until it literally splits apart and frequently provide significant information as to the impacting object. For example, a three-pointed laceration on the forehead is consistent with an impact with the corner of something that is generally cube-shaped (**Figure 5**). Crescent-shaped lacerations on the scalp and underlying skull are consistent with hammer blows (**Figure 6**).

The Concept of Class-Specific and Individual Characteristics

While most observers would appreciate the pattern of a molded boot sole on the side of a victim's head (**Figure 7**), there are potentially thousands of boots that were manufactured with exactly the same sole pattern. The injury may show characteristics of that class of object (size 10 molded boot sole), but it cannot be reasonably matched to a specific boot

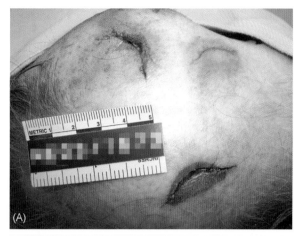

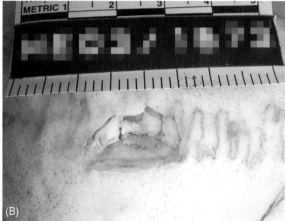

Figure 6 (A) Homicide victim struck multiple times with a hammer. The characteristic crescent-shaped lacerations result from tangential blows. (B) One hammer blow was so forceful that it created an identical crescent-shaped fracture of the skull.

with individual characteristics unique to that boot that would be reproduced on the skin. However, if the commonly available boot sole had a rock stuck in the tread that was also reflected in the skin injury, then both class-specific and individual characteristics would be present in common with both the injury and the boot sole, making a unique match possible.

The Degree of Confidence in Offering an Opinion in an Injury–Instrument Comparison

In providing an opinion as to whether an instrument could have caused a particular injury, the pathologist may offer one of several degrees of confidence. The instrument may be "inconsistent" with the injury, effectively ruling out the instrument as having caused the injury. The instrument may be "consistent" with the injury, meaning that it could have caused the injury, but not necessarily to the exclusion of

any other instrument. This opinion is usually offered when an injury reveals only class-specific characteristics in common with the instrument. Finally, the comparison may be "conclusive," when only that instrument could have caused the injury. Only unique objects or common objects with unique characteristics (like a rock stuck in the shoe tread pattern) causing an injury would lead a pathologist to such a confident opinion.

Documentation of the Patterned Injury

Written descriptions alone are inadequate for the documentation of a patterned injury if any meaningful comparison with a suspect object is anticipated. Diagrams and acetate tracings of the actual wound can offer more information than a verbal description, but the precision of the diagrams and accuracy of the tracings are dependent on the artistic skill of the pathologist. The most efficient and accurate way to document an injury is by photographs. Although articles and books have been written about the technical merits of camera selection, film choice, and lighting conditions, technique is by far of the greatest importance. Photographs are taken at the forensic autopsy for four reasons: first, to provide a visual record for the pathologist to refer to at a later time; second, to allow other professionals to review the pathologist's findings and formulate their own opinions; third, to show to jurors in trial; and finally, for teaching purposes. Most pathologists accomplish the first goal and find whatever photos they have taken useful for their own review. Unfortunately, poor technique often precludes use of the photos for the other purposes.

Specifically with respect to patterned injury documentation, the following technique issues are critical for injury–instrument comparison.

1. The skin surface with the patterned injury must be clean. Extraneous blood, dirt, or foreign material will either obscure relevant details of the injury or erroneously suggest injury details that are not actually present.
2. A ruler and case number or other identifying information must be present in the photograph of the injury (and of a suspect instrument). Optimally, the ruler would be placed on the skin surface adjacent to the injury so that the ruler is at the same height as the injury. Otherwise there is no possibility of judging the true size of the injury later in the photograph.
3. The photograph must be taken with the camera perpendicular to the skin surface. Anything else creates a tangential view and distorts the true

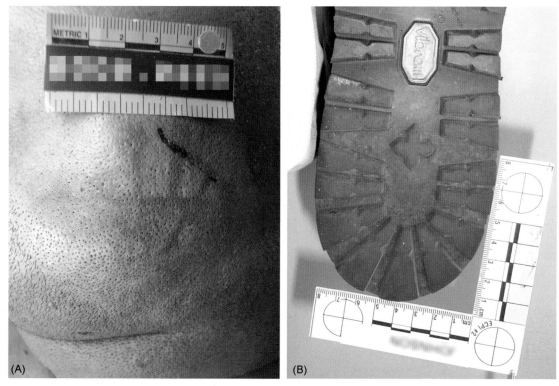

Figure 7   (A) Homicide victim with stomping contusion on the scalp. The straight lines and right angles in the bruise are indicative of a manufactured item causing the injury. (B) A portion of the boot sole used in the stomping attack. The boot sole has class characteristics consistent with the injury.

appearance, shape, and size of the injury in a photograph. Some people make use of the American Board of Forensic Odontology (ABFO) no. 2 scale for just this purpose. If the circles at the corners of the ruler are anything but circular in the photograph, the picture was taken tangentially to the ruler, and presumably to the skin surface, hindering any subsequent injury–instrument comparison.

4. The injury should fill most of the picture area (cropping through the lens). This eliminates having to magnify the area of interest in a more "overall" photo with the inevitable image degradation that occurs with enlargement.

5. The camera used must be capable of taking a close-up (macro) photograph. Some cameras are not capable of providing a macro function and will result in blurry close-up photos. Notorious are the inexpensive, instant picture film cameras used in emergency rooms for quick injury documentation.

The author prefers to use digital cameras for all autopsy photography. The pictures are arguably as good as film pictures (with image sizes in the 3 or 4 megapixel range) and they are immediately available for archiving, review, and digital manipulation.

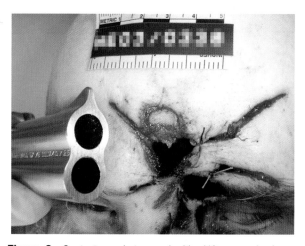

Figure 8   Contact gunshot wound with .410-gauge derringer. Only the lower barrel has been fired. After reapproximating the gas pressure-induced marginal lacerations, a side-by-side comparison reveals the shape of the barrels and sight on the skin.

Making the Injury–Instrument Comparison

The easiest way to make an injury–instrument comparison is to place the suspect instrument next to the injury for visual comparison and photographic documentation. This is commonly performed if the instrument is available for examination at autopsy.

For example, the side-by-side comparison of firearms with self-inflicted, contact gunshot wounds reveals obvious similarities without performing additional effort (**Figure 8**). Actual contact between the suspect instrument and skin surface should be avoided in cases where DNA analysis is anticipated as cross-contamination may occur.

In most instances, however, the suspect instrument will only be available at some later date and must be compared separately. The most convenient way to do this is digitally to arrange photographs of the injury and instrument with image-editing software such that similarities can be appreciated. The author makes frequent use of Adobe Photoshop, but several other suitable image-editing programs are available. The stepwise process is performed as follows (**Figures 9** and **10**):

1. The two photos (instrument and injury) are adjusted so that they are in the same scale.
2. The instrument photo is inverted, thereby creating a mirror image of it. (Instruments provide a

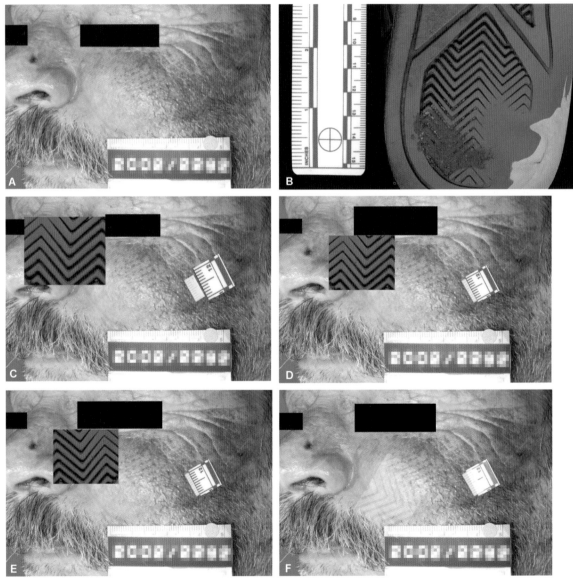

Figure 9   (A) Homicide victim with a patterned contusion on the left face having a series of equidistant parallel, zigzag lines. (B) The suspect instrument (the sole of a tennis shoe) photographed with a ruler. (C) A portion of the tennis shoe sole and ruler layered over the injury image. Note that the rulers are not in the same scale. (D) The shoe sole and ruler are reduced in size so that the two rulers are in the same scale. (E) The shoe sole is inverted left to right as an impression on the skin would be a mirror image of the object. (F) The final comparison image. The shoe sole has been rotated, color spectrum inverted, and aligned to the injury, revealing that the injury is consistent with having been created with the sole of this shoe.

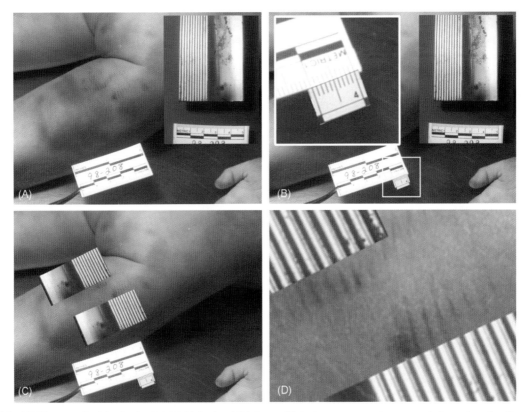

Figure 10 (A) Photograph of the bruised right thigh of a child. Several injuries are present composed of a series of uniform, parallel contusions. The end of the suspect instrument (an extruded aluminum doorway threshold) is visible in the inset. (B) The same scale is present in both the injury and instrument photos and is shown in the left upper inset. (C) A portion of the threshold is inverted, duplicated, and placed next to two of the injuries. (D) Final comparison image revealing that the injury is consistent with having been created with the threshold.

mirror image or rubberstamp impression on the skin surface.)

3. The instrument image is arranged next to or over the injury image.
4. The pathologist determines the likelihood of the instrument having caused the injury.

The most challenging analysis is made with less than perfect starting material. Take the case of a 42-year-old woman (**Figure 11**) who was murdered in her sleep along with three of her four children. She was shot and struck multiple times through a cotton nightgown. A prime suspect who stalked the woman's teenage daughter was arrested the next day driving a stolen car in the area of the murder but he was ultimately released for insufficient physical evidence. The crime remained unsolved for 25 years. Although the victim's firearm injuries were the fatal injuries, one bruise below the right breast showed potential for comparison with a metal bar in possession of the prime suspect when he was arrested in the stolen car. This bar had remained in an evidence warehouse ever since he was arrested for auto theft.

The autopsy photo (**Figure 11A**) seems to suggest that the pathologist is focused on the bruise under the right breast which the photographer documented. Unfortunately, the photo was taken too far away and at a slightly tangential angle. To make matters worse, the pathologist had the ruler in his right hand instead of on the body next to the injury! However, to the pathologist's credit, he recorded in his report that the injury was 2 cm wide, providing scale for the injury in the photograph. The bar was wrapped with a leather-ette steering-wheel cover with multiple ventilation holes. A smooth plastic cord was tightly knotted around the cover at one end. The knot was crudely made with multiple tight throws, making its appear-ance in combination with the characteristics of the steering-wheel cover unique. After photographing the bar, stepwise digital manipulation of the bar and injury photographs was performed using Adobe Photoshop. The author found the comparison conclu-sive for the injury under the right breast having been caused by being struck with the bar, thereby linking the original suspect to the murders. Corroboration for the comparison was later provided during the trial by

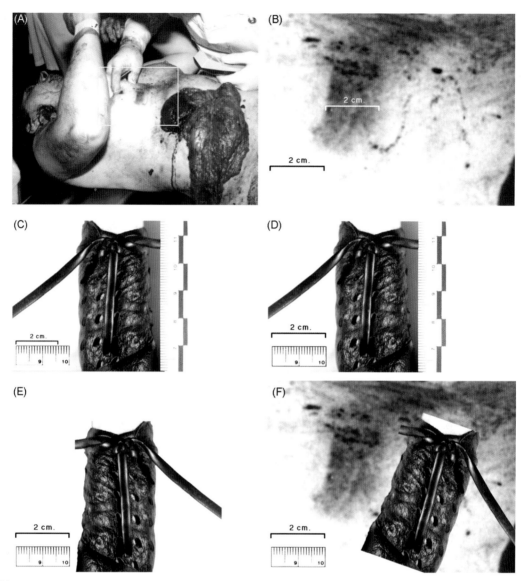

Figure 11 (A) Twenty-five-year-old autopsy photograph of a woman with shotgun wounds of the neck and abdomen, and a patterned bruise just below the right breast (boxed). (B) Enlargement of the bruise with a 2-cm scale applied to the bruise based on the bruise width description in the autopsy report. (C) Photograph of the suspect instrument (a metal bar wrapped in a leatherette steering-wheel cover) with ruler. Notice that the scale of the bar is larger than the scale of the injury. (D) The image of the bar is reduced to match the scale from the injury photograph. (E) The image of the bar is inverted horizontally to provide for the mirror image appearance of the bar. (F) The final comparison image with the bar slightly rotated to align with the bruise. The author concluded that the bar was used to create the injury.

the fact that the surviving son (now in his 30s) was able to identify his childhood toy car that was also among the evidence removed from the stolen car 25 years earlier. The suspect apparently took a souvenir from the crime scene. He was convicted.

See Also

Crime-scene Investigation and Examination: Suspicious Deaths

Further Reading

Burd DQ, Gilmore AE (1968) Individual and class characteristics of tools. *Journal of Forensic Sciences* 13(3): 390–396.

Clark EGI, Sperry KL (1992) Distinctive blunt force injuries caused by a crescent wrench. *Journal of Forensic Sciences* 37(4): 1172–1178.

Rao VJ (1986) Patterned injury and its evidentiary value. *Journal of Forensic Sciences* 31(2): 768–772.

Zugibe FT, Costello JT (1986) Identification of the murder weapon by intricate patterned injury measurements. *Journal of Forensic Sciences* 31(2): 773–777.

PHARMACOLOGY OF LEGAL AND ILLICIT DRUGS

K A Savage and D Wielbo, National Forensic Science Technology Center, Largo, FL, USA

Introduction

The increasing incidence of drug abuse has wide forensic and legal implications, both nationally and internationally. Whether involved in toxicological analyses or drug seizure analyses, forensic practitioners should be aware of the pharmacological effects of the substances they encounter.

Pharmacology is the study of the biochemical and physiological effects of drugs and their mechanisms of action. The magnitude of a pharmacological response correlates to the concentration of drug at the site of action. Drug concentration is in turn affected by how well the drug is absorbed into the systemic circulation after administration, how it distributes throughout the body, and its subsequent metabolism and elimination.

Absorption, Distribution, Metabolism, and Excretion

Most drugs are administered orally and absorbed via the gastrointestinal (GI) tract . The rate and extent of appearance of drug in the systemic circulation depends on a series of processes: rate of release of drug from the dosage form, solubility, absorption across membranes, gastric emptying, and first-pass metabolism.

Biodistribution depends on the lipid solubility of each drug and the rate at which a drug crosses membrane barriers into the peripheral circulation and the central nervous system (CNS). Once absorbed, the drug may undergo significant chemical modification to render it into a water-soluble form that facilitates elimination and excretion by the body.

Most drugs are metabolized by membrane-bound liver enzymes. The cytochrome P450 mixed-function oxidase system catalyzes oxidation and conjugation with glucuronide. Metabolism generally occurs in the liver and, to a limited extent, the plasma, GI tract, kidneys, and lungs. Enhanced drug metabolism creates lower circulating levels of the parent drug and, as a result, higher drug doses are needed to achieve the same blood levels of the parent drug and an equivalent drug response.

The excretion of drugs and metabolites terminates their activity and presence in the body. Drugs may be eliminated by various routes; the kidney plays a major role by facilitating drug excretion into the urine. Some drugs are also excreted in feces, bile, lungs, sweat, saliva, and breast milk.

Similar drug concentrations do not produce the same pharmacological effects in all subjects. These differences may be due to several factors.

Age

The young and elderly have a lowered metabolic capacity. The very young may have enhanced sensitivity to drugs because the microsomal enzymes responsible for metabolism (particularly conjugation) are not fully active until several months after birth. Older children metabolize drugs at a similar rate as adults.

Patients older than 60 years have a decreased capacity for drug metabolism due to a gradual decline in physiological efficiency. In the elderly, protein binding may be decreased and renal excretion reduced, resulting in higher blood levels of a drug compared to younger patients.

Disease

Diseases can affect all drug absorption, distribution, and elimination processes. GI disturbances can decrease drug absorption; cardiovascular diseases affecting peripheral blood flow can decrease the rate at which drugs cross tissue membranes. Endogenous free fatty acids released into the plasma during trauma displace weak acidic drugs from albumin-binding sites. Diseases affecting the liver and/or kidneys probably have the greatest effect on drug concentration by compromising metabolism and excretion. Impaired liver function due to disease or chronic drug use greatly increases blood drug levels.

Weight

A patient's weight determines the volume of distribution of a drug, directly impacting blood drug concentrations. Drug metabolism is also generally faster in males than in females.

Genetic Factors

The genetic control of the number of receptor sites, the extent of protein binding, and the rate and extent of drug metabolism cause variations in drug concentrations and responses. Some drug-metabolizing enzymes are polymorphic, resulting in slow, rapid, or ultrarapid drug metabolizers. The incidence of some polymorphism may be higher in some ethnic groups.

Diet

Diet can influence drug metabolism: changing the diet of an asthmatic patient from high to low protein increases the half-life of theophylline. Patient exposure to other drugs (alcohol) can significantly affect the metabolism of certain drugs.

Drug Classes

Depressants

These substances cause CNS depression and include ethanol, barbiturates, methaqualone, and tranquilizers. They cause relaxation, feelings of well-being, and sleepiness.

Barbiturates   Barbiturates are derivatives of barbituric acid, and **Figure 1** shows the chemical structure of a selection of barbiturates. Generally, barbiturates suppress activity of all excitable tissues in the CNS, peripheral nervous system (PNS), and cardiovascular system (CVS). Barbiturates bind to a site on the GABAA receptor and mediate major CNS effects by depressing neuronal excitability, inhibiting gamma-aminobutyric acid (GABA) binding to its postsynaptic receptor. The GABAA receptor is the main inhibitory receptor in the CNS. Receptor activation opens a Cl^- channel that mediates neuronal inhibition.

Barbiturates were once used to treat anxiety and insomnia, but the side-effects were found to be undesirable and possibly lethal. Since the introduction of

the benzodiazepine anxiolytics, the clinical use, and abuse, of barbiturates has declined. Long-acting barbiturates such as phenobarbital have continued to be used as anticonvulsants and have the least potential for abuse (**Table 1**).

Barbiturates are administered orally or parenterally. As weak acids, they are absorbed rapidly from the stomach and small intestine into the systemic circulation. They rapidly penetrate the CNS and redistribute to other tissues. These drugs are highly bound to plasma proteins.

Long-acting barbiturates have the lowest lipid solubility, are less bound to plasma proteins, and have the shortest onset of action and the longest duration of action, slowly penetrating the CNS and slowly redistributing to other tissues. Biotransformation involves hepatic oxidation and glucuronidation. Metabolism is usually slow and the metabolites produced are generally inactive. Insignificant amounts of barbiturate substances are excreted unchanged. Barbiturates have relatively narrow therapeutic indexes, so there is a high risk of toxicity associated with these drugs, especially when combined with other depressants such as alcohol.

Chronic use induces metabolic and tissue drug tolerance. Cellular tolerance results in diminished tissue response, despite the maintenance of constant plasma drug levels.

Barbiturate withdrawal occurs 12–20 h after the last dose and is characterized by anxiety, irritability, increased heart rate and respiration rate, muscle pain, nausea, tremors, hallucinations, confusion, and seizures. Barbiturates decrease rapid eye movement (REM) sleep, and withdrawal is associated with

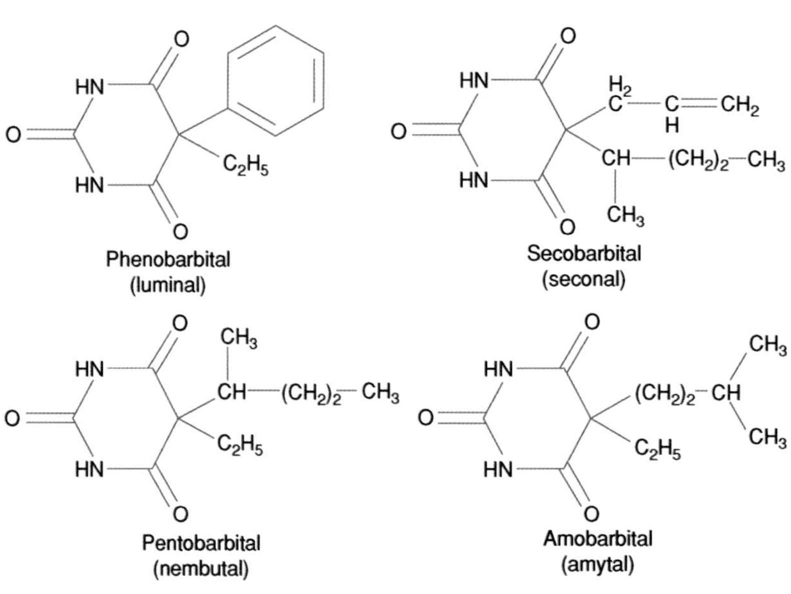

Figure 1 Chemical structures of barbiturates.

Table 1 Pharmacological responses of barbiturates

Peripheral nervous system	Cardiovascular system	Long-term use
Inhibit autonomic nicotinic receptors, causing hypotension and reduced cardiac function Anesthetic properties may inhibit skeletal muscle nicotinic receptors, suppressing neuromuscular transmission and causing slight muscle relaxation	Inhibition of autonomic nicotinic receptors causing mild hypotension Overdose associated with shock, renal failure, and death Associated with decreased cardiac output, cerebral blood flow, and myocardial contractility	Induces cytochrome P450 enzyme systems, increasing barbiturate metabolism; increases the biotransformation of other drugs, decreasing blood drug levels and promoting tolerance

sleep disruptions (nightmares, insomnia, or vivid dreams).

Benzodiazepines Benzodiazepines are synthetic depressant drugs. Their varied chemical structures impart a variety of chemical properties and pharmacological effects. Benzodiazepines are short acting and routinely used as hypnotics and preoperative anesthetics. Benzodiazepines with half-lives greater than 24 h are used as anxiolytics in the treatment of anxiety and insomnia. Unlike barbiturates, a wide range of doses can be used to treat anxiety, making dose determination easier to relieve anxiety without inducing sleep. Rebound insomnia may occur with some short-acting benzodiazepines but the effects are less severe than those seen with barbiturates. Rebound insomnia does not occur with longer-acting benzodiazepines.

Benzodiazepines also have clinical indications as anticonvulsants, antidepressants, and for the treatment of acute alcohol withdrawal. These agents may also reduce stress-induced GI disorders.

The physiological effects of benzodiazepines are similar to those of the barbiturates, but their mechanism of action is slightly different. Like barbiturates, the major effect of benzodiazepines is the CNS depression of neuronal excitability, mediated by the effect of benzodiazepines on the binding of GABA to its postsynaptic receptor. Benzodiazepines are allosteric modulators that bind to the benzodiazepine binding site of the GABA receptor and increase the receptor affinity for GABA. A GABA receptor γ subunit is required for a response to benzodiazepines; variants of this receptor subunit determine receptor selectivity for certain benzodiazepines.

Peak plasma concentrations occur within a few hours of oral administration. Most benzodiazepines are administered orally or intravenously; diazepam and midazolam may be administered rectally, and alprazolam may be administered sublingually. Diazepam and triazolam are more lipophilic than chlordiazepoxide and lorazepam and penetrate the CNS rapidly, providing a fast onset of action. Benzodiazepines are extensively plasma protein-bound (60–95%), so they are susceptible to drug interactions. Displacement of benzodiazepine from plasma proteins increases the amount of free drug and its pharmacological effect. Benzodiazepines undergo microsomal oxidation followed by glucuronidation prior to urinary excretion. Several phase 1 metabolites of benzodiazepines are active, with longer half-lives than the parent drug (e.g., nordiazepam).

Tolerance to the sedative effects of benzodiazepines often develops within about 1 week of treatment; tolerance to the anxiolytic effects does not occur in short-term use. Tolerance occurs more during benzodiazepine abuse, requiring doses many times greater than the therapeutic dose to achieve desired effects. Benzodiazepine use is associated with physical dependence. Mild withdrawal symptoms include anxiety, dizziness, headache, insomnia, tremor, muscle stiffness, and sensitivity to light and sound. Severe symptoms include intense anxiety, nausea, vomiting, delirium, hallucinations, hyperthermia, sweating, panic attacks, paranoid psychoses, increased heart rate, increased blood pressure, and seizures. Short-acting and high-potency benzodiazepines are most likely to result in dependence, although long-term use is probably the major risk factor.

Ethanol The beneficial effects of ethanol have been well documented. Moderate ethanol consumption – less than two drinks per day (a standard drink being 30 ml of 100-proof liquor, 120 ml of wine, or a 10-oz. bottle of beer) – has been associated with lowered risk of coronary heart disease (red wine has been shown to be most beneficial). The hypnotic properties of ethanol have been exploited to induce sleep, and the treatment for methanol and ethylene glycol toxicity is the administration of ethanol. Ethanol is a more effective substrate for alcohol dehydrogenase, the enzyme that produces toxic metabolites (**Table 2**).

CNS effects of ethanol are related to blood alcohol concentration (BAC) (**Table 3**). Effects are more

Table 2 Physiological effects of ethanol

Cardiovascular system (CVS)	Cardiomyopathy, arrhythmia, congestive heart failure; moderate doses associated with higher high-density lipoprotein levels and less cardiovascular disease. Vasodilation causes warm flushed skin, which is why alcohol has traditionally been used to warm the body in cold weather. Vasodilation increases heat loss, leaving the person colder than before. Excessive ethanol consumption may promote hypertension; people consuming more than three drinks per day generally have higher systolic and diastolic blood pressure than those consuming fewer than three drinks per day
Central nervous system (CNS)	Small amounts depress complex CNS pathways promoting relaxation, loss of inhibition, and increased talkativeness. As blood ethanol increases, judgment, decision-making abilities, and reflex reactions are impaired. Very high doses further depress the CNS, inducing sleepiness, coma, and death via respiratory depression
Gastrointestinal (GI) tract	Ethanol stimulates the production of gastric juices and decreased pepsin. At concentrations above 40%, mucosal membranes become irritated, causing hyperemia or gastritis; chronic alcoholics often have chronic gastrointestinal irritation
Kidney	Diuretic effects due to increased liquid intake, and suppression of antidiuretic hormone
Liver	Acute ethanol ingestion has little effect. Long-term consumption causes liver damage and steatosis; hepatic exposure to large amounts of ethanol decreases fatty acid oxidation processes of ethanol metabolism; acetaldehyde accumulation causes lipid peroxidation. Initial effects are reversible; over time liver repair causes collagen deposition, irreversible fibrotic changes; cirrhosis; liver failure, and death

Table 3 Central nervous system effects related to blood alcohol concentration (BAC)[a]

BAC ($g\ 100\ ml^{-1}$)	Stage of impairment	Behavioral effects
0.01–0.05	No noticeable impairment	Apparent normal behavior; impairment detected by specialized tests
0.03–0.12	Euphoric effects	Slight euphoria, increased sociability, talkativeness, and self-confidence; slowed information processing; decreased judgment, attention, and control; sensory motor impairment begins
0.09–0.25	Excitation	Emotional instability, impaired memory, comprehension, and perception; critical judgment decreases. Increased reaction times, decreased visual acuity, impaired balance, drowsiness
0.18–0.30	Confusion	Disorientation, confusion, dizziness, visual disturbances, increased pain threshold, staggering, slurred speech, apathy, lethargy
0.25–0.40	Stupor	Diminished motor functions; decreased responsiveness and inability to stand or walk; vomiting, incontinence, sleep/stupor
0.35–0.50	Coma	Unconsciousness, coma, depressed reflexes, hypothermia, impaired circulation, and respiration, possible death
+0.45	Death	Respiratory arrest

[a]These are guidelines – the effects are altered by a number of different factors.

pronounced with increasing blood levels compared to decreasing blood levels. However, these are only guidelines and the effects, and their correlation with blood alcohol level, depend on a person's regular intake of alcohol and whether he or she is dependent on alcohol. Ethanol mediates its CNS-depressant effects by suppressing the actions of GABA at the GABAA receptor and blocking the N-methyl-D-aspartate (NMDA) glutamate receptor.

After oral ingestion, some ethanol is absorbed directly from the stomach and the rest is absorbed in the small intestine. Absorption of alcohol is affected by a number of factors, including gastric emptying rate, the presence of food in the stomach, and the concentration of ethanol consumed. Higher ethanol concentrations increase alcohol absorption, but very high concentrations decrease absorption by restricting passage through the pyloric sphincter into the stomach.

BAC is also affected by weight and gender. The heavier the person, the larger the volume of body water and the lower the BAC obtained from a given amount of ethanol. Women generally have a higher proportion of fat tissue and a smaller volume of body water than men of the same weight; therefore, women may achieve a slightly higher BAC when consuming the same quantity of ethanol as men of the same weight. Men also have higher levels of gastric alcohol dehydrogenase, causing some ethanol metabolism before it can be absorbed. Ethanol distributes throughout the body, crossing the blood–brain and placental barriers.

Alcohol dehydrogenase, the main enzyme of ethanol metabolism, is abundant in the liver and present in smaller amounts in the stomach and kidney. This enzyme converts ethanol to acetaldehyde, which is further metabolized by mitochondrial aldehyde

Table 4   The three distinct phases of ethanol withdrawal symptoms

Phase	Time after discontinuation	Symptoms
Initial	A few hours	Tremulousness, weakness, headache, perspiration, anxiety, nausea, abdominal cramps, vomiting, mild hallucinations
Seizures	2–3 days	Generalized seizures
Delirium tremens	3–4 days	Auditory, visual and tactile hallucinations, insomnia, agitation, disorientation, restlessness, fever, sweating, tachycardia; death may occur

dehydrogenase to acetate and eventually carbon dioxide. The alcohol dehydrogenase step is the rate-limiting step in alcohol metabolism, becoming saturated at or above a BAC of 0.02 mg per 100 ml. Polymorphisms exist in the mitochondrial aldehyde dehydrogenase enzyme (ADH2), resulting in gain or loss of function. For example, approximately 90% of Asians have a polymorphism in this enzyme, resulting in increased function, which in turn leads to accumulation of acetaldehyde. This acetaldehyde accumulation results in a severe flushing reaction.

Ethanol is also metabolized by the cytochrome P450 system, particularly CYP2E1. CYP2E1 is induced by regular ethanol consumption and may significantly contribute to ethanol metabolism in frequent users. Approximately 5–10% of the ingested ethanol is eliminated in breath, sweat, urine, and feces.

Unlike most drugs, ethanol elimination is a zero-order process: initially, elimination is dose-dependent but, as alcohol dehydrogenase becomes rapidly saturated, elimination becomes almost linear (pseudolinear). Ethanol is normally eliminated from the blood at a rate of $0.01–0.025\,\mathrm{g}\,\%\,\mathrm{h}^{-1}$, but this rate can vary significantly between individuals. The elimination rate may also depend on the amount of alcohol normally consumed. The following are general guidelines:

- nondrinker: $0.012\%\,\mathrm{h}^{-1}$
- social drinker: $0.015\%\,\mathrm{h}^{-1}$
- alcoholic: $0.03\%\,\mathrm{h}^{-1}$.

Pharmacokinetic and pharmacodynamic ethanol tolerance occurs quickly. As a consequence of pharmacodynamic tolerance, some alcoholics can have BACs of up to 0.35 mg per 100 ml without appearing impaired. Cognitive and psychomotor functions remain impaired and the lethal dose of alcohol remains the same even when tolerance occurs to other effects. Cross-tolerance occurs with ethanol and other CNS-depressants (barbiturates and benzodiazepines).

Withdrawal (not hangover) symptoms are characterized into three distinct phases (**Table 4**). Death often occurs during delirium tremens (there is a mortality rate of approximately 10%). Symptom severity

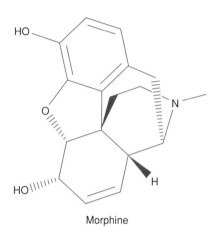

Figure 2   Chemical structure of morphine.

depends on the ethanol dose and the duration and continuity of administration. Psychological dependence may occur with moderate use, manifesting as ethanol cravings before or during social events.

Opioids   Opiate agonists are drugs that produce effects similar to those of morphine (**Figure 2**). Morphine antagonists include naloxone and naltrexone. Partial agonists/antagonists include buprenorphine and pentazocine. These agents behave like morphine but have some antagonist activity. Clinically, opioids are administered orally, transdermally (skin patches), intravenously, or rectally to treat pain, cough suppression, and diarrhea. Side-effects include respiratory depression, nausea and vomiting, constipation, miosis, cardiovascular effects, pulmonary edema, and seizures.

Opioids cross the blood–brain barrier and bind to specific opioid receptors. There are three main opioid receptors: mu (μ), kappa (κ), and sigma (σ).

Receptor distribution varies within the CNS and is species-specific. Stimulation of each of the receptors produces different clinical effects. Many opioid drugs have different affinities to more than one receptor type, producing variations in the observed clinical effect.

There are three main families of endogenous opioid peptides; each elicits analgesic and physiological functions (**Table 5**). Each peptide has a high affinity for one receptor type, but each binds to all the opioid receptors with different affinities. Enkephalins have a high affinity for the δ receptor, dynorphins have a high affinity for the κ receptor, and endorphins have a high affinity for the μ and δ receptors.

Morphine is well absorbed from most routes of administration. Opioids have relatively short half-lives; morphine has a half-life of a few hours, whereas methadone has a half-life of approximately 24 h.

Opioids bind to plasma proteins but rapidly leave the circulation and accumulate in highly perfused tissues (lungs, liver, kidneys, and spleen). Long-term use of high doses of lipophilic opioids (fentanyl) may cause accumulation in fatty tissue. Codeine and heroin cross the blood–brain barrier more rapidly than amphoteric drugs such as morphine.

Opioids are metabolized and excreted via the kidney. Morphine's free hydroxyl groups are glucuronidated at the 3- or 6-positions to form morphine-6-glucuronide (an active metabolite that may have greater analgesic activity than morphine) or morphine-3-glucuronide (**Figure 3**). Morphine glucuronides, with small amounts of unchanged drug, are excreted in the urine, with up to 85% of the dose being recovered in a day. Some opiate–glucuronide conjugates are excreted in the bile.

Significant tolerance to analgesic and euphoric effects occurs rapidly with opiates, especially those with high affinity for μ receptors (heroin, morphine, meperidine, fentanyl, and methadone), resulting in users administering up to 40–50 times the normal lethal dose. Tolerance to the effects of constipation and meiosis occurs more slowly, even after extensive use.

Opiate withdrawal is extremely uncomfortable but not life-threatening. Symptoms tend to be the opposite of the acute drug effect and include muscle aches/pains, joint aches/pains, abdominal cramps, anxiety, diarrhea, pupillary dilation, lacrimation, rhinorrhea, "gooseflesh," sweating, and vomiting.

Withdrawal begins within 12 h of the last dose, peaking at 36–48 h. Symptoms usually disappear within 7–10 days.

Withdrawal is most severe when opioids are displaced from the receptors by the administration of an opioid antagonist. In opioid overdose cases, the drug naloxone competes with the opioid agonist for opioid receptors, reversing the overdose. If the dose of naloxone exceeds the amount required, severe withdrawal symptoms occur. Opiates produce severe psychological dependence, especially heroin, because the euphoria experienced is so intense.

Heroin   Illicit opiate use is usually associated with heroin (diacetylmorphine), a semisynthetic agent produced by reacting morphine and acetic anhydride. Usually encountered in the form of a white to brown powder, or a brown to black tar. It has effects

Table 5   The three main families of endogenous opioid peptides

Endogenous peptide family	Peptides in family	Amino acid structure
Enkephalins	Leu-enkephalin	Tyr-Gly-Gly-Phe-Leu
	Met-enkephalin	Tyr-Gly-Gly-Phe-Met
Dynorphins	Dynorphin A	Tyr-Gly-Gly-Phe-Leu-Arg-Arg-Ile-Arg-Pro-Lys-Leu-Lys-Trp-Asp-Asn-Gln
	Dynorphin B	Tyr-Gly-Gly-Phe-Leu-Arg-Arg-Gln-Phe-Lys-Val-Val-Thr
Endorphins	α-Neoendorphin	Tyr-Gly-Gly-Phe-Leu-Arg-Lys-Tyr-Pro-Lys
	β-Neoendorphin	Tyr-Gly-Gly-Phe-Leu-Arg-Lys-Tyr-Pro
	β_h-Endorphin	Tyr-Gly-Gly-Phe-Met-Thr-Ser-Glu-Lys-Ser-Gln-Thr-Pro-Leu-Val-Thr-Leu-Phe-Lys-Asn-Ala-Ile-Ile-Lys-Asn-Ala-Tyr-Lys-Lys-Gly-Glu

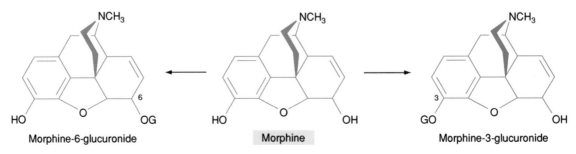

Figure 3   Morphine glucuronidation, forming morphine-6-glucuronide and morphine-3-glucuronide.

similar to those of morphine, lasting 4–6 h, and is significantly more powerful and addictive. Street heroin in the USA is about 2% pure. Other components of the street preparation include cutting agents (sugar, starch, household cleanser, and brick dust) and adulterants (strychnine and quinine). Heroin can be injected intravenously after dissolving in water, lemon juice, or vinegar (the acidity inhibits hydrolysis of heroin and facilitates dissolution). Heroin vapors are often inhaled after heating the drug on aluminum foil. Characteristic effects of heroin and related opiates include drowsiness, euphoria, constricted pupils, and, occasionally, nausea.

Stimulants

Stimulant drugs include cocaine, amphetamine, methamphetamine, caffeine, and methylphenidate (Ritalin). These agents stimulate the CNS, induce a sense of well-being, increase alertness, decrease fatigue, suppress appetite, and can lead to strong psychological dependence.

Cocaine Cocaine (**Figure 4**), derived from the coca plant grown in the Andean mountains of South America, is legitimately used in the USA as a local anesthetic in ear, nose, and throat surgery. Crack is a smokeable form of cocaine produced by combining hydrochloride salt with water and baking soda to make cocaine freebase. The drug is rapidly absorbed through the lungs. The salt form is snorted (insufflated) and absorbed across nasal membranes. Common diluents in street preparations include lidocaine (lignocaine), procaine, sodium bicarbonate, and starch.

At low doses, cocaine increases arousal and motor activity. At moderate doses, heart rate increases. Hypertension results from the increased peripheral resistance (due to vasoconstriction) and the increase in heart rate. Body temperature is increased and the pupils dilate. At high doses, cocaine can induce convulsions. Cardiac arrest is not uncommon due to a direct action of the drug on the heart muscle. Cocaine prevents conduction of sensory impulses by blocking ion channels in the neuronal membrane. This block inhibits the propagation of electrical signals along the axon, inhibiting sensory messages to the CNS (**Table 6**).

Cocaine can potentiate neurotransmission in catecholaminergic neurons using norepinephrine (noradrenaline), dopamine, or 5-hydroxytryptamine as neurotransmitters. In the periphery, this occurs mainly at noradrenergic terminals in the sympathetic component of the autonomic nervous system, and in the brain it occurs at monoaminergic terminals. Cocaine blocks the reuptake of monoamine into the synaptic terminal, potentiating neurotransmitter effects. Potentiation of norepinephrine (noradrenaline) causes mydriasis, vasoconstriction, hypertension, tachycardia, and tachypnea.

The potentiation of dopamine in the brain is largely responsible for the behavioral effects of cocaine, such as intense euphoria, heightened sexual excitement, and self-confidence; paranoia, hallucinations, and dysphoria may also occur. The initial "rush" experienced with cocaine is followed by a "crash" corresponding to respective increases and decreases in brain dopamine levels.

Cocaine hydrochloride is water-soluble and is administered orally, intranasally, or intravenously. Oral administration results in low bioavailability (20%) and less CNS distribution due to first-pass metabolism. Intravenous administration ("mainlining") allows 100% bioavailability and dramatic CNS effects. Insufflation produces less intense effects and is associated with atrophy and necrosis of the nasal mucosa and septum. Freebase cocaine is smoked, producing rapid and intense effects. Cocaine crosses the blood–brain barrier and is concentrated in the spleen, kidneys, and brain.

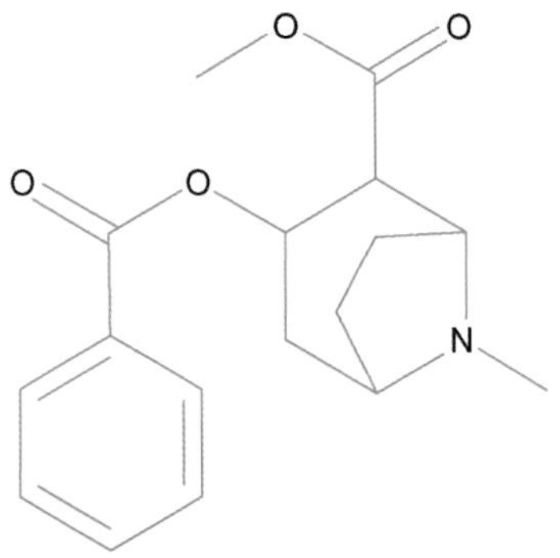

Cocaine

Figure 4   Chemical structure of cocaine.

Table 6   Pharmacological effects of cocaine

	Physiological effect
Cardiovascular system	Increased heart rate and blood pressure; constriction of coronary arteries reduces blood supply to the heart
Central nervous system	Short-lived euphoria, arousal, alertness, tremor, seizures, and dysphoria may occur with higher doses; tactile hallucinations
Local anesthetic	Blocks nerve conduction; effective as a topical anesthetic
Other effects	Rhinitis

Cocaine has two primary metabolites, ecgonine methyl ester and benzoylecgonine. Both are inactive and excreted in the urine. Smaller amounts of ecgonine and the active metabolite norcocaine are also formed. Breakdown of cocaine to ecgonine methyl ester is rapidly catalyzed by cholinesterases present in serum and the liver. Hydrolysis of the other ester linkage to form benzoylecgonine may be nonenzymatic. Demethylation of cocaine to form norcocaine occurs through the hepatic mixed-function oxidase system. Cocaethylene is a metabolite of cocaine formed when taken concomitantly with ethanol. It is an active metabolite and has a longer half-life than cocaine. Cocaine is excreted fairly quickly, with a half-life of about 40 min.

Tolerance occurs rapidly (within days of use) in chronic drug users due to the upregulation of cocaine-binding sites in the brain. Significant tolerance is not associated with occasional or binge users.

Cocaine is not associated with severe withdrawal syndromes. However, reported symptoms include anhedonia, anergia, craving, depression, fatigue, lethargy, hypersomnolence, mood disorders, and suicidal behavior.

Stimulant drugs are associated with very strong psychological dependence; users exhibit extreme drug-seeking behavior, that is often detrimental to their health and lives.

Amphetamine and methamphetamine Amphetamine and methamphetamine drugs are commonly illegitimately produced in clandestine laboratories in the form of white or tan powders that are snorted, injected, smoked, and ingested (**Figure 5**). Ice is a very pure smokeable form of methamphetamine. Amfetamines, including methamphetamine, methylene dioxyamphetamine, and methylenedioxymethamfetamine (MDMA), are similar to cocaine in pharmacological action (**Table 7**). Like cocaine, amphetamines cause restlessness, stimulation, appetite suppression, paranoia, and psychosis. Their effects last 4–12 h.

The following amphetamines are used clinically:

- D-Amphetamine is marketed as Dexedrine and is used to treat attention deficit hyperactivity disorder (ADHD) and narcolepsy.
- Methylphenidate is marketed as Ritalin and is used to treat ADHD and narcolepsy.
- Phentermine is used to treat obesity.

Amphetamine, like cocaine, is a sympathomimetic drug, although its mechanism is slightly different. Amphetamines increase monoaminergic activity by stimulating the release of dopamine and norepinephrine (noradrenaline) from the nerve terminals, increasing their synaptic concentration. Amphetamines inhibit dopamine reuptake at the nerve terminal and inhibit monoamine oxidase, the enzyme that metabolizes monoamine neurotransmitters, prolonging their availability. Amphetamine may also directly activate catecholamine receptors.

Amphetamines are weak bases (pK_a of 9 or 10); ionization in the digestive system after oral administration slows their rate of absorption. Amphetamines

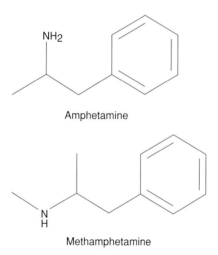

Figure 5 Chemical structures of amphetamine and methamphetamine.

Table 7 Pharmacological effects of amphetamines

	Physiological effects
Cardiovascular system	Increased blood pressure, heart rate, and force of contraction; reflex heart rate decreases are encountered due to increased blood pressure; myocarditis is common and potentially fatal. Vascular effects include vasospasm, edema, necrosis, and paresthesia
Smooth muscle	Increased muscle tone, tremors; contraction of bladder sphincter and difficulty in urination; reduced gastric motility and drug absorption; rhabdomyolysis may cause muscle necrosis and renal failure
Central nervous system	Euphoria, mood elevation, increased alertness; increased confidence and physical strength. Euphoric effects last longer than with cocaine; enhanced concentration and physical performance; appetite suppression
Other effects	High doses produce stereotopy (repetitive fixing of objects, cleaning, bathing, grooming, or repetition of words or sentences)

are more potent when taken intravenously or by inhalation. Amphetamines cross the blood–brain barrier and are concentrated in the spleen, kidneys, and brain. Amphetamine and other similar drugs are metabolized by the liver. Some drug is excreted unchanged in the urine. Methamphetamine undergoes p-hydroxylation and demethylation, generating a small amount of amphetamine; again, some drug is excreted unchanged.

Both the clearance and the half-life of amphetamine depend on urinary pH. In acidic conditions, amphetamine is ionized and reabsorption from the nephron does not occur. The clearance is rapid and the half-life ranges from 7 to 14 h. In basic conditions, the drug is un-ionized and renal reabsorption occurs. Excretion depends on metabolic processes, and the half-life is extended to 16–34 h. Urinary pH can be altered by drug use and diet.

As with cocaine, tolerance to the effects of amphetamine rapidly develops with chronic drug use; no significant tolerance is associated with occasional or binge use. Amphetamine is not associated with severe withdrawal syndromes, but reported symptoms are similar to those experienced with cocaine. The effects of psychological dependence are also similar to those experienced with cocaine.

Hallucinogens

Hallucinogenic agents cause alterations in the normal thought processes, perceptions, and moods. These drugs include marijuana, lysergic acid diethylamide (LSD), phencyclidine (PCP), peyote, and psilocybin.

Marijuana   Marijuana, derived from the plant *Cannabis sativa*, is encountered in different forms, the most common being a smokeable form called cannabis. Its use elicits hallucinations, relaxation, increased appetite, a distorted sense of time, reduced judgment and coordination, and uncontrollable laughter. The high lasts 3 h or more.

The main active component of cannabis is Δ^9-tetrahydrocannabinol (THC). However, cannabis contains an entire family of constituents known as the cannabinoids (more than 60 have been identified). The effects of cannabis result from the effects of each of the cannabinoids.

Cannabis has been shown to have legitimate clinical uses for treatment of nausea and vomiting in cancer patients undergoing chemotherapy and the stimulation of appetite in acquired immunodeficiency syndrome (AIDS) and cancer patients. Nabilone and dronabinol are Δ^9-THC analogs and can be used clinically as antiemetics for cancer patients undergoing chemotherapy and to stimulate appetite in AIDS or cancer patients. Nabilone is marketed for these indications in the UK, whereas dronabinol (Marinol) is marketed in the USA.

Despite being considered a relatively harmless drug, cannabis has a number of significant physiological effects, including tachycardia (heart rate may increase by 20–50%), increased blood pressure (users may experience orthostatic hypotension), decreased body temperature, dry mouth and throat, reddening of the conjunctivae of the eyes, decreased intraocular pressure, decreased pupil size, and hunger.

Smoking cannabis can cause adverse effects such as lung disease, wheezing, and coughing. Cannabis elicits behavioral effects that are dependent on the dose and form of cannabis taken as well as the state of mind, mood, and expectations of the individual prior to use. Moderate doses can cause euphoria, heightening of senses, altered sense of time (time appears to pass much more slowly), and short-term memory impairment. High doses can cause anxiety, aggression, confusion, hallucinations, nausea, and vomiting.

Behavioral effects are not well correlated with plasma THC concentrations since there is a delay before the onset of the long-lasting psychological effects that remain when blood THC levels decrease. Cannabis alters the ability of a user to perform skilled tasks, including driving.

Cannabinoids bind to G-protein-linked (G_i) cannabinoid receptors inactivating adenylyl cyclase, which directly inhibits calcium channel function. CB_1 cannabinoid receptors in the CNS are localized in areas that correspond to the effects of cannabis:

- hippocampus and cortex: memory and learning
- basal ganglia and cerebellum: balance and coordination
- mesolimbic dopamine pathways: reward.

CB_2 cannabinoid receptors located in the PNS may be involved in inflammation and immunity suppression associated with cannabis use.

THC is a weak acid ($pK_a = 10.6$), un-ionized at physiological pH. Cannabinoids are highly lipid-soluble and are slowly absorbed from the stomach and small intestine. Absorption can be increased by adding oil to the plant material before consumption, which is often achieved by baking the material in cookies. Significant first-pass metabolism occurs with oral ingestion of cannabis; a much larger dose must be ingested to achieve the same effects experienced when the drug is inhaled. Bioavailability after oral administration is about 6%, and peak effects occur 1–3 h after ingestion, lasting up to 5 h.

After inhalation, 10–25% of the cannabinoids enter the lungs. Drug effects are experienced within a few minutes, peaking at 30 min. Bioavailability after inhalation is estimated to be 14–50%. Cannabinoids distribute throughout the body but tend to accumulate in the lungs, kidney, and bile. Approximately 1% of a dose crosses the blood–brain barrier.

Some metabolism occurs in the lungs or stomach or intestine, but most occurs in the liver. Δ^9-THC is metabolized extensively to produce the major metabolite, 11-hydroxy-Δ^9-THC (reported to have significant THC-like activity). 9-Carboxy-Δ^9-THC is also produced in significant quantities; it is conjugated with glucuronic acid to form 9-carboxy glucuronide, the major metabolite in blood and urine.

In low to moderate cannabis users, metabolites can be detected in blood for up to 5 days and in urine for up to 12 days after administration. In regular high-dose users, detection times may be up to 25 days after use.

Onset of cannabis tolerance is rapid but short-lived. Both behavioral and physiological tolerance occur. Fewer mood-altering effects are experienced by regular users of cannabis, and regular users experience less of a "high" than naive users. There is significant individual variation in the development of tolerance to the effects of cannabis.

Cross-tolerance occurs between the effects of cannabis and alcohol; regular cannabis users experience reduced effects to alcohol and vice versa. Relatively few substance abusers seek treatment for cannabis addiction, but long-term users may experience withdrawal symptoms that include restlessness, irritability, mild agitation, insomnia, sleep disturbances, and nausea and cramps.

Psychological dependence may occur with cannabis use; users believe they need the drug in order to function in their everyday lives.

Serotonin-like hallucinogenic agents LSD is a semi-synthetic substance produced from ergot alkaloids with serotonin-like properties that was originally developed as a treatment for schizophrenia. Extremely small doses (25 µg) can result in a 12-h high. This drug causes marked mood changes and distortion of sensory perceptions (time and distance). Synesthesia may occur: this is a condition in which colors are "heard" and sounds are "seen." The effects experienced depend on the setting and the user's mental state. Although considered impossible to overdose, LSD-related deaths have been attributed to accidents occurring while under the drug's influence. Flashbacks – spontaneous and fragmentary recurrences of a previous "trip" – have been reported days or months after use. The drug is usually taken orally. It is sold as blotters or sugar cubes, with each hit containing about 100 µg. Other pharmacological effects include

dilated pupils, elevated blood sugar levels, tingling of extremities, drowsiness, nausea, vomiting, diarrhea, and spontaneous abortion due to uterine muscle stimulation.

The CNS effects of LSD may include altered time perception (time appears to pass very slowly) and mood changes; distorted perception of size and shape of objects, movements, color, sound, touch, and body image; and anxiety or depression following use.

LSD resembles the CNS neurotransmitter serotonin (5-HT) and is a serotonin agonist with specific activity for the following receptor subtypes: 5-HT$_{1A}$, 5-HT$_{1C}$, and 5-HT$_2$. LSD is orally and sublingually absorbed with a 2- or 3-h half-life. Effects are felt after 40–60 min, with peak effects occurring after 2–4 h and disappearing after 6–8 h. LSD is distributed throughout the body, but only 1% of a dose reaches the brain. It concentrates in the liver, where it is rapidly metabolized before being excreted in the bile and feces.

N-desmethyl-LSD and 2-oxo-3-hydroxy-LSD are the major metabolites found in the urine (**Figure 6**). Together with the glucuronide of the 13-hydroxy metabolite, they can be detected up to 96 h after drug use. Only a small amount (1–3%) is excreted as unchanged drug.

LSD tolerance occurs rapidly. Within a few days of repeated drug administration, the user stops experiencing drug effects. The tolerance is short-lived and disappears after approximately a week of abstinence, enabling the user to experience all the drug effects. Cross-tolerance occurs between LSD, psilocybin, and mescaline, indicating that these drugs may have a common mechanism of action. There have been no reports of a physical withdrawal syndrome from LSD, but its use is associated with psychological dependence.

Psilocybin Psilocin and psilocybin naturally occur in the *Psilocybe* mushroom. Pharmacological action is similar to that of LSD but the agents are less active. Ten to 15 *Psilocybe* mushrooms induce hallucinogenic effects when taken orally. *Psilocybe* mushrooms are also dried and smoked with tobacco or extracted with boiling water to produce infusions. Abuse was popular at approximately the same time as LSD was popular. Although it is 100 times less potent than LSD, the effects are the same when dosage adjustments are made. Once absorbed, psilocybin is converted to the active agent psilocin, thought to be responsible for behavioral effects.

Dimethyltryptamine Dimethyltryptamine (DMT) is recovered from the bark of certain trees indigenous to

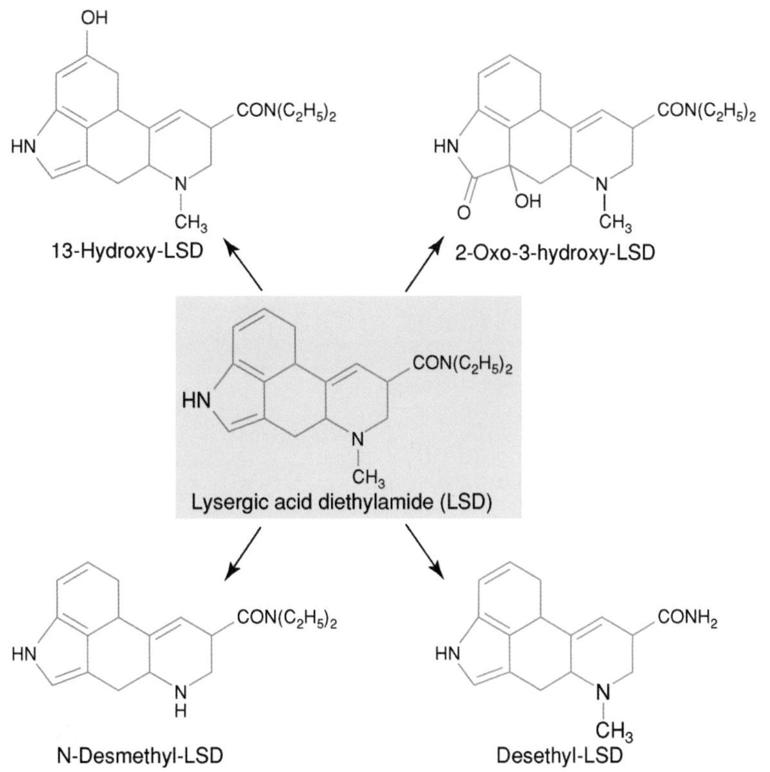

Figure 6   Chemical structure and metabolism of LSD.

the jungles of South and Central America. It is much less potent than LSD and very short-acting. For this reason, it is known as the "businessman's lunch" since the effects disappear within 1 h.

Bufotenine   The chemical name for this agent is 5-hydroxy-DMT, a derivative of DMT. The drug is obtained from the beans of several trees from the genus *Anadenanthera* and the flesh of a fish called the "dream fish." It was originally discovered in the skin of a species of toad from the family Bufonidae, and it is not hallucinogenic when taken orally. The drug must be injected or inhaled for effects to be experienced.

Norepinephrine (noradrenaline)-like hallucinogens
Obtained from the peyote cactus, mescaline's use was legalized by the US Congress in 1970 due to its central use in Native American ceremonies. Today, laws can still be passed against its use at the state level. The drug is readily absorbed when taken orally, and hallucinogenic effects are experienced within about 1 h of consumption, producing effects similar to those of LSD that last for several hours. This drug is approximately 2000 times less potent than LSD.

Ecstasy and other "designer drugs"   Designer drugs encompass a drug group originally synthesized by altering the chemical structure of mescaline to circumvent the law when it only covered specific named drugs. These agents became known as designer drugs and include dimethoxyamphetamine (DMA), 2,5-dimethoxy-4-methylamphetamine (DOM), 2,5-dimethoxy-4-ethylamphetamine (DOET), and others. Many of these drugs have effects similar to those of amphetamine.

Ecstasy refers to MDMA, originally made by Merck in 1914. It was first used as a drug of abuse in the 1960s and is commonly known as X, Adam, E, and XTC. It induces effects similar to those of marijuana or low-dose PCP. Ecstasy causes a heightened sense of emotions and does not cause hallucinations. It is abused for its ability to increase energy and for the sense of euphoria and well-being. It sharpens perceptions and causes users to be more sociable.

Other hallucinogens
Phencyclidine (phenylcyclhexyl, piperidine, and PCP)   This was first used as an anesthetic animal tranquilizer in the USA but is no longer legitimately produced. PCP is produced illegally in clandestine labs as a white powder that is taken orally, smoked (often with marijuana), or snorted in combination with cocaine.

Symptoms rapidly appear that resemble schizophrenia: euphoria, depression, agitation, violence,

Table 8 Absorption rates for different routes of administration of PCP

Route of administration	Time to effect	Time to peak effect
Oral	20–40 min	90 min
Inhalation	1 min	5–30 min
Intravenous	1 min	10 min

hallucinations, paranoia, panic, and suicidal tendencies. As a dissociative anesthetic, the user is aware of what is happening but does not feel involved. The user is insensitive to pain and is able to run on two broken legs or continue to fight after being shot. The drug is smoked, ingested, snorted, or injected; adverse effects include hypertension, tachycardia, coma, cardiac failure, and psychosis.

The effects caused by PCP include tachycardia, elevated blood pressure, sweating, miosis, and vertical and horizontal nystagmus. Other CNS effects include detachment, disorientation, euphoria, a feeling of floating in space, alterations in perception of body image, relaxation, and a warm, tingly feeling. Users may experience a period of depression following use. This drug is associated with violent criminal behavior.

PCP has been shown to have effects on a variety of neurotransmitter systems: dopaminergic system (agonist actions), cholinergic system (complex actions), NMDA receptors (antagonistic effect), noradrenergic system (undefined), and serotonergic system (undefined).

The probable mechanism responsible for the main effects of PCP is its interaction with a PCP receptor. It is thought that the receptor is responsible for the behavioral effects of the drug since other drugs with PCP-like effects have been shown to act at this site. This site has been identified as a site on the NMDA receptor complex.

PCP is absorbed well via various routes of administration (**Table 8**). The effects of PCP can last for up to 8 h. This long duration of action is due to the fact that it is rapidly taken up into the brain and fatty tissues, from which it is then slowly released.

PCP is extensively metabolized by the cytochrome P450 system. The metabolites are not active and do not contribute to the effects caused by PCP. The polar metabolites are excreted in the urine. Also, about 10% of the dose is excreted unchanged, making urine an ideal choice for testing for PCP use. Because PCP is rapidly distributed to fatty tissue, the drug and its metabolites can be detected in urine for a prolonged period after use. In fact, in chronic users, they can be detected for a period of weeks after use.

As with LSD, tolerance occurs rapidly and is short-lived. There have been very few reports of physical dependence associated with PCP use. However, a few cases have reported a withdrawal syndrome consisting of anxiety, nervousness, and depression. As with LSD, psychological dependence may occur such that users experience an intense craving for the drug.

Ketamine This drug, usually taken orally or intravenously, is an anesthetic used in children and animals, and it has a shorter duration of action than PCP. It is available as a drug of abuse (known as K or Special k) and has been reportedly used as a date rape drug.

See Also

Alcohol: Acute and Chronic Use, Postmortem Findings; **Autopsy, Findings:** Drug Deaths; **Substance Misuse:** Cocaine and Other Stimulants; Substitution Drugs; Sedatives

Further Reading

Drummer OH, Odell M (2001) *The Forensic Pharmacology of Drugs of Abuse.* Oxford, UK: Oxford University Press.
Feldman RS, Meyer JS, Quenzer LF (1997) *Principles of Neuropsychopharmacology.* Sunderland, MA: Sinauer.
Goldfrank LR, Flomenbaum NE, Lewin NA, *et al.* (eds.) (2002) *Goldfrank's Toxicologic Emergencies, 7th edn.* New York: McGraw-Hill.
Hardman JG, Limbird LE, and Gilman AG (eds.) (1995) *Goodman & Gilman's The Pharmacological Basis of Therapeutics.* New York: McGraw-Hill.
Katzung BG (ed.) (1995) *Basic and Clinical Pharmacology, 6th edn.* East Norwalk, CT: Appleton and Lange.
McKim WA (2003) *Drugs and Behavior: An Introduction to Behavioral Pharmacology,* 5th edn. New York: Prentice Hall.
Stark MM, Payne-James JJ (2003) *Symptoms and Signs of Substance Misuse.* New York: Greenwich Medical Media.
Winger G, Hofmann FG, Woods JH (1992) *A Handbook on Drug and Alcohol Abuse: The Biomedical Aspects,* 3rd edn. Oxford, UK: Oxford University Press.

POISONING, OVERVIEW AND STATISTICS

A L Jones and P I Dargan, National Poisons
Information Service, London, UK

Introduction

It is difficult to obtain reliable information on the morbidity and mortality resulting from poisoning, even in countries with comparatively advanced population health data collection systems. Despite difficulties in the interpretation of available data, certain general observations can be made on the epidemiology of poisoning. Childhood poisoning is usually accidental, and tends to be associated with low morbidity and mortality. In western Europe and North America it is most often due to household products and pharmaceuticals: in developing countries, pesticides and household products are most commonly involved. In adults, self-poisoning is usually deliberate (suicide or parasuicide) and has higher morbidity and mortality. Analgesics and psychotropics predominate in western Europe and North America as cause of admission to hospital, though carbon monoxide is responsible for most deaths occurring outside hospital. In developing countries accidental and deliberate pesticide poisoning remains the commonest cause of adult deaths by poisoning. The mortality rate for deliberate self-poisoning in developing countries is estimated at 10–20%, largely with pesticides but including all sources, in contrast with the 0.5–1% commonly found in western Europe and North America.

In some countries, the rate of acute poisoning has increased. For example, the number of acute poisoning cases in Moscow and large Russian cities has increased almost twofold in the last 15 years. The main groups of toxic agents causing poisoning are pharmaceutical (up to 63.1%), alcohol and surrogates (up to 49.3%), and corrosives (up to 21.8%); figures vary between different Russian regions. Mortality from poisoning in Russia has also increased in recent years; the main causes of fatalities are alcohol (62.2%), carbon monoxide (15.4%), acetic acid (6.3%), and pharmaceuticals (4%).

The Global Burden of Disease study points to 75% of worldwide deaths during 1990 being due to self-harm, including poisoning, alcohol abuse, smoking, and obesity. It is estimated that 99% of all fatal poisonings occur in developing countries. The incidence and pattern of suicide vary from country to country. Cultural, religious, and social values play some role in this regard.

Acute poisoning is the leading cause of unnatural deaths and third most common cause of emergency admissions in rural India; insecticides were responsible for 35% of clinical and 55.4% of fatal cases. Young married males of rural background with agricultural occupation and failure of monsoon were the identified risk factors associated with poisoning cases. A 25-year autopsy study (1972–1997) of acute poisoning deaths from a tertiary care hospital in Northern India showed a steep increase in incidence of poisoning since 1987. Again, most were 14–30-year-old males. The main victims were students and unemployed youths, followed by agricultural workers and domestic workers. The proportion of suicidal deaths increased from 34% (1972–1977) to 77% (1992–1997), whereas accidental deaths decreased from 63% to 17% in the same period. Barbiturates (37%) and copper sulfate (22%) were the most common poisons causing mortality between 1972 and 1977: organophosphates (46%) became the most common between 1977 and 1982. Since 1982 aluminum phosphide has been the most common poison.

There is a paucity of information on suicide from Pakistan, an Islamic country in which data collection poses challenges as a variety of social, legal, and religious factors make reporting and diagnosing suicide difficult. Thus newspaper reports are just about the only way of having a feel for numbers. Over a 2-year period 306 suicides were reported from 35 cities; more than half used organophosphates, while psychotropics and analgesics were used infrequently. The study challenges the widely held belief that suicide is a rare phenomenon in an Islamic country, and underscores the need for more culture-specific research on this important public health problem.

Childhood poisoning also varies significantly worldwide. Children under 5 years had higher hospitalization rates in New Zealand than adults, but were less at risk of death than any other age group. Similarly, in Finland, children under 6 years were the most frequently hospitalized because of poisoning; the commonest causes were plants, berries, mushrooms, and corrosives. In a study of attendances at a pediatric emergency department in Trieste, Italy, between 1975 and 1994, trends showed a decrease in pharmaceutical poisonings, probably due to the introduction of child-resistant containers, and an increase in domestic poisons. There was also an increase in carbon monoxide inhalation and alcohol poisonings amongst teenagers. In a poisons center study in Spain, 35.2%

of all poisoning occurred in children under 2 years of age. In Bordeaux, France, acute poisoning in children is still a public health problem. The overall mortality rate was 0.33/1000 but most cases of acute poisoning were accidental, benign, and mainly attributed to ingestion of a nontoxic substance. In Tehran, Iran, after drugs (32.1%), hydrocarbons were the most frequent cause of poisoning (19.2%). In a poisons center study in Taiwan, Japan, substances most frequently found to have been ingested by children were household products, benzodiazepines, and pesticides, with a recorded mortality rate of 1.4%. In Costa Rica children under 5 years accounted for 39.2% of cases reported to a poisons center.

Retrospective data on childhood poisoning from eight regional hospitals in India revealed that pediatric poisoning represented 0.23–3.3% of the total poisoning. The mortality ranged from 0.64% to 11.6%. Kerosene was one of the causes of accidental poisoning where wood charcoal is not used. Pesticide poisoning was more prevalent in Punjab and West Bengal, whereas plant poisoning was very common in Shimla. Significant snake envenomation was recorded from rural Maharashtra. Thus, within India, various regions show variation in types and frequency of childhood poisoning. Many of these studies highlight the unacceptably high rate of preventable accidental poisoning of children.

Poisoning Data Collection for Epidemiology

Enquiries made by healthcare professionals (e.g., in the UK) and in some instances by members of the public (e.g., in New Zealand) to poisons centers provide some information on acute poisoning. The best routinely collected epidemiological data on poisoning come from the Toxic Exposure Surveillance System (TESS) in the USA. This recorded telephone calls made for advice from members of the public and healthcare professionals about poisoning across a population of 260 million Americans in 2000.

However, data are collected differently in different healthcare systems. For example, in the UK the National Poisons Information Service only takes calls from healthcare professionals, whereas Australia and the USA offer a combined public and professional access service. In all countries calls to poisons centers tend to overestimate the size of the poisoning problem, because calls are made where significant exposure has not taken place, "for advice" just in case. In contrast, hospital admission data tend to underestimate the size of the real population of poisoned individuals as many do not need or seek medical help. Few centers have the resources to obtain

reliable follow-up data, and thus the clinical course and outcome are often unknown. Toxicological analysis to confirm exposure is rarely performed, except where the results may influence management.

Data on poisoning in developing countries are generally poor and most data are in case series format that gives at best a snapshot of events and may not represent current trends. There is scope for epidemiological studies in developing countries. However, the International Program on Chemical Safety has created a harmonized poisons center call database (Intox) to try to improve data collection across the world.

Recording death as a result of poisoning is not easy because most deaths occur outside hospitals, and more than one toxin may be involved. Even when a toxicological laboratory analysis is performed, only requested substances will be identified. Comparative epidemiology of death by poisoning between different countries is made difficult by differences in the way deaths are investigated, certified, registered, and coded in different countries. The World Health Organization (WHO) has recommended the use of an additional "nature of injury" code, which identifies the mechanism or agent of injury and the intent. The International Classification of Disease (ICD) classification of drugs fails to distinguish between different antidepressant drugs or between heroin and methadone. Deaths registered since January 2001 in England and Wales have been coded to ICD-10, which makes it easier to identify total deaths from drugs of abuse, but the breakdown by type of drug is difficult if only the underlying cause of death is available. Deaths due to carbon monoxide or barbiturates have markedly decreased in the UK over the last 35 years. The number of suicides due to poisons has decreased in recent years in the UK but the total number of suicides remains stable.

In the USA poisoning deaths are recorded by at least two systems: US poisons control centers as reported by the TESS and the National Center for Health Statistics (NCHS). Deaths reported in TESS represent 5% of the poisoning deaths tabulated by NCHS. The concern is that differences observed in the two data sets may lead to differing health policies to address poisoning hazards. For example, cases may not be reported to poison control centers when the death occurred before arrival at hospital or after recognition as a poisoning during an autopsy. Reporting to poison control centers by the public and healthcare professionals is voluntary and a poison control center's participation in TESS is also voluntary. Nevertheless, TESS provides a valuable complement to NCHS data because of the timeliness of reporting, the attempts to integrate clinical information and autopsy findings, its value for detecting sentinel events, and the ability to study specific trends. Short-comings of the NCHS data set are that information available to medical certifiers is often incomplete. The overall rate of agreement on the ICD-9 code for the underlying cause of death in the death certificate with the ICD-9 code after autopsy was 71%, and there was disagreement about the cause of death in one-third of cases, which reflects difficulties of diagnosis *in vivo* as well as differences in product details. The ICD-9 coding system used by NCHS does not have the same level of product detail as the coding system used in TESS, thereby preventing the identification of specific drugs and chemicals involved in poisoning deaths. The potential for coding errors at the point of origin exists in both data sets.

The WHO/Euro Multicenter Project on parasuicide monitors trends in the epidemiology of suicide attempts across 13 European countries. The highest average male age-standardized rate of suicide attempts was found for Helsinki, Finland (314/100 000) and the lowest rate (45/100 000) was for Guipuzcoa, Spain. The highest average female age-standardized rate was found in Cergy-Pontoise, France (462/100 000) and the lowest rate (69/100 000) was for Guipuzcoa, Spain. With only one exception (Helsinki), suicide attempt rates were higher among women than men. In most centers, the highest rates were found in younger age groups. More than 50% made more than one attempt, and 20% of second attempts were made within 12 months of the first attempt. Compared with the general population, those who attempted parasuicide more often belonged to the social categories associated with social destabilization and poverty.

Self-Poisoning with Analgesics

Demography of Overdose with Analgesics

TESS data show that in adults over the age of 19 years analgesics such as indometacin, aspirin, and acetaminophen (paracetamol) are commonly taken in overdose in the USA. Acetaminophen and ibuprofen are most commonly ingested in overdose by children under the age of 6 years. Aspirin, aspirin combinations, and acetaminophen combinations are rarely ingested in childhood, which presumably reflects reduced availability to this age group because of Reye's syndrome for aspirin and the opioid component of acetaminophen.

Outcome Data for all Analgesic Overdoses

The majority of calls made to US poisons centers about analgesics refer to acetaminophen or nonsteroidal antiinflammatory drugs (NSAIDs: ibuprofen

and indometacin), and that aspirin forms the minority of analgesics calls. Most patients have no sequelae after exposure to any analgesic, and 10–20% of those exposed have only minor sequelae, e.g., nausea. Aspirin is one to three times as likely as acetaminophen or NSAIDs to cause mild or moderate sequelae. The rate of major sequelae in aspirin poisoning is approximately the same as in acetaminophen poisoning. The rate of major sequelae in NSAID poisoning (ibuprofen and indometacin data combined) is approximately a third of that of acetaminophen. The major limitation in analysis of the data is the TESS definition of what constitutes minor, moderate, or major outcomes and this is particularly difficult to assess over a telephone, since such effects have a variable time course and are altered by treatment; for example, N-acetylcysteine use is associated with nausea and flushing in some patients. Thus such data can only give an overview.

The death rate for aspirin, both as a percentage of those treated and as a percentage of those exposed, is slightly higher than acetaminophen and the death rate for NSAIDs is about 10-fold lower. These death rates reflect deaths where the analgesic was declared to have been taken – it is not necessarily the cause of death in the patient. In many cases no analytical confirmation of toxin ingested was undertaken.

Acetaminophen Overdose

The main feature of untreated acetaminophen poisoning is hepatotoxicity. Comparative data worldwide on acetaminophen poisoning are remarkably difficult to obtain and it is very difficult making comparisons between countries because poisons centers' functions are different. From telephone call data to poisons centers it appears that 0.02–0.04% of each country's population take acetaminophen in overdose each year. This presumably reflects its widespread availability (e.g., 3.2 thousand million tablets are sold every year in the UK, that is, about 50 tablets per head).

A total of 0.02% of the Australian population and 0.08% of the UK population require admission or assessment at a healthcare facility each year because of acetaminophen poisoning. This is larger than the 0.01% of Americans accessing healthcare and could either reflect differences in access to hospital because of nationalized health services in Australia and the UK, or point to a smaller problem in the USA.

The first cases of liver failure due to acetaminophen were reported in 1966. Definitions of acute liver failure now vary worldwide and may depend on treating physicians. ICD-10-AM coding of acute liver failure is helpful but, due to expansion of codes from the former ICD9-CM to ICD-10-AM more recently, acute liver failure episodes are difficult to distinguish in data from the USA, UK, and Australia from chronic liver failure. In addition, it should be remembered that the ICD-10-AM code is not used purely for acetaminophen poisoning and it may not be due to acetaminophen alone. Acetaminophen is the commonest cause of acute liver failure in the USA and in the UK. Acetaminophen-induced acute liver failure occurs in 0.6% of hospital episodes in Australia, and the same is true for the UK. In contrast, a "major" outcome (including acute liver failure and other major events) is reported for 1.5% of exposures and 3.5% of admissions in the USA. It is possible that the incidence of acetaminophen-induced acute liver failure is higher in the USA than in other countries, but the 3.5% figure may be skewed because of more difficult access to healthcare in the USA, and the "major outcome" data are not subdivided into acute liver failure and other events. In addition, individual patients' risk factors for acetaminophen poisoning are not assessed in any of the data sources and can give rise to differences in data, although in this respect it may be expected that the genetics of the population and alcohol use would be similar between, for example, Australia and the UK.

In all, 99.6% of admissions with acetaminophen poisoning survived according to the AIHW (Australian Institute of Health and Welfare) data; 0.4% died. This compares to USA data of 0.4% of admissions to healthcare facilities, recorded through TESS. More detailed information is available on 47 deaths due to acetaminophen poisoning in the USA from TESS in 2001: 32 were due to "acute," two due to "acute on chronic," and 12 due to chronic overdoses. All deaths were in adults over 17 years of age, except for one death of a 3-year-old.

Acetaminophen is a common poison in some regions of the developing world. Cases of hepatotoxicity have been reported from Bahrain, Chile, Hong Kong, Israel, Kuwait, Malaysia, Singapore, South Africa, and Taiwan.

"Accidental" versus "Deliberate" Acetaminophen Overdoses

An accidental overdose is one with no overt suicidal intent. The USA reports a different pattern of overdoses from that experienced in the UK, Denmark, or Australia; most US overdoses are reported as "unintentional." This may be a real phenomenon or may reflect idiosyncrasies of different healthcare systems.

Lee and coworkers reviewed cases of "acute liver failure" admitted to 17 academic units in the USA from January 1998 to October 2000 and reported 60% as "accidental" overdoses; acetaminophen was

the most frequent cause of acute liver failure (98/258 = 38% of cases). TESS data support this view, suggesting 36 259 unintentional overdoses per year of acetaminophen alone compared with 19 443 intentional ones. In contrast, all acetaminophen calls made to the National Poisons Information Service in the UK were collected over a 14-week period ($n = 280$ calls). Only 19 were "accidental;" all of these were staggered overdoses; 17 received treatment with N-acetylcysteine. Five developed "hepatotoxicity" but all alanine and aspartate transaminase and international normalized ratio abnormalities resolved within 24–48 h, and none developed acute liver failure.

In the UK it is estimated that acetaminophen ± ethanol still accounts for 100–200 deaths annually. Whilst many patients may die relatively quickly due to opioid co-ingestion, death at home from acetaminophen poisoning alone is very unusual. Most acetaminophen-alone deaths occur in hospital from liver failure. Hence, acetaminophen poisoning is the largest cause of death from acute poisoning in hospital, despite the availability of an effective antidote if the overdose has occurred in the previous 12 h, and advances in the treatment of liver failure. The steep rise in dextropropoxyphene-related deaths between 1969 and 1979 prompted the introduction of blister packaging for acetaminophen/dextropropxyphene products. Whilst this probably arrested the sharp increase in deaths, the trend is still upwards in the UK.

Aspirin Overdose

In the UK, in 1985, 22.7% of analgesic overdoses were due to aspirin, but its use in overdose declined to 10.6% in 1997. Salicylate or aspirin poisoning is much less common than 20 years ago but, because of this, doctors may fail to recognize its severity or treat such patients optimally. American TESS data report 27 deaths in 2000 due to aspirin in patients between 15 and 88 years of age. One was due to chronic use, one unknown, and 25 were acute overdoses. One was reported as unintentional and the rest "suicide," with plasma concentrations between 40 and 1450 mg l^{-1} and timing uncertain.

NSAID Overdose

Ibuprofen is very commonly taken in overdose, as the TESS data show. Overdose by most NSAIDs causes little more than mild gastrointestinal upset, including mild abdominal pain. Vomiting and diarrhea may occur and 10–20% may have convulsions. Serious features include coma, prolonged fits, apnea, and bradycardia, but are very rare. Deaths have been reported after massive overdose of ibuprofen, but none so far with mefenamic acid.

Self-Poisoning with Antidepressants

In New Zealand, as in western Europe and North America and Australasia, antidepressant medications remain amongst the commonest classes of drugs taken alone or in combination. An important trend is the increasing use of selective serotonin reuptake inhibitors (SSRIs), and the newer antidepressants are associated with <10% of the risk of death than the older antidepressants. There is a strong association between area deprivation and deaths from antidepressants. Self-poisoning with antidepressants is common in urban areas throughout the tropics, but carries low mortality.

Self-Poisoning with Anxiolytic and Sedative Drugs

Self-poisoning with benzodiazepines is common in urban areas throughout the tropics, western Europe, and North America, but when taken alone carries a low mortality.

Sedative drugs are a common cause of fatal poisoning in the UK. The fatal toxicity index (FTI) is calculated by dividing the number of deaths (in England, Scotland, and Wales in this study) by the total number of prescriptions for the drug. For benzodiazepine anxiolytics the FTI was 3.0. In contrast, chloral hydrate carried an FTI of 46.5 and barbiturates 146. Whilst FTIs largely reflect the inherent toxicity of the drug in question, it is not possible to exclude from the coroner's data used in the calculations that the drug is more frequently taken, or prescribed for or taken in overdose by an at-risk group. Similarly, individual patient variables may alter the risk of poisoning, such as age, gender, other medical conditions, and whether the drugs were prescribed for drug dependence, psychiatric illness, or other indications. Alcohol potentiates the sedative effects of these drugs and these patients also have a disproportionately higher risk of suicide or accidental poisoning, both of which may increase the FTI for these drugs.

There was a marked decline in deaths due to high-toxicity drugs such as barbiturates, chloral hydrate, and betaine between 1983 and 1992 in the UK, with only small further reductions since. The reduction in deaths due to barbiturates directly followed reduced frequency of prescriptions. In contrast, reduction in deaths due to benzodiazepines coincided with a major reduction in prescription of temazepam gelatin capsule preparations in January 1996, showing there is scope for reducing sedative drug overdose mortality if they are being deliberately misused.

In Finland, the rate of psychotropic and sedative drug-poisoning admissions increased from 35%

to 47% during the 1980s. In Poland, almost 25% of drug poisoning reported to the poisons center was due to sedative and to psychotropic drugs.

In Tehran, Iran, drugs were the most common cause of intoxication (60.2%). Of these, benzodiazepines (24.5%) were the most frequent.

Self-Poisoning with Antimalarials

Chloroquine poisoning is prevalent in Africa and the Pacific region and is often fatal. Chloroquine is the most common cause of pharmaceutical poisoning admission at referral hospitals in Zimbabwe. It is most often taken deliberately, especially in women who are pregnant. Quinine is a recognized drug used for self-harm in Europe. Cases have been seen in Casablanca, Morocco, and Thailand.

Drugs of Abuse

Defining drug abuse-related poisoning episodes and deaths is not easy. The EMCDDA (European Monitoring Centre for Drugs and Drug Addiction) has defined a standard list of ICD-9 codes for comparison of drug abuse-related mortality across Europe, but only counts deaths certified as due to a single substance, explicitly certified as "drug abuse/dependence." Thus, deaths due to other drugs that are often abused, such as cocaine and temazepam, are excluded if drug dependence/abuse was not written on the death certificate. EMCDDA data for England and Wales showed that deaths due to drugs of abuse increased from 140 per year in 1979–1981 to 568 in 1999. The Office for National Statistics (ONS) poisons-related deaths data in England and Wales show that deaths involving heroin and morphine, recorded on the death certificate, have risen steadily since 1993 in the UK and, if this trend continues, and deaths from carbon monoxide continue to fall, heroin will shortly be expected to be the leading cause of death by poisoning in England and Wales. Deaths involving methadone in England and Wales peaked in 1997 at 421 and have since fallen, presumably due to measures to limit the leakage of methadone from those to whom its is prescribed into the community, for example, pharmacy-supervised ingestion. Other controlled drugs account for relatively few deaths. In England and Wales, deaths due to amphetamines (including ecstasy) rose from 11 to 28 annually between 1993 and 1999.

Heroin and/or morphine dominated as a cause of fatal poisonings in Norway and Sweden. In Denmark, heroin and/or morphine caused about half of the fatal poisonings only, and nearly one-third of the fatal poisonings were caused by methadone. Except for two cases in Sweden, methadone deaths were not seen in the other Nordic countries. Amphetamine caused one-tenth of the fatal poisonings in Sweden. In Finland only one-tenth of the deaths were caused by heroin and/or morphine and more by codeine and ethylmorphine. In Taiwan, amphetamines are the most frequently ingested poisons.

Self-Poisoning with Volatile Substances

Volatile substance abuse is the largest single cause of death in males aged 14–18 years after road traffic accidents in the UK and accounts for 20% of the deaths in men aged 20–29 years. It is not frequently encountered in the tropics.

Carbon Monoxide

The decline in fatal carbon monoxide poisoning in England and Wales from a peak in the early 1960s has been attributed to the replacement of coal gas with natural gas. This measure reduced both accidental and suicidal poisoning by a particular agent without a corresponding increase in suicide by other means.

In Turkey carbon monoxide deaths represent 27% of all poisoning fatalities. A 5-year (1997–2001) study of carbon monoxide poisoning in France showed domestic source was the commonest, with vented gas heating systems, mobile heaters, and thermal motors being the commonest sources.

Pesticide Poisoning

Pesticides are the most important poison used for self-harm throughout the tropics, being both common and associated with high mortality, and represent a major developing-world public health problem. It is deliberate self-poisoning that causes the majority of deaths rather than occupational exposure.

A recent study in Bangladesh showed 14% of all deaths amongst women aged 10–50 years were due to poisoning, mostly pesticides. Organochlorine compounds were the main cause of death (51.6%), followed by organophosphorous compounds (37.7%); however the trend is toward replacement of organochlorines with organophosphates. Poisoning with organochlorines has recently become an important cause of unremitting seizures in parts of South Asia. Poisoning is common in young children as they explore the environment with their mouths but as the dose ingested is seldom significant, the mortality rate is low.

Organophosphate pesticides were responsible for the majority of deaths in most self-poisoning cases in the developing world, particularly from rural areas, and the fatality rate is as high as 46% in some series. The fatality rate in Sri Lanka is 21.8%. In Sri Lanka in 1995–1996 organophosphate poisoning occupied 41% of the hospital's medical intensive care beds. Carbamate poisoning is widely reported in Brazil, Israel, and Jordan and after ingestion of rodenticides. The most common cause of fatal poisoning in Turkey between 1996 and 2000 was insecticides (43%). Among the insecticides, the organophosphates comprised 78%. Drug-related deaths were very rare.

Aluminum phosphide has recently become the commonest means of self-poisoning in Northern India, with a 61% mortality rate. It is particularly common in 11–15-year-olds.

Nearly 50% of all calls to the poison center in Malaysia related to pesticide poisoning. Pyrethroids were a common source of calls to a poisons center in India.

Where toxicity is well-recognized by the community, paradoxical increases in the rate of poisoning have occurred. Self-harm practices have grown around dimethoate in Zimbabwe, paraquat in Trinidad, Samoa and Fiji, malathion in Guyana, and parathion in Thailand. Compared with the last survey of poisoning in Zimbabwe, the pattern of poisoning at referral hospitals has changed over the last decade, with an increase in pesticide and pharmaceutical cases and a marked fall in cases of traditional medicine poisoning. Organophosphate poisoning is increasing rapidly in Zimbabwe. In Japan, the most frequent cause of poisoning was paraquat with a mortality of 76%. The second most frequent cause was organophosphate/carbamates with a mortality of 24%. When these two pesticides are excluded the mortality was only 3%.

Although there continues to be concern about possible toxicity from environmental and occupational exposure to pesticides in the UK, such compounds are responsible for fewer than 1% of deaths from acute poisoning in England and Wales.

Domestic and Industrial Chemicals

These are responsible for significant numbers of deaths and long-term disabilities worldwide. Domestic chemical poisoning is a major problem in African and Asian communities. Agents that are commonly involved include kerosene (in up to 68% of cases), Dettol (chloroxylenol), sulfuric acid, and bleach. The commonest age group involved is under 6 years and such products are often kept in nonchild-resistant containers. Poisoning was commoner among the lower socioeconomic classes and in males. In Ile-Ife, Nigeria, kerosene was the commonest agent, accounting for

40.9% of all cases; followed by caustic soda (20.4%) and traditional mixtures (19.7%). Oral administration of palm oil is the commonest home remedy. Morbidity was commonest with caustic soda, while a traditional mixture was responsible for 80% of all mortality. Paint thinners were commonly ingested in Delhi, India. Kerosene, pesticides, and medicinal substances remain the commonest agents associated with poisoning in Malaysia.

However, in Hong Kong adults largely take domestic products with the intention of self-harm. Deaths were due to aspiration of Dettol or detergent, or ingestion of sulfuric acid. Potassium permanganate is a common household disinfectant that has been used for self-harm in Hong Kong with fatal hepatorenal complications. Self-poisoning with hydrochloric or sulfuric acid is a major problem in Taiwan, with a 12% case fatality rate. Formic and acetic acids are used in rubber manufacture and self-poisoning with these agents is a problem in rubber plantation regions such as India and Sri Lanka and carries 30% mortality. Car battery acid poisoning was reported in Cape Town, South Africa, with fatalities.

Copper sulfate is widely used for self-harm in Southeast Asia. Death results in 25% of cases from hepatorenal failure, hemolysis, and gastrointestinal hemorrhage. In Seoul, South Korea, potassium cyanide represented 62% of all suicides from poisoning. Reports of cyanide self-poisoning have also been seen from India and Taiwan. Other chemicals that have been used for self-poisoning include turpentine, chromic acid, and ethylene bromide in India; sodium chlorite, ferric chloride, and methylene chloride in Taiwan; xylene in Jordan; and arsenic and cyanide in Zimbabwe.

Alcohols

Alcohol is second only to drugs for frequency of poisoning in Poland. It is also very common in Russia.

Plants

Plant poisoning is globally uncommon but locally popular in some areas. For example, in Sri Lanka there are thousands of cases each year of yellow oleander (*Thevetia peruviana*) poisoning and it causes 4.1% of deaths due to poisoning. Ingestion of oduvan (*Clistanthus collinus*) is a common self-harm practice in India. *Datura strammonium* poisoning has been reported in the tropics and is increasing in prevalence in the West because of the known hallucinogenic properties. In India, plant poisoning accounts for 1.5% of calls to a poisons center; *Datura* is the most commonly ingested plant being reported.

Herbal or Traditional Medicines

Traditional medicines are a common cause of accidental poisoning, but a rare cause of intentional self-poisoning. In South Africa, a study of 1306 cases of poisoning found 16% of admissions were due to traditional remedies but carried a mortality rate of 15%. Nonspecific effects, including vomiting, abdominal pains, and diarrhea, were most commonly encountered. A large proportion of patients also suffered from hematuria and dysuria.

Chinese medicines have been reported to be commonly used for self-poisoning in Hong Kong and Taiwan and are an increasing problem in the UK.

Rare Poisons

Thallium-containing rodenticides were banned in the USA during the 1960s, but they are still used in some tropical countries. Deliberate self-poisoning has been reported in Mexico and Thailand. All but two of 50 patients in the Mexican series made a full recovery. Of 19 patients poisoned with avermectin in Taiwan, seven showed significant signs of toxicity and one died.

Long-acting "superwarfarin" compounds such as brodifacoum cause long-term coagulopathies and have been used for self-poisoning in Hong Kong. Dapsone is a common cause of accidental poisoning in children in India, but not worldwide.

Poisoning by cosmetic products is rarely serious but 46 cases of hair dye (paraphenylenediamine) poisoning resulted in 12 deaths in Khartoum, Sudan, and Casablanca, Morocco.

Possible Interventions to Change the Epidemiology of Poisoning

Availability

Banning common poisons, such as pesticides, may be effective in particular regions. Improved storage of pesticides and medicines may also reduce the incidence of poisoning. However, locking pesticides away safely is difficult in rural areas where farmers live in huts without beds, furniture, or cupboards. While it may be possible to ban the more toxic pesticides and replace them with safer ones, safer pesticides are expensive and therefore unaffordable in the developing world. Banning some pesticides has led to the adoption of other, equally dangerous ones.

Pack-Size Restrictions

There are some UK data to support efficacy of legislation on pack sizes. Hawton and coworkers showed that the annual number of deaths from acetaminophen poisoning decreased by 21% (confidence interval 5–34%) after legislation. Liver transplant rates decreased by 66% (55–74%) and the rate of acetaminophen overdosage decreased by 11% (5–16%). The average number of tablets taken in overdose decreased by 7% (0–12%). However, the mean blood concentration of acetaminophen did not change. Corresponding data for aspirin showed that the annual number of deaths from salicylate poisoning decreased by 48% (11–70%) but the average number of tablets taken did not decrease. Irish data on 2020 cases suggest no impact from a voluntary scheme of restriction in pack size and Scottish data are similarly negative. Whilst the incidence of acute liver failure is falling, this may reflect the absolute incidence falling but the ratio of acetaminophen to acute liver failure may be the same.

Packaging

Every encouragement should be given to manufacturers to provide better labeling and packaging of potentially harmful products, if necessary by legislation, but there is a need for industry to be self-regulating. The packaging should not require the user to have a PhD in chemistry or toxicology to understand the information provided. Because of the inconvenience and longer time required to punch out the tablets, strip packaging may reduce the number of tablets that can be readily swallowed by adults with self-poisoning and studies have shown that large overdoses were mainly from loose tablets.

As a result of child-resistant closures, a greater emphasis on safety in the home, improved access to poisons information, improved management, and the introduction of blister packaging, fatal poisoning in children less than 10 years of age is now rare in some countries such as the UK.

Dilution of Products

To reduce instances of paraquat/diquat poisoning, for example in Japan, dilution of the available product or formulation in other than liquid form would be desirable.

Putting an Antidote, e.g., Methionine, into Acetaminophen Tablets?

Methionine is an effective antidote in acetaminophen poisoning. However, if used as a prophylactic it would need to be put in all acetaminophen tablets to be effective. Methionine metabolizes to homocysteine, which is an independent risk factor for CAD (coronary artery disease) and stroke. There was therefore concern that regular acetaminophen and methionine

use may induce hyperhomocysteinemia. However, a recent study with 16 volunteers demonstrated no difference in endothelial-dependent vascular responses after acute (250 mg methionine orally) 1 month of 250 mg per day or 1 week of $100 \, \mathrm{mg \, kg^{-1}}$ g per day, although a 1-week regime significantly increased plasma homocysteine concentrations. Other concerns around methionine are that it is a carcinogen, and may reduce serum folate, and hence is of concern in pregnancy. Inconveniences are that combination tablets have a fishy taste and cost eight times more than standard acetaminophen tablets.

Banning Drugs

During criminal extortion of a company making acetaminophen in Australia, where a batch had been contaminated with strychnine and all acetaminophen products were then removed from over-the-counter sales, a switch to therapeutic use of aspirin and NSAIDs took place. There was a concurrent significant increase in accidental ibuprofen overdoses and increase in deliberate aspirin overdoses. A switch to aspirin may claim excessive deaths in overdoses and increased adverse effects from therapeutic use. A switch to NSAIDs would not be expected to increase death from overdose, but again would be expected to result in increased adverse effects from therapeutic use.

Making Certain Drugs Prescription-Only

There are no data to support a view that removing, for example, acetaminophen or aspirin from over-the-counter use would necessarily limit the number of overdoses, since significant overdose with prescription-only products occurs, such as tricyclic antidepressants. Australian data showed that, during the acetaminophen extortion, when acetaminophen became prescription-only, there was a substantial cost/time resource perspective for prescriptions.

Monitoring Use of Drugs

As more medicines become available over-the-counter, healthcare professionals have less control over use. It is important therefore that some control is maintained. Better monitoring will be needed in terms of adverse therapeutic events and overdose and increased collaboration with pharmacists will be needed, together with better databases for recording information. Surveillance work is important in identifying problems and allowing appropriate remedial action to be taken as new products emerge or changes in packaging or sales affect the incidence of poisoning by certain products. The poisons centers of each country should form an important part of this work.

Improved Care of Poisoned Patients

Lack of evidence-based guidelines, lack of resources such as drugs, intensive therapy unit facilities, and staff are key variables altering outcome in poisoning.

Striking at the Core of the Problem

The practice of deliberate self-harm is open to programs to reduce its incidence. Such interventions to prevent recurrence of self-harm behavior might include postcards from the edge, education in schools, and increased availability of counseling.

Conclusions

There are no agreed best-practice guidelines to govern collection of toxicology data worldwide and these require to be developed. The prevalence of drug-related hospital admissions in North America and western Europe point to preventive strategies to decrease the availability of toxic doses of drugs (including illicit drugs) for ingestion as the key to reducing hospital admissions for poisoning. Measures to reduce carbon monoxide deaths still further need to be employed. In less well-developed countries, support is needed to develop effective prevention and medical management strategies and resources, to deal with pesticide and household poisoning in particular. The efficacy of any intervention can only be assessed if adequate methods of recording data are employed. There remains an enormous challenge to reduce the incidence, morbidity, and mortality of poisoning worldwide.

See Also

Alcohol: Acute and Chronic Use, Postmortem Findings; **Deliberate Self-Harm, Patterns**; **Drug-Induced Injury, Accidental and Iatrogenic**; **History of Toxicology**; **Internet:** Toxicology; **Pharmacology of Legal and Illicit Drugs**

Further Reading

Baker SP (2000) Where have we been and where are we going to in injury control? In: Mohan D, Tiwari G (eds.) *Injury Prevention and Control*, pp. 13–26. London: Taylor and Francis.

Balit C, Isbister GK, Peat J, Dawson A, Whyte I (2001) Pharmaceutical terrorism: a natural experiment influencing analgesic poisoning. *Clinical Toxicology* 9: 530.

Buckley NA, Whyte IM, Dawson AH, *et al.* (1995) Correlations between prescriptions and drugs taken in self-poisoning: implications for prescribers and drug regulation. *Medical Journal of Australia* 162: 194–197.

Clemessy J-L, Taboulet P, Hoffman JR, *et al.* (1996) Treatment of acute chloroquine poisoning: a 5 year experience. *Critical Care Medicine* 24: 1189–1195.

Eddleston M (2000) Patterns and problems of deliberate self-poisoning in the developing world. *Quarterly Journal of Medicine* 93: 715–731.

Eddleston M, Rezvi-Sheriff MH, Hawton K (1998) Deliberate self harm in Sri Lanka: an overlooked tragedy in the developing world. *British Medical Journal* 317: 133–135.

Flanagan RJ, Rooney C (2002) Recording acute poisoning deaths. *Forensic Science International* 128: 3–19.

Jones AL (2002) Over-the-counter analgesics: a toxicologic perspective. *American Journal of Therapy* 9: 245–257.

Jones AL, Hayes PC, Proudfoot AT, *et al.* (1997) Should metionine be added to every paracetamol tablet? *British Medical Journal* 315: 301–303.

Litovitz T, Klein-Schwartz W, White S, *et al.* (2001) 2000 AAPCC annual report; TESS surveillance. *American Journal of Emergency Medicine* 19: 337–395.

Matthew H (1970) Acute poisoning. *Community Health* 2: 18–22.

Sam-Lai NF, Saviuc P, Danel V (2003) Carbon monoxide poisoning monitoring network: a five-year experience of household poisonings in two French regions. *Journal of Toxicology and Clinical Toxicology* 41: 349–353.

Stewart MJ, Steenkamp V, Zuckerman M (1998) The toxicology of African herbal remedies. *Therapeutic Drug Monitoring* 20: 510–516.

Townsend E, Hawton K, Harriss L, Bale E, Bond A (2001) Substances used in deliberate self-poisoning 1985–1997: trends and associations with age, gender, repetition and suicide intent. *Social Psychiatry and Psychiatric Epidemiology* 36: 228–234.

POSTMORTEM CHANGES

Contents
Overview
Electrolyte Disturbances
Postmortem Interval

Overview

M Tsokos, University of Hamburg, Hamburg, Germany

Introduction

The changes and underlying biologic processes that a human body or its remains undergoes after death are complex and, as with other biologic phenomena, there is a broad range of variables influencing postmortem changes by altering the underlying progress of tissue destruction. As a general rule, changes in ambient (environmental) temperature tend to alter the rate but not the underlying biological mechanisms of postmortem changes. A summary of the main intrinsic and extrinsic factors accelerating or decelerating the onset and extent of postmortem changes is given in **Table 1**.

It is generally impossible to draw any definite conclusions concerning the time of death from the appearance of a single postmortem change, or to predict what postmortem changes are to be expected after a particular postmortem interval has elapsed. Despite this, in the early postmortem interval (approximately within 24 h of death), in some cases the presence of several postmortem changes may, when analyzed together with the deceased's rectal temperature, give the death investigator valuable hints concerning the timeframe in which the subject probably died. An experienced forensic entomologist can occasionally narrow the date-of-death window even in the very late postmortem period, whereas the forensic pathologist or medical examiner, respectively, working with the signs of putrefaction, adipocere, mummification, or skeletonization will only be able to give broad estimations in such cases. However, this article does not focus on detailed aspects of estimation of the time elapsed since death but rather concentrates on the morphology and conditions in which different postmortem changes may present.

While most postmortem changes discussed in this article are, at least to a certain degree, frequently observed in the death investigator's practice, some postmortem changes shown here may occur only occasionally and under specific intraindividual or environmental conditions. The inexperienced or unwary may interpret such unusual postmortem changes incorrectly, especially in curious death scene scenarios and when found in fatalities with additional signs of external violence preceding death. In such cases, hasty conclusions may lead the investigative enquiries in the wrong direction or, in the worst case, to a miscarriage of justice. Therefore, apart from giving a synopsis of common and uncommon postmortem changes seen in the death investigator's daily practice, it is also the aim of this article to draw the reader's attention to potential differential diagnoses between postmortem changes and vitally acquired body alterations and the pitfalls they may contain.

In the following context, death is defined as the irreversible cessation of blood circulation.

Table 1 Intrinsic and extrinsic factors influencing the onset and extent of postmortem changes

Acceleration of onset and extent of postmortem changes
Death occurred in a hot, moist environment/under high ambient temperatures
Subject is overweight/has a high fat content
Subject suffered/died from underlying infection or sepsis
Subject was intoxicated (e.g., with illicit drugs such as heroin)
Subject suffered/died from open wounds (perforating/penetrating traumatic injuries such as stab wounds, gunshot wounds, impalement injuries) or during surgical procedures
Body surface is insulated by warm clothing or other covering
Considerable time interval elapsed after death until artificial cooling of the body
Deceleration of onset and extent of postmortem changes[a]
Death occurred in a cool (cold), dry environment/under low ambient temperatures[b]
Subject was scantily dressed/naked/undressed shortly after death
Subject was stored in a cooling apparatus shortly after death

[a]All these factors slow the rate of postmortem changes but in general do not alter the underlying postmortem biologic processes.
[b]In addition to slowing the onset and extent of postmortem changes, low ambient temperature has a considerable impact on a delayed manifestation of odor of the body and thereby on the attraction of insects to the body, thus making the human remains less olfactorily absorbing for carnivores and rodents.

Livor Mortis

Livor mortis (synonyms: livores, postmortem lividity, postmortem hypostasis) is visible as a usually bluish-violaceous to purple coloration appearing on lower (dependent) parts of the body within 30 min to 3 h after death.

After the cardiovascular system has ceased to function, under the influence of gravity, movement of blood into the dependent parts of the body occurs (**Figure 1**). Livores correspond to hypostasis (gravitational pooling of blood) into the capillaries within the dermis (consisting of the papillary and reticular layer) in the dependent parts of the body. Therefore, when a subject has died in a prone position, livores will spread over the front of the body, while when death has taken place in a supine position, livores will spread over the back of the body (**Figure 2**).

Patterned Appearance and Contact Blanching of Livor Mortis

Livor mortis is frequently patterned since the appearance of livores is hindered when the vessels in dependent parts of the body are obstructed due to outer-surface compression, for example, when prominent parts of the body such as areas over bony structures firmly adhere to a rigid surface due to the weight of the body or when tight clothing compresses the involved vessel lumina (**Figures 3** and **4**). In such areas, livor mortis is absent: the involved outer-body surface appears pale to white, in contrast with the surrounding livor mortis. This contact blanching may image the exterior of objects that were in contact with the dependent parts of the body surface during livor mortis formation and occasionally the distinctive morphological appearance of contact blanching may give the death investigator valuable hints about the case in question (**Figure 5**).

Creasing of the skin or tight clothing may produce contact blanching on the neck which may resemble ligature marks (**Figure 6**). Therefore, knowledge of the position of the head and neck as well as the cloth worn at the time of death is important for the death investigator.

Chronological Sequel of Livor Mortis Formation

After a first patchy development of livor mortis within 30 min to 3 h after death, livores become confluent. Under moderate to cool climatic conditions, livores are usually fully developed within 4–8 h postmortem, reaching their maximum intensity after an average of 10 h postmortem (**Table 2**). Livor mortis is most intense in cases of sudden death with a short agonal period and a great circulating blood volume.

In the early postmortem interval, roughly until 12–18 h after death, livor mortis is not yet fixed. Nonfixation of livor mortis means that it can be blanched when a blunt object such as a finger, the hand, or an instrument is pressed against the skin in areas of livores formation (**Figure 7**). This selective pressure forces the blood from the engorged capillaries, resulting in a pale to white blanching which quickly refills. A similar phenomenon results if the body is moved into a new position. Livor mortis will then shift to the dependent parts of the body as a result of body movement. The capability of livores to shift as a result of the gravitational movement of blood is assumed to depend on a prevailing number of intact erythrocytes within the vascular system: selective pressure moves the blood cells within the vessels. However, this assumption has been questioned more than once by different authorities.

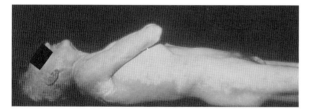

Figure 1   Livor mortis in dependent areas of the body.

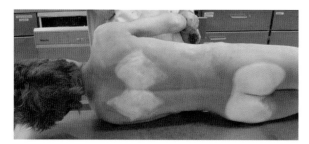

Figure 2   Intense livor mortis formation on the posterior parts of the body surface with typical contact blanching over the scapular region and buttocks.

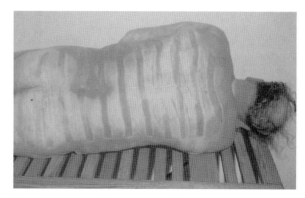

Figure 3   Patterned appearance of livor mortis on the back of the body.

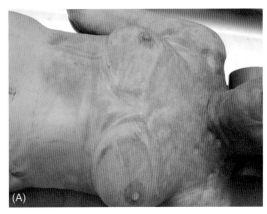 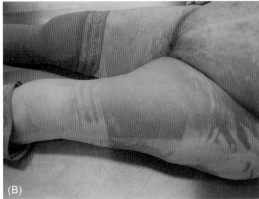

Figure 4 (A), (B) Contact blanching of livor mortis induced by tight clothing.

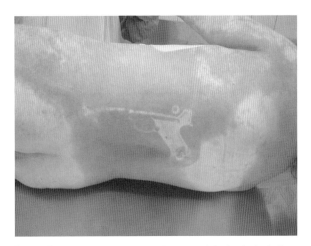

Figure 5 Contact blanching on the back of the body depicting a pistol.

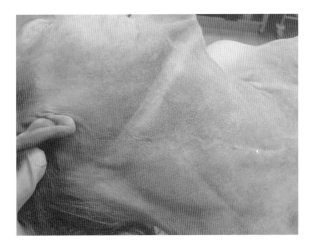

Figure 6 Contact blanching upon the skin of the anterior neck that should not be confused with a ligature mark.

After 18–24 h, livor mortis becomes fixed: livores cannot be blanched by selective pressure on the body surface and the effect of gravity does not move

Table 2 Sequential order of usual appearance of the different states of livor mortis under moderate to cool climatic conditions

Finding	Earliest appearance	General appearance	Latest appearance
Patchy beginning of development	0.5 h p.m.	2 h p.m.	3 h p.m.
Full development, confluence	4 h p.m.	6 h p.m.	8 h p.m.
Reaching maximum of intensity	6 h p.m.	10 h p.m.	16 h p.m.

p.m., postmortem.

livores. The time of onset of fixation of livores mostly depends on the ambient temperature to which the body has been exposed: high ambient temperatures are positively correlated with an early onset of fixation of livor mortis. When livor mortis is fixed, a change in body position will have no effect on the original pattern of livores. Fixation of livor mortis is considered a result of hemolysis of the blood serum: with the breakdown of erythrocyte membranes during autolysis, the erythrocytes become pervious for hemoglobin and its derivates: subsequent diffusion of hemolytic blood serum through the walls of the vessels is involved in livores formation. In this case, selective pressure over an area of livor mortis will have no noticeable effect on the movement of blood cells within the vessels or on the hemolytic coloration of the surrounding tissue. This theory has also been doubted, but the underlying pathophysiological mechanisms that are decisive for nonfixation or fixation of livores have so far shown no real practical value.

It should be mentioned that cases have been reported where shifting of livores has been observed, even after 48 h or more but this phenomenon is mostly restricted to cases with cold ambient temperatures.

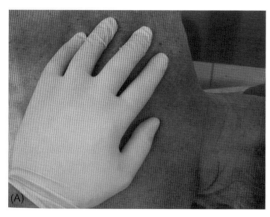 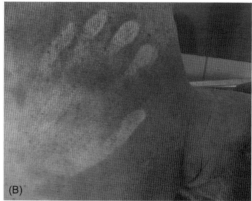

Figure 7 (A), (B) Contact blanching of livor mortis (within the state of nonfixation of postmortem lividity six hours after death of this individual). Selective pressure with the hand leads to a pale to white area of blanching which quickly refills.

Color of Livor Mortis

In the early phase of their formation, livores have a reddish color, due to the prevailing number of erythrocytes carrying oxygenated hemoglobin. With an increase in the length of the postmortem interval, livores become darker, and when fully developed, the normal color of livor mortis is bluish-violaceous to purple. This is a result of oxygen dissociation from both the postmortem hemoglobin of erythrocytes and continuous oxygen consumption from cells that initially survive the cessation of cardiovascular function (e.g., skeletal muscle cells survive cessation of the cardiovascular system for 2–8 h). The resulting product is deoxyhemoglobin, which is bluish-violaceous to purple in color.

Light reddish/pink livores Light reddish or pink livores are frequently seen in carbon monoxide poisoning, fatal hypothermia, cyanide poisoning, or in bodies deposited postmortem in cold ambient temperatures.

A light reddish or pink, sometimes described as "cherry-red," coloration of livores is classically seen in carbon monoxide poisoning as a result of carboxyhemoglobin formation (**Figure 8**). The assumption that a bluish-violaceous color of the matrix of the nails, when found together with a light reddish color of livores, refutes carbon monoxide poisoning as being responsible for the reddish coloration of livores must be vehemently contradicted. Tsokos and coworkers have seen cases of fatal carbon monoxide poisoning where the matrix of the nails showed a bluish-violaceous color despite carbon monoxide hemoglobin concentrations of 50% and more. In such doubtful cases, laboratory testing of heart blood samples should be carried out immediately to avoid exposing other individuals to danger at the scene of death.

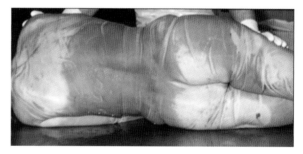

Figure 8 Pink ("cherry red") coloration of livores in carbon monoxide poisoning.

Light reddish or pink livores are also frequently seen in fatal hypothermia cases since cold ambient temperature inhibits dissociation of oxygen from the hemoglobin. Oxygenated hemoglobin has a lighter red color than deoxyhemoglobin. Under cold ambient temperatures (roughly below 15 °C), reoxygenation of hemoglobin slowly occurs postmortem, and this is the explanation for the light red color of livores seen in bodies after storage in a cooling apparatus postmortem (**Figure 9**).

In cyanide poisoning, the cyanide inhibits dissociation of oxygen from the hemoglobin by blocking cytochromoxidase activity, leading to a light reddish or pink coloration of livor mortis.

Brownish color of livores A brownish, sometimes described as "chocolate," color of livor mortis is seen in poisoning with nitrates, nitrites, or sodium chloride (**Figure 10**). The reason for this brown coloration is the formation of methemoglobin.

Greenish color of livores Livores often turn partly green under the influence of putrefaction processes due to hemoglobin conversion into sulfhemoglobin.

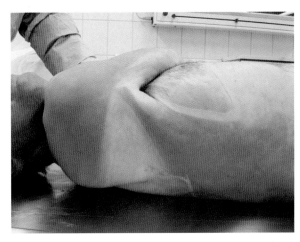

Figure 9 Light reddish/pink livores due to reoxygenation of hemoglobin after storage of the body in a cooling apparatus. Note the bluish-violaceous marginal zone next to the contact blanching over the scapular region which is a result of anewed oxygen dissociation from the hemoglobin of erythrocytes after the body was brought into the relatively warmer temperatures of the autopsy room.

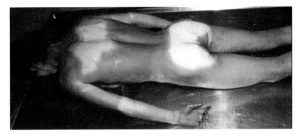

Figure 10 Brownish color of livor mortis in nitrate poisoning.

Livor Mortis in Internal Organs

Comparable with the development and their location of appearance on the outer body surface, livores are found in dependent parts of internal organs such as the lungs, heart, liver, and kidneys.

In the lungs, blood and transudation accumulation, the latter due to circumscribed hypostasis, may occasionally be confused with edema of the lungs or pneumonia.

In the heart, internal livores, demonstrated by a reddish discoloration zone in the myocardium, may mimic fresh infarction. The exact location of livores in the myocardium depends on the posture of the body after death.

In the liver, when livores have developed in a right-sided position of the body, contact blanching deriving from the ribs may be observed.

Difficulties arising from the presence of livor mortis in internal organs and their differentiation from underlying diseases are easily solved by microscopic examination.

Absence of Livor Mortis

Livores may be sparse or even absent in fatalities where there was considerable blood loss before death, whether from internal sources (e.g., gastrointestinal bleeding) or as a result of external hemorrhage (e.g., stab wounds, traumatic amputation of limbs). In most such cases, the external examination will explain inconspicuous or absent livores by revealing the source of bleeding (e.g., blood smears resulting from hematemesis or melena (**Figure 11**), external injuries). The total absence of livores necessitates a blood loss of at least 65% of the circulating blood volume in adolescents and 45% in infants. In cases with antemortem anemia (e.g., aplastic anemia, autoimmune hemolytic anemia, anemia secondary to malignancy, malnutrition, or infection) livor mortis will be unnoticeable, depending on the hemoglobin count in the circulation before death.

In sun-tanned or dark-skinned individuals, livores may be difficult to establish or unnoticeable.

In drowning deaths, depending on the depth and time the body was under water, livores may not develop since the vessels beneath the outer surface of the body that are normally involved in livor mortis formation are obstructed due to compression by surrounding hydrostatic water pressure. If the body is recovered from the water within roughly 24 h, livores may develop in the then dependent parts of the body, but this will depend on the water temperature. In bodies recovered from cold water, this phenomenon may be observed even after a postmortem interval of 48–72 h.

Criminalistic Aspects

When a subject has died in a supine position, livores will spread over the posterior side of the body, and when death took place in a prone position,

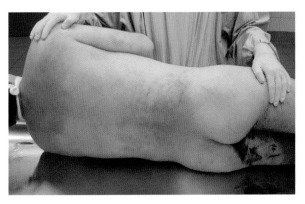

Figure 11 Sparse postmortem lividity due to fatal anal blood loss from a carcinoma of the rectum. Note blood smears around the anal orificium.

livores will spread over the anterior side of the body. However, the reverse assumption, that a deceased who has livores on the back of the body has died in a supine position or that livores found on the front of the body indicate that this person died in a prone position, may be misleading since, as mentioned above, livores have the ability to shift when the body is moved to a new position before livor mortis has become fixed.

In hanging deaths, livor mortis will be apparent in the dependent parts of the body (e.g., glove-like and stocking-like appearance of livores on the lower parts of the arms and legs, respectively). However, the finding of livores in the dependent parts of the body corresponding to hanging does not unequivocally exclude that this body has been transferred into this posture postmortem, for example, to conceal a homicide.

If a body is found in a supine position but livor mortis is seen on the anterior side of the body, this implies that the body has been moved a considerable time after death, after fixation of livor mortis.

Differential Diagnoses

Livor mortis may be confused with bruising by the inexperienced, although this is rare. Within the first 24 h after death, evidence of contact blanching caused by selective pressure to the outer body surface will help to differentiate between bruising and livores, since application of surface compression to an area of bruising will not cause blanching. In the later postmortem interval, the incision of a doubtful skin area will make a clear distinction since no hemorrhage will be apparent in the soft tissue beneath livores formation.

Frost erythema, hypothermia-induced red-purple spots seen over prominent bony parts of the body such as the shoulder, knee, or elbow joints, may occasionally be mistaken for livores by the unwary (**Figure 12**). Bearing in mind that frostbite is regularly found on nondependent parts of the body and often shows no confluence, its differentiation from livores should not present any difficulties.

Vibices

Vibices (synonyms: death spots, postmortem ecchymoses) are tiny, often spot-like, sometimes confluent, oval to round, bluish-blackish hemorrhages of postmortem origin exclusively limited to areas of livor mortis (**Figure 13**). Vibices result from postmortem mechanical rupture of subcutaneous capillaries and smaller vessels (predominantly veins) due to an increase in intravascular pressure arising from pooling

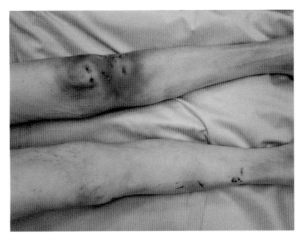

Figure 12   Frost erythemas over the left knee joint.

of erythrocytes in this vascular compartment under the influence of gravity during livor mortis formation. Histologically, erythrocytes appear intact within the vibices in the early postmortem interval (**Figure 14**). With increasing length of postmortem interval, under the influence of autolysis and putrefaction processes, vibices diminish in number and intensity due to the breakdown of erythrocyte membranes, with subsequent hemolysis and diffusion of hemoglobin and its derivates into the surrounding tissue.

When livores are sparse, vibices are usually absent. The formation of vibices depends on the total amount of circulating blood volume antemortem and is therefore more often seen in obese than in underweight decedents. The duration of the agonal period has no influence on whether vibices manifest or not.

Differential Diagnoses

Vibices should not be confused with petechial bleeding as a result of traumatic asphyxia or spot-like or more confluent cutaneous bleedings due to septic disseminated intravascular coagulation. As a general rule and helpful in the differential diagnosis is the fact that the appearance, intensity, and extent of vibices are positively correlated with that of livor mortis and therefore vibices are strictly limited to the body parts where livores are existent.

Rigor Mortis

Rigor mortis (synonym: postmortem rigidity) is the stiffening of muscles after death. Rigor mortis is preceded by a total (primary) relaxation of the musculature immediately after death. Shortly thereafter, rigor mortis begins to appear in the muscles of the eyelids and the jaw (at the earliest 20 min postmortem); the jaw tightens due to stiffening of the masticatory

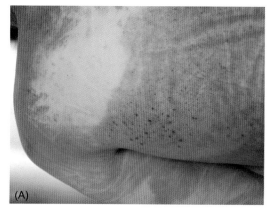
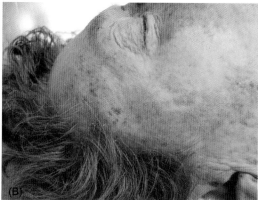

Figure 13 Vibices seen on the skin of the (A) back of the body and (B) temple.

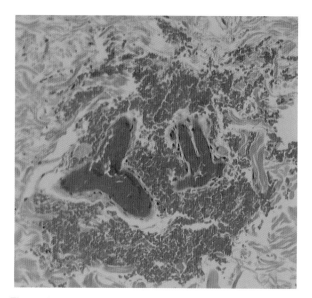

Figure 14 Histological appearance of vibices 8 hours postmortem. A zone of postmortem "bleeding" with intact erythrocytes lacking any surrounding inflammatory cellular response is seen next to two subcutaneous venules.

muscles. After that, postmortem rigidity begins to affect larger muscle groups with stiffening of elbow and knee joints 2–6 h after death. However, the rate of onset and time of full development of rigor mortis are highly variable and, as with all postmortem changes, for the most part are particularly dependent on the ambient temperature (high ambient temperatures accelerate the onset and intensity of rigor mortis, although extremes of cold have also been reported to produce a rapid onset of rigor mortis). In forensic pathological practice, the intensity of rigor mortis is assessed on a purely subjective basis by scrutinizing whether joints can be moved (flexion/extension) and if muscle stiffening offers resistance. As a result, determination of the state of rigor mortis varies greatly from one investigator to another. In addition,

numerous intrinsic and extrinsic factors affect the development of rigor mortis and therefore using the state of rigor mortis to estimate the postmortem interval is of no real value.

Pathophysiology of Rigor Mortis Formation

Muscles are composed of myofibrils, which are again composed of myofilaments. Two types of myofilaments can be distinguished: actin and myosin. Under the influence of adenosine triphosphate (ATP), actin and myosin form a contractile compound, actomyosin, which is the basic source of energy for muscle contraction. After death, ATP formation terminates and ATP is continuously consumed (to be precise, some ATP is still generated by anerobic glycolysis for a short period of time postmortem but this can be overlooked in the present context). With a decrease in ATP levels, actin and myosin enter into a nonshiftable and rigid state of adhesion until, under the influence of autolysis and putrefaction, protein disintegration of myofibrils leads to loosening of rigor mortis.

In mechanical terms, postmortem rigidity is characterized by a loss of muscle elasticity and plasticity, an increase in stiffness, and shortening of muscle length.

Experimental investigations have shown that the onset of rigor mortis is earlier and more rapidly progressive in red than white muscles, which has been attributed to ATP levels falling more rapidly after death in red than white muscles. However, this observation is highly academic and of no value for practical forensic casework.

Chronological Sequel of the Development and Disappearance of Rigor Mortis

In cool and temperate climate zones, rigor mortis is usually fully developed after 6–18 h (**Figure 15**). In high ambient temperatures the onset of rigor mortis is accelerated and postmortem rigidity may even be fully developed as early as 1–2 h after death.

Any forceful physical exertion before death leads to a decrease in ATP levels within the musculature and therefore also accelerates the time of onset of rigor mortis (e.g., in death by drowning where there is a violent struggle during the drowning process). The onset of rigor mortis may also be rapid in babies and children or in deaths due to electrocution. When the onset of rigor mortis is rapid, its duration is usually shorter than in cases with delayed onset under equal ambient (environmental) temperatures.

Rigor mortis develops in all muscles at the same time and at the same speed. However, due to the different diameters of the muscles involved, postmortem rigidity becomes noticeable at first in smaller muscle groups. When fully developed, rigor mortis may lead to such a rigidity of the body that it may be capable of supporting the whole body weight (**Figure 16**). In such cases, even the most forceful efforts to break down rigor mortis may be fruitless.

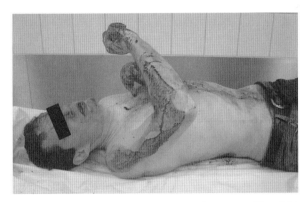

Figure 15 Fully developed rigor mortis in a case of homicide due to stabbing. At the death scene, the deceased was found in an upright to forward body posture leaning against a chair.

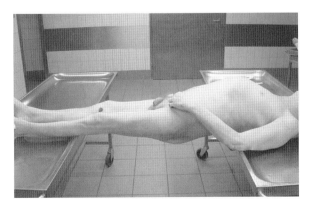

Figure 16 When fully developed, rigor mortis may lead to such a rigidity of the body that it may be capable of supporting the whole body weight.

The development of postmortem rigidity is usually progressive from the head down to the shoulder girdle and arms and then to the legs, a phenomenon that has been known since 1811 as "Nysten's rule." This finding can be explained by the greater diameter of the muscle groups located at joints that are farther down the body. But the exception proves the rule: after heavy physical exertion of the leg muscles, rigor mortis will develop earlier in the lower parts of the body than in the upper parts due to muscle activity in the legs with a resulting decrease in ATP levels.

When rigor mortis is broken, which means by forcefully stretching the joints against their fixation by rigor mortis, it will not return if it is fully developed. When only partly set, rigor mortis may redevelop again after having been broken.

In cool and temperate climates, loosening of rigor mortis reflected by a secondary relaxation of the muscles (in other words, a decrease in tension after full development of rigor mortis) begins 24–36 h postmortem, a finding that is again highly dependent on the ambient temperature (high ambient temperatures accelerate the time of onset of loosening of rigor mortis and therefore shorten its duration). Usually, rigor mortis disappears in the order in which it appeared but the finger joints usually remain stiff the longest.

In putrefied bodies, rigor mortis is absent. Rigor mortis may be weak or even unnoticeable in subjects who were suffering from a debilitating illness before death, in cachectic individuals, or those who died in an advanced state of multiple sclerosis, amyotrophic lateral sclerosis, or Duchenne muscular dystrophy.

Table 3 gives an overview of intrinsic and extrinsic factors that influence the onset of postmortem rigidity.

Table 3 Intrinsic and extrinsic factors influencing the onset of postmortem rigidity

Factors accelerating the time of onset of rigor mortis
Physical exhaustion before death (e.g., forceful muscular exertion during a fight or violent struggle during drowning)[a]
High body temperature/fever at the time of death[a]
Convulsions before death (e.g., due to underlying epilepsy or drug-induced)[a]
High ambient temperatures
Factors delaying the time of onset of rigor mortis
Debilitating diseases
Cachexia
Cool/cold ambient temperatures
Death following a short agonal period

[a]The accelerated onset of rigor mortis is mediated by a decrease of adenosine triphosphate concentration in such constellations.

Cadaveric Spasm

Reports of an instanteous appearance of full rigor mortis of the whole body immediately after death ("cadaveric spasm") occasionally appear in the literature. The true existence of cadaveric spasm is highly doubtful from an academic point of view since a satisfactory biological explanation for this phenomenon is lacking. When personal belongings or leaves are found grabbed in the hands (**Figure 17**), the logical explanation is that they were actually located under the palms when postmortem rigidity set in. Most reports of cases of cadaveric spasm derive from observations on the battlefields of World Wars I and II. In the overwhelming majority, the phenomenon of cadaveric spasm is easily explained by postmortem movement of the affected bodies due to blast waves from explosives hitting the battlefield. After blast wave-induced movement of the bodies, they were found in unreasonable positions that would not have been maintained during primary relaxation of the muscles after death. Another logical explanation in some cases is the fixation of tetanic convulsion in rigor mortis, which has been observed in rare cases.

Rigor Mortis in Internal Organs

Postmortem rigidity not only affects the skeletal muscles, it is also found in the myocardium as well as in internal organs such as the uterus, the gallbladder, or urinary bladder. As with the skeletal musculature, rigor mortis is preceded by a total primary relaxation of all muscles of internal organs. This muscle relaxation immediately after death explains leaking of urine or seminal fluid from the urethral orifice due to flaccidity of the urinary bladder and the pelvic diaphragm, respectively.

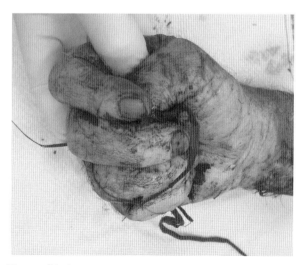

Figure 17 Leaves found grabed within the hands of a body recovered from water (no "cadaveric spasm"!).

The finding of "gooseflesh" after death is the result of postmortem contraction of the erector pili of the skin.

Criminalistic Aspects

Rigor mortis is occasionally helpful in determining whether a body has been moved after death. If a body is found in an illogical posture, such as a body position that would not have been maintained under the influence of gravity during primary relaxation of the muscles after death, this position implies that the body has been moved after the development of rigor mortis.

Rigor mortis may make examination of the palms and the inside aspects of the fingers difficult so that current marks or defense injuries located here may be overlooked.

Particularly in children, a marked anal dilatation may be observed postmortem. As mentioned before, immediately as death occurs and preceding the onset of rigor mortis, the whole body musculature loses its tone. In children, rigor mortis may fix a dilated anal orifice and this finding may persist after rigor mortis has faded. Therefore, anal dilatation alone is not a sufficient marker for penetrative anal abuse before death.

Muscle relaxation immediately after death with opening of the eyes and the mouth and subsequent fixation in rigor mortis often occurs after death, giving the face the appearance of grimacing. However, despite common belief, the face of a deceased does not reflect whether the individual's last moments were of fear or fright.

Algor Mortis

Algor mortis (synonym: postmortem cooling) is the normal cooling of a body after death as the result of equilibration of the body with the ambient (environmental) temperature.

The normal rectal temperature in life is 36.9 °C (range 34.2–37.6 °C) but the assumption that a "healthy" person had a "normal" body (rectal) temperature at the time of death is often erroneous since many factors influence body temperature at the time of death (**Table 4**).

The heat exchange between the body and the surroundings is mediated by conduction, convection, radiation, and evaporation. The main factors influencing a drop in body temperature after death are conduction and convection. Radiation can usually be disregarded, but evaporation may be important if the body or clothing is wet.

The rate of cooling of a body after death depends on the following factors:

Table 4 Individual factors potentially influencing body temperature at the time of death

Rise in body temperature at the time of death due to:

Infectious diseases (e.g., pneumonia, sepsis)[a,b]
Psychic ("emotional") stress
Physical activity (e.g., sports, fight, escape)
Central fever (e.g., stroke, intracranial hemorrhage)
Hyperthyroidism
Malignant hyperthermia
Exsiccosis
Administration of neuroleptic medication
Intoxication with illicit drugs (e.g., heroin, cocaine)

Lowering of body temperature at the time of death due to:

Hypothermia (e.g., prolonged exposure of the subject to a natural cold environment, artificial hibernation)
Hypothyroidism
Administration of muscle relaxants
Peripheral arterial occlusive disease

[a]Note that in elderly people infectious diseases may present without fever.
[b]When estimating the time since death using temperature-based methods, the error due to fever is greatest during the first hours postmortem and decreases with progression of the postmortem interval.

- body weight (the heavier the body, the slower the rate of cooling)
- temperature gradient between the core temperature of the deceased and the ambient temperature (the higher the temperature gradient, the faster the cooling; heat exchange between the body core and surface is exclusively mediated by conduction)
- gender (females have a higher fat content than males and thus males cool more rapidly postmortem when compared to females of identical weight)
- body mass index in relation to surface area (the lower the body mass index and surface area, the faster the cooling)
- environmental conditions and surrounding medium (e.g., still or flowing water, draft, wind, sun radiation on the body (with potential rewarming of the body days after death); water immersion cools a body much faster by convection than does exposure to air of the same temperature)
- surface insulation of the body by clothing or other covering such as blankets
- wet clothing
- body posture (the body cools faster in a stretched-out than in a crouched-down position).

After death, the body temperature stays relatively constant – this is referred to as the "postmortem temperature plateau." In moderate to cool climates, this temperature plateau lasts for 1–3 h and this is then followed by a linear rate of cooling (between 0.5 and 1.5 °C per hour) for the next 10–16 h. Then, as the body temperature approaches ambient temperature, the hourly cooling rate slows down. Estimating the time since death based only on body (rectal) temperature is often inaccurate since the length of the temperature plateau is generally unknown and such an assessment is useless when the body temperature has approached the ambient temperature.

Criminalistic Aspects

Temperature-based nomogram methods to estimate the time since death that are founded on: (1) measurements of rectal temperature and mean ambient temperature at the death scene; (2) determination of body weight; and (3) the use of an empirical corrective factor are considered the most reliable methods by leading authorities in the field. Such temperature-based methods and their related formulas are most useful in temperate and cool climates in industrialized countries where most people die indoors where there is heating; they are often useless in warm or tropical climate zones and outdoor deaths.

Autolysis

Autolysis is "self-digestion" of tissue resulting from the breakdown of cell function postmortem. When the continuous oxygen supply stops after death and the cytoplasmic pH decreases, loss of cell membrane integrity results. As a result, lysosomes and their digestive enzymes (mainly hydrolases) are released from the cells. Self-protective mechanisms of cells and tissues from endogenous noxae break down. Lysosome-rich organs express signs of autolysis earlier than do organs with less hydrolytic enzyme content. Autolysis develops faster in warm and hot ambient (environmental) temperatures than in cool or cold conditions and is accelerated by fever antemortem.

On external examination of the body, the earliest sign of autolysis is detectable as a whitish, cloudy appearance of the cornea. At autopsy, autolytic changes are manifest as a doughy consistency of the parenchyma of the pancreas with loss of its normal macroscopic architecture on cut surfaces. Liquefaction of the splenic pulp is another early phenomenon of autolysis that may be confused with softening of the spleen as a sequel of acute splenitis (septic spleen). The lung parenchyma contains a large number of macrophages whose lysosomes release hydrolytic enzymes, leading to a dim appearance of the outlines of cellular structures under the microscope. The adrenal glands normally retain their macroscopic appearance but appear flabby, with loss of cohesion of the medulla. In the stomach, where mucus secretion has stopped after death, gastric acid affects the mucosal surface with resultant loss of relief of the gastric mucosa. Postmortem leakage of gastric juice within the peritoneal cavity due to autolytic self-digestion has been reported to take place in rare cases. As a result of breakdown of erythrocyte membranes, hemolysis of the blood serum occurs. The intima of larger and smaller arteries becomes reddish to light brownish, and this is referred to as "imbition." This imbition is a result of a hemolytic discoloration of the inner vessel layer.

By definition, autolysis is a pure result of endogenous enzyme activity and bacterial processes play no role. However, destruction of tissue by autolysis and by bacterial processes runs a parallel course and their products overlap. Therefore, it is more an academic question than a matter of practical relevance whether superficial skin slippage is a result of pure autolysis (as considered by some authors) or whether putrefaction processes play the major part in its development.

Maceration

Maceration is sterile autolysis of an unborn fetus who has died *in utero* enclosed within the amniotic cavity. The most prominent finding at the external examination is skin slippage with underlying brownish-blackish discoloration of tissue (**Figure 18**). If the amniotic cavity has been opened prior to the delivery of a stillborn fetus, bacterial putrefaction will alter the appearance of maceration. The presence of maceration without any putrefactive changes in a recently delivered child is indicative of stillbirth.

Putrefaction

Putrefaction is the bacterial degradation of soft tissue. After death, when homeostasis ceases, anaerobic bacteria (mostly *Clostridium* and *Proteus* species) migrate from the gut into blood vessels and into tissue where they multiply and spread through the whole body.

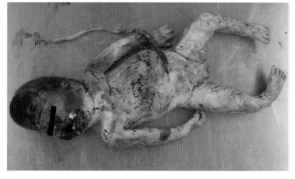

Figure 18 Manifestation of maceration in a stillbirth.

The terms "putrefaction" and "autolysis" are often used synonymously in the Anglo-American literature but these processes must be strictly differentiated since, by definition, bacterial processes play no role in the development of autolytic changes. In addition, autolysis paves the way for bacteria to spread through the body by the breakdown of cell integrity of the gut mucosa. The term "decomposition" is also often used synonymously with putrefaction. By strict definition, decomposition is the product of soft-tissue degradation by aerobic bacteria (originating from outside environmental sources), but for practical purposes this differentiation seems far too academic since both processes cannot be distinguished adequately.

Factors Accelerating the Onset of Putrefactive Tissue Changes

Many variables affect the onset, extent, and time course of putrefaction but temperature is the most decisive factor. Putrefactive tissue changes develop faster under warm and hot ambient (environmental) temperatures than under cool or cold conditions. Putrefaction is accelerated in individuals who die of systemic infections (e.g., gas gangrene, sepsis) because blood and organs have already been invaded by bacteria before death on the one hand and on the other hand, body temperature is usually raised in such fatalities at the time of death. The administration of antibiotics before death often slows down putrefaction processes. Since open wounds are a portal of entry for microorganisms from the outside environment, those who die with or from wounds that are wide open and extending far down within the subcutaneous tissue show accelerated rates of putrefaction. Obesity also accelerates the onset of putrefaction. Putrefaction is delayed in individuals with a considerable loss of blood before death since hemoglobin as well as other proteins from blood cells are a main source of energy for the bacteria involved in putrefactive processes.

Underlying Mechanisms of Putrefaction

The process of putrefaction is catalyzed by autolysis-induced breakdown products of proteins, carbohydrates, and lipids that serve the bacteria as a source of energy.

Hydrogen sulfide is the main product of reductive catalysis by endogenous bacteria. The compound of hydrogen sulfide with hemoglobin released from autolytic erythrocytes leads to the formation of sulfhemoglobin, which is responsible for the characteristic greenish discoloration of putrefied human skin and tissue.

Venous marbling, the outlining of superficial epidermal blood vessels, is the result of a combination of autolysis of erythrocytes (postmortem hemolysis) and intravascular multiplication and growth of intestinal bacteria that use blood vessels as "through roads" to spread over the entire body. Whether marbling manifests with a greenish or a more violaceous to muddy-brownish color depends on the total amount of sulfhemoglobin formation within the affected vessels.

The characteristic bloating of a putrefied body as reflected by the swelling of the face, distension of the abdomen, and, in males, scrotal swelling is a result of bacterial gas formation. On palpation, crepitus is noticed. Putrefactive gas has an offensive foul odor and is the volatile final product of bacterial reductive catalysis. It is mainly composed of methane, hydrogen sulfide, carbon dioxide, ammonia, mercaptanes, and primary amines. The purging of putrefactive fluid from mouth and nostrils as well as eversion of the lips and protrusion of the tongue are also a result of bacterial gas formation with subsequent increase in intrathoracic pressure.

Morphology of Putrefaction

The exact chronological order of the appearance of putrefactive changes is highly variable and depends on a broad variety of individual as well as environmental conditions. Therefore, it is beyond the scope of this article to give a satisfactory overview of all morphological findings and the timeframes in which they may have developed in different seasons and climatic zones. However, putrefactive body changes usually follow a sequential order.

The earliest sign of putrefaction is a greenish skin discoloration of the abdomen, usually visible first in the right lower abdominal quadrant (**Figure 19**). While this greenish skin discoloration becomes more prominent and spreads over the whole body, skin slippage with glove-like peeling of the horny skin layer of the hands, formation of gaseous or putrefactive fluid-filled skin blisters, marbling (**Figure 20**), purging of putrefactive fluid from mouth and nostrils (**Figure 21**), swelling of the face with bulging of the eyes, eversion of the lips, and protrusion of the tongue between the teeth and lips (**Figure 22**), bloating of the abdomen under tension, and, in males, scrotal swelling develop. Hair and nails become loose and can be easily pulled out. In advanced states, the skin has a brownish-blackish appearance.

Changes of internal organs as a result of putrefactive processes are dilatation of the renal pelvis and the ventricles and vestibules of the heart as a result of bacterial gas formation. Muddy-brownish putrefactive fluid is found within the pleural and peritoneal cavity. So-called "putrefaction crystals," yellowish particles composed of tyrosine and leucine, are found

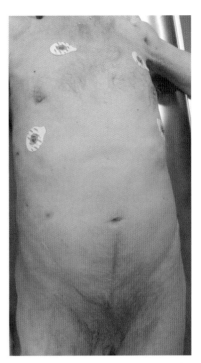

Figure 19 Greenish skin discoloration more prominent in the right than the left lower abdominal quadrant.

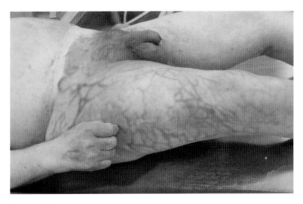

Figure 20 Marbling.

on the surface of the internal organs, especially on the surface and bottom side of the liver, adhering loosened to Glisson's capsule, as well as on the capsule of the spleen. The liver shows a spongy consistency, giving both cut sections and histologic sections in more advanced stages a Swiss-cheese-like appearance (**Figure 23**). The intestinal loops are distended due to gas formation. The myocardium appears muddy-brownish to blackish and hence, myocardial infarction easily escapes macroscopic detection. The brain appears soft to liquefied with loss of the cortical-surface structures and a dark grayish to green discoloration of cortex, caudate nucleus, and putamen. Gaseous bubble formation is seen under the mucosal surfaces of internal organs. In advanced stages of

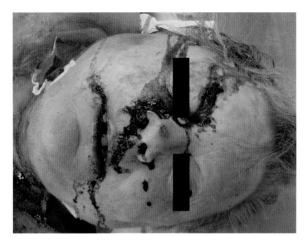

Figure 21 Purging of putrefactive fluid from mouth and nostrils.

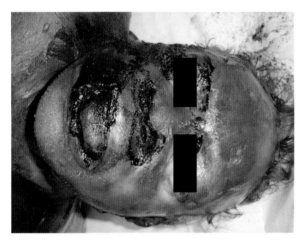

Figure 22 Marked swelling of the face with bulging of the eyes, eversion of the lips, and protrusion of the tongue. Note also purging of putrefactive fluid. It is easily understood from this photograph that visual identification of a deceased is rendered difficult in an advanced state of putrefaction.

putrefaction, the volume of bacterial gases produced is usually enough to float solid organs such as liver, kidneys, or spleen when brought into a water bowl at autopsy. The prostate gland is usually the organ offering most resistance to putrefaction and may occasionally be used to determine the gender of otherwise totally putrefied human remains.

Criminalistic Aspects

The manifestation of putrefaction may cause problems of interpretation of autopsy findings, and accordingly, death may seem suspicious. Putrefaction may mask the traumatic injuries an individual sustained before death. In addition, purging of putrefaction fluid from the mouth and nostrils is frequently confused with blood deriving from

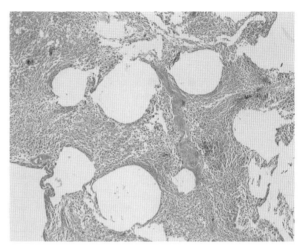

Figure 23 Swiss cheese-like appearance of the liver at histological examination (original magnification × 10, hematoxylin-eosin).

antemortem facial injuries by individuals unfamiliar with the phenomenon.

Putrefactive tissue changes may also render visual identification difficult.

Differential Diagnoses

A major problem in forensic autopsy practice is the broad variety of a number of artifacts produced in more advanced states of putrefaction as well as the possible overlapping of putrefactive tissue changes with underlying diseases, the latter being lost at gross inspection of the affected organ. Examples are the presence of froth in the heart in a putrefied body that must not be misinterpreted as air embolism, a flabby appearance of the heart due to bacterial gas production that may mimic dilatation of the ventricles and vestibules of the heart, venous marbling seen under the mucosa of the esophagus that may be mistaken for esophageal varicosis, or putrefactive liquefaction of the lung parenchyma that may be misdiagnosed as edema of the lungs. Putrefactive fluid within the pleural cavity may be mistaken for hemothorax.

Coma blisters, bullous lesions occasionally found in the setting of coma, for example, due to intoxication with barbiturates, benzodiazepines, theophylline, or in carbon monoxide poisoning, may be mistaken for skin blistering as a result of putrefaction and, vice versa, coma blisters may be overlooked when putrefactive changes of the body have begun. Concerning the differential diagnosis, coma blisters are most often seen at sites of dermal compression and appear histologically as subepidermal blister formation without any epidermal necrosis but with eosinophilic necrosis of the eccrine sweat gland coils.

Adipocere

Adipocere (synonyms: grave wax, corpse wax) is the product of the decomposition of adipose tissue formed by the hydrolysis of triglycerides into glycerine and free fatty acids. Adipocere is a grayish-white, at first waxy mass that over time becomes a crumbly to solid consistency when fatty acids crystallize, leading to the solidification of the affected body parts.

Adipocere forms in both surface and subsurface conditions as well as in embalmed and unembalmed bodies.

Various bacteria, especially *Clostridium perfringens*, seem to be involved in the formation of adipocere by playing a key role in the formation of fatty acids postmortem. The presence of water is essential for the bacterial and enzymatic processes involved in adipocere formation. However, it is now well apprehended that the formation of adipocere does not necessarily depend on the presence and persistence of moisture since the water content of adipose tissue is sufficient for the bacterial and enzymatic activity involved in adipocere formation. The presence of oxygen (e.g., exposure of the body or parts of it to air) in general inhibits adipocere formation.

Since its formation requires lipids, adipocere is more frequently seen in females, the well nourished, and the obese than in individuals with a lower adipose tissue content such as individuals who are underweight or cachectic. Apart from the external manifestation of adipocere, internal organs may be involved in adipocere formation: this finding is independent of the lipid content of the affected organs since, through the hydrolysis of triglycerides into glycerine and free fatty acids, neutral fats liquefy and penetrate into the surrounding tissue. The finding of an involvement of skeletal muscles in adipocere formation can be attributed to the same underlying mechanism.

Depending on the environmental conditions, adipocere formation may be observed as early as 1 month after death. However, the presence of adipocere usually indicates a postmortem interval of at least several months. Once formed, adipocere may remain unchanged for hundreds of years.

Adipocere formation is most often seen in corpses that have been submerged in water for a long period of time, for example, bodies recovered from shipwrecks. The rate of development of adipocere in immersed corpses has been related to the water temperature and it was long assumed that adipocere formation is accelerated by higher water temperature. However, recent investigations do not regard the temperature of the water as essential for speed of adipocere development.

Apart from the resting time, the manifestation of adipocere in buried human remains depends on a variety of individual factors such as the geographical location of the burial site, season of burial, vegetation of the burial site, depth of the grave, insect colonization of the corpse before burial, and other anthropogenic influences (for example, if a body is easily accessible to insects, adipocere is unlikely to form), the composition of the coffin used, and the texture of the soil (chemical and physical soil properties).

Mummification and skeletonization may accompany adipocere formation but usually adipocere formation is accompanied by an increase in the volume of the affected body. A preferential formation of adipocere has been observed in body parts with open wounds, thus paving the way for clostridial colonization.

Mummification

Mummification is the product of desiccation, the drying-up process of soft tissue. Mummification may affect the entire body or only parts of it when only distinct portions of the body have been exposed to the proper environmental conditions. Natural mummification occurs in dry, usually hot climatological conditions. However, mummification also occurs in bodies located in frozen environments; mummified human bodies found in polar regions or in glaciers after hundreds of years are of special interest from the archeological and anthropological points of view.

Artificial mummification for the purpose of soft-tissue preservation has been practiced throughout time in prehistoric cultures, especially in regions in which climatological conditions favor natural mummification.

During the process of mummification, soft tissue undergoes considerable shrinkage by losing body fluids via evaporation, resulting in considerable loss of body weight (up to 60–70%). The skin turns hard and has a brown to black leathery appearance (**Figure 24**), forming a thick shell over the body. Eventually all the hair disappears. In mummified bodies, the arms are often found abducted in the shoulder joints, flexed in the elbow joints, and the hands are clenched into fists in most cases. This flexion is also often recognizable in the lower limbs. The reason for this phenomenon is the shrinkage of muscles and tendons, causing flexion in the joints of the extremities due to predominance of the flexor muscles.

Despite dehydration of the body surface, the internal organs become dark, viscous, and paste-like. With the increase in the postmortem interval and under the

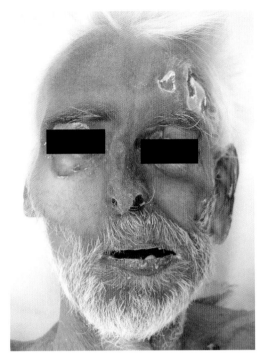

Figure 24 Natural mummification. Brown to black leathery appearance of the skin.

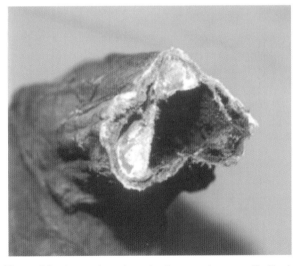

Figure 25 Cut sections through a forearm of a mummified body with total loss of muscles and soft tissue.

influence of putrefaction and maggot activity, the internal organs undergo considerable shrinkage and may vanish totally. On cut sections through the limbs, a total loss of muscles and soft tissue may be seen in advanced stages of mummification (**Figure 25**). Although some authors consider that microscopic examination of remnants of internal organs in bodies presenting in advanced states of mummification is unrewarding, this author has more than once seen cases where a precise histologic diagnosis relating to underlying diseases (e.g., bronchopneumonia, liver cirrhosis, carcinoma) could be established in mummified human remains even after postmortem intervals of up to several years.

Artifacts caused by insects on mummified corpses (e.g., holes made by maggots) may appear greater than they were before mummification due to the shrinkage of tissue; they should not be confused with stab wounds or shotgun pellet holes.

The appearance of mummified corpses may be modified by scavenger activity and bones may be lost due to animal activity. Occasionally, rodents nests may be found inside body cavities in mummified corpses.

Primary and Secondary Mummification

Two types of mummification are of general forensic interest: primary and secondary mummification. Primary mummification is generally not accompanied by relevant putrefaction processes of the affected body and will therefore predominantly occur in environmental conditions that favor a rapid drying of soft tissues, preventing enteric bacteria and microorganisms from outside causing relevant putrefaction. Secondary mummification by definition follows considerable putrefaction of the body. Secondary mummification of human bodies found in open spaces is seen more often than in bodies in indoor settings.

Skeletonization

Skeletonization (synonym: skeletalization) is the total or partial loss of soft tissue (complete or incomplete skeletonization, respectively) with resultant exposure of bones. Incomplete skeletonization may proceed to complete skeletonization but this does not necessarily take place since only discrete portions of the body may be exposed to the proper environmental conditions (**Figure 26**).

The length of the postmortem interval needed for skeletonization of a body or parts of it is highly variable and mainly depends on the ambient temperature, insect colonization of the body, and scavenger activity. Under warm to hot environmental conditions, and increasingly under the influence of moisture, aerobic bacterial activity from the outside is accelerated with resultant advanced manifestation of odor of the body, attracting insects and scavengers to the body. Skeletonization and mummification often occur together in different or identical parts of the body (**Figure 27**).

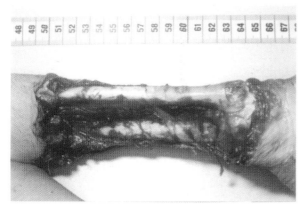

Figure 26 Incomplete skeletonization of a forearm due to postmortem animal scavenging by a domestic German Shepherd.

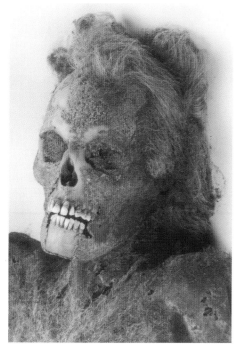

Figure 27 Co-occurrence of skeletonization and mummification.

Usually all skin, soft tissue, and muscles are lost before a skeleton becomes disarticulated. Disarticulation of bones in skeletonized bodies is more often seen to take place from the head downward and from central to peripheral than in the reverse way.

Postmortem Preservation by Freezing

Artificial Postmortem Preservation by Freezing

If a body has been frozen immediately after death, for instance in a freezer with the aim of hiding the corpse, the rate of postmortem changes slows virtually to zero. When a corpse is first frozen, for example, before dumping the body to conceal the time of death and confuse the investigating authorities, and then exposed to warm ambient temperatures, more advanced putrefaction is usually observed on the outer body surface than internally. The reason for this phenomenon is that in such cases the enteric flow has most often been put to death before any relevant putrefaction of the viscera could occur. Accordingly, anaerobic bacteria from the outside will have a greater effect on putrefaction of the exterior surface of the body than on the inside within the same time span after the corpse is defrosted. In addition, ice crystal artifacts may be seen in histological sections of the myocardium, corroborating such an assumption.

Freeze-Drying

Freeze-drying, the process of body preservation mediated by sublimation, is predominantly seen in bodies recovered from polar regions and permafrost zones in Siberia or the Middle East. Such bodies are usually well preserved externally and internally, or may show mummification. When freeze-dried bodies are mummified, the internal organs are usually better preserved than in cases where mummification occurred under hot environmental conditions.

Miscellaneous

Postmortem Changes and Injuries to the Skin

Injuries due to handling, transportation, and storage of the body   Abrasions and lacerations on the skin may be produced by manipulation of the body during postmortem handling, transportation, and storage. When arising in the early postmortem interval (but only in cases where the epidermis is still intact and no postmortem skin slippage has occurred as a result of autolysis and/or putrefaction), these postmortem injuries are relatively easily distinguished from vitally acquired injuries by their light yellowish-brownish to golden, shiny appearance (**Figure 28**). They result from loss of the barrier function of the epidermal layer with subsequent evaporation of tissue fluid. In doubtful cases, incision of cutaneous injuries of postmortem origin will reveal a hardened, slightly flattened area on cut sections without any hemorrhage in the underlying soft tissue.

In skin areas where the epidermis is very thin (e.g., the tip of the nose and the scrotum), drying as a result of postmortem evaporation of tissue fluids occurs.

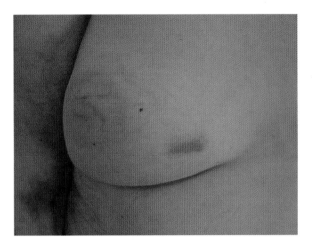

Figure 28 Superficial postmortem injury upon the skin with a light yellowish-brownish to golden, shiny appearance.

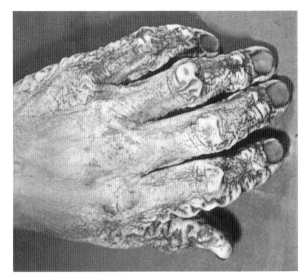

Figure 29 Washer-woman's skin in a drowning victim.

The result is a hardened, light-brownish appearance of the affected epidermal surfaces (sometimes referred to as the earliest stage of mummification).

Skin changes produced by corrosives Corrosives such as acids or alkalis may lead to loss of the epidermal layer of the skin. In particular, gastric juice running out during handling or transportation of the body may produce pale, sometimes band-like, cutaneous alterations that should not be confused with ligature marks when located on the neck.

Skin changes produced by postmortem urine leaking Postmortem urine leaking may cause extensive skin damage to a child on the perigenital skin areas that were in contact with a urine-soaked diaper postmortem. Such postmortem skin changes should be differentiated from vitally acquired alterations and not interpreted uncritically as signs of child neglect before death.

No vital reaction will be detected in any of the aforementioned skin alterations by microscopic examination.

Washerwoman's skin In bodies recovered from water or moist environments, the skin of the palms of the hands and the feet has whitish discoloration of the epidermis associated with swelling, wrinkling, and vesicular detachment up to glove-like peeling, mainly as a result of soaking of the horny layer of the epidermis. This finding, referred to as washerwoman's skin, that is especially seen after prolonged exposure to water in drowning deaths (**Figure 29**), should not be confused with another form of skin change seen on the palms of the hands and the soles of the feet and caused by heat. In the latter case,

histological examination shows fluid-filled blisters in the stratum germinativum, hyperchromasia, and palisade arrangement of the nuclei as well as clumping of the erythrocytes corresponding to a morphological variation of a second-degree burn due to the special anatomy of friction skin.

Drying of Mucosal Surfaces

Postmortem evaporation of tissue fluids and hypostasis after cessation of circulation leads to drying of mucosal surfaces, for example, of the lips, the tip of the tongue, the glans of the penis, the glans of the clitoris, or the pudendal lips, resulting in a hardened, light to dark brownish appearance of the affected mucosal surfaces.

External Changes of the Eye after Death

As with most postmortem changes, alterations of the eye after death are accelerated in their onset and intensity under warm ambient temperatures and in dry climates.

Under moderate to cool ambient temperatures, 3–9 h after death, the cornea has a whitish, cloudy appearance as a result of autolysis. With further increase in postmortem interval, the cornea loses its turgor.

If the eyes remain open after death, the areas of the sclera exposed to air dry out; this results first in a yellowish discoloration that subsequently turns into a brownish-blackish band-like zone called "tache noire" (**Figure 30**).

The conjunctivae soften and become a light grayish color. In states of advanced putrefaction, conjunctival petechiae, for example, as a result of asphyxia, may not be distinguished due to hemolysis and

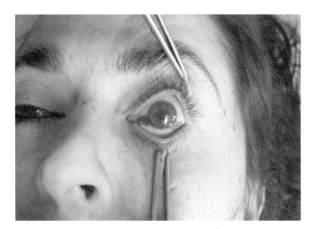

Figure 30   Tache noir.

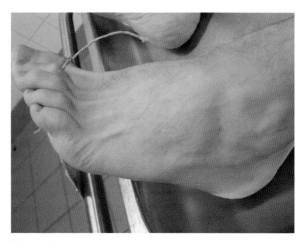

Figure 31   Postmortem hypostasis in the lateral sub-malleolar muscles.

sulfhemoglobin production, giving the conjunctivae a homogeneous grayish to light greenish appearance.

Pink Teeth and Nails Phenomenon

Pink discoloration of teeth and nails is a rare postmortem finding that is thought to derive from hemolysis after exudation of hemoglobin and hemoglobin derivates. This phenomenon seems to depend on the anatomical presence of porous structures, an anatomic feature that is found in the dentine tubules of the crowns and roots (but not in the enamel, which is more compact and therefore not colored) of the teeth as well as in the fingernails and toenails. The overwhelming majority of observations of this phenomenon have been described in association with premortem cranial blood congestion, particularly in asphyxial deaths such as strangulation, death in a head-down position, and drowning. Pink discoloration of teeth and nails has been reported even after postmortem intervals of several months.

Submalleolar and Thenar Eminence Hypostasis

Postmortem hypostasis in the muscles located in the lateral submalleolar region (**Figure 31**) and the thenar eminence may mimic antemortem bruising. An incision will show lack of hemorrhage within the muscle tissue.

Fungi

Fungi may colonize the body in every possible location and at all times during the postmortem interval. However, the eyes are more often affected by fungal colonization under dry conditions and the mouth and nose are more often colonized with fungi in moist to wet environments (**Figure 32**). Fungi may mimic antemortem pouring of chemical substances over the body.

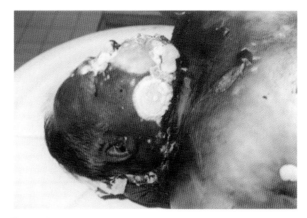

Figure 32   Fungi colonization most prominent around nose and mouth in a body exhumed 4 months after death.

Arthropods

A large number of arthropod species are attracted to human bodies after death, primarily flies (Diptera), beetles (Coleoptera), and their larvae. The arthropods feed, live, or breed in and on the corpse, depending on their biological preferences, and on the state of body decomposition. Most arthropod species colonize a corpse for only a limited period of time ("faunal succession").

Criminalistic aspects   By calculating their developmental stages, arthropods are useful in estimating the time that a corpse has been inhabited by animals ("colonization interval"), and this opens up a wide range of applications for forensic entomology embedded in a criminalistic context. Apart from useful information concerning the estimation of time since death or the time a body was stored in particular environmental conditions at a specific place, additional information can be obtained from arthropods, that is, found on or in corpses, at a scene of crime, at the place where a body had been dumped, or on the clothing of a suspect. In specific cases, a suspect may be linked to the scene of crime as a result of arthropods found on the soles of the shoes. Arthropods that live in restricted areas and are found on a corpse in a different area may prove that the body was moved after death, while blowfly larvae can give information on how long children or elderly people were subjected to neglectful care. An experienced forensic entomologist can make such conclusions, but regularly requires at least baseline data concerning the local area such as the time of appearance of arthropods and data on temperature ranges.

Cutaneous holes and soft-tissue defects, for example, made by maggots, especially when overlapped by tissue shrinkage due to mummification with resulting enlargement of the defects, can mimic gunshot wounds or other mechanical tissue defects sustained antemortem, for example, as a result of stabbing with pointed instruments such as knives or scissors.

Animal Depredation

The phenomenon of postmortem animal interference with human bodies or their remains is a substantial part of the taphonomic processes a body undergoes after death and animal depredation occurring after death is routinely encountered in forensic pathology. Postmortem injuries can be inflicted by all kinds of animals, irrespective of their size or environmental origin, whether from land, sea, or air. The discrimination between antemortem injury versus postmortem artifacts generally presents no difficulties because of the total absence of hemorrhages and reddening in the tissue adjacent to the wound margins (**Figure 33**) and the lack of any vital reaction under the microscope.

The most effective tissue removers are insects and rodents. Skin and soft-tissue artifacts caused by rodents may occur as early as within the first hour postmortem. In the majority of injuries inflicted postmortem by rodents, the wounds have a circular appearance (**Figure 34**) and the wound margins are finely serrated, showing irregular edges. Distinct parallel series of cutaneous lacerations deriving from the biting action of the upper and lower pairs of the rodent's incisors are diagnostic of rodent activity (**Figure 35**). However, the determination of a distinct rodent species (e.g., rats, mice) by the morphological appearance of the damage to skin and soft tissue is often unconvincing.

A broad range of carnivores may be involved in the postmortem destruction of corpses located in open

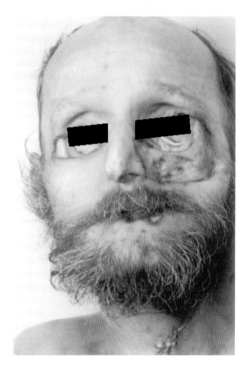

Figure 33 Circular defects around both eyes due to mixed rodent activity. Note the total absence of hemorrhages and reddening in the tissue adjacent to the wound margins indicative of postmortem origin of the wounds.

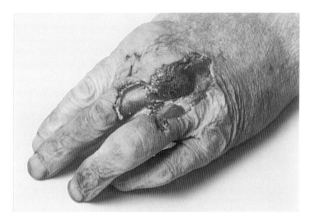

Figure 34 Circular skin and soft tissue defect on the back of the hand caused postmortem by mice.

spaces or indoors (e.g., wild animals such as foxes and big cats or domestic animals such as dogs or cats). The wound margins caused by carnivores often appear more regular than those caused by rodents (**Figure 36**). V-shaped to rhomboid punctured wounds are often seen in the intact skin in the immediate vicinity of the actual wound margins (**Figure 37**). Such stab-wound-like defects represent canine tooth marks of carnivore origin. An additional criterion of animal depredation by carnivores is

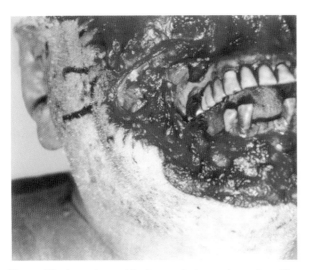

Figure 35 Irregular and finely serrated wound margins with a series of parallel cutaneous lacerations deriving from the biting action of the upper and lower pairs of rodents. This large tissue defect in the face was caused postmortem by rats.

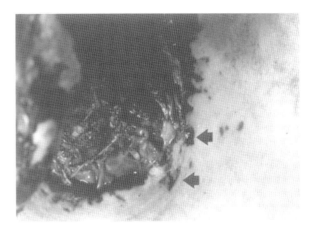

Figure 37 V-shaped to rhomboid punctured wounds are seen in the intact skin next to the wound margin. Such stab wound like defects represent canine tooth marks of carnivore origin (same case as **Figure 36**).

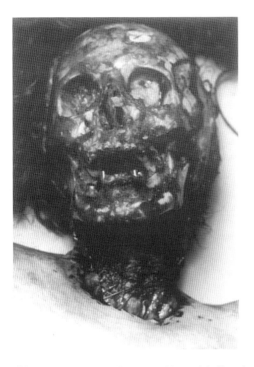

Figure 36 Postmortem injuries caused by a pit bull terrier.

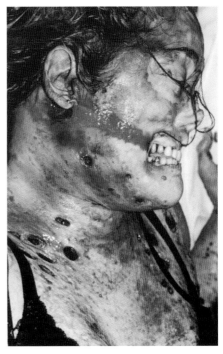

Figure 38 Oval to round cutaneous defects caused by crustaceans postmortem on the neck and upper trunk in a drowning victim. Such injuries should not be confused with stab wounds or gunshot holes.

the presence of claw-induced linear scratch-type abrasions in the vicinity of the damaged skin areas.

In drowning victims or persons whose death led to their deposition in water or when a body has been dumped in an aquatic environment, postmortem artifacts on the body surface due to aquatic living structures are often observed, too, and should not be confused with vitally acquired injuries (**Figure 38**).

See Also

Autopsy: Procedures and Standards; **Autopsy, Findings:** Postmortem Drug Sampling and Redistribution; Organic Toxins; Drowning; **Carbon Monoxide Poisoning:** Incidence and Findings at Postmortem; **Postmortem Changes:** Postmortem Interval; **Toxicology:** Methods of Analysis, Postmortem

Further Reading

Benecke M (2004) Forensic entomology: arthropods on corpses. In: Tsokos M (ed.) *Forensic Pathology Reviews*, vol. 2, pp. 207–240. Totowa, NJ: Humana Press.

Byard RW (2004) Medicolegal problems with neonaticide. In: Tsokos M (ed.) *Forensic Pathology Reviews*, vol. 1, pp. 171–185. Totowa, NJ: Humana Press.

Clark MA, Worrell MB, Pless JE (1997) Postmortem changes in soft tissues. In: Haglund D, Sorg MH (eds.) *Forensic Taphonomy. The Postmortem Fate of Human Remains*, pp. 151–164. Boca Raton, FL: CRC Press.

DiMaio VJ, DiMaio D (2001) *Forensic Pathology*, 2nd edn. Boca Raton, FL: CRC Press.

Fiedler S, Graw M (2003) Decomposition of buried corpses, with special reference to the formation of adipocere. *Naturwissenschaften* 90: 291–300.

Gill-King H (1997) Chemical and ultrastructural aspects of decomposition. In: Haglund D, Sorg MH (eds.) *Forensic Taphonomy. The Postmortem Fate of Human Remains*, pp. 93–108. Boca Raton, FL: CRC Press.

Kahana T, Almog J, Levy J, *et al.* (1999) Marine taphonomy: adipocere formation in a series of bodies recovered from a single shipwreck. *Journal of Forensic Science* 44: 897–901.

Knight B, Nokes L (2002) Temperature-based methods I. In: Knight B (ed.) *The Estimation of the Time Since Death in the Early Postmortem Period*, 2nd edn., pp. 3–42. London: Arnold.

Nokes L, Madea B, Knight B (2002) Changes after death. In: Knight B (ed.) *The Estimation of the Time Since Death in the Early Postmortem Period*, 2nd edn., pp. 209–243. London: Arnold.

Rutty GN (2001) Post-mortem changes and artefacts. In: Rutty GN (ed.) *Essentials of Autopsy Practice*, vol. 1, pp. 63–95. London: Springer-Verlag.

Tsokos M, Matschke J, Gehl A, Koops E, Püschel K (1999) Skin and soft tissue artifacts due to postmortem damage caused by rodents. *Forensic Science International* 104: 47–57.

Electrolyte Disturbances

L M Al-Alousi, Leicester Royal Infirmary, Leicester, UK

Introduction

Brief Historical Consideration

The postmortem chemistry of the blood and some other body fluids has been the subject of extensive and often elaborate and tedious investigations for a century or so. As early as the mid-1920s, Paul as well as Pucher and Burd had published on the "postmortem chemical determinations" of the blood and the cerebrospinal fluid (CSF). Among the earliest substances studied were electrolytes such as sodium (Na^+), chloride (Cl^-), and potassium (K^+) ions. Primarily, these research works had been clinically orientated especially in relation to the diagnosis of renal diseases. But forensic applications of the postmortem chemistry had soon become an established area for large numbers of forensically tailored studies. In the 1940s and 1950s, Jetter and McLean as well as Naumann, amongst other researchers, had published their classical works on the postmortem analysis of electrolytes in various body fluids such as the blood, CSF, and the vitreous humor. In 1963, Evans published his book "The Chemistry of Death" in which he discussed the chemistry of various tissues in the early and late postmortem periods. Since the late 1960s and early 1970s, Coe had published several papers rightly considered by many as landmarks in this field. This topic does still attract considerable interest from forensic scientists as is evident by the large volume of recent literature that exists today. A number of useful reviews are provided in this article.

Physiological Aspects and Definitions of Terms

An electrolyte is a substance that when dissolved in water separates into ions and is able to conduct electricity by movements of ions. Thus, electrolyte disturbances cannot be discussed without an understanding of the body fluid balance. Electrolytes are measured in milliequivalents per liter ($mEq\,l^{-1}$). For ions having a single charge, e.g., Na^+, K^+, Cl^-, or HCO_3^-, the number of $mEq\,l^{-1}$ equals the number of $mmol\,l^{-1}$ and for ions having two charges such as Ca^{2+}, Mg^{2+}, or phosphate HPO_4^{2-}, the number of $mEq\,l^{-1}$ is twice the number of $mmol\,l^{-1}$. Two-thirds of body fluid is within the cells and called intracellular fluid (ICF) and the rest is outside the cells and called extracellular fluid (ECF). Interstitial fluid (ISF), i.e., fluid in between the cells, constitutes about 80% of the ECF and plasma (blood) forms the other 20% of the ECF, which also includes many other body fluids, such as the CSF, aqueous and vitreous humors, and lymph and pleural, pericardial, peritoneal, and synovial fluids. During life, cell membranes separate the ICF from the ISF and blood vessel walls divide ISF from plasma although at the level of capillaries, plasma and ISF may exchange with each other, as the capillary wall is thin and permeable. In life, the amounts of water and solutes (electrolytes and inorganic ions) in various body fluids are continuously corrected so that the volume of each fluid type remains fairly stable. This is called fluid balance, which depends on electrolyte balance and vice versa. By the same token, acid–base balance means that the amounts of acids and bases, determined by H^+ and HCO_3^- (i.e., another form of electrolyte balance), are continuously corrected during life so as to keep the pH of each body fluid within a fairly stable range; the pH of arterial blood in a healthy adult is usually 7.35–7.45. This is regulated by various buffer systems, which means the mechanisms that enable the body to convert strong acids and bases to weak acids and bases. During life, water constitutes about 45–75% of total body mass depending on age and gender. Under normal conditions, water and electrolyte gain and loss are regulated hand in hand, i.e., "water follows salt." The ultimate source of water and electrolyte gain is via ingestion (about 2300 ml of water daily) although metabolism produces a small amount called "metabolic water" (about 200 ml daily). On the other hand the body loses about 2500 ml of water daily by kidneys (1500 ml), skin (600 ml), lungs (300 ml), and via feces (100 ml). Most electrolytes are absorbed through the small intestines by active transportation, passive diffusion, or both. For example, sodium is absorbed first by diffusion into the intestinal epithelium then transported out by active sodium pumps (Na^+/K^+ ATPase). Chloride and most anions can passively follow sodium, whereas potassium, calcium, phosphate, and many other electrolytes are absorbed by active transportation. The electrolyte contents of ECF and ICF are different: sodium and chloride are most abundant in the former and potassium, magnesium, and phosphate are most abundant in the latter. During life, this is maintained via active Na^+/K^+ pumps at the cellular membrane. Homeostasis is the condition in which the contents of the body fluid compartments are maintained relatively constant within physiological limits.

Disease, Death, and Electrolytes

During life, when electrolyte contents of body fluids are disturbed beyond homeostatic limits, pathological conditions (with or without signs and symptoms), diseases, or even death may follow (Table 1). In fact, many think that the mechanism of almost any death is basically biochemical in origin, which is largely due to electrolyte disturbances. This effectively means that every death is associated with at least some electrolyte disturbances. This complicates the interpretation of postmortem results and restricts the usefulness of electrolyte analysis after death. At and after the somatic death, i.e., when the body ceases to function as a whole entity, body cells are confronted with three

Table 1 Blood electrolyte disturbances and associated diseases

Electrolyte (Normal adult values)	Pathological condition	
	Deficiency	Excess
Sodium (Na^+) 136–148 mEq l^{-1}	Hyponatremia E.g., starvation, neglect, sun stroke, vomiting, diarrhea, burns, alcohol and/or drug intoxication, diuretic abuse, renal disease, water intoxication (a form of child abuse)	Hypernatremia E.g., high sodium diet and salt intoxication (a form of child abuse); decreased sodium loss due to renal impairment, hyperthermia, drug and alcohol intoxication, low water intake in dehydration and starvation
Chloride (Cl^-) 95–105 mEq l^{-1}	Hypochloremia E.g., excessive vomiting, over-hydration, aldosterone deficiency, congestive heart failure and therapy with some diuretics (e.g., furosemide (frusemide)).	Hyperchloremia E.g., dehydration, starvation, neglect, severe renal failure, hyperaldosteronism, and excessive chloride intake
Potassium (K^+) 3.5–5.0 mEq l^{-1}	Hypokalemia E.g., vomiting or diarrhea, hyperaldosteronism, kidney disease or some diuretics therapy	Hyperkalemia E.g., renal failure, crushing injuries to body tissues, severe burns, or hemolyzed blood transfusion
Calcium (Ca^{2+}) Total = 9–10.5 mEq l^{-1}	Hypocalcemia E.g., hypoparathyroidism, elevated phosphate levels or low calcium intake	Hypercalcemia E.g., hyperparathyroidism, some cancers, excessive vitamin D, and Paget's disease of bone
Magnesium (Mg^{2+}) 1.3–2.1 mEq l^{-1}	Hypomagnesemia E.g., alcoholism, congestive cardiac failure, diabetes mellitus, and some diuretics therapy	Hypermagnesemia E.g., some antacids high intake, aldosterone deficiency, and hypothyroidism
Phosphate (HPO_4^{2-}) 1.7–2.6 mEq l^{-1}	Hypophosphatemia E.g., disturbances in gastrointestinal and renal functions and aldosterone	Hyperphosphatemia E.g., renal failure and hemolytic anemias

Data from Tortora GI and Grobowski SR (2000) *Principles of Anatomy and Physiology*, 9th edn., pp. 613, 856, and 965–973. New York: John Wiley & Sons, Inc.

major events or phenomena, which have profound effect on the ability of the body to maintain its homeostatic contents. First, hypoxia or anoxia, i.e., lack or deficiency of oxygen (O_2) at the tissue or cell level, increases the permeability of the cell membrane and blood vessel wall leading to leaking of the ICF, ECF, ISF, and the plasma to each other. Also, the lack of O_2 causes changes in the pH of the blood and other body fluids leading to further disturbances in fluid contents including electrolytes. Second, lack of energy due to the death process leads to the abrupt or gradual cessation of the active electrolyte pumps across the cell membrane including that of the alimentary system and vascular wall cells. Therefore, electrolyte movements through various body compartments are not maintained according to the physiological requirements but rather follow physical laws governed principally by gravity and simple physical diffusion leading to drastic pH and electrolyte disturbances. Third, the processes of autolysis and cell disintegration in general cause breakdown of the cell membrane leading to virtually complete mix-up of various body fluids. The end result is a dramatic and unpredictable change of electrolyte contents of body fluids.

Limitations of Postmortem Electrolyte Interpretations

The analysis of electrolytes (and in fact, other chemicals) of body fluids after death has been used for the following purposes: estimation of the postmortem interval (PMI); diagnosis of the cause of death; and evaluation of certain anatomical disorders. Practically, it is virtually unviable to find a meaningful way for the analysis of postmortem electrolyte contents of ICF and ISF. Therefore, most or all studies of electrolytes after death are conducted on a small ECF fraction, namely, the vitreous humor, CSF, and the blood. However, because of the hemolysis of the red cells, a postmortem blood sample is, in reality, a mixture of intravascular ICF and ECF. Moreover, due to general breakdown of the cell membrane after death, body fluid compartments ooze into each other and fluids are mixed up together to extents that vary with tissue temperature and pH, environmental temperature, time, cause and mode of death, and other factors. Also, as electrolyte movements after death follow almost pure physical laws such as the gravity laws, the electrolyte contents of a postmortem sample are understandably site-related. For example, in recent years, several workers such as Balasooriya and Hill, Madea and coworkers, and Pounder and coworkers have pointed out significant quantitative between-eye electrolyte differences. Regardless of the

type of body fluid and the location of sampling, individual variations in electrolyte contents are known to exist during life and continue to exist or even widen after death. Besides these individual variations, there are other factors that tend to add uncertainties to the already highly erratic and unpredictable postmortem electrolyte levels. Examples of these factors and uncertainties are the subtle biochemical conditions that exist in life (**Table 1**) and pass unnoticed or undiagnosed after death so that the subject or the sample is marked as normal or a control. Other examples include the mysterious effect of the agony of the moment of death and the uncontrolled influence of the conditions and length of sample storage.

Forensic Applications

It follows from the above discussion that a postmortem electrolyte level found in a given body fluid roughly indicates the value of that electrolyte in that body fluid during life ± the net effect of various factors such as:

- the length of the interval of death or the PMI
- cellular pH and temperature
- environmental temperature
- mode and cause of death
- individual variations
- effects of the agony of death
- presence or absence of undiagnosed minor biochemical conditions during life or at the moment of death
- the pathological conditions that existed antemortem.

Therefore, the overall picture is rather complex, which is reflected in the many inconsistencies and irregularities found in the results of most postmortem electrolyte studies. This remark together with the observation that most chemical methods are cumbersome, expensive, time-consuming, require special machinery, and yet, in most instances yield difficult results to interpret or practically unreliable conclusions have made many leading field workers consider that chemical methods are of limited practical value and the postmortem electrolyte analysis is not an exception to this.

Nevertheless, the study of electrolyte changes after death is, at least from theoretical and academic points of view, of some value in the following situations.

Assessment of certain antemortem conditions or disorders In renal disease, Coe has used hypernatremia accompanied with mild degrees of urea retention as "good" evidence of dehydration. Most patholo-gists, however, would be reluctant to use such an inference in medicolegal reports prepared for a court of law. In cases of electrolyte imbalance, Coe has studied a large number of cases and suggested four patterns:

1. "Dehydration pattern" is characterized by increased vitreous sodium and chloride (>155 and $>135\,\mathrm{mEq\,l^{-1}}$ respectively) and moderate increase of urea nitrogen ($40–100\,\mathrm{mEq\,l^{-1}}$). This pattern may be found in cases of neglect, salt intoxication, and starvation (all can be rare forms of child abuse).
2. "Uremia pattern" is characterized by marked increases of vitreous urea and creatinine without significant increases in sodium or chloride. This can be seen in renal disease.
3. "Low-salt pattern" is characterized by low vitre-ous sodium, chloride, and potassium (<130, <105, $<15\,\mathrm{mEq\,l^{-1}}$ respectively) associated with some increase of serum bilirubin and urea nitrogen $<5\,\mathrm{mg\,100\,ml^{-1}}$. This pattern is most likely seen in chronic alcoholics.
4. "Decomposition pattern" is characterized by low vitreous sodium and chloride but high potassium indicating a long postmortem interval (<130, <105, and $>20\,\mathrm{mEq\,l^{-1}}$ respectively).

In cases of asphyxia vs. cardiac arrhythmia, studies of blood gases are not consistent and must be viewed with caution. Although many modern neuro-researchers would like to link epilepsy with abnormalities of $Na^+/K^+/Ca^{2+}$ channels (channelo-pathies), this is largely a molecular genetic problem and, therefore, the implication on forensic post-mortem chemistry is of no or little consequence. Recently, Delva has described trends to link various forms of congestive heart failure and some cardio-myopathies to magnesium deficiency. He also em-phasized the important role played by magnesium in the operation of the sodium/potassium pumps (Na^+/K^+ ATPase).

Confirmation of the cause of death The only exam-ple in forensic medicine is that of drowning in salt water and river water. "Biochemical tests" of the blood obtained from the right and left sides of the heart have been postulated to differentiate be-tween these two types of drowning, but, unfortunate-ly, most results of the so-called "biochemical tests" have been shown to be unreliable. Recently, Zhu and coworkers described new serum markers for the differentiation between fresh and salt water drown-ing. They reported that the characteristic feature

of salt water drowning was a low left–right blood urea nitrogen (BUN) ratio and marked increase in the serum chloride, magnesium, and calcium levels of the left heart blood. Azparren and coworkers stud-ied the left–right ventricular blood strontium (Sr) concentration as a marker for drowning and claimed that this test had yielded a highly significant positive result.

Estimation of the time of death Chemical approaches for the timing of death form the second most commonly investigated techniques after the temperature-based methods. However, many of these studies are made on substances other than electro-lytes. Nonetheless, one of the electrolytes, i.e., the vitreous K^+, is correctly considered as the most reli-able of all chemical methods. It is worth noting, that, in general, the chemical methods for estimating the time since death are widely considered as the least reliable and the least practicable of all other methods. Almost all types of electrolytes have been studied for the purpose of the estimation of PMI. The most notable of these are Na^+, Cl^-, K^+, Ca^{2+}, P^{3-} or P^{5-}, S^{2-}, and Mg^{2+}.

Sodium (Na^+)
Blood Blood or serum sodium was shown to de-crease quickly after death but the rate of decrease involved large individual variations and although it was estimated at $0.9\,\mathrm{mEq\,l^{-1}\,h^{-1}}$, visualizing the plot of the scattered Na^+ values indicates that the least-square regression used was meaningless. Recently, Singh and coworkers claimed a highly significant relationship between logarithms of serum Na^+ and K^+ concentrations, Na^+/K^+ ratio, and PMI within the first 3–58 h after death. Yet they noted that these variables were significantly affected by other factors, such as environmental temperature, cause of death, age, and gender.

Cerebrospinal fluid (CSF) Naumann showed that the concentrations of many of the CSF electrolytes including sodium, chloride, potassium, calcium, mag-nesium, and phosphorus generally decrease after death. However, this decrease was noticeably erratic to the extent that it could not be used for any sensible timing of death. Fekete and Brunsden made similar observations.

Vitreous humor (VH) Jaffe and Coe demonstrated that vitreous sodium is stable for the first 30 h after death and in a study of 145 normal adults, Coe found that vitreous sodium concentrations ranged from 135 to 151 $\mathrm{mEq\,l^{-1}}$ with an average value at 143 $\mathrm{mEq\,l^{-1}}$.

Synovial fluid Madea and coworkers compared the sodium contents of synovial fluid (SF) with that of VH in 74 normal adults and found that the concentrations in both fluids were comparable. In the SF, they found that Na^+ values ranged from 86 to $164\,mmol\,l^{-1}$ ($=mEq\,l^{-1}$) with the median at $145\,mmol\,l^{-1}$.

Chloride (Cl^-)

Blood Jetter, Schyler and Coe have all reported a decrease in the plasma or blood chloride after death with average concentrations ranging roughly between 80 and $90\,mEq\,l^{-1}$ and a postmortem decrease of 0.25–$0.97\,mEq\,l^{-1}\,h^{-1}$. However, looking at the scatter plot, the so-called least-squares correlation appears meaningless. Recently, Singh and coworkers claimed a highly significant relationship between logarithms of plasma chloride and PMI within the first 3–58 h after death, yielding a standard error of $\pm2.1\,h$. However, they stated that this was significantly influenced by other factors, e.g., environmental temperature, cause of death, age, and gender.

Vitreous humor (VH) Coe reported that vitreous chloride, like sodium, remained constant for the first 18 h after death with a concentration ranging between 104 and $132\,mEq\,l^{-1}$ and an average of $120\,mEq\,l^{-1}$.

Synovial fluid The levels of synovial chloride were reported by Madea and coworkers in 65 cases to range between 49 and 116 with a median value at $100\,mEq\,l^{-1}$.

Potassium (K^+)

Blood Blood or plasma potassium increases so rapidly after death that its use for the estimation of the time of death is virtually impossible. Jetter reported that within the first hour or so after death, serum K^+ increases to $18\,mEq\,l^{-1}$ followed by further albeit gradual increase.

Vitreous humor (VH) Many investigators have noted that the rise in the levels of vitreous potassium after death is the most reliable chemical marker for estimating the PMI. Jaffe was the first to note that vitreous K^+ increases after death at a regular rate. Subsequently, many workers including Adelson and coworkers, Coe, and others had reinforced this observation. Although there was a general agreement that the rise in the vitreous potassium was roughly arithmetic, there were wide variations in the degree of correlation between the vitreous potassium concentration and the PMI. These discrepancies were

reflected in the large differences of the standard deviations (SD) of the time estimates found by various investigators. For instance, while Sturner and Lie reported $\pm5\,h$, Adelson, Hughes, Hanson, and Coe had all reported more than $\pm10\,h$. In fact, Hanson and coworkers, in a series of 203 cases found $\pm20\,h$ (1 SD). Marchenko (cited by Madea) in a series of 300 cases found vast individual variations and he concluded that vitreous potassium was only useful within 3–6 h. Krause and coworkers (cited by Madea) demonstrated even worse correlation than the above and showed a range of scatter between 9 and 107 h for potassium values between 5 and $28\,mEq\,l^{-1}$. In view of these wide variations, many researchers attempted to refine the potassium method. Thus, Adjutantis and Coutselinis claimed to have achieved $\pm1.1\,h$ within the first 12 h of death by analyzing bilateral samples withdrawn at 3 hourly intervals and extrapolating back to the "normal" vitreous K^+ value at the moment of death at $3.4\,mEq\,l^{-1}$. Madea and coworkers used selective methods by analyzing the vitreous humor for both potassium and urea (as an internal standard) so as to exclude the cases where there was, in their view, antemortem K^+ imbalance. They carried out extensive mathematical calculations and attempted several maneuvers only to narrow the confidence limit by $<4\,h$ (from ±25.51 to $\pm21.78\,h$). Recently, Muñoz and coworkers claimed considerable improvement in the potassium to postmortem (K^+/PMI) correlation results simply by repositioning the variables so that the PMI is used (correctly) as the dependent variable and the K^+ as independent, instead of the other way round that, according to them, seemed to have been used (incorrectly) so far. The same workers claimed improved estimations of the PMI by combined analysis of vitreous potassium and hypoxanthine.

Synovial fluid Madea and coworkers found K^+ concentrations of the synovial fluid to range from 2.6 to $23.6\,mEq\,l^{-1}$ with a median value of $9.5\,mEq\,l^{-1}$.

Calcium (Ca^{2+})

Blood According to Jetter and Naumann, serum calcium remains constant in the early PMI. Hodgkinson and Hamblton found that the serum total calcium concentrations elevated in eight samples obtained between 11 and 50 h after death. In two other samples, they found that total serum calcium remained constant for the first 2 h postmortem. However, Fekete and Brundson were not able to establish normal postmortem values, as the scatter they found was unduly wide.

Cerebrospinal fluid (CSF) Naumann found that antemortem and postmortem calcium concentrations in the CSF were comparable.

Vitreous humor (VH) Coe found that in adults, calcium concentrations remain constant in the early postmortem interval and vary from 6 to 8.4 mg $100\,ml^{-1}$ with an average value at 6.8 mg $100\,ml^{-1}$. Naumann studied 211 cases and found an average calcium concentration of 7.2 mg $100\,ml^{-1}$ within an average PMI of 9 h.

Synovial fluid Madea compared total calcium concentrations of vitreous humor and synovial fluid and found the values to range from 1.05 to 2.33 $mmol\,l^{-1}$ with a median of 1.68 $mmol\,l^{-1}$ for vitreous calcium and from 1.51 to 3.58 $mmol\,l^{-1}$ with a median value of 2.36 $mmol\,l^{-1}$ for synovial calcium.

Sulfur (S^{2-})

Blood Jensen found that the level of postmortem sulfate was directly proportional to the level of urea or creatinine in the serum. Coe reported that inorganic sulfate in the serum remained unchanged for the first 24 h after death and then decreased by approximately 20% in the following 2 days.

There are no available reports on the sulfur in the CSF and VH.

Phosphorus (P^{3-} or P^{5-})

Blood Jetter showed that inorganic phosphorus increased in the serum as early as 1 h after death and reached a level of 20 $mEq\,l^{-1}$ at about 18 h postmortem. Both Jetter and Schyler reported an increase in postmortem serum organic phosphorus.

Cerebrospinal fluid (CSF) Naumann reported a significant increase in the CSF postmortem phosphorus (being 5.2 $mEq\,l^{-1}$) compared to its antemortem value (being 0.8 $mEq\,l^{-1}$), but no correlation exists between this and the time of death.

Vitreous humor (VH) Naumann also reported that inorganic phosphorus of the VH varied from 0.1 to 3.3 $mEq\,l^{-1}$ with an average value of 1.2 $mEq\,l^{-1}$. No correlation with postmortem interval was mentioned.

Magnesium (Mg^{2+})

Blood In five of eight cases, where blood or serum samples were obtained from 11 to 38 h after death, Hodgkinson and Hamblton found increases in postmortem serum magnesium concentrations varying from 2.4 to 5 $mEq\,l^{-1}$. Coe's investigations for determining calcium by cresolphthaline complexone demonstrated that magnesium probably begins to move from the intracellular fluid to the plasma well before significant hemolysis occurs. A similar inference was substantiated by Hodgkinson and Hamblton. According to Naumann, when hemolysis starts plasma magnesium increases rapidly to levels up to 20–30 $mEq\,l^{-1}$.

Cerebrospinal fluid (CSF) According to Naumann, who studied 131 cases for about 10.5 h after death, the average CSF magnesium increases slightly during the postmortem interval (being on average 2.9 $mEq\,l^{-1}$) from that of the antemortem level (being 2 $mEq\,l^{-1}$). This appears not to have challenged.

Vitreous humor (VH) Swift and coworkers examined 38 cases of children in relation to postmortem interval and found that two-thirds of these cases showed a slow increase in magnesium concentration of VH varying from 0.003 to 0.09 mg $100\,ml^{-1}\,h^{-1}$. They also showed that postmortem vitreous magnesium varies with the age of the child. Blumenfled and associates substantiated this last finding.

Hydrogen (pH)

Blood Jetter demonstrated that acidity of the blood after death increases as a factor of time (PMI). He found that pH values averaged 6.73 for the first 12 h after death while for the next 12 h period it averaged 6.43. Straumfjord and Butler reported a similar observation and added that there were variations in the pH depending on the source of the blood sample being highest in the blood obtained from the upper extremities and lowest in the right ventricular blood.

Conclusion

In conclusion, the electrolytes of various body compartments undergo profound redistribution after death resulting in significant quantitative changes, which have been used in forensic pathology for three main purposes as described earlier. However, unfortunately, the interpretation of the postmortem electrolyte analysis is very difficult and often futile. Nevertheless, postmortem chemistry of body fluids and tissues still attracts considerable research attention.

See Also

Autopsy: Adult; **Autopsy, Findings:** Postmortem Drug Sampling and Redistribution; Fire; Drowning; **Children:** Emotional Abuse; **Postmortem Changes:** Overview; Postmortem Interval; **Starvation**

Further Reading

Azparren JE, Vallejo G, Reyes E, Herranz A, Sancho M (2000) Study of the diagnostic value of strontium, chloride, hemoglobin and diatoms in immersion cases. *Forensic Science International* 108(1): 51–60.

Coe JI (1977) Postmortem chemistry of blood, cerebrospinal fluid and vitreous humor. In: Tedeschi CG, Eckert WG, Tedeschi LG (eds.) *Forensic Medicine: A Study in Trauma and Environmental Hazards*, vol. 2, *Physical Trauma*, pp. 1033–1060. Philadelphia, PA: W. B. Saunders.

Coe JI (1989) Postmortem biochemistry of blood and vitreous humor in pediatric practice. In: Mason JK (ed.) *Pediatric Forensic Medicine and Pathology*, pp. 191–203. London: Chapman and Hall.

Delva P (2003) Magnesium and heart failure. *Molecular Aspect of Medicine* 24(1–3): 79–105.

Madea B, Henssge C (2002) Eye changes after death. In: Knight B (ed.) *The Estimation of the Time since Death in the Early Postmortem Interval*, 2nd edn., pp. 103–133. London: Edward Arnold.

Madea B, Kreuser C, Banaschak S (2001) Postmortem biochemical examination of synovial fluid: a preliminary study. *Forensic Science International* 118: 29–35.

Muñoz JI, Suárez-Peñaranda JM, Otero XL, *et al.* (2001) A new perspective in estimation of postmortem interval (PMI) based on vitreous [K$^+$]. *Journal of Forensic Science* 46(2): 209–214.

Muñoz JI, Suárez-Peñaranda JM, Otero XL, *et al.* (2002) Improved estimation of postmortem interval based on differential behaviour of vitreous potassium and hypoxanthine in death by hanging. *Forensic Science International* 125: 67–74.

Nokes L, Madea B (2002) Changes after death. In: Knight B (ed.) *The Estimation of the Time since Death in the Early Postmortem Interval*, 2nd edn., pp. 209–243. London: Edward Arnold.

Pounder DJ, Carson DO, Johnston K, Orihara Y (1998) Electrolyte concentration difference between left and right vitreous humor samples. *Journal of Forensic Science* 43(3): 604–607.

Schyler F (1963) Determination of the time since death in the early postmortem interval. In: Lundquist F (ed.) *Methods of Forensic Sciences*, vol. 2, pp. 253–293. New York: John Wiley & Sons, Inc.

Singh D, Prashad R, Prakash C, *et al.* (2002) Linearization of relationship between serum sodium, potassium concentration, their ratio and time since death in Chandigarh Zone of North-West India. *Forensic Science International* 130: 1–7.

Singh D, Prashad R, Prakash C, Sharma SK, Pandey AN (2003) Double logarithmic, linear relationship between plasma chloride concentration and time since death in humans in Chandigarh Zone of North-West India. *Legal Medicine* 5(1): 49–54.

Zhu BI, Ishida K, Taniguchi M, *et al.* (2002) Possible postmortem serum markers for differentiation between fresh-, saltwater drowning and acute cardiac death: a preliminary investigation. *Forensic Science International* 125(1): 59–66.

Postmortem Interval

D J Pounder, University of Dundee, Dundee, UK

This article is adapted from 'Pathology: Postmortem Interval' in *Encyclopedia of Forensic Sciences*, pp. 1167–1172, © 2000, Elsevier Ltd.

Introduction

Evidence of the time elapsed since death, the postmortem interval, may come from three sources: (1) the body of the deceased; (2) the environment in the vicinity of the body; and (3) information on the deceased's habits, movements, and day-to-day activities. All three sources of evidence (corporal, environmental, and anamnestic) should be explored and assessed before offering an opinion on when death occurred. The longer the postmortem interval, the less accurate is the estimate of it based upon corporal changes. As a consequence, the longer the postmortem interval, the more likely it is that associated or environmental evidence will provide the most reliable estimates of the time elapsed.

No problem in forensic medicine has been investigated as thoroughly as the determination of the postmortem interval on the basis of postmortem changes to the body. Many physicochemical changes begin to take place in the body immediately or shortly after death and progress in a fairly orderly fashion until the body disintegrates. Each change progresses at its own rate which, unfortunately, is strongly influenced by largely unpredictable endogenous and environmental factors. Consequently, using the evolution of postmortem changes to estimate the postmortem interval is invariably difficult, and always of limited accuracy.

Body Cooling

Body cooling (algor mortis or "the chill of death") is the most useful single indicator of the postmortem interval during the first 24 h after death. Some authorities would regard it as the only worthwhile corporal method. The use of this method is only possible in cool and temperate climates, because in tropical regions there may be a minimal fall in body temperature postmortem, and in some extreme climates, such as desert regions, the body temperature may even rise after death.

Since body heat production ceases soon after death but loss of heat continues, the body cools. After death, as during life, the human body loses heat by radiation, convection, and evaporation. The fall in body temperature after death is mainly the result of radiation and convection. Evaporation may be a significant factor if the body or clothing is wet. Heat loss by conduction is not an important factor during life, but after death it may be considerable if the body is lying on a cold surface.

Newton's law of cooling states that the rate of cooling of an object is determined by the difference between the temperature of the object and the temperature of its environment. A plot of temperature against time gives an exponential curve. However, Newton's law applies to small inorganic objects and does not accurately describe the cooling of a corpse which has a large mass, an irregular shape, and is composed of tissues of different physical properties. The cooling of a human body is best represented by a sigmoid curve when temperature is plotted against time. Thus, there is an initial maintenance of body temperature which may last for some hours – the so-called "temperature plateau" – followed by a relatively linear rate of cooling, which subsequently slows rapidly as the body approaches the environmental temperature. The postmortem temperature plateau is physically determined and is not a special feature of the dead human body. Any inert body with a low thermal conductivity has such a plateau during its first cooling phase. The postmortem temperature plateau generally lasts between 30 min and 1 h, but may persist for as long as 3 h, and some authorities claim that it may persist for as long as 5 h.

It is usually assumed that the body temperature at the time of death was normal. However, in individual cases the body temperature at death may be subnormal or markedly raised. As well as in deaths from hypothermia, the body temperature at death may be subnormal in cases of congestive cardiac failure, massive hemorrhage, and shock. The body temperature may be raised at the time of death following an intense struggle, in heat stroke, in some infections, and in cases of pontine hemorrhage. The English forensic pathologist Simpson recorded a personal observation of a case of pontine hemorrhage with a temperature at death of 42.8 °C (109 °F). Where there is a fulminating infection, e.g., septicemia, the body temperature may continue to rise for some hours after death.

Thus the two important unknowns in assessing time of death from body temperature are: (1) the body temperature at the time of death, and (2) the length of the postmortem temperature plateau. For this reason assessment of time of death from body temperature cannot be accurate in the first 4–5 h after death when these two unknown factors have a dominant influence. Similarly, body temperature cannot be a useful guide to time of death when the cadaveric temperature approaches that of the environment. However, in the intervening period, over the linear part of the sigmoid cooling curve, any formula which involves an averaging of the temperature decline per hour may well give a reasonably reliable approximation of the time elapsed since death. It is in this limited way that the cadaveric temperature may assist in estimating the time of death in the early postmortem period.

Unfortunately the linear rate of postmortem cooling is affected by environmental factors other than the environmental temperature and by cadaveric factors other than the body temperature at the time of death. The most important of these factors are body size, body clothing or coverings, air movement and humidity, and wetting or immersion in water.

Body size is a factor because the greater the surface area of the body relative to its mass, the more rapid will be its cooling. Consequently, the heavier the physique and the greater the obesity of the body, the slower will be the heat loss. Children lose heat more quickly because their surface area to mass ratio is much greater than that of adults. The exposed surface area of the body radiating heat to the environment will vary with the body position. If the body is supine and extended, only 80% of the total surface area effectively loses heat, and in the fetal position the proportion is only 60%.

Clothing and coverings insulate the body from the environment and therefore slow body cooling. The effect of clothing has a greater impact on corpses of low body weight. A bedspread covering may at least halve the rate of cooling. For practical purposes, only the clothing or covering of the lower trunk is relevant.

Air movement accelerates cooling by promoting convection, and even the slightest sustained air movement is significant if the body is naked, thinly clothed, or wet. Cooling is more rapid in a humid rather than a dry atmosphere because moist air is a better conductor of heat. In addition the humidity of the atmosphere will affect cooling by evaporation where the body or its clothing is wet. A cadaver cools more rapidly in water than in air because water is a far better conductor of heat. For a given environmental temperature, cooling in still water is about twice as fast as in air, and in flowing water, it is about three times as fast.

Simple formulae for estimating the time of death from body temperature are now regarded as naive. The literature is replete with formulae that were enthusiastically recommended at first and later disavowed. The best tested and most sophisticated current method for estimating the postmortem interval from body temperature is that of the German researcher Henssge. Even so, it is acknowledged that the method may produce occasional anomalous results. It uses a nomogram based upon a complex formula, which approximates the sigmoid-shaped cooling curve. To make the estimate of postmortem interval, using this method requires: (1) the body weight; (2) the measured environmental temperature; and (3) the measured deep rectal temperature, and assumes a normal body temperature at death of 37.2 °C. Empiric corrective factors allow for the effect of important variables such as clothing, wetting, and air movement. The use of these corrective factors requires an element of personal experience. At its most accurate this sophisticated methodology provides an estimate of the time of death within a time span of 5.6 h with 95% probability. One of the most useful aspects of the nomogram is the ease with which the effect of changes in the variables can be tested. As a result it is an educational as well as a practical investigative tool.

The assessment of body cooling is made on the basis of measurement of the body core temperature, and, postmortem, this requires a direct measurement of the intraabdominal temperature. In practice either the temperature is measured rectally, or the intrahepatic/subhepatic temperature is measured through an abdominal wall stab. Oral, aural, and axillary temperatures cannot be used because after death these are not reflective of the body core temperature. For the measurement, an ordinary clinical thermometer is useless because its temperature range is too narrow, and the thermometer is too short for insertion deep into the rectum or liver. A chemical thermometer 25–30 cm (10–12 in.) long with a range from 0 to 50 °C is ideal. Alternatively, a thermocouple probe can be used, and this has the advantage of a digital readout or a programmable printed record.

Whether the temperature is measured via an abdominal stab or per rectum is a matter of professional judgment in each case. If there is easy access to the rectum without the need to disturb the position of the body seriously and if there is no reason to suspect sexual assault, then the temperature can be measured per rectum. It may be necessary to make small slits in the clothing to gain access to the rectum, if the body is clothed and the garments cannot be pushed to one side. The chemical thermometer must be inserted about 8–10 cm (3–4 in.) into the rectum and read *in situ*. The alternative is to make an abdominal stab wound after displacing or slitting any overlying clothing. The stab can be made over the right lower ribs and the thermometer pushed into the substance of the liver, or alternatively a subcostal stab will allow insertion of the thermometer on to the undersurface of the liver. If a method of sequential measurements of body temperature is to be used, then the thermometer should be left *in situ* during this time period. Taking sequential readings is much easier with a thermocouple and an attached printout device.

The core body temperature should be recorded as early as conveniently possible at the scene of death.

The prevailing environmental temperature should also be recorded and a note made of the environmental conditions at the time the body was first discovered, and any subsequent variation in these conditions. Temperature readings of the body represent data, which, if not collected, are irretrievably lost. Therefore, the decision not to take such readings should always be a considered one.

Rigor Mortis

Ordinarily, death is followed immediately by total muscular relaxation, primary muscular flaccidity, succeeded in turn by generalized muscular stiffening, rigor mortis. After a variable period of time, as a result of the development of putrefaction, rigor mortis passes off spontaneously to be followed by secondary muscular flaccidity. There is great variation in the rate of onset and the duration of rigor mortis, so that using the state of rigor mortis to estimate the postmortem interval is of very little value. In general, if the body has cooled to the environmental temperature and rigor is well developed, then death occurred more than 1 day previously and less than the time anticipated for the onset of putrefaction, which is about 3–4 days in a temperate climate.

As a general rule, when the onset of rigor is rapid, then its duration is relatively short. The two main factors which influence the onset and duration of rigor are the environmental temperature and the degree of muscular activity before death. Onset of rigor is accelerated and its duration shortened when the environmental temperature is high, so that putrefaction may completely displace rigor within 9–12 h of death. Rigor mortis is rapid in onset, and of short duration, after prolonged muscular activity, e.g., after exhaustion in battle, and following convulsions. Conversely, a late onset of rigor in many sudden deaths can be explained by the lack of muscular activity immediately before death.

Classically, rigor is said to develop sequentially, but this is by no means constant, symmetrical, or regular. Antemortem exertion usually causes rigor to develop first in the muscles used in the activity. Otherwise, rigor is typically first apparent in the small muscles of the eyelids, lower jaw, and neck, followed by the limbs. It involves first the small distal joints of the hands and feet and then the larger proximal joints of the elbows, knees, and then the shoulders and hips. It is generally accepted that rigor mortis passes off in the same order in which it develops. The forcible bending of a joint against the fixation of rigor results in tearing of the muscles and the rigor is said to have been "broken." Provided the rigor had been fully established, it will not reappear once broken down by force. Reestablishment of rigor, albeit of lesser degree, after breaking it suggests that death occurred less than about 8 h before rigor was broken.

The intensity of rigor mortis depends upon the decedent's muscular development, and should not be confused with its degree of development. In examining a body both the degree (complete, partial, or absent joint fixation) and the distribution of rigor should be assessed, after establishing that no artifact has been introduced by previous manipulation of the body by other observers. Attempted flexion of the different joints will indicate the degree and location of rigor. Typically, slight rigor can be detected within a minimum of 30 min after death but may be delayed for up to 7 h. The average time of first appearance is 3 h. It reaches a maximum, i.e., complete development, after an average 8 h, but sometimes as early as 2 h postmortem or as late as 20 h.

The biochemical basis of rigor mortis is not fully understood. Postmortem loss of integrity of the muscle cell sarcoplasmic reticulum allows calcium ions to flood the contractile units (sarcomeres), initiating the binding of actin and myosin molecules and mimicking the normal contraction process. Normal relaxation in life is achieved by energy-dependent (adenosine triphosphate (ATP)-driven) pumping of calcium back across the membrane of the sarcoplasmic reticulum but this fails postmortem because of membrane disruption and lack of ATP. The actin–myosin complex is trapped in a state of contraction until it is physically disrupted by the autolysis which heralds the onset of putrefaction. This process is characterized by proteolytic detachment of actin molecules from the ends of the sarcomeres, and consequent loss of the structural integrity of the contractile units. Although the biochemical basis of rigor mimics that of muscle contraction in life, it does not cause any movement of the body in death.

Livor Mortis

Lividity is a dark purple discoloration of the skin resulting from the gravitational pooling of blood in the veins and capillary beds of the dependent parts of the corpse. Synonyms include livor mortis, hypostasis, postmortem lividity, and, in the older literature, postmortem suggillations. Lividity involves the skin and the internal organs such as lungs, myocardium, and skeletal muscles. Pressure of even a mild degree prevents the formation of lividity in that area of skin, so that a supine body shows contact pallor over the shoulder blades, elbows, buttocks, thighs, and calves. Similarly, tight areas of clothing or jewelry, as well as skin folds, leave marks of contact pallor. Lividity is present in all corpses, although it may be inconspicuous in some, such as

following death from exsanguination. Intense lividity may be associated with postmortem hemorrhagic spots (punctate hemorrhages), that are best not referred to as petechial hemorrhages since they have nothing to do with asphyxia or agonal phenomena. They are easily recognized, occurring only in association with intense lividity and sparing adjacent areas of contact pallor.

The medicolegal importance of lividity lies in its color, as an indicator of the cause of death, and in its distribution, as an indicator of body position. The purple color of lividity reflects the presence of deoxyhemoglobin in the increasingly oxygen-depleted postmortem blood. Death from hypothermia or cyanide poisoning imparts the pink hue of oxyhemoglobin, carbon monoxide poisoning the cherry-red of carboxyhemoglobin, and poisoning from sodium chlorate, nitrates, and aniline derivatives impart the gray to brown color of methemoglobin.

The development of livor is too variable to serve as a useful indicator of the postmortem interval, but the tradition of evaluating it remains entrenched in forensic practice. Most authorities agree that lividity attains its maximum intensity, on average, at around 12 h postmortem, but there is some variation in descriptions of when it first appears, and when it is well developed, i.e., confluent. Hypostasis begins to form immediately after death, but it may not be visible for some time. Ordinarily its earliest appearance, as dull red patches, is 20–30 min after death, but this may be delayed for up to 2 h, or rarely 3 h. The patches of livor then deepen, increase in intensity, and become confluent within 1–4 h postmortem, to reach a maximum extent and intensity within about 6–10 h, but sometimes as early as 3 h or as late as 16 h. Faint lividity may appear shortly before death in individuals with terminal circulatory failure. Conversely, the development of lividity may be delayed in persons with chronic anemia or massive terminal hemorrhage.

After about 10–12 h the lividity becomes "fixed" and repositioning the body, e.g. from the prone to the supine position, will result in a dual pattern of lividity since the primary distribution will not fade completely but a secondary distribution will develop in the newly dependent parts. The blanching of livor by thumb pressure is a simple indicator that it is not fixed. Fixation of lividity is a relative, but not an absolute, phenomenon. Well-developed lividity fades very slowly and only incompletely. Fading of the primary pattern and development of a secondary pattern of lividity will be quicker and more complete if the body is moved early during the first day. However, even after a postmortem interval of 24 h, moving the body may result in a secondary pattern of lividity developing. Duality of the distribution of lividity is important because it shows that the body has been moved after death. However, it is not possible to estimate with any precision, from the dual pattern of livor, when it was that the corpse was moved.

Areas of lividity are overtaken early in the putrefactive process, becoming green at first and later black. The red cells are hemolyzed and the hemoglobin stains the intima of large blood vessels and diffuses into the surrounding tissues, highlighting the superficial veins of the skin, a process referred to as "marbling."

Putrefaction

Putrefaction is the postmortem destruction of the soft tissues of the body by the action of bacteria and endogenous enzymes and is entirely capable of skeletonizing a body. The main changes recognizable in the tissues undergoing putrefaction are the evolution of gases, changes in color, and liquefaction. The same changes seen on the surface of the body occur simultaneously in the internal organs.

Bacteria are essential to putrefaction and commensal bacteria, mainly from the large bowel, soon invade the tissues after death. Colonic anaerobes, such as *Bacteroides* spp., anaerobic lactobacilli, clostridia, and anaerobic streptococci, thrive in the oxygen-depleted tissues of the corpse. Typically, the first visible sign of putrefaction is a greenish discoloration of the skin of the anterior abdominal wall. This most commonly begins in the right iliac fossa, i.e., over the area of the cecum, where the contents of the bowel are more fluid and full of bacteria (about 10^8 to 10^{10} organisms per gram of solid). Any antemortem bacterial infection of the body, particularly septicemia, will hasten the onset and evolution of putrefaction. Injuries to the body surface promote putrefaction by providing portals of entry for bacteria. Putrefaction is delayed in deaths from exsanguination because blood usually provides a channel for the spread of putrefactive organisms within the body. Although putrefaction tends to be more rapid in children than in adults, the onset is relatively slow in unfed newborn infants because of the lack of commensal bacteria in the gut.

Environmental temperature has a great influence on the rate of development of putrefaction, so that rapid cooling of the body following a sudden death will markedly delay its onset. In a temperate climate, the degree of putrefaction reached after 24 h in the height of summer may require 10–14 days in the depth of winter. Putrefaction is optimal at temperatures ranging between 21 and 38 °C (70 and 100 °F), and is retarded when the temperature falls below 10 °C (50 °F) or when it exceeds 38 °C (100 °F). A

high environmental humidity will enhance putrefaction. Heavy clothing and other coverings, by retaining body heat, will speed up putrefaction. The rate of putrefaction is influenced by body build because this affects body cooling. Obese individuals putrefy more rapidly than those who are lean. Whereas warm temperatures enhance putrefaction, intense heat produces "heat fixation" of tissues and inactivates autolytic enzymes, with a resultant delay in the onset and course of decomposition.

There is considerable variation in the time of onset and the rate of progression of putrefaction. As a result, the time taken to reach a given state of putrefaction cannot be judged with accuracy. An observer should not assert too readily that the decomposed state of a body is inconsistent with an alleged time interval. As a general rule, when the onset of putrefaction is rapid, then the progress is accelerated. Under average conditions in a temperate climate, the earliest putrefactive changes involving the anterior abdominal wall occur between 36 and 72 h after death. Progression to gas formation, and bloating of the body, occurs after about 1 week. The temperature of the body after death is the most important factor generally determining the rate of putrefaction. If it is maintained above 26 °C (80 °F), then the putrefactive changes become obvious within 24 h and gas formation is seen in about 2–3 days.

According to an old rule of thumb (Casper's dictum), 1 week of putrefaction in air is equivalent to 2 weeks in water, which is equivalent to 8 weeks buried in soil, given the same environmental temperature. After normal burial, the rate at which the body decomposes will depend to a large extent on the depth of the grave, the warmth of the soil, the efficiency of the drainage, and the permeability of the coffin.

Gases produced by putrefaction include methane, hydrogen, hydrogen sulfide, and carbon dioxide. The sulfur-containing amino acids, cysteine, cystine, and methionine yield hydrogen sulfide, which combines with hemoglobin and ferrous iron to produce green sulfhemoglobin and black ferrous sulfide, respectively. Decarboxylation of the amino acids, ornithine and lysine, yields carbon dioxide and the foul-smelling ptomaines, putrescine (1,4-butanediamine) and cadaverine (1,5-pentanediamine), respectively. These ptomaines are detectable by cadaver dogs. Deamination of L-phenylanaline yields ammonia and phenylpyruvic acid, which forms a green complex with ferric iron. Bacterial and fungal fermentation yields ethyl alcohol, confounding the interpretation of postmortem alcohol concentrations.

Early putrefaction is heralded by the waning of rigor, green abdominal discoloration, a doughy consistency to the tissues, and hemolytic staining of vessels. Localized drying of the lips, tip of the nose, and fingers may be seen. The face swells and discolors and the swollen lips are everted, making facial recognition unreliable. The epidermis separates from the dermis, giving rise to "skin-slip." Distension of the abdominal cavity by putrefactive gases characterizes the bloating stage of decomposition. It is these gases that cause a submerged body to rise to the surface and float. In males, gas is forced from the peritoneal space down the inguinal canals and into the scrotum, resulting in massive scrotal swelling. Gaseous pressure expels dark malodorous fluid, "purge fluid," from the nose and mouth, mimicking antemortem hemorrhage or injury. Similar fluid flows from the vagina; there is emptying of feces from the rectum and prolapse of rectum and uterus may occur. The doughy consistency of the tissues of early putrefaction is replaced by the crepitant effect resulting from gaseous infiltration along necrotic tissue planes beneath the skin and in deeper tissues. Large subepidermal bullae fill with gas, sanguineous fluid, or clear fluid. Gas bubbles appear within solid organs such as liver and brain, giving a "Swiss-cheese" appearance, and the blood vessels and heart are filled with gas. These putrefactive changes are relatively rapid when contrasted with the terminal decay of the body. When the putrefactive juices have drained away and the soft tissues have shrunk, the speed of decay is appreciably reduced.

The progression of putrefaction may be modified by vertebrate or invertebrate animal activity. Wild animals, domestic pets, livestock, fish, and crustaceans may be involved; most commonly it is insects, particularly fly larvae (maggots). In a hot humid environment with heavy insect activity, a corpse may be skeletonized in as little as 3 days. Although this insect activity is destructive of physical evidence, the insects themselves can provide useful information for estimation of time of death. All soft tissues are generally lost before the skeleton becomes disarticulated, typically from the head downward (with the mandible separating from the skull and the head from the vertebral column) and from central to peripheral (from vertebral column to limbs).

Adipocere

Saponification (making soap) or adipocere formation is a modification of putrefaction characterized by the transformation of fatty tissues into a yellowish-white, greasy (but friable when dry), wax-like substance, which has a sweetish rancid odor when its formation is complete. During the early stages of its production, a penetrating and very persistent ammoniacal smell is emitted. Adipocere, also known as "grave wax" or "corpse wax," develops as the result of hydrolysis of fat with the release of fatty acids which, being acidic, inhibit putrefactive bacteria. Fatty acids take on sodium or potassium to form hard soap (sapo durus) or soft soap (sapo domesticus) respectively. Replacement of sodium and potassium by calcium gives an insoluble soap, which contributes a more brittle quality to the adipocere. However, fat and water alone do not produce adipocere. Putrefactive organisms, of which *Clostridium welchii* is most active, are important, and adipocere formation is facilitated by postmortem invasion of the tissues by commensal bacteria. A warm, moist, anaerobic environment thus favors adipocere formation.

Adipocere develops first in the subcutaneous tissues, most commonly involving the cheeks, breasts, and buttocks. Rarely, it may involve the viscera such as the liver. The adipocere is admixed with the mummified remains of muscles, fibrous tissues, and nerves. The primary medicolegal importance of adipocere lies not in establishing the postmortem interval but rather in the preservation of the body, which aids in personal identification and the recognition of injuries.

The presence of any adipocere indicates that the postmortem interval is at least weeks and probably several months. Under ideal warm, damp conditions, adipocere may be apparent to the naked eye after 3–4 weeks. Ordinarily, this requires some months and extensive adipocere is usually not seen before 5 or 6 months after death. Some authorities suggest that extensive changes require not less than a year after submersion, or upwards of 3 years after burial. Once formed, adipocere will ordinarily remain unchanged for years.

Mummification

Mummification is a modification of putrefaction characterized by the dehydration or desiccation of the tissues. The body shrivels and is converted into a leathery or parchment-like mass of skin and tendons surrounding the bone. Mummification develops in conditions of dry heat, especially when there are air currents, e.g., in a desert. Newborn infants, being small and sterile, commonly mummify. Mummification of bodies of adults in temperate climates is unusual unless associated with forced hot-air heating in buildings or other artificial favorable conditions. The forensic importance of mummification lies primarily in the preservation of tissues, and this aids in personal identification and the recognition of injuries. The time required for complete mummification of a body cannot be precisely stated, but in ideal conditions mummification may be well advanced by the end of a few weeks.

Maceration

Maceration is the aseptic autolysis of a fetus, which has died *in utero* and remained enclosed within the amniotic sac. Bacterial putrefaction plays no role in the process. The changes of maceration are only seen when a stillborn fetus has been dead for several days before delivery. Examination of the body needs to be prompt since bacterial putrefaction will begin following delivery. The body is extremely flaccid with a flattened head and undue mobility of the skull. The limbs may be readily separated from the body. There are large moist skin bullae, which rupture to disclose a reddish-brown surface denuded of epidermis. Skin-slip discloses similar underlying discoloration. The body has a rancid odor but there is no gas formation. Establishing maceration of the fetus provides proof of a postmortem interval *in utero*, and therefore proof of stillbirth and conclusive evidence against infanticide.

Vitreous Potassium

Several researchers have studied the relationship between the potassium concentration of the vitreous humor of the eye and the postmortem interval. However, within 100 h postmortem, the 95% confidence limits of the different researchers vary from ± 9.5 h up to ± 40 h. Cases with possible confounding antemortem electrolyte disturbances can be excluded by eliminating all cases with a vitreous urea above an arbitrary level of 100 mg dl^{-1}. (High urea values in vitreous humor always reflect antemortem retention and are not due to postmortem changes.) Having eliminated these cases, there is a linear relationship between vitreous potassium concentration and time elapsed after death up to 120 h. However, the 95% confidence limits are ±22 h, so that the method has no real practical application. There are also sampling problems in that the potassium concentration may differ significantly between the left and right eye at the same moment in time.

See Also

Decomposition, Patterns and Rates; **Postmortem Changes:** Overview

Further Reading

Haglund WD, Sorg MH (1997) *Forensic Taphonomy. The Postmortem Fate of Human Remains.* Boca Raton, FL: CRC Press.

Henssge C (1988) Death time estimation in case work: I. The rectal temperature time of death nomogram. *Forensic Science International* 38: 209–236.

Henssge C, Knight B, Krompecher T, Madea B, Nokes L (2002) *The Estimation of the Time Since Death in the Early Postmortem Period*, 2nd edn. London: Edward Arnold.

Madea B, Henssge C, Honig W, Gerbracht A (1989) References for determining the time of death by potassium in vitreous humor. *Forensic Science International* 40: 231–243.

PREPARATION OF WITNESSES

Contents
Scotland
United States of America

Scotland

C G M Fernie, University of Glasgow, Glasgow, UK

In Scotland a system known as precognition has arisen in the preparation of witnesses before a trial. Before considering what precisely this means, it is useful to outline the ethical and legal issues that have to be taken into account in releasing information for court purposes. Also, we will consider how these principles have developed in recent years as there is an apparent paradox between what actually happens in practice as opposed to guidance formulated by regulatory bodies and statutes originating from the UK parliament.

The UK-wide regulatory body for the medical profession, the General Medical Council (GMC), publishes guidance within its document *Confidentiality:*

Protecting and Providing Information on disclosure of information in specific circumstances where the doctor may require ethical advice. One such situation is where a doctor is likely to be cited to give evidence in court. Indeed, a failure to adhere to the GMC constraints may constitute serious professional misconduct, in which case it is possible for the ultimate sanction of erasure to apply.

The principle espoused here was enshrined within the Hippocratic oath, which was probably written in the fifth century BC. A modern restatement of this oath was produced by the World Medical Association, when formed in 1947, and this became known as the Declaration of Geneva. Specific reference was given to this issue:

> I will respect the secrets which are confided in me, even after the patient has died: I will maintain by all the means in my power, the honour and the noble traditions of the medical profession.

This is one of the earliest references to the concept of professional secrecy and one can see the derivation of current ethical guidance and legislation in the series of statutes that flowed from this principle.

Parliament saw fit to legislate on this subject, commencing with the Data Protection Act 1984 that only applied to computerized records. There was progression through the Access to Medical Reports Act 1988 relating to preemployment matters, the Access to Health Records Act 1990, encompassing written notes, and culminating in the Data Protection Act 1998. These acts were all designed to enhance the rights of individuals to ensure that accurate data were retained by healthcare professionals and that there was a legislative right for individuals to view their records and have any mistakes remedied. Although the primary purpose was to allow people to know what information was contained within their medical records, parliament also wished to have statute-based law to prevent unauthorized release of sensitive information.

There are, however, specific circumstances when a doctor may breach a professional confidence without either ethical or legal ramifications as a consequence. Such a situation arises, for example, when giving evidence in court. Unlike the solicitor–client relationship, the medical profession along with the priesthood does not enjoy absolute privilege. Therefore, the doctor should answer truthfully and fully while testifying in court. Whilst the GMC does guide the doctor to question the presiding officer of the court if a matter of confidence appears irrelevant to the proceedings, there is no doubt that the doctor must bow to the court's authority if told to do so as otherwise he/she would be in contempt of court. The

example given by the GMC is where attempts are made to compel the medical practitioner to disclose information relating to relatives or partners of the patient, who are not parties to the proceedings, and the doctor has reservations about the appropriateness of the disclosure.

Consequently, it appears quite clear that a doctor may not release such information, unless (1) a patient gives informed consent to a doctor divulging information or (2) is ordered to do so by the presiding officer of the court (magistrate, sheriff, or judge). In the latter situation the doctor should assess whether there are necessary criteria to breach confidentiality without patient consent, such as with a public-interest disclosure.

Despite the foregoing explanation, in Scotland the system of precognition has arisen historically in the preparation of witnesses before a trial. In fact, although this has traditionally been associated with criminal cases and this article deals with that context, this approach is now also used in civil cases and representation has even been made to the GMC to allow this in preparation for a hearing of the Professional Conduct Committee involving a case that took place in Scotland.

It is interesting that there is no statutory definition as to what constitutes a precognition, but it is generally accepted that this is to know before (the trial) the evidence that an individual is likely to give if called upon to do so. The Defence's right to take precognitions is a matter which is enshrined in the common law (1987, *Stair Memorial Encyclopaedia*). Although Lord Thomson's *Second Report on Criminal Procedure in Scotland* (1975) devotes a whole chapter to the subject of precognitions, it deliberately makes no attempt to define them.

Precognition of a witness may be undertaken by either the Crown or the Defence and it is through the process of precognition that the Defence is made aware of the strength of the Crown's case. Having had the benefit of this process, the Defence can offer clients full advice on their position and prepare cases for trial if necessary.

Precognition-taking is a distinctive feature of the Scottish system. In contrast, with other jurisdictions such as England and Wales, there is disclosure of the Crown's case which virtually does away with the need for independent investigation by the Defence.

Precognitions differ from other statements in the sense that they cannot be put to witnesses during the course of a trial. Whereas a witness statement is essentially an account of what the witness has said, a precognition is a precognoscer's account of the witness's evidence, i.e., the statement subsequently produced has been filtered through the mind of the precognoscer. This is perhaps a subtle distinction but it is an important one given the exclusion of precognitions from the court process.

In fact, witnesses are under no direct legal obligation to agree to be precognosced by the Defence. There is some authority for the view that they have a civic duty to do so, but that is all.

In *Her Majesty's Advocate* v. *Monson* [1893] 1 Adam 114, the Lord Justice-Clerk expressed the view that:

> every good citizen should give his aid, either to the Crown or to the Defence in every case where the interests of the public in the punishment of crime, or the interests of a prisoner charged with a crime, call for ascertainment of facts.

In *Wilson* v. *Tudhope* [1985] SCCR 339 (Sh Ct), Sheriff Gordon took the view that this duty is merely a moral one and cannot be enforced.

Because witnesses are under no legal obligation to agree to be precognosced, this clearly may pose a problem for the Defence. In 1967, the Grant Committee considered the issue of whether the Defence should have the power to compel witnesses to attend for precognition. They recommended against it, apparently taking the view that if defense solicitors were granted these powers of compulsion, there was a danger that the powers might be overworked. The Grant Committee was also concerned about the difficulties that might arise where accused parties chose to defend themselves. The solution recommended was that it should be possible for the Defence to cite witnesses for precognition under oath before a sheriff.

This procedure was first introduced by the Criminal Justice (Scotland) Act (1980) and is currently set out in section 291 of the Criminal Procedure: Scotland Act (1995). It is exceptional for medical witnesses to be precognosced in this way, but it is not totally unknown, should they be unwilling to cooperate with the process.

Although some writers believe that evidence given at precognition is as privileged as that spoken in court as far as breach of confidentiality is concerned, the GMC may not share that interpretation, as they state unequivocally: "You should not disclose personal information to a third party such as a solicitor, police officer, or officer of a court without the patient's express consent," except in the specific circumstances outlined and there is no consideration here of precognition.

Finally, what was said by a witness when she/he was precognosced prior to giving evidence cannot be put to her/him whilst giving testimony in court, the exception being the unusual situation where that precognition was given under oath in front of a Sheriff.

An unsworn precognition such as that normally provided to a solicitor or their agent is excluded on the basis that this is only what the witness is alleged to have said to the precognoscer.

See Also

Preparation of Witnesses: United States of America

Further Reading

Declaration of Geneva (1948) Adopted by the General Assembly of World Medical Association at Geneva Switzerland, September 1948.
Gee DJ, Mason JK (1990) *The Courts and the Doctor*, vol. 6, p. 85. Oxford, UK: Oxford Medical Publications.
General Medical Council (2000) *Confidentiality: Protecting and Providing Information.* London: General Medical Council.
Raitt F, Green W (2001) *Evidence*, 3rd edn, vol. 1, p. 8. Edinburgh, UK: W Green & Son.

United States of America

M M Houck, West Virginia University, Morgantown, WV, USA

Introduction

The Role of the Witness

The forensic expert has two duties of equal importance: first, to perform scientific investigations, either in the field or laboratory, to reach a conclusion about evidence; and, second, to communicate those results and their meaningfulness to a judge or jury through testimony. Testimony in part is what makes forensic science unique; no other scientific discipline has this legal requirement. Like peer-reviewed journal articles, presentations at meetings, colloquia, and other forms of interaction in which scientists engage, testimony is a structured method of communicating scientific results, but with one significant difference.

The duties of a forensic scientist take place in two very different environments. The first duty occurs under the rules, methods, and norms of science at the crime scene or in the scientist's laboratory. Forms of communication between peers are the articles and presentations mentioned above. The second duty, however, takes place in a locale that is foreign to most scientists: the courtroom. And very few, if any, of scientists' rules of operation travel with them into the legal arena – some may even be detrimental. Attorneys have no such professional portmanteau: they always play by their rules in their home field. The friction thus created between attorneys and scientists results from two conflicting cultures with different norms. Furthermore, testimony is peer-to-layperson, not peer-to-peer, and the expert must adjust his/her speech, vocabulary, and thoughts appropriately.

The Difference between Reports and Testimony

Scientific articles are the canonical form of communication for scientists and researchers but the articles originally had a very different form than they do today. The style, presentation, and argumentation of a seventeenth-century scientific article had many of the components of good story-telling: strong active verbs, first-person narrative, expressive vocabulary with a lack of technical jargon, and few, if any, abstractions. By contrast, twentieth-century scientific articles demonstrate just the opposite with their passive, third-person voice, technical terminology, high quantitative components, increased cognitive complexity, and higher volumes of data.

Forensic scientists are caught in a stylistic dichotomy that goes largely unnoticed: While they write reports in a twentieth-century style, testimony is presented in what could be considered a seventeenth-century style. Therefore, "the fibers were examined by polarized light microscopy, Fourier transform infrared spectroscopy, and microspectrophotometry" in a report translates to, "I examined the fibers by placing them on a glass microscope slide and analyzing them with various microscopes and instruments that tell me about the fiber and measure its color" during testimony. Experts and attorneys alike should pay attention to this phenomenon as it pertains to the nature of scientific writing and legal testimony.

Voir Dire/Qualifications

An expert is qualified in two steps. First, the attorney who issued the subpoena to the expert asks questions that establish the witness' expertise. These questions are designed to demonstrate facts about the witness' background to meet with the judge's and opposing attorney's approval; this is sometimes referred to as "qualifying a witness." Second, the opposing lawyer challenges those qualifications through additional questions; this is called the *voir dire* (French for "speaking the truth") of the witness. If the judge determines that the witness is qualified to speak as an expert on a subject, the proponent attorney begins direct examination of the witness.

All of the work the forensic expert completed – collection, examination, and testing of the evidence, writing of reports, and pretrial conferences – is merely preparatory to testifying in the trial. The most important role of the forensic scientist is interpreting a complicated scientific discipline to a judge or jury. In this light, the expert should not testify only as to conclusions, but should also explain how those conclusions were reached and what they mean to the facts of the case (*Bethea* v. *United States* 537 F.2nd 1187. (D.C. Ct. App. 1976)). Otherwise, why testify? Experts are not fact witnesses – they are called to court because they can provide their expert opinions and should do so.

Most people confuse resumés and curriculum vitae (CV). A CV is the complete description of a career, including employment, education, training, teaching, publications, presentations, awards, and professional associations. All this information should pertain to the expert's professional life; hobbies such as archery and needlepoint should not be included. Other items to exclude from a CV are any personal information other than the expert's name (no home address or phone number), social security number, or other non-work-related contact information. A CV may be entered into evidence and therefore becomes a public document, available to anyone who obtains a copy of the case file.

A resumé, on the other hand, is a condensation of the most pertinent facts about a career. Resumés are brief – generally one page – and to the point: employment, education, and perhaps professional affiliations are stated. Resumés are for employment applications. Experts should provide CVs prior to testifying in court to both attorneys; additional copies should be brought to court just in case. Resumés are too incomplete to be useful to court officials.

It may be helpful for the expert to have his/her *voir dire* qualifications written in a question-and-answer format. The answers should not be written down completely, however, as this may lead an onlooker to decide that the witness doesn't even know his/her own qualifications; brief outlines, notes, and obvious abbreviations should be used to guide the attorney. If the witness is qualified in a variety of disciplines (hairs and fibers, typewriting, and handwriting), then he/she should have a different set of qualifying questions for each specialty.

Getting through *voir dire* should be the time for the expert to demonstrate his/her expertise, qualifying him/her for the testimony he/she is about to offer. The last thing an attorney wants is a surprise during *voir dire*, for example, that the expert failed an introductory chemistry course – twice. A prepared attorney has reviewed the expert's CV and cleared any embarrassments or impeachments ahead of time.

For an expert who has testified rarely, *voir dire* builds confidence; it reminds him/her that he/she is an expert and has extensive knowledge in the current topic. If an expert has never testified before, the attorney should be direct: "How many times have you testified previously?" Everyone has a first time. A good answer to this is, "This is the first time I've been required to testify." For an expert who testifies often, the danger resides in sounding either bored or pompous. If a particular publication or training class in the expert's CV is relevant, the attorney may ask about it to break the routine.

Prepared attorneys can save themselves in the courtroom by taking time to review the CV of all experts, not just their own. Much can be hidden in a CV, as any human resources person can attest. Time gaps between jobs, lack of or restricted professional development (only receiving training from one agency), job-hopping, and similar deficiencies are all potentially fertile ground for investigation. The more competent attorneys will discover as much as possible about an expert before the trial. It can be useful to order transcripts of previous trials if the expert testified on the same or similar topics.

Direct Testimony

Direct testimony is the expert's first chance to demonstrate his/her demeanor and command of the subject matter. The expert must lay the foundation of the science, the examinations conducted, and the significance of the results. The proponent attorney should not be an obstacle to this process – it is the expert's moment to shine; the opposing attorney will be enough of an obstacle on cross-examination. During direct examination the expert develops a rapport with the jury. This is facilitated with a conversational tone and relaxed approach. The expert educates the jury without being condescending. The expert should look at the attorney during questioning but look at the jury (or judge) when answering; they are the trier of fact and the answers are for their benefit.

Direct testimony builds the attorney's argument and the expert provides the relevant facts. The attorney and the expert should decide in advance on format – go question-by-question in a tight script, an open question-and-exposition format, or a combination. Courts may grant leeway with direct testimony, so the attorney could ask, "How are forensic hair examinations conducted?" to which the expert can give a discursive answer. For attorneys who are unfamiliar with the science employed and who are willing for a seasoned expert to pace him/herself, this may work best. Other attorneys favor an orderly approach, which can be effective if the case or the evidence is complex.

Cross-Examination

The US adversarial system of justice allows the accused to question the testimony of a witness against him/her. Cross-examination is not a necessary evil but a required part of the justice process. Experts who correctly performed their tests and examinations, came to valid and legitimate conclusions, and prepared properly for trial have nothing to fear from a cross-examination. Some attorneys may have knowledge of science or a particular forensic specialty and may present a challenge to the inexperienced expert. Experts must remember they have been "asked to be in the courtroom because the justice system requires their expertise." Cross-examination is not, or should not be, a personal attack.

Experts should present the same demeanor and temperament with both attorneys. Being solicitous on direct but defensive or aggressive on cross-examination will make the expert seem biased. Tempo is also important and should remain the same regardless of the questioner; the experienced witness controls the speed and flow of testimony. This gives the jury time to listen to both questions and answers.

Attorneys are not scientists, and vice versa. An attorney may use a term in a sense other than what the scientist understands. A good example is "error." To a scientist, every measurement contains some error and this is a quantity to be evaluated and understood – "standard error of the mean" is a statistical value, for example. To a lawyer, however, "errors" are bad, they are mistakes, and they mean the expert has done something wrong. Therefore, experts should not hesitate to clarify terms or questions presented to them. If the attorney happens to misstate the facts as the scientist knows or has established them, the scientist should also not hesitate to correct the attorney first and then answer the question.

Although "error" was used as an example above, everyone makes mistakes. Admitting a mistake or an apparent lack of thoroughness in testing may tarnish the expert's reputation but not as badly as if the expert covers it up. Admitting to a mistake demonstrates honesty and integrity; it also shows the jury that the expert is human.

Too few attorneys pay close attention during the cross-examination of their witnesses. Much can be learned about strategy, tactics, and the quality of the expert from a careful consideration of this trial phase. Experts, in many ways, are sitting ducks – they cannot question, object, or defend themselves other than through answering the questions they are asked.

Preparation for Attorneys

"The importance of the pretrial conference for the attorney cannot be overstated." Attorneys must take time to prepare their witnesses properly. The significant aspects of the upcoming testimony should be reviewed by both parties. The pretrial can be thought of as a dress rehearsal and the attorney and the expert should review their notes and be prepared to discuss the case before coming to the pretrial conference. The attorney should thoroughly familiarize the expert with all exhibits which will be entered into evidence that pertain to the expert's testimony. Preparation prior to the pretrial conference and the trial itself is essential for both the expert and the attorney.

It never hurts to be informed. An attorney should read about the expert's discipline, even if it is only a chapter in an introductory textbook. Terminology and concepts are key to familiarization and this leads to a smooth and comfortable delivery. The expert will also appreciate this effort because it makes his/her job easier than working with an attorney who steadfastly remains ignorant or who is cavalier and breezy about the subject.

The majority of forensic experts in the USA work for a government agency (local, state, or federal), although many work for private firms or are self-employed. An attorney may question an expert about having a bias or preference for whom they testify ("Isn't it true that you've never testified for the prosecution/defense?"). Experts should not be ashamed that they work for the government or are only employed by the defense – these situations are outside their control. Government agencies rarely accept defense work (it's not their mandate) and defense attorneys typically cannot employ government workers (it's against their mandate). Nevertheless, employment by the government, testifying only for the prosecution or the defense, or failure to meet with opposing counsel before trial are issues that can be used to effect by attorneys. The prepared expert should be ready for questions of this nature. An attorney may ask, "Aren't you being paid [by the federal, state, local government/opposing counsel] for your testimony today?" implying that your testimony has been purchased. A gentle reminder that nearly everyone appearing in court today, including the attorneys, judge, and jury, are being compensated for their time should close down that line of questioning. Another type of question similar to this is, "You've spoken with the government's/defendant's attorney, haven't you?" There is no secret about the fact that

you have talked with the attorney who subpoenaed you. There is nothing improper about talking to the attorney before the trial. Wise attorneys, unless they suspect something is amiss, steer clear from these baiting questions.

Preparation for Witnesses

If an expert isn't prepared to testify, he/she doesn't belong in the courtroom. Preparation entails reviewing reports, understanding the fundamental theories of the discipline, familiarity with the science (not what exams the expert performed – that is the method or protocol) of the discipline, and the timing and names involved in the case. The prepared expert is also familiar with the courtroom, the prosecutor, and all the parties involved.

Dress, Demeanor, and Diplomacy

Courts are very conservative environments and a good witness blends in. It is a courtroom, not a theater. Dress appropriately. Tattoos, piercings (other than earrings on women), and anything that might distract a jury (a shiny brooch that dangles) should be removed or covered.

At some point during testimony, an attorney may ask a question that angers an expert. An expert should never show his/her anger and never answer a question in anger. When experts lose control of their emotions, they will not do what they are in court to do: give truthful answers. They should remain calm, be polite, and answer the question. The more an attorney attempts to aggravate the expert, the more courteous and professional the expert should become. Experts themselves are not on trial in a case, no matter what may be asked. If questions are too insulting, the proponent attorney may object, but the expert must remain calm and handle questions without help. It is important to keep in mind that nothing a lawyer says is evidence unless it is answered affirmatively by the witness.

The expert should remain dignified at all times, from the moment he/she enters the courtroom and takes the oath until he/she leaves the courtroom. Do not chew gum, fidget, or groom (scratch, pick, or preen). A slim briefcase and the necessary documents are all that should be taken to the witness stand.

How to Listen to Questions

Listening is critical to successful testimony. Experts should be responsive and simple in their answers. Don't embellish. If the question is not understood, clarification can be requested. This is especially important if the question is vague or contains a value judgment, such as "Isn't it a fact that your laboratory has had problems?" If the question is not clarified, the answer may be misleading.

Whenever a person tells the same story twice, no matter how carefully, inconsistencies are possible. Previous inconsistent statements can be reconciled by the expert with his/her best recollection of what happened, and explaining the inconsistency ("If I said the evidence was returned on April 7th, I misspoke. It was returned on April 17th").

How to Answer Questions

Attorneys have an absolute right and sometimes a duty to object and the expert must give them that opportunity. The judge must rule on the objection before the expert can answer. Experts should wait until the objections and ruling are over before answering.

Hypothetical questions are just that – questions that offer a hypothesis containing only facts that have been testified to in the trial, but asking the expert to offer an opinion based solely on those facts. The facts must be clearly understood and sufficient for an opinion to be made. Hypotheticals can be dangerous because the expert has conducted examinations and rendered expert opinions based on much more data than are offered in any hypothetical question. To ask a hypothetical on only a verbal surmise of a situation may be misleading and the expert must pay close attention to any such question.

Some experts have the notion that all questions should be answered "yes" or "no." Many questions cannot be answered accurately with only "yes" or "no" because either the question is, or the answer would be, incomplete or ambiguous. If the attorney asks the expert to "only answer 'yes or no,'" the expert is entitled to tell the attorney that the question cannot be answered "yes or no" without the answer being misleading. The court should not direct you to answer "yes or no," unless the question permits that kind of answer. If the court does direct you to answer "yes or no," the comment regarding the need for an explanation, with luck, will flag the question or area of inquiry as something to be covered in redirect questioning.

The expert should beware of compound questions. If several questions are rolled into one, it may be difficult, if not impossible, to answer each one accurately unless they are broken down. In such a case, the expert may say, "I will try to answer your questions one by one." If the question is too long, the expert could ask, "Can you break those questions down for me and ask them one at a time?"

What to Do if You Are Alone

An expert can be alone in two ways: near the courtroom and on the stand. The first typically happens when the expert is waiting to testify. Someone may try to strike up a conversation that may segue into talking about the case. The expert should not discuss the case with anyone except the attorneys or the judge. Attorneys have been known to use investigators (who do not identify themselves) to elicit comments from experts that are then used against them in the courtroom. If someone identifies him/herself as related to the case on trial and tries to start a conversation about the case, the expert should not do it alone. For example, if the opposing attorney introduces him/herself and asks questions about your impending testimony, an appropriate response might be, "I'd be glad to discuss this but I'd feel more comfortable if both attorneys were present for this conversation." Otherwise, the expert may enter into *ex parte* (away from one party in the case) conversation that could become part of the attorney's questioning in the courtroom ("Didn't you just tell me in the hallway..."). No stenographic transcript will be available to establish what was said or not said.

Regrettably, experts are often alone on the stand as well. The proponent attorney may not pay attention and not object or be ignorant of rehabilitating questions on redirect. The prepared expert knows this and is ready to go it alone.

Leaving the Courtroom

When an expert is finished testifying, the judge will excuse him/her; this release may be liable for recall for future or rebuttal testimony. If the expert is excused (and no indication of further testimony is given), he/she should collect his/her briefcase and notes, stand, and calmly leave the courtroom. He/she should not speak, gesture, wink, smile, or do anything else at or to either attorney, the jury, bailiff, or onlookers – no one. If an investigator or attorney follows the expert to ask or tell him/her something, the expert should listen or answer and then leave. Nothing should be said until the courtroom is left behind. Experts who have no further business in the courthouse should leave; experts who have no further business with the attorney who subpoenaed him/her should go home or back to work.

See Also

Expert Witness: Qualifications, Testimony and Malpractice; Medical; Daubert and Beyond

Further Reading

Bell S (2004) *Encyclopedia of Forensic Science*. New York: Facts on File.

Brown PM (1987) *The Art of Questioning: Thirty Maxims of Cross-Examination*. New York: Macmillan.

Faigman DL (2000) *Legal Alchemy: The Use and Misuse of Science in the Law*. New York: WH Freeman.

Foster KR, Huber PW (1999) *Judging Science: Scientific Knowledge and the Federal Courts*. Cambridge, MA: MIT Press.

Gross AG, Harmon JE, Reidy M (2002) *Communicating Science: The Scientific Article from the 17th Century to the Present*. Oxford, UK: Oxford University Press.

Houck MM (ed.) (2001) *Mute Witnesses: Trace Evidence Analysis*. San Diego, CA: Academic Press.

Houck MM (ed.) (2003) *Trace Evidence Analysis: More Cases from Mute Witnesses*. San Diego, CA: Academic Press.

Martel M (1989) *Mastering the Art of Q&A: A Survival Guide for Tough, Trick and Hostile Questions*. Homewood, IL: Business One Irwin.

Pritchard FN (2002) *Attorney Versus Engineer: Who Controls the Making of Product Litigation?* PhD dissertation. Los Angeles, CA: Department of Sociology, University of California.

Reference Manual on Scientific Evidence (2005) Federal Judicial Center, available online at http://www.fjc.gov/newweb/jnetweb.nsf.

PROFESSIONAL BODIES, FRANCE – FORENSIC MEDICAL AND SCIENTIFIC TRAINING

L Martrille and E Baccino, Centre Hospitalier Universitaire de Montpellier, Montpellier, France

Introduction

Forensic work is undertaken by various scientific specialists (physicists, chemists, biologists, medical professionals, anthropologists, and odontologists), who provide evidence in investigations for trials in civil or a criminal courts.

The forensic community in France shares the same goal as those elsewhere, but there are certain differences, which can be summarized as follows:

1. Medicolegal doctors are independent experts, working in the justice system on a case-by-case basis; their salaries are paid by the Ministry of Health. Forensic scientists, however, are generally employees of the police or gendarmerie (see below for a description of the difference between these two organisations).
2. Autopsies account for a small percentage of medicolegal activity, with clinical forensic medicine making up the majority; both are undertaken by the same physicians.
3. There is close control by the magistrates on forensic activity, from the scene of the crime, throughout the investigation, until the end of the trial.

Medicolegal Activity and Forensic Medicine in France

Heterogeneity characterizes medicolegal activity and forensic medicine in France. This is due to the large variety of applications, the uneven density of specialists in the country and the existence of several courses of study to become a forensic specialist.

Medicolegal Activity: Qualitative and Quantitative Data

A minority of teams undertake the whole range of medicolegal activity, including forensic pathology and "clinical forensic medicine", similar to the role of police surgeons/forensic physicians in the UK (i.e., examining both alleged victims and assailants).

These teams are based in the Centre Hospitalier Universitaire (University Hospital Centres; CHU) of which there are 25 in France and where the following services are also usually available: forensic toxicology, DNA analysis, physical anthropology, and forensic histology. Entomology and diatom identification are only performed in single centers. Several of these teams are also in charge of medical care of detainees.

Forensic Pathology

Statistics for several years from the French Ministry of Justice show that about 7000 forensic autopsies a year are performed nationally, for a population of more than 60 million. This statistic is due to a low crime rate but also to French judicial peculiarities, including strongly enforced medical confidentiality with regard to the cause of death, and decision-making left in the hands of the magistrates on a case-by-case basis, as there is no statute-defined policy.

In 75–80% of cases, these autopsies are performed in well-equipped autopsy rooms in large hospitals. In only four cities is more than one autopsy performed per working day.

Whenever possible a forensic doctor is called to the scene of a crime. No statistics are available for body examination at the scene, but personal research in three cities (Brest in northwestern France, Montpellier in the south, and Créteil in the southern suburbs of Paris) has shown that the ratio of autopsy/scene examination varies between one in two and one in four. Consequently, it can be hypothesized that, on a national level, between 1400 and 2500 scene examinations are performed every year.

Clinical Forensic Medicine

This includes the examination of people in custody (~250 000 per year nationally) and of living victims (victims of child abuse, battered women, victims of assault or rape). The clinical forensic medical examination involves the determination of the period of total temporary incapacity (known as the incapacité totale de travail [ITT]). The length of an ITT will affect legal proceedings: an ITT of fewer than eight days is a minor contravention of the law; a criminal offense has occurred where the ITT is longer than this.

Again, no national statistics are available. However, data from the same three cities mentioned above suggest that the number of living victims examined each year is between three and seven times higher than the number of autopsies (20 000–45 000 living victims are examined each year by forensic physicians). These data are open to question as Les Urgences Médico-Judiciaire de Paris (a hospital-based clinical forensic medicine unit) claimed it carried out 25 000 cases (including people examined in custody) in 1997.

Forensic Doctors: Number, Origin, and Training

La Société de Médecine Légale et de Criminologie de France (a nationwide forensic medicine society) has 400 members; the majority are forensic doctors, but some with only part-time involvement in forensic medicine. According to a recent estimate, nationwide 250 physicians were involved full-time in forensic medicine.

As a result of this limited number, it is only in some university hospitals that it is possible for a forensic doctor to be on duty around the clock year-round to perform all the clinical forensic activities mentioned above. In smaller cities and rural areas, forensic doctors focus on serious criminal cases, such as rape, homicide, child abuse, and other cases are dealt with by a general practitioner (GP). To improve this situation, emergency room doctors are being trained in forensic medicine.

Curricula

Most forensic doctors are now trained through a national diploma called Capacité des Pratiques Médico-Judiciaires, created in 1997, which requires students to receive practical instruction for 30 days a year over 2 years in an accredited hospital unit (usually a forensic medicine unit in a university hospital). They must also attend 200 h of lectures, including 30 h on medical law, 50 h on forensic pathology (scene examination, autopsy techniques, cause, and mode of death), 60–70 h on clinical forensic medicine (medicolegal and psychological aspects of rape, child abuse, battered women, and other types of violence). The rest of the teaching concerns the care of those in custody and detainees, and the biological aspects of forensic medicine (e.g., odontology techniques for identification, forensic anthropology, toxicology, and DNA analysis).

This is appropriate for most clinical forensic medicine and crime-scene examination, but, in most centers, students are not experienced enough to perform an autopsy alone. Fortunately, in most centers (but not all, as it rests on the decision of the magistrate) autopsies are performed by two physicians (usually the physician who attended the scene of the crime and the senior physician).

Another route to becoming a forensic doctor is the Complementary Specialized Study Diploma (DESC Diplôme d'étude spécialisée complémentaire), reserved for medical interns. In France, to become an intern, a selective examination must be passed at the end of general medical studies, i.e., 8 years after secondary school. After 4 years of internship in any specialty, a candidate who aspires to become a forensic medicine specialist needs two more years of practical and full-time training in a medical forensic unit plus 200 h of lectures. The graduate is then expected to be able to perform all forensic medicine activities, including autopsies.

As expected, this exclusive and demanding process has resulted in an output of fewer than 40 graduates nationally in 1996. This is why the Capacité diploma was initiated: the DESC route is chosen by those who intend to become academics (researchers and/or professors) in forensic medicine.

A recent survey has shown that only approximately 750 forensic doctors are needed to provide each local judicial court with the appropriate basic emergency forensic medicine services (clinical and crime-scene examination).

With regard to autopsies, due to the low French activity (in comparison with international standards), concentration in a regional and, sometimes, distant autopsy center (hospital-based) seems to be the only solution, for the sake of quality.

Research and Teaching

Research To summarize the state of research in forensic medicine in France, one only needs state that, within the long list of the sections of the National Institute of Medical Research (INSERM, Institut National de la Santé et de la Recherche Médicale), there is none about forensic medicine (or forensic science). As a result, state-funded research programs in forensic medicine are limited to scattered projects (fewer than 10 so far).

There are also regionally funded (lower-budget) programs and, several years ago, the Société Nationale de Médecine Légale et de Criminologie de France created the Prix Louis Roche (with limited funding), designed to encourage a researcher in this field. There is no Masters or PhD program in forensic medicine. However, a PhD program in forensic anthropology and bioethics has recently been created: these two specialties are of course very useful in forensic activity but are very specialized (4–5 students per year nationally).

Teaching In GP medical training, in medical schools nationally, 20–40 h of lectures are dedicated to forensic medicine, in particular to enable students to provide appropriate medical certificates for living victims, and death certificates, and also to familiarize them with the principles of medical law, especially medical liability and medical confidentiality. To date there is only one city where it is possible for all students to spend a week in a hospital forensic medicine unit. In addition to forensic medicine lectures, during the first year of medical school, a few hours are spent on bioethics.

Forensic medicine lectures are much more popular among GPs, once they are faced with practical problems, such as an examination of a child abuse case,

or the understanding of a growing and burgeoning medicolegal legislation.

In addition, at postgraduate level, professors of forensic medicine are often in charge of several courses (1–2 years), such as training future experts in the evaluation of bodily damage for the civil court or insurance companies; courses in victimology (how to take care of a victim properly from a judicial, medical, and psychological point of view); social security medicine; and teaching at the law school.

Summary

Even though not all needs are presently fulfilled with regard to the number of physicians and research and teaching, there has been a general increase in the role of forensic medicine in France since the 1980s.

Forensic doctors are heading a new specialty, called "violence medicine," which encompasses the effects of violence and the care of the perpetrators (in custody or in jail), allowing a better knowledge of the complex interconnection between victims, perpetrators, and crime.

The main problem in France remains financial, as the body that makes the decision as to the choice of expert and whether or not to perform an autopsy is the Ministry of Justice, where salaries are so low that it is impossible to make a living from penal activity alone. The Ministry of Health is therefore in charge of funding this activity, on a goodwill basis, resulting in too many parttime forensic physicians having to do another, more lucrative, medical activity to compensate.

Forensic Scientists Specializing in Criminalistics

Definition

The Police Technique et Scientifique (PTS) is the body of forensic scientists tasked with investigating criminal activities. Its history extends back to that of Bertillon (who described bertillonage – an anthropometric technique) and to the Professor of Legal Medicine, Edmond Locard, founder of the first French crime laboratory, in Lyons, in 1910.

Criminalistics encompasses all the techniques used to reconstruct a crime and to identify the perpetrator. This requires the use of all accessible chemical, physical, and biological methods to analyze material evidence from collection until the release of the report.

The border between forensic medicine and forensic science is sometimes unclear, as forensic medicine is a significant provider of pieces of evidence for the crime laboratories, and the victim, whether dead or alive, is part of the crime scene.

Moreover, some forensic crime laboratories and forensic medicine units have developed comparable technical capacities in DNA fingerprinting, toxicology, entomology, physical anthropology, and diatom identification.

Organization

The current approach is multidisciplinary, as crime-scene technicians work in close collaboration with the crime laboratories, which sometimes send scientists to the crime scene. As a result, there is a need for a crime-scene technical adviser to the crime laboratories.

In France, as in some other Mediterranean countries, there is a dual organization of law enforcement agencies, i.e., police (Ministry of the Interior) for urban areas and gendarmerie (Ministry of Defense) for suburban and rural areas.

National Police   Within the division of judicial police, there is a subdivision of forensic sciences (PTS), which has two levels: central (judicial identity, forensic laboratory, crime documentation, computer and technological traces and external services), including five crime laboratories (in Paris, Lyons, Marseille, Lille, and Toulouse), 19 regional and 11 local departments of judicial identity, 19 regional departments of crime documentation, and 167 local departments of forensic police.

Paris and its *prefecture de police* has its own organization. This has 2400 police officers, 1700 of whom are dedicated to forensic science, i.e., evidence collection and analysis.

In addition, 6000 field police officers trained in basic evidence collection techniques for minor crimes complete this national network.

National gendarmerie   The subdivision of judicial police has several forensic sciences services under its control:

1. One central crime laboratory in Rosny sous Bois, a Paris suburb, that is organized into 12 departments and has 200 employees. This laboratory can send scientists to the crime scene on request from magistrates or investigators, to help the gendarmerie crime-scene technicians, who are trained at the Corps National Centre in Fontainebleau (another Paris suburb).
2. A technical unit of judicial intelligence and documentation.
3. Local units with over 500 officers trained in crime-scene investigation methods.

All the officers of the 3500 gendarmerie units throughout the country receive basic training and equipment for simple crime investigation.

Both police and gendarmerie have mass-disaster units for identification purposes, and these have, already had to be involved in several cases.

They also work together in managing national databases, such as those for fingerprints, DNA ballistic features, drug chemical profiling), missing persons, stolen vehicles, and criminal offenses. These databases, used at a national level, constitute a powerful tool in forensic intelligence, revealing serial crimes, identifying criminals, and matching suspects with already known and classified criminals.

In 1992, the Conseil Superieur de la Police Technique et Scientifique (high council for forensic sciences), presided over by the Minister of the Interior, and incorporating representatives from defense, police, and justice, was formed. This has played an important role in encouraging all forensic sciences agencies to work together.

Only the police provide an integrated forensic science capacity and a multidisciplinary approach, which is increasingly needed in complex crimes and as new, sophisticated technologies become available. There are, however, a few private laboratories and experts in single techniques, such as DNA analysis, ballistics questioned documents, toxicology, fire, and explosions.

It is impossible to assess the level of activity of these private structures. The choice between state (police or gendarmerie) or private experts will depend mainly upon geographical considerations and the choice of investigators; however, the magistrate, who controls the entire investigation process in France, can, by law, choose whomever he or she wants to work with.

Personnel and Training

Within police and gendarmerie crime laboratories, there are two types of personnel: those in charge of the organization (the leadership of the laboratory being undertaken by the gendarmerie or the police), and the technicians. The technicians may come from civil sources, as the scientific and technical skills needed for these positions are not always available within the gendarmerie and police forces.

Even though this situation could be a potential source of conflict, it seems to work fairly well, especially as the numbers of personnel increased dramatically in the early 1990s, after a report from the Ministry of the Interior showed that the level of finance and personnel in France was 5–7 times lower than that in the UK.

Training

In France, there is no national board certifying a diploma or curriculum for becoming a technician in a crime laboratory. There are a couple of specialized training courses in Lyons and Paris, but these diplomas are not a prerequisite for obtaining a position in a crime laboratory. Therefore, it is not surprising that there is no PhD program in France for forensic science, and that senior officers who wish to obtain a PhD have to go to other countries. Considering the highly technical equipment used within a crime laboratory and the fast-moving science involved, such a lack is, in the medium term, a concern for the efficiency of French crime laboratories, especially with regard to the progress made during the 1980s.

Conclusion

There is an apparent clear separation between crime laboratories and forensic medicine in France. However, they have common fields (DNA analysis, toxicology, forensic anthropology, entomology) that provide opportunities for fruitful collaboration. This collaboration should be increased, as physicians require the technical skills and equipment provided by the crime laboratories, and the crime laboratories must rely on the academic background and possibilities provided by the university hospital.

Grouping all the experts (medical and scientific) within the same organization, independent of the judicial process, should be in the interest of the forensic personnel, improving the quality of expertise, and therefore being in the best interests of justice for the public.

See Also

Professional Bodies: United Kingdom; Rest of the World

PROFESSIONAL BODIES

Contents
United Kingdom
Rest of the World

United Kingdom

J Payne-James, Forensic Healthcare Services Ltd, London, UK

Introduction

Regulation of standards of different healthcare professionals varies widely in the UK. There are a number of specific "professional regulators" responsible for several professions. These are listed in **Table 1**. Other organizations are involved in the monitoring and assessment of standards and these are listed in **Table 2**. **Table 3** indicates the number of health professionals registered in the UK. Some professions are controlled by statute and others by codes of practice or guidelines set by other bodies established for that purpose.

Most regulatory bodies have a role in setting or defining standards of practice and provide the means by which practitioners who have deemed to have failed to achieve such standards can be disciplined. Sanctions vary depending on the regulating body and may, for example, allow for the removal of a practitioner from a register or for the supervision of that practitioner when working, or make requirements for training.

The roles and functions of the General Medical Council (GMC) will now be considered in detail as an example illustrating the principles of some professional regulatory bodies in the UK.

General Medical Council

The GMC was first established by statute by the Medical Act 1858 in part to enable "persons requiring medical aid ... to distinguish qualified from unqualified practitioners." To do this a register was created. Subsequent Medical Acts – the most recent being the Medical Act 1983 – expanded the role and workload of the GMC. Recently its activities have come under unprecedented external scrutiny and

Table 1   Professional regulators

Dental Practice Board
General Chiropractic Council
General Dental Council
General Medical Council
General Optical Council
General Osteopathic Council
Health Professions Council
Nursing and Midwifery Council
Royal Pharmaceutical Society of Great Britain

Table 2   Organizations involved in monitoring quality and standards

Audit Commission
Clinical Standards Board for Scotland
Health Quality Service
National Audit Office
National Care Standards Commission

Table 3   Number of registrants with the Health Professions Council (at April 1, 2003) (www.hpe-uk.org)

Profession	Registrants
Art therapists	1992
Chiropodists/podiatrists	9013
Clinical scientists	3408
Dietitians	5782
Medical laborarory technicians	21 895
Occupational therapists	24 576
Orthoptists	1328
Prosthetists and orthotists	786
Paramedics	9334
Physiotherapists	35 643
Radiographers	21 484
Speech and language therapists	8900
Total	144 141

critical examination from the public and within the profession itself. The GMC's role is limited to the powers and duties conferred by statute. It is not a general complaints body and can only act where there is evidence that a doctor may not be fit to practice. As such its actions may be subject to public law challenge by the route of judicial review. The GMC explains its role thus:

> Protecting the public: We have strong and effective legal powers designed to maintain the standards the public have a right to expect of doctors. We are not here to protect the medical profession – their interests are protected by others. Our job is to protect patients.
>
> The public trust doctors to set and monitor their own professional standards. In return doctors must give their patients high-quality medical care. Where

any doctor fails to meet those standards, we act to protect patients from harm – if necessary, by striking the doctor off the register and removing their right to practice medicine.

We are a charity whose purpose is the protection, promotion and maintenance of the health and safety of the community.

These principles apply to all doctors, whether working within the National Health Service (NHS) or in other areas such as private practice. The majority of the GMC's income is derived from the registration of new members and from the annual retention fees of existing members.

Structure and Functions of the GMC

In December 2002, the Privy Council approved new legislation, which allowed the most comprehensive and wide-ranging reform of professional regulation since the establishment of the GMC in 1858. The three main elements are

1. reducing the membership of Council from 104 to 35 and increasing lay membership
2. reform of "fitness to practice" procedures and how complaints about doctors are dealt with
3. reform of registration procedures, with the introduction of revalidation, a regular demonstration by doctors that they meet standards required for continued registration.

The new changes are set out in the Medical Act 1983 (Amendment Order) 2002.

Registration

The GMC is a body that sets standards for undergraduate, preregistration, and postgraduate medical education. Doctors must be registered with the GMC to practice medicine in the UK. To register with the GMC, they must have a recognized medical qualification. The medical register shows who is properly qualified to practice medicine in the UK. Registration confers certain privileges, allowing doctors to undertake certain procedures or functions. Examples of statutes that specifically refer to medical practitioners as having a role or function are given in **Table 4**. The type of work that requires doctors to be registered includes: employment in the NHS; prescribing certain drugs; and issuing medical certificates required for statutory purposes.

Various groups of doctors may be considered for the purposes of registration, including doctors qualifying from a UK medical school who are eligible for provisional and full registration. Doctors qualifying in another European Economic Area (EEA) member

Table 4 Examples of statutes with defined roles/functions for medical practitioners

Abortion Act 1967
Access to Medical Records Act 1990
Air Force Act 1955
Armed Forces Act 1981
Army Act 1955
Births and Death Registration Act 1953
Cancer Act 1939
Children Act 1989
Children and Young Persons Act 1969
Chiropractors Act 1994
Courts-Martial (Appeals) Act 1968
Crime and Disorder Act 1998
Crime (Sentences) Act 1997
Criminal Appeal Act 1968
Criminal Justice Act 1967
Local Government Finance Act 1992
Magistrates' Courts Act 1980
Marriage Act 1949
Medicines Act 1968
Mental Health Act 1983
Misuse of Drugs Act 1971
National Health Service and Community Care Act 1990
Opticians Act 1989
Public Health (Control of Disease) Act 1984

Table 5 Duties of a doctor

As a doctor you must:
- make the care of your patient your first concern
- treat every patient politely and considerately
- respect patients' dignity and privacy
- listen to patients and respect their views
- give patients information in a way they can understand it
- respect the rights of patients to be fully involved in decisions about their care
- keep your professional knowledge and skills up-to-date
- recognize the limits of your professional competence
- be honest and trustworthy
- respect and protect confidential information
- make sure that your personal beliefs do not prejudice your patients' care
- act quickly to protect patients from risk if you have good reason to believe that you or a colleague may not be fit to practice
- avoid abusing your position as a doctor
- work with colleagues in the ways that best serve patients' interests

state and who are nationals of an EEA member state (or non-EEA nationals with European Community (EC) rights) are eligible for full registration (they are also eligible to apply for provisional registration if their medical education includes a period of postgraduate clinical training); doctors from other countries can find out their situation by contacting the GMC (www.gmc-uk.org).

Full registration is required for unsupervised medical practice in the NHS or private practice in the UK. Specialist registration may be required for a consultant post within the NHS. Provisional registration allows newly qualified doctors to undertake the general clinical training needed for full registration and such doctors are only entitled to work in resident junior house officer posts in hospitals or institutions. Limited registration requires an appropriate primary qualification. Applicants for limited registration must provide evidence of their current capability for practice in the UK either by passing a linguistic skills test or by providing other evidence.

Registration carries both privileges and responsibilities. The duties of a doctor – which the GMC describes as the "contract between doctor and patient which is at the heart of medicine" – are listed in **Table 5**. The GMC gives clear guidance on the principles of good medical practice and standards of competence, care, and conduct expected of doctors in all aspects of their professional work. Serious or persistent failures to meet these standards may put a doctor's registration at risk.

Fitness-to-Practice Procedures

The GMC's fitness-to-practice procedures and powers are linked to licencing doctors and maintaining the medical register. The GMC can take action against doctors if the doctor has been convicted of a criminal offense; there is evidence of conduct that appears to be so serious that it is likely to call into question the doctor's fitness to continue in medical practice (serious professional misconduct (SPM)); there is evidence of a repeated departure from good professional practice, whether or not it is covered by specific GMC guidance, sufficiently serious to call into question a doctor's registration (seriously deficient performance); or there is evidence that a doctor is not fit to practice medicine because of the state of his/her health. **Table 6** illustrates examples of cases where the GMC may need to intervene. Any doctor whose "fitness to practice" is questioned should seek advice from his/her own medical defense organization (MDO).

Following a complaint, one of the GMC's caseworkers will assess whether concerns should be investigated further. The doctor concerned will be given an opportunity to comment on the allegations. Once all the evidence is available, the case will be considered by one or more GMC members appointed as "screeners" who will decide whether a case needs to be referred to the next stage of the GMC's fitness-to-practice procedures. All cases will initially be reviewed by a medical member, and if either the medical member or a lay member decides that the case does raise serious concerns, it will be placed under one (or more) of the following procedures: conduct, performance, or health. If both agree that there is no need for any further action against the doctor, the

Table 6 Examples of when the General Medical Council may need to intervene

- Serious or repeated mistakes in carrying out medical procedures or in diagnosis, for example, incorrect dosages on prescriptions, prescribing inappropriate drugs
- Failure to examine patients properly or respond reasonably to patient needs
- Fraud or dishonesty in financial matters or in dealings with patients or research
- Serious breaches of a patient's confidentiality
- Treating patients without making sure that they know what is involved and agree to it
- Making sexual advances towards patients
- Misusing alcohol or drugs

GMC will write to the complainant and to the doctor explaining the decision. The GMC aims to be able to take a screening decision within 6 months of receiving a complaint. If there is evidence that the doctor poses an immediate risk to patients the GMC will ensure that the case is dealt with quickly, and will ask the Interim Orders Committee to decide whether the doctor should be suspended or have conditions imposed on his/her registration while inquiries continue.

Conduct Procedures

The GMC's conduct procedures consider allegations of SPM, and deal with doctors convicted of criminal offenses (excluding minor motoring offenses). The Preliminary Procedure Committee (PPC) is a panel of medical and lay members which meets in private to decide whether a case should be referred to the Professional Conduct Committee (PCC) for a full formal inquiry in public. Criminal cases involving custodial sentences can be fast-tracked to a full hearing of the PCC. If the PPC decides there is no need to refer the case to the PCC they may still provide the doctor with advice about his/her future conduct. The rules which govern the GMC's procedures do not allow for an appeal against a PPC decision. If either screener decides that a case raises a possible issue of SPM, the GMC will write formally to the doctor setting out the allegations against him/her. The doctor then has a further chance to comment before the case is considered by the PPC. The GMC will ask the doctor if he/she agrees to these comments being disclosed to the complainant.

The PCC is the final stage of the GMC's conduct procedures. The inquiries are conducted in public and the doctor, the complainant, and other witnesses will need to give evidence under oath, with questioning from the panel hearing the case, and lawyers representing both sides. If a doctor is found guilty of SPM the PCC can: (1) erase the doctor from the register;

(2) suspend the doctor's registration; (3) impose conditions on the doctor's registration; or (4) give the doctor a warning. If the PCC finds that the doctor is not guilty of SPM it may decide to take no action against the doctor or may issue advice about future conduct. If the Committee orders that a doctor is suspended or struck off, and believes others could be put at risk, or that it would be in the doctor's interest to stop medical work at once, suspension of registration can be imposed immediately. Application to the High Court can be made to have that order lifted. There are 28 days to appeal to the Judicial Committee of the Privy Council against the decision to suspend registration or impose conditions. These appeal procedures apply for all fitness-to-practice decisions.

Performance Procedures

The GMC's performance procedures assess doctors whose performance appears to be seriously deficient. There is initial consideration by a screener. The screener does not have to notify the doctor at this stage. If the screener considers there is a case to be answered the GMC will invite the doctor to undergo an assessment of his/her skills and knowledge – a performance assessment. If the doctor refuses to participate or undergo an assessment he/she will be referred to the Assessment Referral Committee (ARC). The ARC has the power to direct the doctor to undergo an assessment within a fixed period of time. The assessment is carried out by a team of trained assessors. The assessment will cover the doctor's attitudes, knowledge, clinical and communications skills, and clinical records and audit results. After the assessment the team will report to the case coordinator. The case coordinator will decide on the next step. This may be: (1) to take no further action if the assessment has revealed no serious performance problems; (2) to ask that the doctor takes action to improve his/her performance (if the problems have been identified but they pose no risk to patients); and (3) to refer the doctor to the Committee of Professional Performance (CPP) if serious problems have been identified. The CPP may, if necessary, suspend or place conditions on the doctor's registration.

Health Procedures

Health procedures can be utilized if a doctor is attempting to practice despite being seriously affected by ill health. The most serious cases are reported to the Health Committee (HC), which can suspend or place conditions on the doctor's registration. The central feature of the health procedures is a medical assessment by experts. Any issues raising questions about health are referred to a "health screener" – a GMC member who is a psychiatrist. The health screener decides whether patients are being put at risk, and whether there is enough evidence to suggest that the ability to practice may be seriously impaired by a physical or mental condition. The health screener may decide not to get involved if he/she believes that local measures, which are already being taken, will prevent harm to patients. If the screener decides on further action, examination will be proposed by at least two medical examiners chosen by the GMC, but who are not GMC members. Recommendations will be made about treatment required, medical supervision, and support advised, which might be limitations, including avoiding single-handed practice, practicing only if supervised, or not practicing medicine at all.

If the doctor is considered fit for medical work, the screener will close the case. If it is believed that the ability to practice is seriously impaired by a condition, the screener will ask the doctor to accept recommendations for medical supervision and for restrictions on medical work. Once agreement has been reached about medical supervision, the health screener will choose a doctor to supervise and to arrange necessary treatment.

In most cases, doctors under the health procedures cooperate. However the HC will become involved in some circumstances, for example, if the doctor does not agree to be medically examined or refuses to accept recommendations for medical supervision or limitations on medical work.

The HC meets in private and adopts legal rules of procedure. All the HC members are GMC members. The main evidence at the hearings is the written medical reports. The Committee must decide whether ability to practice is seriously impaired by a health problem. If it is, they may suspend registration for up to 12 months; or put conditions on registration for up to 3 years. The Committee will consider the case again at the end of the period of suspension or when the conditions are due to be reviewed, and another medical examination will generally be undertaken before the hearing. The Committee will decide whether there is any risk to patients on the basis of the evidence, including up-to-date reports from the medical supervisor. If they then decide to close the case, the doctor can return to medical work, without any restrictions. If the case is kept under review, further conditions can be imposed, or registration suspended for up to a year at a time. If the Committee has suspended registration for 2 years, registration can then be suspended indefinitely. There would then be no need for further hearings unless requested by the doctor.

Interim Orders Committee

The GMC has the powers either to suspend or place conditions on a doctor's registration at any stage in its procedures. This can be done: (1) when the doctor may be a risk to patients; (2) when the doctor may be a risk to him/herself; and (3) when it is in the public interest. The Interim Orders Committee's (IOC's) role is to consider the application of interim measures on a doctor's registration while fitness-to-practice procedures continue. This is a very severe sanction that is only applied when there is evidence of a clear need to act immediately to suspend or restrict a doctor.

Other Relevant Bodies

The National Clinical Assessment Authority (NCAA) was set up by government to deal with underperforming doctors and aims to reduce the number and length of suspensions. The NCAA is a special health authority established on April 1, 2001. The GMC has agreements (Memoranda of Understanding) with the NCAA to ensure they work together effectively to protect patients. The aim of the NCAA is to provide a support service to NHS primary care, hospital and community trusts, the Prison Health Service, and the Defence Medical Services when they are faced with concerns over the performance of an individual doctor. In order to help doctors in difficulty, the NCAA provides advice, takes referrals, and carries out targeted assessments where necessary. The NCAA's assessment involves trained medical and lay assessors. The NCAA is established as an advisory body, and the NHS employer organization remains responsible for resolving the problem once the NCAA has produced its assessment (www.ncaa:nhs.uk).

Appraisal and Revalidation

Appraisal has been introduced by the Department of Health in the UK for doctors working in the NHS. The aim is to give doctors regular feedback on past performance and continuing progress and to identify education and development needs – it is part of a doctor's career development. Concurrently the GMC made proposals to license and revalidate all registered doctors. The aims of appraisal are shown in **Table 7**. Details of appraisal may be found at www.appraisaluk.info.

For NHS doctors, appraisal will also be the method for gathering revalidation evidence. All doctors must have a license to practice to treat patients or prescribe for them. Every 5 years all doctors who want to remain in practice must present evidence to the GMC that they are competent in their field of practice and

Table 7 Aims of appraisal

- to set out personal and professional development needs, career paths, and goals
- to agree plans for them to be met
- to review the doctor's performance
- to consider the doctor's contribution to the quality and improvement of local healthcare services
- to optimize the use of skills and resources in achieving the delivery of high-quality care
- to offer an opportunity for doctors to discuss and seek support for their participation in activities
- to identify the need for adequate resources to enable service objectives to be met

have kept up to date. This will allow the doctor's license to practice to be renewed.

To simplify matters, the UK Department of Health and the GMC agreed that a single set of documentation would be used for appraisal and revalidation. For doctors within managed organizations, five sets of completed annual appraisal forms can be submitted to the GMC as evidence to support revalidation. Alternatively, the evidence gathered for the appraisal process could also be submitted to the GMC as evidence to support revalidation.

If a doctor in the future wishes to continue to practice (including prescribing and signing statutory certificates), a license to practice will be required. The GMC will grant doctors a license to practice by the end of 2004, unless they tell the GMC they don't want one. To maintain a license to practice, doctors must take part in revalidation when requested by the GMC. From January 1, 2005, by law, a doctor is unable to practice without a license.

To keep a license to practice, the GMC will ask all doctors, normally once every 5 years, to show them that they have been practicing medicine in line with the standards set out in the publication *Good Medical Practice*. Doctors will need to be able to show the GMC that they have followed the standards that are relevant to their specialty and their practice. It is the doctor's own responsibility, not that of others.

The GMC will tell doctors the result of their own revalidation as soon as is possible. The license will, of course, remain valid until they have made the final decision about the revalidation. A doctor will have the right of appeal against any decision to withdraw, or refuse to restore, their license to practice. Further and regularly updated information on revalidation is located at www.revalidationuk.info. Both appraisal and revalidation will continue to modify, change, and evolve substantially in the next few years.

Clinical Governance

Clinical governance as a concept can be defined as "a framework through which NHS organizations are accountable for continuously improving the quality of their services and safeguarding high standards of care by creating an environment in which excellence in clinical care will flourish" and is seen as a means by which better monitoring and safer clinical practice can be achieved.

Emphasis is now placed on integrated quality improvement systems incorporating clinical audit, risk management, evidence-based practice, adverse incident reporting, and a whole range of other processes that are designed to identify and disseminate areas of good practice and areas where improvements in patient care and safety can be made. Although labeled as "clinical" governance, the term covers any system or process within the NHS that has a direct impact on the quality of patient care, therefore management decisions can constitute a clinical governance issue and be reportable as such.

The principles of clinical governance apply to all those who provide or manage patient care services in the NHS and are thus inextricably linked to those underpinning professional self-regulation. Thus all registered practitioners have a responsibility to themselves, their colleagues, and their patients to contribute and respond to the clinical governance framework of their organization. It is no longer possible to ignore concerns about one's own performance or that of fellow healthcare professionals.

See Also

Professional Bodies, France – Forensic, Medical and Scientific Training; **Professional Bodies:** Rest of the World

Further Reading

Department of Health (1998) *A First Class Service. Quality in the New NHS*. London: Department of Health.

General Medical Council (1998) *Seeking Patients' Consent: The Ethical Considerations*. London: GMC.

General Medical Council (2000) *Confidentiality: Protecting and Providing Information*. London: GMC.

General Medical Council (2001) *Good Medical Practice*. London: GMC.

General Medical Council (2002) *Research: The Role and Responsibilities of Doctors*. London: GMC.

www.ncaa.nhs.uk

www.hpc-uk.org

www.gmc-uk.org

Rest of the World

S Cordner and H McKelvie, Victorian Institute of
Forensic Medicine, Southbank, VIC, Australia

Introduction

As with many medical and scientific disciplines, there
are a number of forensic organizations and associations that are established to support the work and
further education of practitioners, and to create valuable opportunities to meet and share information and
experiences. An internet search of any popular forensic website will reveal links to long lists of such
entities: many are based at universities, within states
or provinces, while others have national membership.
Some organizations have international coverage, or
at least names that imply it. What follows is a brief
list of a selection of international and regional orga-
nizations/associations that are considered by the
authors to be important contributors to the promotion of regional and international exchange in
forensic science disciplines. It is by no means an
exhaustive list.

It is to be noted that most of the information
provided about these organizations is directly derived
from their constituting documents and/or official
websites.

Organizations

Indo-Pacific Association of Law Medicine and Science (INPALMS)

In 1978, Professor Chao, the first president of
INPALMS, and Professor Salgado acted on a suggestion that a forensic medicine and science organization
be established to cater to the needs of the Indo-Pacific
region. There were already two existing international
associations in this field: the International Academy of
Legal Medicine and Social Medicine, founded in 1938
and the International Association of Forensic Sciences
(IAFS), founded in 1957. INPALMS aimed to cover
regions outside Europe and the USA and to maintain
permanent national and individual members in regular
communication through newsletters. The association
was initially known as the Asian Pacific Association of
Law, Medicine, and Sciences and was established in
1983 at the congress held in Singapore. INPALMS
was formally inaugurated in 1986 in Colombo,
Sri Lanka at the Second Indo-Pacific Congress on
Legal Medicine and Forensic Sciences. The change in
name from Asian-Pacific to Indo-Pacific came about to
include Africa.

The association was primarily set up to promote
national and international cooperation in matters of
education and research in the fields of legal medicine,
forensic science, and law enforcement; to organize
and sponsor conferences, workshops, and seminars;
and to publish material in connection with the
subjects of legal medicine, forensic science, and law
enforcement. It also aimed to hold an international
congress on legal medicine, forensic science, and law
enforcement at least once every 3 years, in a country
in the Indo-Pacific region.

Triennial Congresses Up to 500 registrants from as
many as 37 different countries have attended each of
the eight congresses: (1) 1983 Singapore; (2) 1986
Colombo, Sri Lanka; (3) 1989 Madras, India;
(4) 1992 Bangkok, Thailand; (5) 1995 Bali, Indone-
sia; (6) 1998 Kobe, Japan; (7) 2001 Melbourne,
Australia and (8) 2004 Manila, Philippines.

Newsletter A newsletter is distributed to all
INPALMS members on a semiregular basis. Enquiries
and contributions can be made to the editor at
sal@sltnet.lk.

Web access INPALMS does not yet have a dedicated website, but details of the forthcoming Congress are normally posted on a website established for
this purpose. A web search using the search term
"INPALMS" will be successful in locating current
Congress information.

International Association of Forensic Sciences

Inaugurated in 1957, IAFS is a worldwide association
that brings together academics and practicing professionals of various disciplines in forensic science,
including forensic scientists: those working in police,
government, or private forensic laboratories, dealing
with fingerprints, biochemical grouping, drug
analysis, toxicology, ballistics, trace evidence examination, and accident reconstruction, and those working in other branches of forensic science, such as
forensic psychiatry, physical anthropology, medical
law and bioethics, and forensic odontology.

The aims and objectives of IAFS are: (1) to develop the forensic sciences; (2) to assist forensic scientists and others to exchange scientific and technical
information; and (3) to organize meetings.

According to its constitution, IAFS organizes a
world meeting every 3 years. Since 1957, a total of
16 triennial meetings have been organized in major
cities around the world.

The governing body of the association is the council, which comprises all living past-presidents and is

chaired by the president in office. Elected by council, the president in office is responsible for organizing in the final year of office an international meeting of the association.

Information about and contact details for IAFS can be found at the website established for the forthcoming meeting. Currently, the relevant website is www.iafs2005.com.

Australian and New Zealand Forensic Science Society

The Australian and New Zealand Forensic Science Society (ANZFSS) was formed in 1971 with the aim of bringing together scientists, police, criminalists, pathologists, and members of the legal profession actively involved in the forensic sciences. The society's objectives are to enhance the quality of forensic science by providing both formal and informal lectures, discussions, and demonstrations encompassing the various disciplines within the forensic sciences. In addition, the society holds an international symposium every 2 years. The meetings and symposia cover the major areas of forensic science, such as toxicology, biology, odontology, pathology, crime scene, firearms, arson, explosions, fingerprints, homicide, disasters, documents, and drug-associated crime. Currently the society has members from all states and territories in Australia and New Zealand. There is a branch of the society in each state of Australia, in Australian Capital Territory, and in New Zealand. The Victorian branch of the ANZFSS holds regular meetings and organizes visits to places of forensic interest. These meetings usually involve lectures by experts in their field and provide opportunities for members and guests to meet in an informal atmosphere. The meetings are organized by the committee. The committee is elected at the annual general meeting and comprises the president, vice president, secretary, treasurer, and other general members.

Membership Membership is open to all residents of Australia or New Zealand who have a genuine interest in forensic science. The society always welcomes new members.

Contacts Contact details are available for Australian states and New Zealand on the ANZFSS website at www.nifs.com.au/ANZFSS/ANZFSS.

International Organization of Forensic Odonto-Stomotology (IOFOS)

The objects of the IOFOS are: (1) to provide liaison between societies of (legal) forensic odontology on

a global basis; (2) to promote good will, advancement, and research in forensic odontology; and (3) to publish a newsletter on a regular basis.

Membership is open to any society, provided its regulations accord with the objectives of the IOFOS. Member societies have the obligation to send to IOFOS an annual report of their activities in forensic odontology. There are currently 27 member societies.

The IOFOS also maintains the *Journal of Forensic Odonto-Somatology.*

Details about the newsletter, journal, and membership of the IOFOS can be found on its website at www.forodont.se/iofos/.

European Network of Forensic Science Institutes (ENFSI)

ENFSI was founded in October 1995, with the aim of ensuring that the quality of development and delivery of forensic science throughout Europe is at the forefront of the world. The means of achieving this aim are through membership meetings (held triennially), open forensic science meetings, and the work of a board, expert working groups, and committees. Meetings are held annually, with the activities of the board and expert working group and committees taking place throughout the year. The activities of the standing committees include developing policies and providing advice to the expert working groups and ENFSI members to help the laboratories of ENFSI members (ENFSI laboratories) comply with best-practice and international standards.

Membership

Eligibility for membership is confined to directors (or their nominees) of the institutes in Europe, where the majority of the workload consists of forensic science casework in a broad area of crime investigation. In addition, directors of other institutes involved in forensic science are considered for membership if this is beneficial to the aims of ENFSI. There are currently about 50 members.

ENFSI has a website at www.enfsi.org.

Interpol Disaster Victim Identification (DVI) Committee

An Interpol working party on DVI composed of police officers, forensic pathologists, and forensic odontologists was set up in 1980. The working party, subsequently recognized as the Interpol Standing Committee on DVI, was responsible for overseeing the development of a DVI form and guide, which has been formally adopted by the Interpol General Assembly. These documents aim to contribute to the efficiency and effectiveness of disaster handling in general and of identification procedures in particular. It is designed to encourage the compatibility of procedures across international boundaries, which is essential in these days of ever-increasing world travel. The recommendations in the guide cannot address every possible eventuality but they give sound practical advice on major issues of victim identification, underlining the importance of preplanning and training. Such preparation, and an awareness of the many potential demands and difficulties with which police services may be faced, will undoubtedly contribute to successful operations, and thus benefit all involved, including victims, relatives, and the other agencies with which the police cooperate when disasters occur.

The standing committee recognizes the basic human right of individuals to be properly identified after death and that the identification of disaster victims continues to be of increasing international importance with regard to police investigations, in addition to other legal, religious, and cultural requirements. To this end, it recommends that all the organizations' member countries use the DVI form in all appropriate circumstances, including cases in which there is only one victim to be identified. The form and guide are disseminated to all Interpol member countries.

The standing committee's ongoing responsibilities are to:

- coopt specialists from other organizations as appropriate (e.g., United Nations Department of Humanitarian Affairs, airline operators, forensic science services)
- consider relevant previous incidents, identifying technical developments and experience from which improvements to procedures and standards in DVI matters, including documentation, technology, computerization, education, and training may be made
- ensure that the DVI forms and guide to DVI procedures are maintained so as to provide the best possible practical assistance and advice to member countries
- make recommendations to enhance cooperation, liaison, information exchange, and practical assistance between member countries and with other relevant national and international agencies and organizations when planning for, or responding to, disasters

- meet regularly to achieve these aims and disseminate advice and recommendations on good practice promptly to member countries.

Information about the Interpol DVI Committee can be found at www.interpol.int/Public/DisasterVictim. Contact for the standing committee is through dvi@interpol.int.

Latin American Forensic Anthropology Association (ALAF)

ALAF is a not-for-profit association that was established in 2003 by a group of Latin American anthropologists. It has the following aims:

- to establish ethical and professional criteria for the practice of forensic anthropology that will ensure the quality of the practice
- to promote the use of forensic anthropology and archeology amongst the forensic disciplines utilized in judiciary investigations in Latin America
- to promote the accreditation of professionals working in forensic anthropology through the creation of an independent accrediting board that will certify the quality of practitioners
- to promote mechanisms that provide families of the deceased with access to the procedures and results of forensic investigations, in accordance with international treaties and recommendations
- to promote the protection of ALAF members and their families, considering the risks associated with working in forensic anthropology in some Latin American countries
- to defend the scientific and technical autonomy of forensic anthropology investigations in Latin America and the Caribbean.

The association organizes congresses for its members and associates. Its patron is Dr. Clyde Snow.

There is currently limited information about the ALAF available on the internet at www.eaaf.org/docs/annualreport/2002/16ALAF.pdf.

See Also

Professional Bodies, France – Forensic, Medical and Scientific Training; Professional Bodies: United Kingdom

RECOVERED MEMORY

B Tully, Psychologists at Law Group, London, UK

Introduction

Following trends in North America, there has been a steady trickle of criminal prosecutions in England based upon recovered memories of childhood sexual abuse. The forensic mental health assessor involved in these cases faces a wide range of difficulties. The science is controversial. Definitions of "recovered memory" and the language of complainants are inconsistent and ambiguous. Cases are complex and eccentric, with no typical pattern. Some complainants affected by the controversy present strategically. There are legal and professional barriers to obtaining historical documentation. Newly recognized phenomena of recovered memories arising from adult-onset psychopathology are sparsely reported. In general there is professional agreement that there is no infallible way of discriminating possibly true recovered memories from false memories. The science of how false memories can and do arise has developed considerably. This has led most medical and psychological associations to draw up guidelines specifying the dangers of "memory work" in psychotherapy. The grounds for determining questionable recovered memories, which are possibly or probably false, has been much developed in the course of the debate within the last decade, and to some extent the intensity of that debate has thus begun to fade. A range of practical guidelines is offered for any mental health practitioner thinking of carrying out such assessments in a specifically forensic context.

Emergence of a Controversy

During the 1980s in the USA there emerged reports of truly extraordinary cases entailing extensive memories returning to adults concerning childhood abuse, predominantly of a sexual nature. Often the newly remembered abuse was said to be traumatic, extensive, and repeated. These cases appeared neither to be recognizable or explainable by the standard accepted mechanisms of human memory, and acquired a special terminology, "recovered memories." The implication was that these memories must have been repressed or amnestically dissociated in a way that differed from ordinary forgetting. Such amnesia would have to have covered all the events, all subjective reactions and efforts to cope, and all attitudes to the perpetrator prior to the belated realization that he or she was such, and would have been resistant to all relevant reminders until the point of eventual "recovery." The return of this "repressed" material often seemed to occur in a staggered fashion over a period of time, especially if the person was psychologically troubled and undertaking psychotherapy. An early example of this was Michelle Smith's account, recovered from apparently complete amnesia, of grotesque repeated sexual abuse at the hands of a satanic cult. Michelle Smith described the ritual sexual sacrifice of stillborn babies and her being forced to undergo surgery to have tails and a horn attached to her body. This and other extraordinary cases, most somewhat less lurid, have been documented by historians of this phenomenon.

First Criminal Trial Relying on Recovered Memories and Expert Testimony

In 1990 in California came the first documented and much publicized case of a prosecution of a man based on an alleged completely recovered memory. Eileen Franklin claimed that she had developed a clear memory, which had occurred whilst watching her own child's face, of her father, George Franklin, smashing the skull of her childhood friend Susan Nason. Little Susan was indeed murdered when she was 8 years old, but no one was found responsible at the time. Ms Franklin's testimony was challenged as not being in accord with how memory is known to work normally. The prosecution called Professor Lenore Terr, a psychoanalytical psychiatrist. She told the court that her research with children indicated that they had very great difficulties forgetting or avoiding thinking of single traumas. However, if trauma occurred repeatedly, then they would learn a cognitive maneuver to dissociate or repress each event as it occurred, and so they could psychologically survive. This, she asserted, explained why Ms Franklin had repressed a real and true memory. For the first time, the court accepted this scientific testimony and convicted. As will be seen to be often the case with the English proceedings, the full facts about the course and fluctuations of the recovered memories were only discovered later. In Eileen Franklin's case it became clear that even her story of how her recovered memories had come back to mind, and the precise contents of those, varied very considerably on different occasions. They could not be reliable, stable long-term memory of actual events, which requires a single true version of a single set of actual events. It took 5 years before George Franklin's conviction was set aside by a federal court. Since that time some courts have excluded recovered memories on the grounds that repressed memory syndrome had not been established to a sufficiently consensual degree in the scientific community. Other courts in other states of the USA have taken a different view.

Definitions: Loosening and Blurring of Language

The psychological expert witness instructed to give evidence in criminal trials on the matter of recovered memories of (usually) childhood sexual abuse faces many difficulties. The first concerns the issue of definitions. Since the early days in the 1980s when the idea of massive repression of repeated, highly traumatic childhood abuse was first floated, there has been a steady loosening and broadening of what are currently referred to as recovered memories. Sometimes they are referred to as simply "delayed" or "inhibited" or "cognitively avoided" memories. In some surveys clients have simply been asked if there had ever been a time when they didn't recall as much as they do currently. Many of these instances are not theoretically controversial. Some writers have used the phrase "recovered memories" in a loose sense. They have conducted surveys where such ordinary remembering is not differentiated from the disputed recovery of memory from what must have been substantial, dense, and perfect amnesia. Their finding of a certain percentage of cases where there may be some corroboration of some of the recalled material confounds the issue and puts mud in the water. There are many instances of remembering where there has been a simple failure to remember, or ordinary forgetting, until a reminder or other circumstance

provides the adequate retrieval cues. Anyone taking a professional examination is likely to have had this experience. Once the adequate reminder is established, the material is recognized as a personal memory which was "forgotten" and is recalled in its central and most memorable detail generally as adequately as it can be. Indeed, using the term "recovered memory" in this looser sense, one major researcher wrote "recovering previously inaccessible information on a later occasion represents the normal state of affairs, rather than an exception to be explained by special mechanisms such as repression and the return of the repressed."

Conflicting Interpretations of Research on Evidence for Repression or Dissociative Amnesia, and Memories Recovered Therefrom

The second problem for the forensic assessor is that the psychological and psychiatric profession remains at least somewhat divided on whether scientific research supports the possibility that recovered memories of traumatic and extensive childhood abuse can be completely lost to memory access for years and even decades, and then be recovered in a more or less reliable form. Major reviews of the psychological literature have been completed concerning scientific attempts to detect and demonstrate repression (in the more-or-less Freudian sense). To date, none of the studies reviewed has provided satisfactory evidence to support this hypothetical mechanism. Such experimental approaches have been criticized as being low in "ecological validity." Others point to the fact that it is hard to think of any other topic in mainstream psychological research (outside psychoanalytic theories and their derivatives) where a proposed mechanism, having failed to be demonstrated by over half a century of resourceful scientific research, still manages to survive with a significant support for its merits. The working party of the British Psychological Society put much weight on the frequency with which subjects who recollected traumatic events in their past then stated that there had been a time in their life when they recalled little or less of those matters which they were now recalling. This metamemorial judgment had already been questioned but it took some time before leading Canadian researchers, in a landmark study, established the control study which had hitherto been missing. They asked university students to recall in various degrees of detail summer camps and high-school graduation days, which were neither traumatic nor difficult to remember. Different groups of students were asked to put differing amounts of effort into this task. Once such effortful memory work was done, the students were asked about their state of memory before the study. Many reported their memory had been less or lacking altogether for specific recollections they had produced in the course of the study. Overall, these were similar in rates to the studies where retrospective judgments of past memory for trauma had been reported lacking. Most importantly, the more effort the students put into recollecting specific past events, the more they biased their judgments of their previous memory as being poorer or lacking. The effortful acts of remembering (mimicking such work in psychotherapy, for example) biased that retrospective report. Therefore such judgments could not be assumed to be a demonstration of preexisting amnesia.

Prospective Studies of Children and Adults Known to Have Been Traumatized

Major comprehensive reviews of studies of prospective follow-ups of cases of repeated trauma have generally failed to find anywhere where only dissociative amnesia could reasonably explain such future omissions in the reporting of past traumatic events. The issue of whether repetition of traumatic experience over extended periods of time was more likely to lead to the complete loss of memory for those events has also been examined. To date such reviews have not supported Terr's expert evidence given in the case of Franklin, referred to earlier.

Case Reports Versus Case Studies

There are perhaps between 100 and several hundred case reports in the literature which are summaries of cases which seem to be examples of repressed/dissociated and then recovered memory. The problem with all of these is that they are case reports, rather than case studies. They are brief summaries of cases, where further background information is needed for a proper consideration and resolution of competing explanations. There are a mere handful of case studies in the literature where a case has been studied with a view to drawing pertinent conclusions arising from that. Perhaps the most outstanding is that of "Jane Doe," reported by David Corwin, a child psychiatrist, in 1997. A child was first interviewed about abuse by Corwin in 1984. She reported abuse, and then was interviewed again by the same psychiatrist 11 years later. She then reported making allegations about different incidents (involving pornographic film-making, among other things). She did not state that there was a time she was oblivious about these events.

She had grown up with the belief that her mother had abused her but she often questioned herself about the extent and her mother's intentions. Several eminent psychologists read the selected transcripts and could not fail to notice just what an incompetent witness this sad daughter of a mother with 14 personalities appeared to be. One psychologist, working with the help of a journalist, discovered that the actual history of the case included the girl's father coaching and threatening her to make up stories of abuse against her mother. Of course this underpins the weakness of case studies where the reporting of the facts is selective.

False Memories

There is practical unanimity in the professional literature as to the fact that false memories can occur and have occurred. Researchers have frequently demonstrated the production of false memories in the laboratory "with trivial ease." Many real-life false or impossible memories have been documented elsewhere. There is less agreement as to whether these are rare and occasional in life outside the laboratory, or whether there is a culturally sponsored epidemic of false memories.

Forensic Experience with Recovered Memory/False Memory Cases

Another problem facing the forensic assessor is that, whilst there is a steady trickle of such cases involving questionable recovered memories, they are hardly numerous. The recovered memory controversy lies at a crossroads of issues concerning trauma, memory, and child abuse. In England, there are few practitioners with knowledge of all these areas who are also available for expert witness work. The sheer eccentricity and atypical nature of each individual case also work against common areas of expert knowledge being established.

Use of Colloquial English by Complainants: What do People Mean by "Blocking out" and Memories "Coming Back"?

Yet another problem for the forensic assessor arises from the inexact expression of colloquial English. Terms such as memories becoming "clearer," or having been "blocked out" or "buried" until recently may refer to nothing questionable at all, but only to the fact that such memorization had been cognitively avoided until that point. The other side of the coin, which poses more problems, is where these same inexact

English expressions really do refer to completely re-covered memories (i.e., from what must have been previous amnesia), which may be very questionable, and the investigators and prosecution have ignored this, believing that a bit of "blocking out" is all too understandable.

Strategic Presentations by Complainants

A fifth problem for the forensic assessor arises from the realization that complainants' testimony is not passively sitting there just waiting to be collected. Owing to the public nature of the controversy, some complainants who have genuinely produced recov-ered memories have been tempted strategically to mask and downplay the full novelty of their "mem-ories." Another complainant swore on oath she had only pretended to have recovered memories as a way of persuading her mother to believe her.

Discovery and Disclosure

Another area of difficulty for the forensic assessor concerns the barriers and problems in obtaining the data needed to arrive at a competent opinion. The failure of police investigators and the prosecution to realize they are dealing with a matter where memory is a probative issue often leads to inadequate investi-gation. It also leads to a failure to safeguard what precarious memories there may be, and maintain an appropriate memory audit trail, in a parallel way to sensitive physical forensic evidence. Prosecutors in England sometimes try to deny the defense access to the information which is relevant to demonstrating possible psychological disorder, questionable memo-ry recovery experiences, and the laying-out of all the evidence for the provenance of memories to be estab-lished. It is not unfair to state that the forensic asses-sor currently rarely gets all the information it is desirable to have.

Recovered Memories Arising in the Context of Adult-Onset Psychopathology

Sometimes recovered memories seem to arise during an adult-onset psychiatric disorder. These mostly ap-pear to be anxious or depressive states. Care must be taken not to use such as retrospective indications or forensic proof of the abuse (as per the warning in the *Diagnostic and Statistical Manual IV* of the American Psychiatric Association). There is no single patho-gnomonic postabuse psychological disorder profile. Nevertheless, the continuity of psychopathological difficulties which fits and is coherent with the

complainant's account of abuse, and his or her attempts to cope or avoid that abuse, and concomi-tant subjective thinking and emotional reactions, may be probative in pointing to an overall coherent narra-tive of a real history of the abuse and its aftermath. That leads to greater confidence that psychopatholo-gy has not jeopardized the veracity of the account, but indeed is a part of the narrative. The alternative sce-nario is that the psychopathology arises in adulthood when there is no continuity from the period of alleged traumatic abuse. Some strong advocates of recovered memories consider that psychopathology itself is re-pressed or rendered inoperable until the recovery of the associated memories. This permits the adult presentation to be classified as a delayed form of posttraumatic stress disorder (PTSD) caused by the childhood abuse. This is extreme delay, by any stan-dards. Prospective studies of PTSD (arising from documented road accidents) show that those who will eventually attract a diagnosis of delayed PTSD are in fact traumatized initially but do not meet the full PTSD criteria. Their trend of deterioration takes more than 6 months and thus they attract the diag-nostic outcome of delayed PTSD. PTSD was not found to be a latent condition waiting to emerge years later in otherwise well people.

Guidelines for Forensic Psychological Assessors Instructed as Expert Witnesses

A forensic assessor should not offer the court a per-sonal opinion as to whether memories are true or false, since typically the assessor will not know all the facts or the status of others. A forensic assessor may offer reasons based on examined significant fea-tures of a case, which render certain memories ques-tionable or likely jeopardized and different from the way ordinary memory is expected to function in the circumstances. The scientific debate is not over (al-though it has quietened down) and there is a duty to inform the court about the range of opinion that exists. Forensic assessors should have a sufficient background in human memory research, the recov-ered memory controversy, trauma recovery, and child sexual abuse. They should be aware of the differences between recovered memories and the victimology entailed in simply belated reporting. Justice requires a full evaluation. Assessors should ask instructing lawyers to procure all healthcare background and therapy notes, and all letters and journals kept by the complainant which refer to the issues. Consent should be sought for the forensic assessor to discuss matters with any mental health professional involved. If both sides appoint experts, the forensic assessor should ask to discuss issues with the other expert and ideally arrange a joint assessment of the complainant. The purpose of the forensic psychological assessor is to discover the provenance and the process of the remembering on which complainants rely when making their accusations. If the data are adequate, then the careful and methodical presentation often speaks for itself.

An initial question is often whether in all the circumstances the memorization process appears to be one of the strictly defined recovered memories, which are questionable, or whether it is the case that the colloquial use of English only suggests it might be so. In questionable recovered memories, the experiences of extensive, traumatic, repeated abuse over a lengthy period of time, the aftermath, coping reactions, and attitudes to the alleged perpetrator all appear to have been completely barred from conscious awareness, no matter what reminders have existed. Normal memory for a dreadful early life history may be lesser or greater, but entails a continuous (if fluctuating) awareness of what has happened which affects the autobiographical sense of self and attitudes to the alleged perpetrator and the abusive activity as it happens to others. Some remembering of attempted or failed coping and avoiding acts and/or intrusive subjective thinking is to be expected.

In cases of questionable recovered memories an emergent awareness that some terrible events happened in childhood often develops before initial imagery or flashbacks, which may come in staggered or fragmented bursts. Early imagery may be questioned or doubted by the subject, but over time it may become clearer, with more horrible events following on over days, or months, and the subject feeling more confident about the veracity of the same. This can be contrasted with normal autobiographical memory where, if all that exists is a knowing awareness that something did happen, then that awareness will have been lifelong, and if specific incidents are reminded later they tend to be limited. If there is less than full confidence in these fragments of old memory, that confidence does not markedly increase as further time passes by, although the intensity of that recollected feeling may increase in the face of another negative life event or depression.

Questionable cases of recovered memories are sometimes characterized by a mushrooming of new material over days and months, with apparently more memorable, more serious, and detailed or even bizarre events evolving over time. Normal memory for long-term autobiographical events recalls the most memorable and likely accurate relatively easily and early, once purposeful remembering begins. Further efforts may retrieve additional material, but such efforts bring diminishing returns.

Questionable recovered memories may completely transform the person's attitude to him/herself, the alleged perpetrator, and those who support or doubt him/her. People with normal long-term memories (even if fluctuating in awareness, avoidance, or denial) may change their behavior once they make a decision to report belatedly, but that is usually based on a circumscribed set of circumstances. It is not usually transformative.

Questionable recovered memories arising in the process of recalling increasing volumes of memory often reach further and further back in time, sometimes going into the period of infantile amnesia during the first 2 years of life. Adults recall almost nothing of their first 2 years and limited fragments from the next 2 or 3 years. There is no research showing adults can recall their own specific thinking with veracity when 3 years old or so. Gradual reaching back earlier and earlier, session after session, is not characteristic of normal remembering.

Questionable recovered memories often have a history of a person making repeated efforts to recall early life material, which itself may be associated or facilitated by counseling, psychotherapy, reading of survivor books, writing of journals, recalling dreams or television programs, or a period of distressing psychological breakdown. Normal, generally accurate autobiographical memory requires none of these special efforts, although specific and relevant reminders may act as an ambush trigger if the person is trying to put certain life events behind him/her, to avoid thinking about them, and engaging with alternative life issues.

Questionable recovered memories of early life are sometimes not stable or consistent, simply because they are newly manufactured. Tellingly, even the more recent memories of the process by which the alleged recovered long-term memories came to mind may be unstable and inconsistent, and give rise to a feeling of the "knew-it-all-along" phenomenon, i.e., the belief about knowing reaches further back than the documented evidence reflects.

Some questionable recovered memories arise for the first time within the context of a serious psychiatric disorder. Psychiatric disorder in people with normal stable long-term memories of childhood abuse does not prevent such patients from still having accurate recollections, but neither does it improve memory hugely. Normal memory of events from the past may be experienced with greater intensity or there may be difficulty thinking at all, depending on the disorder. Where the emergence of recovered memories follows the onset of psychiatric disorder, then there is no research indicating that this makes it more likely true.

Further Reading

Alpert J, Brown L, Ceci S, *et al.* (1996) *Working Group on Investigation of Memories of Childhood Abuse: Final Report.* Washington, DC: American Psychological Association.

Blanchard E, Hickling E (1997) *After the Crash.* Washington, DC: American Psychological Association.

Conway M (ed.) (1997) *Recovered Memories and False Memories.* Oxford, UK: Oxford University Press.

Howe ML (2000) *The Fate of Early Memories.* Washington, DC: American Psychological Association.

Lindsay DS, Read JD (1995) "Memory work" and recovered memories of childhood sexual abuse: scientific evidence and public, professional and personal issues. *Psychology, Public Policy and Law* 1: 846–908.

McNally RJ (2003) *Remembering Trauma.* Cambridge, MA: Belknap Press of Harvard University Press.

Morton J, Andrews B, Bekerian D, *et al.* (1995) *Recovered Memories: The Report of the Working Party of the British Psychological Society.* Leicester, UK: British Psychological Society.

Pendergrast M (1996) *Victims of Memory.* London: HarperCollins.

Pope H, Hudson J, Bodkin JA, Oliva P (1998) Questionable validity of 'dissociative amnesia' in trauma victims. *British Journal of Psychiatry* 172: 210–215.

Read JD, Lindsay DS (2000) "Amnesia" for summer camps and high school graduation: memory work increases reports of prior periods of remembering less. *Journal of Traumatic Stress* 13: 129–147.

Tully B (2001) Special legal requirements for competent forensic assessments of questionable "recovered memories" of childhood sexual abuse in criminal trials. In: Farrington D, Hollin C, McMurran M (eds.) *Sex and Violence*, pp. 123–137. London: Routledge.

REFUGEE MEDICINE

A Aggrawal, Maulana Azad Medical College, New Delhi, India

Introduction

Throughout history wars, battles, civil strife, and in general human conflict of all kinds have caused death and permanent disability for millions of people. A number of people who survive are displaced from their homeland, because of widespread destruction and devastation. Many of them flee to neighboring regions or countries as refugees. A number of others are forced to flee, because of persecution in their own country for reasons of race, caste, creed, or political affiliation.

These displaced persons or refugees face a unique set of ethnic, sociocultural, medical, and medicolegal problems within their host country. These problems arise not only because of overcrowding, ethnic and sociocultural differences, lack of sanitation, water, shelter, nutritious food, and medicines, but also because refugees are sometimes seen as potential threats to citizens of the host country. Instances of human rights violations and various kinds of physical, mental, and psychological trauma including sexual assaults by the citizens, enforcement officials, and army personnel of the host country are not entirely unknown. Sometimes these insults also come from fellow refugees. To deal with various medicolegal and sociocultural problems of refugees effectively, there is a need for medical and paramedical personnel, who are specifically equipped and trained to deal with them. Over the years, the branch of medicine that caters specifically to the medical needs of refugee populations, has become highly specialized and can be referred to as "refugee medicine."

History of Refugee Movements

Refugee Movements due to Religious Persecution

Movements of homeless people across frontiers during and after wars have occurred throughout human history. Many such migrations occurred as a result of religious and racial intolerance. For instance, more than 400 000 French Huguenots (Protestants) were forced to leave France after Louis XIV pronounced the revocation of the Edict of Nantes in 1685. Jews have perhaps suffered the most from such forced migrations. The first significant Jewish Diaspora was the result of the Babylonian Exile of 586 BC. Since then Jews have suffered forced expulsion regularly from several countries and regions, including England (1290), France (fourteenth century), Germany (1350s), Portugal (1496), Provence (1512), and the Papal States (1569). Intensifying persecution in Spain in 1492, culminated in the forced expulsion of that country's large and long-established Jewish population. More recently, Jews were expelled again from Germany, Austria, and Sudetenland (now in the Czech Republic) in the 1930s.

Refugee Movements due to Wars and Political Persecution

Refugee problems intensified in the late nineteenth century after the boundaries of states became more or less fixed, and citizens of a neighboring country were more often than not made to feel unwelcome. The twentieth century saw the movement of people more on political grounds than on religious grounds as had occurred earlier.

The Russian Revolution of 1917 and the postrevolutionary civil war (1917–21) caused the exodus of 1.5 million opponents of communism. Between 1915 and 1923 over 1 million Armenians left Turkish Asia Minor. In the wake of the 1936–39 Spanish Civil War, several hundred thousand Spanish Loyalists fled to France. When the People's Republic of China was established in 1949, more than 2 million Chinese fled to Taiwan and to the British Crown Colony of Hong Kong.

Four major conflicts during the 1950s caused the flight of more than 1 million refugees. These were (1) the Korean War (1950–53), (2) the Hungarian Revolution (1956), (3) the Cuban Revolution (1959), and (4) the Chinese invasion of Tibet (1959). In 1961 the Communist regime of East Germany erected the Berlin Wall to stop these very migrations, but before the creation of that wall – between 1945 and 1961 – over 3.7 million refugees from East Germany found asylum in West Germany. During the 1970s a large number of Vietnamese refugees and during 1980s a still larger number of Afghan refugees left their homes due to wars in their countries.

The Persian Gulf War of 1990–91 created 1.4 million Iraqi refugees who took shelter in Iran; the unresolved Arab–Israeli conflict produced more than 2.5 million Palestinian refugees in the early 1990s; and the political upheavals of eastern Europe produced a large number of refugees throughout the 1990s. The break-up of Yugoslavia produced more than 2 million refugees by mid-1992.

Wars and civil strife in various African countries resulted in a number of refugees. By 1992, there were 6 775 000 refugees within Africa. War in Rwanda created more than 2 million additional refugees in 1994. When the USA and its allies attacked the erstwhile Taliban regime in Afghanistan after the September 11, 2001 attacks, it caused a movement of about 200 000 Afghan refugees to Pakistan (2001). The latest conflict between USA and Iraq (2003) also created a large number of Iraqi refugees.

Refugee Movements due to Territorial Partitions

Several major refugee movements have been caused by territorial partition. After the defeat of Germany in World War II, about 12 million Germans were dumped on the truncated territory of Germany, which was split into east and west regions. Nearly 10 million people were temporarily made refugees by the creation of Bangladesh in 1971. However, the event that has caused the greatest population transfer in history was the partition of the Indian subcontinent in 1947, which resulted in the exchange of as many as 18 million Hindus from Pakistan and Muslims from India. Most of them resided for many months in refugee camps in cramped and overcrowded conditions with limited food, water, medicines, and proper sanitation.

International Action for Refugees

Excellent international work on refugee problems and refugee healthcare has earned as many as four Nobel Peace Prizes – in 1922, 1938, 1954, and 1981. The first significant step addressing the refugee problem was taken in 1921, when the Norwegian explorer and statesman Fridtjof Nansen (1861–1930) was appointed by the League of Nations as High Commissioner for Refugees.

The Nansen Passport

Being aware of the problems of refugees, Nansen devised a so-called "League of Nations Passport", a travel document that gave the holder the right to move more freely across national boundaries. This document later came to be known as the "Nansen Passport." For his work on the refugees of World War I, he was awarded a Nobel Peace Prize in 1922. After his death in 1930, the protection of refugees was entrusted by the League of Nations to the Office International Nansen pour les Réfugiés (Nansen International Office for Refugees, Geneva), whose mandate lasted from 1930 to 1938. In 1938, this office won the Nobel Peace Prize for its work on refugee problems. The majority of refugees at that time were Russians and Armenians, who had become refugees during and after World War I.

Three other major refugee assistance organizations have been the Intergovernmental Committee on Refugees (1938–47), the United Nations Relief and Rehabilitation Refugee Organization (1947–52), and the Intergovernmental Committee for European Migration. The latter was founded in 1951 and was renamed the Intergovernmental Committee for Migration in 1980.

United Nations High Commission for Refugees

The International Refugee Organization (IRO) was a temporary specialized agency, established by the United Nations in 1946. It continued work till

January 1952, and was finally succeeded by the Office of the United Nations High Commission for Refugees (UNHCR) established by the United Nations General Assembly. The UNHCR had however started work much earlier (on January 1, 1951) and it assisted refugees and displaced persons in many countries of Europe and Asia who either could not return to their countries of origin or were unwilling to return for political reasons. Among its main functions was the healthcare and maintenance of refugees in camps. It remains the largest and most significant refugee assistance organization. It has helped an estimated 50 million refugees around the world. For its excellent work on refugees, it earned two Nobel Peace Prizes – in 1954 and 1981.

1951 Refugee Convention

Following the increasing problem of refugees arising as a result of World War II, the General Assembly of the United Nations, by Resolution 429 (V) of December 14, 1950, decided to convene in Geneva a Conference of Plenipotentiaries to complete the drafting of, and to sign, a Convention relating to the Status of Refugees and a Protocol relating to the Status of Stateless Persons. The Conference held at the European Office of the United Nations in Geneva from July 2 to 25, 1951, approved the convention on July 28, 1951, now widely known as the "1951 Refugee Convention."

The Convention consolidated previous international instruments relating to refugees and provided the most comprehensive codification of the rights of refugees yet attempted on the international level. It laid down basic minimum standards for the treatment of refugees, without prejudice to the granting by states of more favorable treatment. The Convention was to be applied without discrimination as to race, religion, or country of origin, and contained various safeguards against the expulsion of refugees. It also made provision for documentation, including a refugee travel document in passport form, a modern version of the older "Nansen Passport." It also defined the term "refugee" for the first time – in clear and unambiguous terms.

1967 Protocol

This Convention was limited to protecting mainly European refugees in the aftermath of World War II, but a 1967 Protocol (signed and adopted on January 31, 1967) expanded the scope of the Convention as the problem of displacement spread around the world.

1969 Africa Refugee Convention

The Organization of African Unity (OAU) was formed in 1963, and since its very inception it was concerned with the refugee problem on the continent of Africa, which had tended to foment trouble between member states. On September 6 to 10, 1969, 41 heads of African states assembled in Addis Ababa, and signed the Convention governing the Specific Aspects of Refugee Problems in Africa, which became effective on June 20, 1974. It was mostly based on the 1951 Refugee Convention, but with some changes and modifications taking into account the specific problems related to African refugees.

1984 Cartagena Declaration on Refugees

During the 1980s serious conflicts occurred in Central American countries, giving rise to an alarming refugee problem in Latin America. To address their specific problems, heads of 10 Latin American States met in Cartegena, Colombia from November 19 to 22, 1984 and adopted the Cartagena Declaration on Refugees, which specifically addressed the problems of Latin American refugees.

Women's Commission for Refugee Women and Children, 1989

Realizing that refugee women face special problems, the Women's Commission for Refugee Women and Children was founded in 1989, as an independent affiliate of the International Rescue Committee.

Declaration on the Protection of Refugees and Displaced Persons in the Arab World, 1992

From November 16 to 19, 1992, a group of Arab experts met in Cairo at the Fourth Arab Seminar on "Asylum and Refugee Law in the Arab World." It was organized by the International Institute of Humanitarian Law in collaboration with the Faculty of Law of Cairo University, under the sponsorship of the UNHCR. It noted the suffering which the Arab World had endured from large-scale flows of refugees and displaced persons. Considering that asylum and refugee law constituted an integral part of human rights law, respect for which should be fully insured in the Arab World, it adopted a declaration that aimed at protecting refugees and other displaced persons within the Arab world.

Who is a Refugee?

The term refugee may mean different things to different people, but the most widely accepted definition of a refugee is that provided by the 1951 Refugee Convention. Article 1A(2) of this Convention defines a refugee as:

> a person who is outside his/her country of nationality or habitual residence; has a well-founded fear of

Table 1   Numbers of people (in millions) of concern to UNHCR (1985–2001)

Year	Africa	Asia	Europe	Latin America	North America	Oceania	Total
1985	3.0	5.1	0.7	0.4	1.4	0.1	10.7
1990	4.6	6.8	0.8	1.2	1.4	0.1	14.9
1995	11.81	7.92	6.52	0.20	0.92	0.05	27.4
1996	9.1	7.7	7.7	0.2	1.3	0.05	26.1
1997	8.09	7.9	5.7	0.1	0.7	0.07	22.7
1998	7.4	7.4	6.0	0.1	1.3	0.07	22.3
1999	6.3	7.5	6.2	0.1	1.3	0.07	21.5
2000	6.3	7.3	7.3	0.09	1.2	0.08	22.3
2001	6.1	8.4	5.6	0.6	1.0	0.08	21.8

Reproduced with permission from UNHCR (2001) *Helping Refugees – An Introduction to UNHCR*. Geneva, Switzerland: Office of the United Nations High Commissioner for Refugees.

persecution because of his/her race, religion, nationality, membership in a particular social group or political opinion; and is unable or unwilling to avail himself/herself of the protection of that country, or to return there, for fear of persecution.

The 1969 Africa Refugee Convention holds this definition (via Article 1(1)), but makes an addition to it via Article 1(2). Article 1(2) says:

The term 'refugee' shall also apply to every person who, owing to external aggression, occupation, foreign domination, or events seriously disturbing public order in either part or the whole of his country of origin or nationality, is compelled to leave his place of habitual residence in order to seek refuge in another place outside his country of origin or nationality.

Internally Displaced Persons (IDP) are people who have been forced to flee their home for the same reasons as refugees, and also because of natural disasters such as famines, cyclones, floods, etc. but have not crossed an internationally recognized boundary.

Table 1 describes the official statistics provided by the office of the UNHCR.

The office of the UNHCR categorizes "people of concern" into four subcategories. They are: (1) refugees, (2) internally displaced persons, (3) asylum seekers or asylees (refugees who have applied for asylum in the host country), and (4) returnees (refugees who have returned to their country, but are still living precariously). Out of a total of 21 793 300 people of concern to the UNHCR in 2001, there were 12 071 700 refugees, 8 021 500 internally displaced persons, 914 100 asylum seekers, and 786 000 returnees, and all face similar problems.

Legislation Related to Refugee Medicine

Several countries have specific legislation related to refugees and their healthcare. In 1980, the USA passed the Federal Refugee Act. It created a uniform system of services for refugees resettled in the USA. The Act entitled all newly arriving refugees to a comprehensive health assessment, to be initiated as soon as possible following arrival. One agency in each state was designated to monitor the provision of these health assessment services.

Health Problems of Refugees

Refugees face unique health problems as a result of overcrowding, lack of shelter, food, water, blankets, sanitation, and medicines and also physical and mental trauma arising from their past experiences and current precarious situation.

Conditions that account for most deaths in refugees and displaced populations are malnutrition, diarrhea, malaria, and acute infections such as measles. Other conditions of concern are hepatitis B, sexually transmitted infections including human immunodeficiency virus (HIV), tuberculosis and other pulmonary infections such as melioidosis and paragonimiasis, parasitic diseases such as hookworms, *Ascaris lumbricoides*, *Strongyloides stercoralis*, *Giardia lamblia*, *Opisthorcis viverrini*, and *Trichuris trichiura*, and psychological disorders such as posttraumatic stress disorder (PTSD).

At the center of refugee medicine lies primary healthcare and prevention. After supplying water, food, and shelter, the number one health priority in a refugee camp is vaccination. Vaccination for hepatitis A and B, cholera, typhoid, and measles must be considered in all refugee camps.

Some Important Considerations in Refugee Medicine

Refugee medicine and healthcare present unique challenges to the medical practitioner. Healthcare providers of the host country may not be fully aware and conversant with the disease pattern of the regions refugees may be coming from. Their languages and

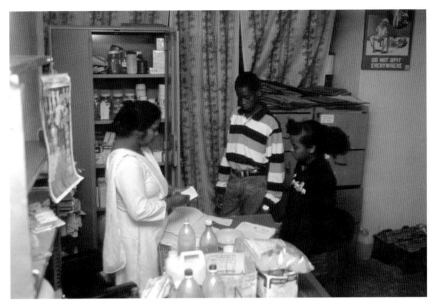

Figure 1 Dispensing medicine to Somali refugee children in New Delhi at the Primary Health Center, run by the Voluntary Health Association of Delhi, supported by UNHCR. (Reproduced with permission of UNHCR/S. Akbar.)

sociocultural codes and mores may be so completely alien that serious difficulties may arise in proper and adequate communication. A professional interpreter may be required. At times – as in cases of female refugees explaining some of their intimate diseases – not only a female interpreter may be necessary, but even a female healthcare provider (**Figure 1**).

Sometimes while healthcare providers may distribute western-style medicines, the refugee population – due to their beliefs in their own local and herbal remedies — may not want to take prescribed medicines and these may be secretly discarded (**Figures 2** and **3**).

Healthcare officials may have to build a personal relationship with refugee patients (**Figure 4**). Many of them may be ignorant or mistrustful of the healthcare system of the host country, be highly traumatized, or suffering from grief, depression or feelings of guilt for surviving. They also may feel shame and rejection for having a communicable disease such as tuberculosis or HIV or may be stigmatized by their community for having a mental illness.

Before a refugee or asylum seeker is admitted in a host country, it is desirable to screen him or her for some basic infections and harmful behaviors that may prove detrimental to the host population. Screening for the following conditions is recommended before admitting a refugee into a host country:

1. Communicable diseases of public health significance:
   a. infectious tuberculosis
   b. HIV
   c. Hansen's disease (leprosy)
   d. syphilis and other sexually transmitted infections
   e. parasitic diseases
2. Physical and mental disorders with associated harmful behaviors
3. Psychoactive substance abuse and dependence
4. Other physical or mental abnormalities, disorders, or disabilities.

Tuberculosis and Associated Pulmonary Disorders

According to the World Health Organization (WHO), about one in three persons worldwide is infected with tuberculosis. The incidence has increased due to the current HIV pandemic. It is typically high in undernourished, starved, and deprived persons living in overcrowded conditions. It is important to realize that many refugees may have come from such conditions and that conditions in refugee camps are not very different. Chest X-rays and Mantoux test must be done in all refugees, and if tuberculosis is suspected, the patient must immediately be referred to antitubercular treatment (ATT). The physician must keep in mind that many patients having an active disease may already have been taking ATT in their home country, and may have developed single-drug or multidrug resistance. It is also important to appreciate that many patients may be suffering from extrapulmonary tuberculosis. It has been said that tuberculosis can mimic everything except pregnancy and if the physician finds that symptoms do not fit in any coherent clinical picture, tuberculosis must be considered.

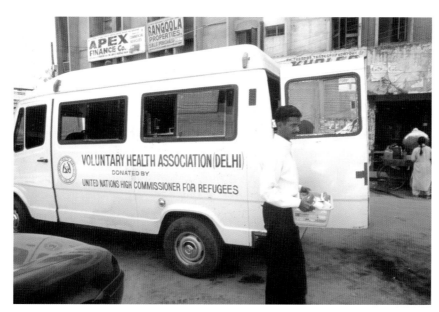

Figure 2 The mobile van for refugees run by the Voluntary Health Association of Delhi which goes to areas where refugees live in New Delhi, dispensing free medicine. The project is supported by UNHCR. (Reproduced with permission of UNHCR/S. Akbar.)

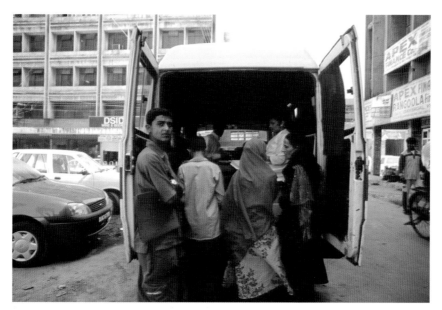

Figure 3 Afghan refugees lining up for medicines from the mobile van run by the Voluntary Health Association of Delhi which goes to areas where refugees live in New Delhi, dispensing free medicine. The project is supported by UNHCR. (Reproduced with permission of UNHCR/S. Akbar.)

In several regions of the world where refugees come from, tuberculosis is considered a stigma, and it is not uncommon for family and friends of the patient to ostracize him or her. Thus education of the patient and their families may be of utmost importance.

Two conditions that may mimic tuberculosis, and which may be quite common in refugee populations, are melioidosis and paragonimiasis. Melioidosis is caused by a Gram-negative motile bacillus *Burkholderia* (formerly *Pseudomonas*) *pseudomallei*. This

bacillus is a saprophyte which can be isolated from ponds, soil, rice paddies, and market produce in endemic areas. Humans contract it by soil contamination of skin abrasions, and less commonly through ingestion and inhalation. The latency period is more than 25 years; the disease was once called the Vietnamese time bomb, reflecting both its origin and long latency period. The symptoms can be remarkably similar to those of tuberculosis, with productive cough, fever, weight loss, and upper-lobe cavitary lesions. The disease is

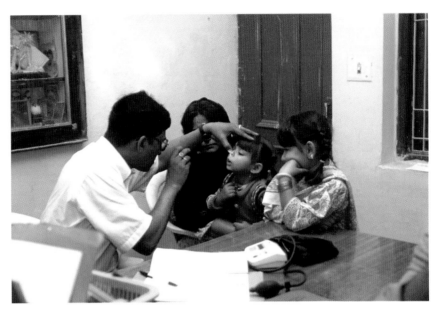

Figure 4 A family of Afghan refugees being examined in New Delhi at the Primary Health Center, run by the Voluntary Health Association of Delhi, supported by UNHCR. (Reproduced with permission of UNHCR/S. Akbar.)

endemic in Southeast Asia. Cases have been reported from Madagascar, Chad, Central West Africa, Iran, and Turkey. If a refugee comes from an endemic area, has a febrile illness, shows a radiographic pattern similar to that of tuberculosis, but from whom *Mycobacterium tuberculosis* cannot be isolated, melioidosis should be considered. Treatment includes antibiotic therapy with levamisole as an adjunct.

Paragonimiasis or endemic hemoptysis is caused by the trematode *Paragonimus westermani* (lung fluke), and is common in countries where raw or partially cooked crab, shrimp, or crayfish (the second intermediate hosts) are consumed. According to one estimate, close to 3 million people worldwide are infected with this disease, the vast majority of them in Asia, particularly China, Korea, Japan, Taiwan, the Philippines, and Southeast Asia. Patients with paragonimiasis may present with cough and hemoptysis. Serology and sputum testing for ova and parasites would confirm the diagnosis. The drug of choice is praziquantel.

Parasitic Diseases

Intestinal parasites are very common in refugee populations. All inmates of refugee populations should be screened for intestinal and other parasites, even if they are asymptomatic. Because of unsanitary and crowded conditions in most refugee camps, this condition can spread rapidly, if not controlled early.

Most parasites cause eosinophilia; a differential blood count is thus essential along with a vigorous stool examination, this may include more than 10 examinations of stools, even if they are found repeatedly negative. In one study of Southeast Asians with

eosinophilia and three negative screening stools for ova and parasites, 95% were found to have a pathogenic parasite on further evaluation. Laboratory investigation schedule for a patient with eosinophilia must include stool microscopy for ova and parasites (repeated several times); day (*Loa loa*) and night (*Wuchereria bancrofti*) blood samples for microfilariae; skin snips for *Onchocerca volvulus*; rectal snips for *Schistosoma mansoni*, *S. japonicum*, and *S. haematobium*; terminal urine for *S. haematobium* ova; and duodenal juice test for *Strongyloides stercoralis*.

The most common pathogenic parasites seen in refugee populations are hookworm, *Clonorchis sinensis*, *S. stercoralis*, *G. lamblia*, *A. lumbricoides*, *T. trichuria*, and *O. viverrini*. Many patients may have multiple parasites. It is important to realize that some helminth infections (strongyloids, opisthorchis, schistosomiasis) may be asymptomatic and persist for many years before causing serious disease. Documented length of infection is more than 20 years in hydatid disease, 32 years in schistosomiasis, and more than 60 years in strongyloidiasis.

HIV Infection and Other Sexually Transmitted Diseases

Refugee camps typically have high rates of HIV and sexually transmitted diseases (STD). Several recent mass population migrations have taken place in areas where HIV infection prevalence rates are high, for example, in Burundi, Rwanda, Malawi, Ethiopia, and Zaire. Conditions that may increase the spread of HIV and other STDs in refugee camps are the high prevalence of infection among commercial sex workers living in the vicinity of camps, prostitution, high rates of blood transfusions due to increasing violence-related trauma, and shortages of laboratory reagents to test blood for HIV.

Furthermore, HIV is generally regarded as a source of shame and fear among most refugee groups. For this reason, many refugees choose not to tell anyone in their community that they are HIV-positive. They therefore live with an enormous burden of silence and a constant fear of exposure and ostracism. Even disclosure to spouses can be difficult, and presents a challenge to healthcare providers. Secrecy increases the potential for spreading HIV infection. Women are particularly vulnerable if partners who are HIV-positive resist the use of condoms.

Mental Health Issues

Most refugees arriving in host countries will have been exposed to traumatic events. These may include threats to their own lives or those of their family or friends, witnessing death squad killings and mass murder and other cruelties inflicted on family or friends, disappearances of family members or friends, perilous flight or escape with no personal protection, separation from family members, extreme deprivation – poverty, unsanitary conditions, hunger, lack of healthcare, forced marches, persistent and long-term political repression, deprivation of human rights and harassment, removal of shelter or forced displacement from homes, refugee camp experiences involving prolonged squalor, malnutrition, physical, psychological, and sexual abuse, absence of personal space, and lack of safety. These psychological burdens are complicated not only by the demands of adjustment to a new country including lack of social codes, mores, and the new language, and concomitant loss of homeland, sociocultural ties, and economic status, but also can be affected by other disease states and malnutrition. This can give rise to several psychological conditions such as anxiety, depression, posttraumatic stress disorder (PTSD), and psychosomatic disorders, which can lead to substance abuse.

Modern research on refugees began after World War II, with studies of Jewish victims of Nazi concentration camps. They suffered from a constellation of symptoms including fatigue, irritability, restlessness, anxiety, and depression. This has been termed as the "concentration camp syndrome" and is often seen in refugee populations, who live in almost identical conditions.

Intervention may include standard western style therapies such as pharmacotherapy, psychotherapy, and counseling. One must also consider community approaches and traditional healing. It is important to realize that the traumatized patient may not want to tell his or her story because of fears of exacerbation of symptoms or breach of confidentiality. A cautious approach on the part of the healthcare provider, where the patient is allowed to narrate at his or her own pace with or without an interpreter, may be very helpful.

Other Disease Entities

Apart from the above, certain other disease entities may be seen more commonly in refugee populations. These include dental caries, pterygium significant enough to interfere with vision, chronic otitis media resulting in partial hearing loss, hematologic disorders such as α- and β-thalassemias, glucose-6-phosphate dehydrogenase (G6PD) deficiency, and hemogloblin E trait (HbE). These conditions should be diagnosed and properly addressed.

General Medical Care

Finally there may be certain medical conditions that are not directly related to a person's refugee status, for example, asthma, cardiac disease, diabetes. It is possible that the patient was deliberately delaying their treatment in their homeland for lack of finances or simple nonavailability of healthcare. The availability of free medical care in the new host nation may mean those problems can be addressed. The need to treat these conditions on a priority basis in a refugee population, where the host nation's citizens themselves may urgently be in need, presents challenging ethical issues. The situation appears more paradoxical when we take into account that several citizens of the host nation may be paying hefty taxes for those very services.

Ethical Issues

Ethics is the application of values and moral rules to human activities. Bioethics is the application of ethical principles and decision-making to solve actual or anticipated dilemmas in medicine. Refugee healthcare raises a number of ethical issues. Some ethically difficult decisions include life-ending triage choices, allocation of scarce and meager resources, and the paradox of preferentially treating refugees in a land where residents of the host country may be equally in need. Using such appropriate ethical standards, one cannot differentiate between the health needs of a refugee and those of the citizens of the host country in the event of refugee status being granted by the host nation. A host nation may perhaps be able to apply some discretion in granting refugee status. But once it has been granted, all refugees must be treated at par with the nation's own citizens, as far as basic health needs are concerned.

It is obvious that the impact of refugees would most strongly be felt in countries with limited resources. Therefore a proper assessment of burden or responsibility sharing should take into account the national resources of countries hosting refugees and displaced persons. Two key indicators of national capacity are (1) the gross domestic product (GDP) per capita and (2) national population. By considering these factors in relation to the scope of displacement, an indication of the relative capacity of countries to host refugees is obtained. **Table 2** lists the top 10 countries in terms of spending the most on refugees in relation to their own GDP. A significant amount of assistance is granted by UNHCR.

Table 3 lists the top 10 countries in terms of hosting the greatest number of refugees in relation to their own population. This could be an indication of the additional burden placed on the citizens of the host country.

Another important ethical issue to consider is the employment of a female practitioner in the examination of female patients. Merely the presence of a female chaperone may not be enough. Many refugees may come from countries where touching of a female by a male other than her husband may be an anathema. The moral and ethical values held by the refugee must be respected. A careless approach in this regard may invite needless allegations of sexual misconduct or even molestation. The patient may be encouraged to use diagrams and charts, if she is uncomfortable pointing to some sensitive areas of her own anatomy.

It is important to appreciate that some refugees may need a professional interpreter. Failure to use their services may result in wrong interpretations.

Many refugees may not be comfortable with the western system of medicine. In such cases, alternative therapies as those prevalent in the refugee's own homeland may be more useful.

Medical research on refugees raises ethical issues too. Refugees are vulnerable as subjects of medical research for several reasons. First they inherently

Table 2 Top 10 countries hosting refugees in relation to their own GDP per capita 1997–2001

2001		1997–2001	
Country	*Rank*	*Country*	*Rank*
Pakistan	1	Sierra Leone	1
Democratic Republic of the Congo	2	Pakistan	2
United Republic of Tanzania	3	Democratic Republic of the Congo	3
Ethiopia	4	United Republic of Tanzania	4
Islamic Republic of Iran	5	Ethiopia	5
Burundi	6	Burundi	6
Zambia	7	Rwanda	7
Federal Republic of Yugoslavia	8	Eritrea	8
Sudan	9	Islamic Republic of Iran	9
Azerbaijan	10	Federal Republic of Yugoslavia	10

Reproduced with permission from *Statistical Yearbook 2001*, published by the office of the UNHCR.

Table 3 Top 10 countries hosting in relation to their own national population, 1997–2001

2001		1997–2001	
Country	*Rank*	*Country*	*Rank*
Bosnia and Herzegovina	1	Bosnia and Herzegovina	1
Liberia	2	Cyprus	2
FYR Macedonia	3	Sierra Leone	3
Federal Republic of Yugoslavia	4	Liberia	4
Azerbaijan	5	Federal Republic of Yugoslavia	5
Kuwait	6	Azerbaijan	6
Armenia	7	Guinea-Bissau	7
Afghanistan	8	Armenia	8
Georgia	9	Kuwait	9
Congo	10	Eritrea	10

Reproduced with permission from *Statistical Yearbook 2001*, published by the office of the UNHCR.

possess lesser political rights. Since they are outside their own country, they are liable to arbitrary action on the part of host country. Second, little technical guidance is available from the usual international instruments on biomedical ethics, such as the Declaration of Helsinki or guidelines from the Council for International Organizations of Medical Sciences (CIOMS).

One of the excuses offered by medical researchers is that the research is directed towards refugees' own welfare (e.g., cause of a diarrhea outbreak, percentage of the population vaccinated for measles, etc.). While this may be correct to some extent, it cannot be denied that all medical research on refugees must observe the key principles of bioethics, namely, informed consent, confidentiality, the principle of "do no harm," and beneficence.

The WHO Advisory Group on Research in Refugee Populations proposed the following guidelines for research in refugee and internally displaced populations:

- undertake only those studies that are urgent and vital to the health and welfare of the study population
- restrict studies to those questions that cannot be addressed in any other context
- restrict studies to those that would provide important direct benefit to the individuals recruited to the study or to the population from which the individuals come
- ensure the study design imposes the absolute minimum of additional risk
- select study participants on the basis of scientific principles without bias introduced by issues of accessibility, cost, or malleability
- establish highest standards for obtaining informed consent from all individual study participants and where necessary and culturally appropriate from heads of household and community leaders (but this consent cannot substitute for individual consent)
- institute procedures to assess for, minimize, and monitor the risks to safety and confidentiality for individual subjects, their community, and for their future security
- promote the well-being, dignity, and autonomy of all study participants in all phases of the research study.

Medicolegal Considerations

Refugee populations consist of people who are terrified, and are away from familiar surroundings. There can be instances of exploitation at the hands of enforcement officials, citizens of the host country,

and even United Nations peacekeepers. Instances of human rights violations, child labor, mental and physical trauma/torture, violence-related trauma, and sexual exploitation, especially of children are not entirely unknown. In many refugee camps in three war-torn West African countries, Sierra Leone, Guinea, and Liberia, young girls were found to be exchanging sex for money, a handful of fruit, or even a bar of soap! Most of these girls were between 13 and 18 years of age. This happened as recently as in 2001. Parents tended to turn a blind eye because sexual exploitation had become a "mechanism of survival" in these camps.

After the civil war restarted in Congo–Brazzaville in December 1998, about 250 000 people fled into the forests of the neighboring Pool region. A total of 1600 cases of rape were reported between May and December 1999, from the hospitals of Brazzaville, which highlights the high prevalence of sexual violence directed against women and girl refugees.

Children and women in refugee camps may be forced to resort to prostitution because of poverty. The clients may include fellow refugees, or more commonly citizens of the host country residing in peripheral areas to the camps, or visiting in order to obtain cheap sex. Besides having legal connotations, the situation can lead to the rapid spread of HIV and other sexually transmitted infections.

Female genital mutilation is common in many African countries. If the refugee population is from these countries, female genital mutilation may still be practiced in refugee camps by local doctors (refugees themselves). In most countries this is a penal offence and may attract relevant penal provisions.

It would be useful for the practitioner to keep in mind the practice of body modification/alteration in several cultures. It is very easy to mistake these "normal" body modifications for injury. One of the most common instances causing misinterpretation is the practice of "cao gio" or "coin rubbing" among several Southeast Asian cultures. This refers to a form of traditional healing where the edge of a coin is rubbed over the skin. It produces a red stripe that may easily be mistaken for child abuse by someone who is not aware of this phenomenon.

Similarly, amputation of the uvula and producing scars or lesions in some African groups is a traditional healing practice. These scars are found on the trunk or face, and other parts of the body. The cutting or burning procedures producing the scars or lesions are usually done for ritual reasons, body enhancement, or for traditional healing. The physician would do well to ask the patient discreetly about those lesions – perhaps with the help of an interpreter – rather than jumping to conclusions.

Another finding that one may encounter during examination of refugees is the finding of artificial penile nodules especially in Southeast Asian men. In these cultures foreign bodies are often implanted under the skin of the penis to enhance sexual performance.

Instances of bribery are known to occur. In 2001, five employees of UNHCR (Nairobi office) were charged with taking money from refugees in exchange for resettlement in western countries. Three of these were Kenyans and one Italian. They were either assigned new duties, or their contracts with UNHCR were not renewed.

There are instances of several people injuring themselves (deliberate selfharm) in order to gain admission in more affluent countries as refugees. In the past, Cubans were allowed to immigrate relatively easily to the USA. But in November 1994, Attorney General Janet Reno issued a policy allowing entry to only those under age 18, pregnant women, or anyone who had a medical condition that could not be treated in Cuba; several Cuban detainees attempted to gain a "medical parole" by injuring themselves. Most of the time, a detainee copied another who had legitimately become ill or injured and who was consequently evacuated to the USA.

In one case, a young man was granted medical parole after he suffered genuine severe burns on his hands after burning himself with melted plastic while molding a sculpture. Seeing this, several other people burned themselves with melted plastic. Similarly, when patients with severe prolapsed hemorrhoids were given medical parole, several people produced bleeding from their rectums by deliberately injuring themselves.

Several other unique cases show that individuals go to any extent to gain illegal entry to a western country as a refugee. One man swallowed a large, metal hog ring, another injected diesel fuel into his scrotum, and five men cut their Achilles' tendons when faced with deportation back to Cuba because of criminal activity. The doctors also reported that so many Cubans presented with symptoms of angina that a cardiologist was brought in for a 3-month term to conduct tests.

All these conditions raise medicolegal issues that must be considered by the healthcare providers. Forensic physicians may be required to differentiate genuine cases of injury from those related to deliberate self-harm. Violations of law and human rights must be reported to the local law enforcement agencies, and to the Human Rights Commission.

Future of Refugee Medicine

The importance of refugee medicine is increasingly being recognized. Several medical universities are now starting postgraduate training courses in refugee medicine. In 1999, the Medical School of University of Pécs in Hungary in association with the International Organization for Migration (Geneva, Switzerland) started one of the first postgraduate courses in migrational medicine. The 1-year course focuses on the health needs of refugees, immigrants, and victims of civil war.

As political and social upheavals increase around the world, the numbers of the refugee population around the world are also on the increase. With close to 12 million refugees currently found across the globe, more specialists in refugee medicine could do much to mitigate refugees' suffering. The introduction of techniques such as telemedicine may be useful in delivering appropriate care.

See Also

Children: Sexual Abuse, Overview; **Deliberate Self-Harm, Patterns; Female Genital Alteration; Human Rights, Controls and Principles; Torture:** Physical Findings; Psychological Assessment

Further Reading

Dorkenoo E (1994) *Cutting the Rose: Female Genital Mutilation – The Practice and its Prevention.* London: Minority Rights Group.

Friedman AR (1992) Rape and domestic violence: the experience of refugee women. *Women and Therapy* 13: 65–78.

Gavagan T, Brodyaga L (1998) Medical care for immigrants and refugees. *American Family Physician* 57(5): 1061–1067.

Herman J (1992) *Trauma and Recovery: From Domestic Abuse to Political Terror.* London: Pandora Press.

Leaning J (2001) Ethics of research in refugee populations. *Lancet* 357: 1432–1433.

Mansella AJ, Friedman M, Gerrity XY, et al. (1996) *Ethnocultural Aspects of Post Traumatic Stress Disorder: Issues, Research and Clinical Applications.* Washington, DC: American Psychological Association.

Ong A (1995) Making the biopolitical subject: Cambodian immigrants, refugee medicine and cultural citizenship in California. *Social Science and Medicine* 40(9): 1243–1257.

Rutter J (1994) *Refugee Children in the Classroom.* London: Trentham Books.

Sandler RH, Jones TC (eds.) (1987) *Medical Care of Refugees.* New York: Oxford University Press.

Sideris T (2003) War, gender and culture: Mozambican women refugees. *Social Science and Medicine* 56: 713–724.

Simmonds S, Vaughan P, Gunn SW (1983) *Refugee Community Medical Care.* Oxford, UK: Oxford University Press.

Toole MJ, Waldman RJ (1997) The public health aspects of complex emergencies and refugee situations. *Annual Review of Public Health* 18: 283–312.

Walker PF, Jaranson J (1999) Refugee and immigrant health care. *Medical Clinics on North America [Special on Travel Medicine]* 83(4): 1103–1120.

Woodward CL (1980) Refugee medicine in Thailand. *Transactions of the American Clinical Climatology Association* 92: 23–27.

Wulf D (ed.) (1994) *Refugee Women and Reproductive Health Care: Reassessing Priorities.* New York: Women's Commission for Refugee Women and Children.

RELIGIOUS ATTITUDES TO DEATH

J E Rutty, DeMonfort University, Leicester, UK

Introduction

Religion is significant for the majority of individuals internationally, offering a system of beliefs about the cause, nature, and purpose of the universe and values with reference to God or gods. Death has a tendency to lead religious customs, as it is exceptionally unusual for funerals not to be associated with religious rites, such customs being found as long ago as 50 000 BC. However, the world's religions are so varied that in such a mixed multicultural civilization it is not astounding that it is simple to cause offense unintentionally. The intention of this article is not to propose a theological examination, but to present an explanatory description that can be simply accessed and employed for reference purposes on the subject of spiritual care after death by healthcare professionals. For ease, the article has been separated into the three broad groupings of contemporary faiths: (1) Abrahamic; (2) Vedic; and (3) other major traditions (**Table 1**). Each section provides brief information on the key beliefs concerning death and care after death, including information on funerals, organ donation, and autopsies.

The Abrahamic Faiths

The three faiths that are closely connected historically are Judaism, Christianity, and Islam, being traceable back to Abraham (around 2000 BC).

Judaism

Judaism holds that individuals have a special relationship – the Covenant – with the one God, Creator and Lord of the universe, and this Covenant guides their way of life. Jews believe that life is sacred and death is under the control of the omnipotent one.

Two of the most important commandments are to honor the dead and comfort the mourner and so deep religious meaning is invested in death and dying rituals. There are diversities within this faith, namely, the orthodox tradition, conservative Judaism, and reform Judaism.

Care after death The body must be handled as little as possible, as considerable importance is attached to the ritual cleansing and clothing of the body. This is undertaken by Jews who are specially qualified and of the same sex as the deceased. Hence, limited laying out should be performed by healthcare staff. Once death has been established, the eyes and mouth of the deceased must be closed by a child, a relative, or a close friend, in that order of preference. The jaw is supported and limbs are straightened with the arms placed by the sides. The body is then labeled and covered with a white sheet. The immediate family will contact the local Jewish undertaker and synagogue and put the ritual proceedings in motion. Very importantly, between the time of death and burial the body is guarded or watched as it is believed to be vulnerable and unable to watch over itself until it has "come home" to its final resting place within the grave. Judaism believes it to be a humiliation to the dead to leave them unburied. Therefore, arrangements are made to bury the deceased ideally within 24 h, and only delayed for the Sabbath and other major festivals. Cremation is most unusual, as historically it is frowned upon as an unnatural means of treating the human body. The preservation of life is an important guiding principle in Judaism and so there is no objection to the principle of organ donation. With regard to autopsies, Jewish law requires that after someone has died the body should be buried in its entirety. According to Judaism, humans were created in God's image and so any mutilation of the body is strongly disapproved of. Therefore, autopsy examinations are not permitted in Jewish law unless required by civil law.

Table 1 Summary of religious beliefs in relation to death

Religion	Care after death	Organ donation and autopsies
Afro-Caribbean community	Routine last offices carried out preferably by a nurse from a similar ethnic background. Body ideally embalmed. Burial preferred. Body may be viewed at home and/or in church	Unlikely to agree. Younger members may have different views
Atheism	Routine last offices are appropriate. Burial or cremation. Humanist funeral	No objection
Baha'i	Last offices are appropriate. The deceased is always buried and never cremated. The place of internment should be within 1 h journey from the place of death	No objection to organ donation or autopsies
Buddhism	Last offices are appropriate. Most Buddhists prefer cremation to burial	No objection to organ donation or autopsies
Christianity	Routine last offices are appropriate. Traditionally UK and Eire Catholics are buried, but there are no religious objections to cremation	No objection to organ donation or autopsies
Church of Jesus Christ of Latter Day Saints	Routine last offices are appropriate; however the sacred garment, if worn, must be replaced on the body afterwards. It is believed to be proper to bury the dead in the ground. Cremation is discouraged, but not forbidden	Individuals are encouraged to evaluate the pros and cons, to implore the Lord for inspiration and guidance, and then to take the course of action that would give them a feeling of peace and comfort
Confucianism	May prefer to be washed by the family. Burial is preferred	No objection, but traditionalists may be superstitious
Hinduism	Non-Hindus should not touch the body. Do not wash the body. This will be carried out by relatives. Jewelry, sacred threads, and other religious objects should not be removed. The body is cremated, as it is only the continuation of the soul that is needed for reincarnation	There is no objection to organ donation. Autopsies are disliked. Ritual preparation will begin after the autopsy. Do not remove jewelry, sacred threads, or other religious objects
Islam	After death the body should not be touched by non-Muslims and so disposable gloves should be worn if this is necessary. Do not wash the body, nor cut hair or nails. Turn the head to the right shoulder, so the body can be buried with the face towards Mecca. The body is ritually washed and wrapped in a white shroud by the family. The funeral should preferably take place within 24 h. Bodies are not cremated as it is believed that there will be a bodily resurrection	Strict Muslims will not agree to organ donation and so do not initiate the discussion, unless the subject is raised by the family. Autopsies are forbidden unless ordered by the coroner. The body is considered to belong to God, hence no part of it should be cut out, or harmed, or donated to anyone else
Jainism	Last offices are appropriate if relatives are unavailable. The body is cremated ceremonially	No objection to organ donation or autopsies: it is considered a good thing to donate organs
Jehovah's Witnesses	Routine last offices are appropriate. Both burial and cremation are acceptable	There is no definite statement related to this issue. Neither organ donation nor autopsies are encouraged; however it is believed to be a matter for the individual conscience. All organs and tissues must be completely drained of blood before transplantation
Judaism	The body must be handled as little as possible as considerable importance is attached to ritual cleansing and clothing. The family will contact the local Jewish undertaker and synagogue and put the ritual proceedings into motion. Very importantly, the body must be guarded until burial. Burial will take place within 24 h, delayed only for the sabbath and other major festivals. It is considered a humiliation not to bury the dead. Cremation is unusual	No objection to organ donation, as preservation of life is an important guiding principle. Autopsies are not permitted under Jewish law unless required by civil law. Any body parts removed for examination must be returned to the body for burial. Ritual preparations of the body will begin after the autopsy
New Age Spirituality	Dependent on underlying religion followed	
Raelians	Dependent on individual beliefs	
Rastafarianism	Routine last offices are appropriate. Burial is preferred, but cremation is not forbidden	Both organ donation and autopsy are considered distasteful and so few would agree. Orthodox members may not permit their hair to be cut

Table 1 Continued

Religion	Care after death	Organ donation and autopsies
Shintoism	The body is prepared by close family members, beginning with a bath of warm water and followed by purification rites before the body is wrapped in a white kimono. Cremation has virtually replaced earth burial. A Shinto funeral is held for Shinto priests. In other cases a Buddhist funeral is appropriate	No objections, although some traditionalists may be superstitious. Considered to be a matter for individual conscience
Sikhism	Normal last offices can be performed by health workers, but normally families will wish to do this themselves. It is imperative to give consideration to the five Ks, particularly the kesh (uncut hair), which must be left intact and kept covered at all times. Additionally a peaceful expression is desired as the face may be displayed on numerous occasions before the funeral. The body is cremated	No objections to organ donation or autopsies. However, special attention should be given to suturing to prevent wound dehiscence, as ritual bathing and dressing will commence after the autopsy
Taoism	The body should be wiped with hot water while it is still warm. If it is a child, he/she should also be dressed in new clothes either shortly before or after death by family or health staff. Burial or cremation is performed: both are highly ritualized so that the ancestors are placated	No objections to organ donation or autopsies, although some traditionalists may be superstitious
Vodun	Dependent on individual beliefs, which will vary according to roots, background, and family upbringing. Burial is preferred	Dependent on individual beliefs which will vary according to roots, background, and family upbringing
Zoroastrianism	Routine last offices are appropriate before being dressed in white clothing. Burial or cremation is acceptable	Probably unwilling to donate organs. Autopsies are forbidden in religious law

(Adapted from Rutty JE (2001) Religious attitudes to death: what every pathologists needs to know. In: Rutty GN (ed.) *Essentials of Autopsy Practice*, vol. 1, pp. 1–22. London: Springer; and Rutty JE (2003) Religious attitudes to death: what every pathologists needs to know, part 2. In: Rutty GN (ed.) *Essentials of Autopsy Practice*, vol. 2. London: Springer (in press).)

Christianity

Christians are followers of Jesus Christ (first century AD), who was born a Jew in the Roman province of Palestine (now known as Israel, Palestine, and Jordan). Christianity is practiced all around the world: there are many differing traditions as a result of disagreements over doctrines through the last two millennia, in turn placing varying significance on death and dying. The three chief forms of Christianity are: (1) Roman Catholicism; (2) the Anglican Communion; and (3) the free churches.

Roman Catholicism About half of all the Christians in the world are Roman Catholics, and Catholicism is the single largest religion. Catholics believe they are in communion with the bishop of Rome, the Pope, the true successor to St. Peter, who was the apostle appointed by Jesus Christ to be the head of his church. The church teaches that life is only a beginning and that death is a move to the fullness of life. The sacrament of baptism is of great significance for Catholics, even more so for children, who should be baptized before or even at death if necessary. At the point of death and up to 3 h after death, extreme unction may

be given. This entails the priest anointing the person with consecrated oil on the forehead and hands in a ceremony symbolizing forgiveness, healing, and reconciliation. Hence, in these circumstances a Catholic priest should always be called.

Care after death Routine last offices are appropriate. Traditionally, Catholics are buried rather than cremated, but there are no religious objections to cremation. However, within Irish communities especially, it is traditional to exhibit the body after death before the funeral. Therefore, particular thought should be taken if the next of kin consent to organ donation or autopsies.

The Anglican Communion Discarding the power of Rome, although agreeing with many Roman Catholic doctrines, the Anglican church represents 4% of the world's Christians. Anglicans believe that those baptized into the Christian faith will share in Christ's resurrection and eternal life after death. Similarly to Catholics, if an infant dies unbaptized, the family may feel that the child has been excluded from the family of God; however, baptism can be performed soon after death by an Anglican priest. At or after death, prayers may be said by the minister offering thanks for the life and entrusting the soul to God's care.

Care after death Last offices are appropriate and burial or cremation is likewise acceptable; there is no opposition to organ donation or autopsies.

The free churches The free churches are Christian groups not tied to Rome or the state and that do not conform to Catholic or Anglican traditions. A number of believers will declare themselves to be Protestants or Chapel. Free churches include: Methodists, Baptists, Salvation Army, Quakers, Seventh Day Adventists, and United Reform Church. Regarding death, it is more likely that the minister will be invited to pray with the patient and family as less importance is put on the administration of sacraments compared to Catholics and Anglicans: several groups do not see baptism of a sick or dead infant as critical.

Care after death Routine last offices are appropriate: burial and cremation are similarly acceptable. There is no religious disapproval of organ donation or autopsies.

New Religions Arising from Christianity

Examples of new religions that have arisen out of Christianity include: Afro-Caribbean community, Church of Jesus Christ of Latter Day Saints (Mormons), and Jehovah's Witnesses.

Afro-Caribbean community The Caribbean Islands' main religion is some form of Christianity; however, there is a wide variation in ritual practices, depending upon the island. The main Christian churches in this population are Anglican, Methodist, or Pentecostal. These communities are more expressive in their practice of religion than their Caucasian counterparts. The extended-family influence can be quite complex, but strong, good relations are maintained, with the family coming together when one of its members dies. There may be more than the usual number of visitors for the dying or deceased, as family members may wish to be near at the time of death.

Care after death It may be ideal that a nurse from a similar ethnic background performs last offices and if the funeral is to be delayed it is preferably embalmed, with burial being the favored means of disposal. The whole community may go to the funeral, which is deemed a significant and elaborate event for the extended family and friends. Before the funeral service and during the church ceremony the body may be viewed. At the graveside the family will fill in

the grave themselves. It is unlikely that traditionalists will agree to organ donation, although younger relatives may hold different beliefs. Concerning autopsies, the older generation may consider that the body must be intact for the after-life and so will be extremely upset by any disfigurement. As a result, it is unlikely that they will consent to an autopsy except for coroner's cases.

Church of Jesus Christ of Latter Day Saints The Church of Jesus Christ of Latter Day Saints has over 11 million members worldwide. By 2080 it is predicted that it will have 265 million members – it is the fastest-growing religion in the world. Mormons embrace the idea that they have reinstated the church as created by Christ. Mormons trust that we have an eternal life extending both sides of our life on earth, resulting in three stages of life: (1) preexistence as a spirit child; (2) a time of probation on earth; and (3) eternal life with the Heavenly Father. At some time after death, the spirit and the body will reunite and be resurrected to the spirit world, which is separated into two: Paradise, where the good spirits wait for resurrection, and Spirit Prison, where the unrighteous spirits live in darkness. The good spirits are able to visit the Spirit Prison and preach the gospel. If one of the unrighteous spirits accepts the gospel and repents, it is able to progress to Paradise. Death is thought to be a blessing and a purposeful role to eternal existence. Spiritual contact is essential, although there are no formal procedures for the dying.

Care after death There are no formal procedures relating to dying and death. Routine last offices are fitting, but the sacred garment, if worn, must be replaced on the body. Cremation is discouraged, though not prohibited, as burial is thought to be proper. The Bishop will offer comfort and practical assistance with funeral arrangements. At the church meetinghouse, the body may be viewed before the funeral. Concerning organ donation and autopsies, Mormons are expected to assess the "for" and "against," asking the Lord for inspiration and guidance before making a decision.

Note Mormons prefer their church to be referred to as the Church of Jesus Christ of Latter Day Saints or the Church of Christ, not the Mormon church.

Jehovah's Witnesses Jehovah's Witnesses aim to live their lives according to the Old and New Testament and are intensely devout. They believe that Jehovah is the Supreme Being and that Jesus is the Son of God, who was a created being who was formerly in a prehuman state as the Archangel Michael. In 1914, the Heavenly Kingdom resulted in the invisible enthronement of Christ as King: the Heavenly Kingdom is presently occupied by an Anointed Class of 135 400 people, the selection of which was concluded in 1935, leaving to date 8600 still living on earth. In the near future Jehovah's Witnesses believe that the battle of Armageddon will commence, where Jesus under Jehovah's divine rage will perform retribution on supporters of all other religions, i.e., false religions, cleansing the world and creating God's Kingdom on earth for 1000 years. Currently, Jehovah's Witnesses regard the world as being under the control of Satan and so will not run for public office, vote in elections, or join the Armed Forces.

Care after death   Routine last offices are appropriate as no official last rites are practiced when death occurs. Both burial and cremation are acceptable. There is no formal written service; instead each is prepared on an individual basis. Organ donation or autopsies are not encouraged, but considered to be a matter of individual conscience. Nevertheless, all organs and tissues must be completely drained of blood before transplantation.

Note   Many traditional faith groups do not grant equal opportunity for women and so the authority in the family tends to be reserved for men. Blood represents life itself and must be handled with respect: such groups do not agree for it to be stored or reused.

Islam

Muslims observe the official conception of their religion in the seventh century AD, deeming that Islam is the belief of all God's prophets from Adam onwards. In Arabic Islam means "to submit," and a Muslim is "one who submits." Muslims believe that God has sent prophets, for instance, Moses, Abraham, and Jesus, to protect this way of life in human society, but their messages have repeatedly been mistaken, forgotten, or distorted. Muslims hold that Mohammed was the very last of these prophets. His message was written down virtually as soon as it was revealed and it has been passed on as God intended through the *Quran*. Muslims worship one God (Allah in Arabic), the creator and ruler of the universe, who is all-powerful and with no equal. The three main branches of Islam are the Sunni, Shi'ite, and Sufi. Muslims hold there will be a Day of Judgment when all the dead will be raised and judged by God. Those whose good prevails over their bad will go to Paradise and the others to the Fire. Death is said to be determined by God and is an element of his plan

and so not to be feared. Extreme grief is suppressed as it is supposed that someone who dies as an observant Muslim will go to Paradise.

Care after death   Following death enormous respect should be shown. The body is ceremonially washed no less than three times with soap and wrapped in a special way with three pieces of white cotton cloth (kafan) along with scent or perfume. If the family is unavailable then last offices by healthcare staff should be minimized as far as possible, while always wearing disposable gloves. This involves closing the eyes, bandaging the lower jaw to the head so that the mouth does not gape, straightening the body by flexing the elbows, shoulders, knees, and hips (thus enabling washing and shrouding of the body later), and turning the head toward the right shoulder (so the body can be buried with the face towards Mecca, south-east). Do not wash the body, or cut hair or nails. Cover the deceased with a sheet, ensuring the whole of the body is covered.

Muslims trust that there will be a bodily resurrection and so bodies are buried, not cremated. The funeral should take place within 24 h: delays cause anguish to families. As the body is believed to belong to God strict Muslims are against organ donation, so the matter should not be discussed unless the family initiates the conversation, or if the deceased has consented in writing beforehand. If organ donation is approved the organs must be transplanted instantly and not kept in organ banks. Except when ordered by the coroner, autopsies are prohibited within the Islamic faith. However, if required, ceremonial preparations in caring for the body will begin after the autopsy.

The Vedic Faiths

Hinduism, Buddhism, and Jainism are three Vedic faiths that began in India. Veda means "sacred knowledge" and is the name of the ancient sacred texts that produced the first clear written traditional religion in India.

Hinduism

Hinduism came to be the term used to describe people who lived east of the river Indus. Hindus refer to their religion as Sanatana Dharma (ancient religion). Very importantly, like many other religions, Hinduism is not just a religion, but also a way of life incorporating countless sects and practices. Its uniqueness stems from the fact that it cannot be traced back to its beginnings: it is seen as a religion that has always existed, and is eternal and unchanging in its essence. Followers of Hinduism believe in one ultimate

Supreme Being who has unlimited forms and who can be understood and worshipped in many different forms. After the death of each physical body, the spirit returns again and again in differing forms, otherwise known as reincarnation. Such forms depend on how faithful people have been in their religious duties. For instance, those who have neglected their duties may be reborn into a lower caste. The spiritual aim is to break free from this cycle of reincarnation. Where possible, just before the soul leaves the body, a few drops of Ganges water, the leaves of the sacred tilsi plant, and a piece of gold are placed in the mouth of the dying person. Death in a hospital can cause great distress, as there is religious significance to dying at home.

Care after death   The relatives should be consulted before the body is touched by anybody after death, because the body should not be washed by non-Hindus. Washing is part of the funeral rites and will typically be carried out by relatives who bathe, dress, and wrap the body in a piece of new cloth. Jewelry, sacred threads, and other religious objects should not be removed. Nevertheless, if the family is unavailable then, while wearing disposable gloves, the eyes should be closed, the limbs straightened, and the body wrapped in a plain sheet with no religious emblems. The body is cremated, as it is just the continuation of the soul that is required for reincarnation. In India, the funeral rites are performed by the eldest son who would light the funeral pyre. Outside India, he may stand by the coffin and watch it pass into the furnace, ensuring the deceased of a good rebirth. On the third day, the ashes are thrown into a river, if possible the river Ganges. After a prearranged number of days, depending on the caste of the deceased, a ceremony known as shradda marks the end of the family's mourning period and the journey of the deceased's soul. Preferably, funerals should take place within 24 h, as in India. There is no opposition to organ donation or autopsies, though these would be unpopular. The ritual preparation of the body will begin following the autopsy.

Buddhism

Buddhism was established in India as a nonconformist system outside Hinduism, during the sixth and fifth centuries BC by Siddhartha Gautama, a Hindu prince who was given the name of Buddha, meaning "Enlightened One." Buddhists openly abandoned the Vedic rites and refused to recognize the caste system as authoritative. Yet, Buddhism shares numerous basic values with Hinduism, together with the notion of reincarnation. There is no god as such in Buddhism

or divine judgment, though the law of "dharma" (cause and effect) affects an individual's destiny. Instead, Buddha is revered as a model of everyday life. Today there are three formal schools: Theravada Buddhism, Mahayana Buddhism, and Tibetan Buddhism. Buddhists believe that death is not the end, but a time to develop into something better. Hence, huge significance is ascribed to the frame of mind at death, which should be tranquil, so chanting may also be performed to create peace of mind, which would be hoped to affect rebirth.

Care after death   There are no official requirements following death and thus routine last offices are suitable. However a Buddhist minister or monk of the same school should be notified of the death immediately. The customary period between death and disposal of the body is 3–7 days. Cremation is favored since there is no belief in the resurrection of the body, but burial is practiced. Any funeral service can be utilized providing there is no mention of Christian doctrine or the Deity. Pregnant women will not attend the service, as Buddhists believe this could cause bad luck for the baby. There is no objection to organ donation or autopsies, given that serving others is elemental in Buddhism and demonstrates compassion. However, if the death was sudden or concerned a small child, Buddhists will be troubled about the deceased's rebirth as the person's mind will not have been prepared before death.

Jainism

"Jain" means those who conquer their inner feelings of hate, greed, and selfishness. The fundamental principle of Jainism is that the world is a place of evil where a countless quantity of souls are trapped, tied to it in a cycle of reincarnations because of "karma" – spiritual residue accrued from immoral behavior in earlier lives. Good conduct eliminates this karma and permits the soul finally to transcend the world and achieve a state of "moksha," eternal spiritual bliss. There are more than 8 million Jains worldwide, 98% of whom live in India, with the biggest Jain communities outside India being within the UK and USA. Jainism is especially unlike other religions in that it accepts that those who are superior spiritually will hasten their own death, typically through starvation. Crucially, Jains do not cry for the deceased, as this will prohibit the dead from rising.

Care after death   Last offices by health staff are suitable, although relations may wish to wash the body after death. If so, Jains will need to wash themselves before eating and drinking. In the UK the body will be dressed in new clothes, but in India a white cloth will shroud the body and new clothes will be given to the poor. A service on the day of the deceased's death will take place in the temple, but the body will be taken home in its coffin to allow close relatives and friends to pray for the soul before the funeral service and look at the deceased's face for the last time. Jains cremate their dead ceremonially, preferably within 24 h. A flower will be positioned on the top of the coffin to resemble life, although it will be removed before cremation as it is thought immoral to harm living things. There is no objection to organ donation or autopsies, as Jains believe it is virtuous to help other people's lives and assist in the creation of new knowledge.

Other Major Traditions

There are a vast assortment of faiths that rest outside the Abrahamic and Vedic religions that have arisen in extremely diverse ways, e.g., atheism, the Baha'i community, Confucianism, New Age spirituality, Raelians, Rastafarianism, Shintoism, Sikhism, Taoism, Vodun, and Zoroastrianism.

Atheism

There are numerous forms of atheism, including: humanism, secularism, rationalism, Buddhism, humanistic Judaism, Christian nonrealism, postmodernism, and unitarianism universalism. Atheism is not a religion or a particular philosophical system, but the absence of a belief in God, trusting that people can formulate appropriate moral codes by which to live devoid of gods. Atheists nonetheless do display sound family ideals, with research illustrating that they have the smallest divorce rate compared to other religious groups.

Care after death For atheists last offices are suitable: there are no rites at death. Many atheists will feel uneasy with religious funerals if religion had no importance for them. As an alternative a humanist funeral will recollect the life of the deceased, exposing their role in humanity, but there are no hymns or prayers included, instead: music; a nonreligious reflection on death; readings of poetry and prose; reminiscences; a eulogy; and ritual actions such as candle lighting; and formal words of goodbye. It is the individual's decision to choose burial or cremation, organ donation, and autopsies.

The Baha'i Community

Established in the nineteenth century by the Persian Mirza Husayn Ali, the Baha'i community was formed

in present-day Iran. Recognized now as Baha'u'llah, which means "the Glory of God," Mirza Husayn Ali was believed to be a prophet sent by God. The Baha'i faith arose from Islam endeavoring to bring together all religions in the belief that there is simply one God who is the creator of all life. Currently, roughly 5 million people follow the Baha'i faith in more than 175 countries. Concerning death, the Baha'i believe that everyone has an eternal soul that is not subject to decomposition and is distinct to everything else in life. At death, the soul is freed to journey throughout the spirit world, that is perceived as an eternal and placeless extension of our own universe. When death occurs no official last rites are practiced.

Care after death Last offices are appropriate and cremation is held to be undesirable as opposed to burial. Significantly, the burial site should be within 1 h journey from the place of death. The body should be placed so that the feet face the Baha'i qibla (the tomb of Baha'Allah near Acre). As the Baha'i faith does not see a discord between modern medicine and religion, there is no objection to organ donation or autopsies.

Confucianism

Confucianism is a major system of thought in China concerned with the principles of good conduct, practical wisdom, and proper social relationships. Confucianism has influenced the Chinese attitude toward life, set the patterns of living and standards of social value, and provided the background for Chinese political theories and institutions. It has spread from China to Korea, Japan, and Vietnam and has aroused interest among western scholars. There are about 6 million Confucians in the world. Several attempts to deify Confucius and to proselytize Confucianism failed because of the essentially secular nature of the philosophy. After the death of Confucius in the early fifth century BC, various schools of Confucian thought have emerged through the centuries, including Mencius, Hsun-tzu, Han Confucianism, and Neo-Confucianism. Beliefs about death will vary depending upon the school of Confucian thought followed.

Care after death At death, relatives cry out loud to inform the neighbors and the family starts mourning and puts on clothes made of a coarse material. The corpse is washed and put in a coffin where food and objects significant to the deceased are placed. Mourners bring incense and money to offset the cost of the funeral. A Buddhist or Taoist priest (or even a Christian minister) performs the burial ritual. Friends and family follow the coffin to the cemetery, along with a willow branch, which symbolizes the soul of the person who has died. The willow branch is carried back to the family altar where it is used to "install" the spirit of the deceased. Liturgies are performed on the seventh, ninth, and 49th day after burial and on the first and third anniversaries of the death. There is no objection to organ donation or autopsies, though conservatives may be extremely superstitious.

New Age Spirituality

The New Age movement has no holy scripts, principal organization, membership, formal clergy, or doctrine. It is a complex system of advocates who share similar philosophies, which they incline to add to whatever other religion they respect. Beliefs embrace astrology as a means of projecting the future, crystals as a basis for healing, and tarot cards for life decisions. They trust moreover that God is a state of higher consciousness and that a person may reach a total understanding of personal human potential. There are a number of essential values, although individuals are supported to decide which agree with them best, e.g. monism, pantheism, panentheism, reincarnation, karma, aura, personal transformation, and holistic health. Viewpoints about death depend on the underlying religion New Age spiritualists abide by.

Care after death Specific care of the body, organ donation, and consent for autopsies are dependent on which underlying religion New Age spiritualists follow.

Raelians

On December 13, 1973, French journalist Claude Vorilhon (named Rael by an extraterrestrial) alleged he was contacted by another planet appealing to establish an embassy to greet his people back on earth. The message described how the extraterrestrials had consciously created life using DNA and cloning to create human beings in their own image: they then left earth, leaving the humans to mature on their own Nevertheless, the extraterrestrials retained contact through prophets, including Buddha, Moses, Jesus, and Mohammed. Now that humans had reached the moon and created life through DNA cloning, the extraterrestrials considered that human beings were ready to understand their alien creators rationally. Raelians believe that today humankind is engrossed in eternal pain caused by the rules of our society. As an alternative we should commit ourselves to reflect, create, blossom, love, and seek pleasure with the highest admiration for others. Viewpoints about death are very individualized; even with the primary faith there is an option of eternal life as a result of the scientific development of human cloning.

Care after death Care after death depends on individual beliefs. Nevertheless, organ donation and autopsies are considered a virtuous act as they may promote or save somebody's life.

Rastafarianism

Rastafarianism is often associated with dreadlocks, smoking marijuana, and reggae music. However, it is much more than simply a religion of Jamaica. It began in the Jamaican slums and spread throughout the world, and currently has a membership of over 700 000 worldwide. Rastafarianism began in the 1930s in the West Indies, among the descendants of slave families who had come from Africa. One of the key doctrines of Rastafarians is that they will eventually be redeemed by repatriation to Africa, their true home and heaven on earth. However, an important historical event occurred when Haile Selassie visited Jamaica on April 21, 1966, convincing Rastafarians not to seek to emigrate to Ethiopia until they had liberated the people of Jamaica. Since then April 21 has been celebrated as a special holy day among Rastafarians.

Rastafarianism is a personal religion with no churches, set services, or official clergy. All members share in the religious aspects, have a deep love of God, and believe that the yemple is within each individual. Visiting the sick, often in groups, is important. The family may pray by the bedside of a dying member, but there are no last rites. Rastafarians believe in the resurrection of the soul, but not of the flesh, after death.

Care after death Routine last offices are appropriate. Burial is preferred, but cremation is not forbidden. The funeral is plain and simple and attended only by intimate family and friends. Both organ donation and autopsy are considered distasteful and few agree to either, except when ordered by the coroner. Members of the faith are readily identified by their distinctive hairstyles. "Dreadlocks" or "locks" are a symbol of faith and a sign of Black pride. Orthodox members do not permit their hair to be cut.

Note There is a taboo on wearing secondhand clothing and orthodox patients may even be unwilling to wear hospital garments; disposal gowns may be preferred. Marijuana is considered to be the "holy herb" and its smoking is a holy sacrament to many. It is believed to be the key to a new understanding of the self, the universe, and God and to be the vehicle to cosmic consciousness.

Shintoism

The traditional religion of Japan is Shinto, meaning "the way of the gods" or "kami." The Japanese do not regard the kami just as divine gods, as it is believed that many of the kami are ancestors who remain close to the earthly world. Ceremonies ask kami, the mysterious powers of nature, for protection and good care. Shintoism is best seen as an animistic religion that reflects the importance to the Japanese of perfection, cleanliness, and harmony with nature and the world of spirits. Death is considered to be an evil that must be accepted as inevitable and irreversible and heart-breaking for everyone involved, including the kami. After death there is no judgment or consignment to heaven or hell: the spirits of the dead merely move into a land that is no longer pure, but a place of decay and corruption, where they are finally released from all physical limitations and again become part of the universal life force. Just as heaven and the underworld are close to the middle land (earth), so the dead remain close to the living. Following death, the spirit of the deceased is held to move into a land that is no longer pure. Shinto rituals provide the dead with a means of escape from decay and corruption, enabling them to grow into exalted beings and become part of the world of kami.

Care after death   Physical contact by healthcare staff should be avoided as the deceased is prepared by the family, first with a bath of warm water and purification rites, before being wrapped in a white kimono. Customarily, family and friends will visit with the deceased for 2 days. Buddhist funerals are appropriate: a Shinto funeral is only held for Shinto priests, important Shinto devotees, and the Emperor and his family. Cremation is favored over burial and no reference should be made to Christian doctrine or the Deity. There is no opposition to organ donation or autopsies, but some purists may be superstitious. However it is critical after death to use respectful words, avoiding the word "body" ("shitai" in Japanese) to relatives. As a substitute, use Japanese comparables for the deceased: "itai" and "go-itai" (go is a prefix, which further raises itai). Furthermore, when discussing the deceased, use flattery, particularly if he/she died in a tragic accident; the only exception to this should be if the deceased performed vicious offenses. Additionally the souls of those who died violently are believed to be restless and potentially hazardous to the living unless they are calmed by food and purification.

Note   Physical contact should be avoided with those who follow Shintoism. The Japanese customarily prefer not to gaze into another person's eyes, since this is considered offensive in their culture. Also, a Japanese person may from respect say "no" three times before giving you a genuine reply. Do not presume that a nod or a smile means agreement, but ask the person if he/she understands what you have said.

Sikhism

In the fifteenth century, Sikhism set aside the religious traditions of the Muslim and Hindu faiths. Sikhism was established by Guru Nanak in what is now Pakistan. Today there are 16 million Sikhs worldwide; more than 80% of the world's Sikh population still live in the Punjab region and the bordering regions of Haryana and Delhi. The UK has the leading community of Sikhism outside Pakistan and India. Sikhs believe that God created everything, so all life is virtuous; however attachment to material things leads to reincarnation and rebirth. After death God judges each soul, and if pure enough that soul will rest with him instead of being reborn. Sikhism places immense importance on the protection of religious freedom, and Sikh men wear five signs of their faith: (1) kesh, uncut hair; (2) kanga, a comb to keep the hair in place; (3) kara, a steel bangle; (4) kirpan, a small sword or dagger; and (5) kacchera, short trousers or breeches. Regarding death, Sikhs retain it is wrong to mourn excessively for the deceased, because they exist in a different body. After death, it is understood that behavior during life is judged by God, resulting in the soul either being in eternal union with God or being reborn.

Care after death   Last offices are appropriate, although occasionally families like to do this themselves. If that is the case, Sikhs who have been touching the body may well take a bath or wash their faces, hands, and feet before returning home. After death, the body is washed and dressed in the five Ks if the person was a member of the Khalsa. The deceased's face may be shown on many instances before the funeral and so a peaceful appearance is desired. The body is cremated as soon as possible, preferably within 24 h. The ashes, and the kirpan and kara, are scattered on running water, i.e., a stream or a river. There is no objection to organ donation or autopsies, but incisions should be carefully sutured, so that subsequent bathing and dressing do not cause wound dehiscence. Ritual proceedings will commence after the autopsy.

Taoism

Beginning in the first century AD, Taoist traditions are followed today by Chinese communities all over the world. Taoism refers to the Way of the Universe; the Tao being the natural force that guides all life, offering well-being and the power to converse with the deities (gods). Taoism is linked to the Chinese concept of "yin" and "yang," that is, the continual balancing and interacting of masculine (yang) and feminine (yin) principles, giving order to life. Supporters of Taoism trust that an individual has no less than one soul, with more than one being male and one female (yang and yin). At death the souls separate. The female soul sinks into the earth as a ghost (kwei) while the male soul rises and becomes a spirit (shen). After death, souls are judged and punished and one of the souls will go to Hell before being able to go to its allotted place. Here souls can bribe keepers to receive better care. It is important therefore that the living family supply their deceased with liberal resources. In response, spirits will pledge victory in life if they are content, or tragedy if not. Traditionally the Chinese who follow Taoism have an aversion to death.

Care after death   The deceased is washed ritually and cleansed with incense. Occasionally embalming may be contemplated. Layers of white paper money or talismans are put over the deceased, representing purification and protection from influences after death. If the decedent is a child then s/he will be dressed in new clothes either just before or after death. Funeral rituals are critical to the welfare of the existing family and are consequently extremely ritualized. For instance, it is inappropriate to bury the deceased immediately, as it is better to wait for the most auspicious date and place for burial. During the funeral special Bank of Hell notes, paper houses, and other goods are burnt to enable the soul to pay for an early release from the various Hells, of which there are 10. Customarily, the bones are exhumed around 10 years later, when they are cleaned and reburied at a site chosen by a feng shui expert. More modern supporters of Taoism favor cremation over burial. When a child has died, occasionally families will not be present at the funeral, nor will they know where the body is buried so that reincarnation can occur early. Usually there is no objection to organ donation and autopsies, but traditionalists may be superstitious, due to the belief that the heart is the center of all life and that it is vital to placate the evil spirits and ghosts who are everywhere; this makes it hard for relatives to give consent.

Vodun

The term Vodun (voodoo) is traceable to an African word for "spirit." Voduns have been traced to the West African Yoruba people more than 6000 years ago. Now there are over 60 million people who practice Vodun worldwide. A religion of numerous traditions, each group respects a distinct spiritual direction and reveres a somewhat dissimilar pantheon of spirits, called loa (mystery). Supporters of Vodun judge that everyone has a soul that has two parts: a gros bon ange (big guardian angel) and a ti bon ange (little guardian angel). The ti bon ange leaves the body during sleep and when the person is possessed by a loa during a ritual. The purpose of rituals is to make contact with spirits, to gain their favor by offering them animal sacrifices and gifts, and to obtain help in the form of more abundant food, higher standard of living, and improved health. A conviction exclusive to Vodun is that the deceased can be revived after burial as, following resurrection, the zombie has no will of its own, remaining under the control of others. In reality, a zombie is a living person who has never died, but is under the influence of drugs administered by an evil sorcerer.

Care after death   This is dependent on individual beliefs that will vary according to the upbringing of the deceased, although burial is preferred.

Zoroastrianism

Originating in the sixth century BC, Zoroastrianism was the dominant religion of Persia (now Iran) until the rise of Islam. Today the largest communities are in India (92 000) and Iran (around 30 000), and it is estimated that there are about 7000 Zoroastrians in the UK, about 5000 of whom live in London. Its scriptures are known as the "Avesta," maintaining a dualistic doctrine, contrasting the force of light and good in the world with that of darkness and evil. Offshoots of Zoroastrianism include Mithraism and Manichaeanism. After death, the soul is allowed 3 days to meditate on its life, when the soul is then judged. If the good thoughts, words, and deeds outweigh the bad, then the soul is taken to heaven, otherwise the soul is led to hell. There are no last rites before death, but Zoroastrians would wish to have their loved ones near at the time of death. Relatives, friends, or rarely, a Zoroastrian priest may say prayers.

Care after death   Last offices are fitting, yet it is imperative that the body is washed before being clothed in white garments. Generally families will supply a "sadra," which is to be worn next to the skin under the shroud, with the sacred "kusti." The family may wish the head to be covered with a cap or scarf. Funerals should take place as soon as possible after death, on the same or next day. In the UK both burial and cremation are accepted, but

Zoroastrians consider that earth burial, cremation, or disposal by water pollutes the sacred elements of the earth, fire and water. Orthodox Zoroastrians believe the body is hostile to the will of God and so will be averse to blood donation and transfusion, as well as organ transplantation. Autopsies are prohibited in religious law and would be declined, excluding coroner's cases.

Conclusion

To conclude, the ultimate choice about whether or not to consent to an autopsy lies at all times with the family except when an autopsy is necessary under a legal authority. Even so, we all attach different meanings to our life and ultimately our death and subsequently it can be obstructive and damaging to take for granted anything concerning the meaning of life events and death for another individual. Knowledge of other people's religion can help us to explain their beliefs and behaviors. Unfamiliarity with another religion or culture can create misunderstandings and communication breakdowns, leaving the healthcare practitioner as a stranger and an outsider rather than someone the family can have faith and confidence in. Compassion and empathy will succeed in earning the gratitude of families.

See Also

Consent: Treatment Without Consent; **Legal Definitions of Death**; **Medical Definitions of Death**; **Organ and Tissue Transplantation, Ethical and Practical Issues**

Further Reading

Berling EA, Fawkes WC (1983) A teaching framework for cross-cultural health care. *Western Journal of Medicine* 139: 934–938.

Boyce M (2002) Zoroastrian faith and philosophy. http://www.religion-info.net.

Braswell GW (1994) *Understanding World Religions.* Nashville: Broadman & Holman.

Char DFB, Tom KS, Young GCK, Murakami T, Arnes R (1996) A view of death and dying among the Chinese and Japanese. *Hawaii Medical Journal* 55: 286–290.

Cytron BD (1991) To honour the death and comfort the mourners: traditions in Judaism. In: Irish DP, Lundquist KF, Nelson VJ (eds.) *Ethnic Variations in Dying, Death, and Grief*, pp. 113–124. London: Taylor & Francis.

Eshleman MJ (1992) Death with dignity: significance of religious beliefs and practices in Hinduism, Buddhism, and Islam. *Today's O.R. Nurse* 14: 19–22.

Gates E (1995) Culture clash. *Nursing Times* 91: 42–43.

Green J (1991) *Death with Dignity: Meeting the Spiritual Needs of Patients in a Multi-cultural Society.* London: Macmillan Magazines.

Green J (1993) *Death with Dignity*, vol. II: *Meeting the Spiritual Needs of Patients in a Multi-cultural Society.* London: EMAP Healthcare.

Green J, Green M (1992) *Dealing with Death: Practices and Procedures.* London: Chapman & Hall.

Gudmundsdottir M, Martinson PV, Martinson IM (1996) Funeral rituals following the death of a child in Taiwan. *Journal of Palliative Care* 12: 31–37.

Hallenbeck J, Goldstein MK, Mebane EW (1996) Cultural consideration of death and dying in the United States. *Clinics in Geriatric Medicine* 12: 393–406.

Hays C, Mitchell J, Harding J (1996) Death and the day of the dead: a Mexican fiesta. *Journal of Multicultural Nursing and Health* 2: 29–33.

Hughes S, Henley A (1990) *Dealing with Death in Hospital: Procedures of Managers and Staff.* London: King Edward's Hospital Fund for London.

Irish DP, Lundquist KF, Nelson VJ (eds.) (1991) *Ethnic Variations in Dying, Death, and Grief*, London: Taylor & Francis.

Levine E (1997) Jewish views and customs on death. In: Parkes CM, Laungani P, Young B (eds.) *Death and Bereavement Across Cultures*, pp. 98–130. London: Routledge.

Mulhall A (1996) The cultural context of death: what nurses need to know. *Nursing Times* 92: 38–40.

Musgrave C (1995) Rituals of death and dying in Israeli Jewish culture. *European Journal of Palliative Care* 2: 83–86.

Nishimoto P (1996) Venturing into the unknown: cultural beliefs about death and dying. *Oncology Nursing Forum* 23: 889–894.

Orlowski JP, Vinicky JK (1993) Conflicting cultural attitudes about autopsies. *Journal of Clinical Ethics* 4: 195–197.

Parkes CM, Laungani P, Young B (eds.) (1997) *Death and Bereavement Across Cultures.* London: Routledge.

Pearson R (1982) Understanding the Vietnamese in Britain. Part II: marriage, death and religion. *Health Visitor* 55:477, 480–481, 483.

Rees D (1997) *Death and Bereavement: The Psychological, Religious and Cultural Interfaces.* London: Whurr.

Reference Services, Central Office of Information (1992) *Aspects of Britain: Religion.* London: HMSO.

Robinson BA (2001) Atheism, agnosticism, free thinking, humanism, etc. http://www.religioustolerance.org.

Robinson BA (2002) New Age spirituality. http://www.religoustolerance.org

Rutty JE (2001) Religious attitudes to death: what every pathologist needs to know. In: Rutty GN (ed.) *Essentials of Autopsy Practice*, vol.1, pp. 1–22. London: Springer.

Rutty JE (2003) Religious attitudes to death: what every pathologist needs to know, part 2. In: Rutty GN (ed.) *Essentials of Autopsy Practice*, vol. 2. London: Springer.

Thompson D (ed.) (1995) *The Concise Oxford Dictionary of Current English*, 9th edn. Oxford: Clarendon Press.

Toropov B, Buckles L (1997) *The Complete Idiot's Guide to the World's Religions*. New York: Alpha Books.

Turner-Weeden P (1995) Death and dying from a Native American perspective. *Hospice Journal – Physical, Psychological and Pastoral Care of the Dying* 10: 11–13.

Varza B (2002) Zoroastrian faith and philosophy. http://www.religion-info.net.

Woo KT (1992) Social and cultural aspects of organ donation in Asia. *Annals of the Academy of Medicine* 21: 421–427.

www.yahoo.com/Society_and_Culture/Religion/Faiths_and_Practices/.

RELIGIOUS EXCEPTION DEFENSE

S M Asser, Hasbro Children's Hospital, Providence, RI, USA

Introduction

An exclusive reliance on faith to treat a minor or self-limited condition may be benign. However, for serious disorders or injury the result is often preventable disability or death.

A few religious denominations practice faith healing to the exclusion of medical care. In some jurisdictions politics, law, and other factors may be enabling this dangerous behavior. In most places it remains possible to prosecute when children are harmed or killed. This is an essential method of placing these groups on notice that parents must provide their children with the necessities of life regardless of their religious beliefs.

By looking at the history of the sects involved along with illustrative cases, investigators, medical examiners, and prosecutors can gain an understanding of both the need to bring criminal charges and the strategies required. This article describes cases from the United States. While laws may vary among jurisdictions, cases similar to these are found worldwide. The focus of authorities should be to understand the issues involved within the context of local laws in order to best protect children.

Background

In its infancy in the nineteenth century, the science-based medical model of healthcare found competition from a range of modalities such as homeopathy, folk practices, and so-called mind cures. Mind cures partially inspired the development of some faith-healing sects. These sects also drew upon cultural inclinations to seek healing by divine intervention, vitalism, and notions that illness could be caused by sin. If illness was due to sin, then acceptance of salvation through faith could remove disease and restore health.

Modern medical and public health advances improved health and dramatically increased life expectancy in the twentieth century. Nevertheless, we begin the twenty-first century with much public interest in traditional practices. Some of these, such as homeopathy, have been scientifically disproved. Others, such as herbal potions, have yet to yield results that are commensurate with their claimed benefits. None has had such a profoundly damaging effect on children's health as an exclusive reliance on faith healing for serious disorders.

Faith-Healing Sects

Groups that use prayer or religious ritual as their only response to illness fall predominantly into two types. Several Pentecostal churches, sometimes called "full gospel" or "word" churches, interpret passages in the New Testament to command them to seek healing through faith. Some claim medicine to be demonic and physicians to be agents of Satan. Others insist that accepting healing through divine intervention is a required demonstration of faith. These sects tend to be small and without a centralized hierarchy, although a few have been responsible for dozens and possibly hundreds of deaths. Examples of denominations with exclusive reliance on faith healing are given in **Table 1**.

The other type is Christian Science, whose members follow the principles of founder Mary Baker Eddy. In the late nineteenth century, Eddy claimed to have discovered a method of healing that was revealed exclusively to her. Unlike other faith healers who accept that disease is real, Eddy's followers maintain that symptoms, and all physical matter, are an illusion. Illness is caused by sin or improper thoughts, and these thoughts can be corrected through the method of prayer exclusively taught in Eddy's church. Diseases of infants and toddlers are attributed to sins or thought errors of the parents, who must pray to

Table 1 Groups that refuse medical care for children

Christ Assembly
Christ Miracle Healing Center
Church of God Chapel
Church of God of the Union Assembly
Church of the Firstborn
Faith Tabernacle
Faith Temple Doctoral Church of Christ in God
First Church of Christ, Scientist (Christian Science)
Followers of Christ
Jesus through Jon and Judy
Northeast Kingdom Community Church
The "No Name" Fellowship
The Believer's Fellowship
The Body
The End Time Ministries
The Faith Assembly
The Source

correct these. Older children are often told that their complaints are not real or scolded for their inability to correct their thinking and improve their health.

In addition to calling their religious practices "scientific," they have co-opted medical terms and claim a system of healthcare based on their faith. Church-trained "practitioners" charge fees for prayers that they refer to as "treatments;" these prayers are typically offered in response to telephone calls.

Christian Science "nurses" offer custodial care. These unlicenced individuals self-certify their credentials. They must state that they accept the tenets of the church as the only requirement for being listed in official church publications. They have no medical training or even first-aid training. Furthermore, their theology prohibits any reliance on material means to heal, prevent, or monitor disease or relieve discomfort. The nurses do not take a pulse or blood-pressure reading or use a fever thermometer. They will not carry out even simple nonmedical measures to relieve pain, such as applying heat or ice to injured areas of the body or giving massage.

In a wrongful-death lawsuit in the case of a boy with untreated diabetes, one Christian Science nurse testified that cutting sandwiches into interesting shapes was all she had been taught specific to the care of children.

The church also runs unregulated "sanatoria" for the ill, staffed by its nurses. While many denominations operate hospitals and clinics, all others do so with qualified and licenced providers.

Once a thriving religion, membership in the Christian Science church has declined markedly in the past 60 years. Despite waning membership, this church has been successful in advancing its political agenda. In the early 1900s, when licencing and regulation were established for physicians, the church succeeded in gaining exemption from such oversight in the USA.

Fees for the church's practitioners are considered a tax-deductible medical expense.

The US government pays Christian Science sanatoria millions of dollars annually for what is, by statute, called "religious non-medical health care." The church has also obtained reimbursement for its practitioners and nurses from many private health insurers.

Exemptions to Child Abuse Charges

In 1974 the US Congress passed the Child Abuse Prevention and Treatment Act (CAPTA) to help states enhance or create child protection systems. In response to requests from Christian Science lobbyists, government regulators required that states receiving CAPTA funds have exemptions to child abuse or neglect laws for parents relying on spiritual healing. These requests were successful, in part because of the previous accommodations for the church's practices in medical licencing statutes. The result has been a wide variety of such exemptions in civil codes concerning child welfare as well as criminal child abuse laws.

In response to many preventable deaths and the concerns of child advocates, the federal government dropped the requirement for exemption laws in 1983, but still allowed states to keep those already passed. By then, nearly all states had such exemption laws and most still have them today. In the 1996 reauthorization of CAPTA, Congress codified states' option to enact exemptions, despite hundreds of reported child deaths in faith-healing sects. Congress did require that states maintain mechanisms to seek court-ordered treatment for children, but many do not come to the attention of authorities in time. Most professionals are familiar with cases of Jehovah's Witnesses who refuse blood transfusions and with court orders for medical treatment of their children. However, unlike the Witnesses, who do avail themselves of medical care, children of members of faith healing sects are generally out of contact with medical providers or child welfare authorities.

Death Statistics

A study of autopsy records by a medical examiner in the state of Washington found that Christian Scientists died earlier, sometimes from treatable disorders, than others in the community. William Simpson studied death rates of graduates of a Christian Science college. They were compared with those from a secular institution and from a Seventh Day Adventist college. The latter group has similar lifestyle prohibitions against caffeine, tobacco, and alcohol as Christian Scientists. Death rates were significantly higher among Christian Scientists. Most notably, rates were up to fourfold higher in cohorts 30 or more years following graduation.

At the other end of the age spectrum are children. A study of perinatal events among the Faith Assembly showed a threefold increase in infant mortality and an 80-fold increase in maternal mortality compared with surrounding populations. Older children have also been affected.

In an investigation of the deaths of 172 children from 21 faith-healing sects during the two decades following the passage of CAPTA, 140 had conditions with expected survival rates exceeding 90% with medical care. All but three children would have clearly benefited in some way from such care.

Many of the deaths occurred after prolonged illnesses, sometimes lasting months, from disorders such as diabetes or leukemia. Others occurred after shorter but no less agonizing periods with conditions such as appendicitis, pneumonia, or dehydration. It can be recognized how readily salvageable these children were by their diagnoses. Examples of the diagnoses from this series are given in **Table 2**.

Massachusetts Citizens for Children has studied testimonial claims of healings through Christian Science and found no credible scientific evidence of efficacy. They estimated that death rates from diabetes were 70-fold higher while death rates from meningitis were over 100-fold higher among Christian Science children than in the general population.

In 1998, an Oregon newspaper reported on deaths of children from the Followers of Christ Church in Oregon City. Reporters documented over 70 headstones of children in the private church cemetery in just over 40 years. Several mothers also died during childbirth. Many cases had evidence or documentation that the fatalities were from readily treatable or preventable disorders. Church Elders were interviewed and responded that they put their children in God's hands, not doctors' hands. Based upon the size of the congregation, a comparison of crude death rates to those in Oregon overall shows a risk of death that was three- to fivefold higher for neonates, infants, and children in this group. Similar to the data from the Faith Assembly from the 1970s, maternal death rates were more than 100 times higher in this sect.

Not only are the numbers of children dying of otherwise treatable conditions intolerable, but the pain and suffering that the children endure in the process are also abhorrent.

Illustrative Cases

Case histories illustrate the suffering involved and also suggest strategies for investigators and prosecutors. While exemption statutes in some jurisdictions may prevent charges for minor offenses, in most states charges for serious crimes such as felony neglect, manslaughter, child endangerment, or murder are appropriate and sustainable.

An eight-month-old girl with several days of fever became increasingly unresponsive. During her final 24 h her parents phoned a Christian Science practitioner 20 times. She succumbed to bacterial meningitis. A two-year-old female suffered partial airway obstruction from aspirating a bite of banana. Her parents frantically called for members of their prayer circle who arrived to pray. She gasped and attempted to breathe for an hour before she died.

A physician left his residency to join a church so opposed to modern medicine that they would not allow members to wear eyeglasses or use canes. His five-month-old son had several respiratory arrests on the last day of a five-day febrile illness that was later determined to be meningitis. The father performed mouth-to-mouth rescue breathing, claiming the action was to rebuke the spirit of death, but he did not summon an ambulance nor take the child to a hospital.

Many parents and others attending these deaths have represented to authorities that they were not aware of the gravity of the child's condition. However, the record generally belies this claim. Examination of

Table 2 Cause of death in medical neglect cases from 21 faith-healing sects

Appendicitis (7)
Birth trauma (5)
Dehydration (6)
Diabetes (12)
Diphtheria (3)
Epilepsy
Ewing's sarcoma
Foreign-body aspiration
Hemorrhagic disease of newborn
Intussusception (3)
Leukemia, acute lymphocytic (3)
Measles (7)
Meningitis (14)
Neonatal asphyxia (22)
Neonatal respiratory failure (3)
Osteogenic sarcoma (3)
Pericarditis
Pertussis
Pneumonia (22)
Renal failure (3)
Small-bowel obstruction
Ventricular septal defect, small (2)
Volvulus (2)
Wilms tumor

Data from Asser SM, Swan R (1998) Child fatalities from religion motivated medical neglect. *Pediatrics* 101: 625–629.

phone records may reveal the timing and frequency of attempts to seek prayer or religious ritual for the child. The presence of fellow church members or sect leaders in the home is another indication that they recognized the seriousness of the illness. Friends, neighbors, and relatives are often aware of the practices of sect members, and also aware of the duration or severity of symptoms. Proper investigation into the timeline of events can establish the degree of parental concern as well as intent to avoid timely medical attention.

A 12-year-old girl from Arizona was kept home from school because of "a problem with her leg." Her school arranged for a teacher to visit her at home. The teacher went to visit a number of times over a 3-month-period, but was always denied entrance. Finally, when the girl's mother told the teacher at the door that they placed God before their own lives, the school alerted child protection services. A court-ordered medical evaluation was too late. The osteogenic sarcoma on her leg had grown to a circumference of over 105 cm. She was in heart failure from severe anemia and her buttocks and genitals were covered with bedsores.

Despite her complaints to hospital nurses about the agony she endured and the recommendation of her physician to amputate her leg to alleviate pain, child services officials came to an agreement with the parents that allowed her transfer to a Christian Science residential facility. There, receiving no medication, she was told by her attendants to suppress her cries so as not to disturb the other residents. She died shortly thereafter.

Mandated reporters of child abuse have often cited religious exemption statutes or parental prerogative as rationale for inaction. While most courts would order life-saving treatment over parental objections if notified in time, laws that fail to define all medical neglect as child abuse in effect discourage reporting of such cases and thus need to be changed.

After a 36-h labor attended by unlicenced midwives, a father became so disturbed by his wife's persistent screaming that he summoned an ambulance. At the hospital, the mother delivered a macerated, decomposing stillborn infant and died shortly thereafter from sepsis. The medical examiner noted that the infant was so foul-smelling that it would have been inconceivable for those in attendance not to be concerned.

Dozens of other infants have died near or at birth. Almost all were term, well-developed infants who died for no reason other than lack of trained assistance. Typically, local authorities performed little or no investigation of these tragedies as infants who had not yet taken a breath were called "stillborn" and

thus not legally persons. However the unlicenced midwives may still be liable for the death.

Other church agents may also be liable. In the case of a 13-year-old girl with diabetes, the church pastor who anointed her with oil and was at her bedside as she lay dying pled guilty to manslaughter (*State* v. *Davis* (1994) Cause #13038, Monroe Cty. Circ. Ct., Miss.). While clergy have a First Amendment right to express their religious beliefs, their conduct may be actionable if they know the child is seriously ill and contribute to the child's demise. In some states they can be charged as accessories to a crime or participants in a conspiracy.

Civil liability may also accrue. The father of an 11-year-old Minnesota boy called the boy's mother, the custodial parent and a practicing Christian Scientist, and asked to speak to his son. The mother told him that the boy was sleeping. In fact, the child was in a diabetic coma and died shortly thereafter. Criminal charges were filed, but the court dismissed them because of fair notice problems created by a religious exemption law (*State* v. *McKown* (Minn. 1991) 475 NW 2d 63, *cert. denied*, 328 US 833 (1992)).

However, the father filed a wrongful-death action in civil court, naming the mother, stepfather, Christian Science practitioner, nurse, and the Christian Science church as defendants, and won a multimillion-dollar jury award. While the church itself was dismissed from the case on appeal, the cause of action against the practitioner, nurse, mother, and stepfather was upheld (*Lundman* v. *McKown* (Minn. 1995) 503 NW 2d 807; *cert. denied* US (1996)).

Investigation and Prosecution

The first obstacle to be overcome is the reluctance to blame otherwise law-abiding and well-meaning parents for an unfortunate outcome. The lack of intent to cause harm is not a requirement for prosecution. Most physically abusive parents do not intend the level of injury that results from their assaults. Medical neglect can lead to results as devastating to children as other forms of abuse. Authorities must treat medical neglect with all due gravity.

Most parents who have been convicted of medical neglect because of their reliance on faith healing have not been incarcerated unless they simultaneously physically abused their children or if there was a prior conviction. However, conditions of probation have generally included a requirement to get medical care for other children in the family.

The purposes of prosecutions, in addition to punishment for law-breaking, are to prevent future neglect and to put the community on notice that medical neglect of children is not acceptable. A number of families and sects have lost multiple children. Without legal consequences, the deaths will continue. In England and Canada, where there are no religious exemptions from child abuse laws, Christian Science church officials counsel their members to take ill children to doctors.

Elements of Successful Prosecution

1. Look for the generally present evidence that caregivers knew that something was amiss with the child and had sufficient opportunity to act. This will often contradict statements by caregivers denying the gravity of the illness. Even the most ardent Christian Scientists, known for their detachment from the reality of pain and suffering, frequently begin to panic when faced with a seriously ill child. Examination of phone records and interviews with neighbors, relatives, and even other members of the sect will provide appropriate evidence.

2. Compare the victim's care with the standard in the community at large. Investigate all of the parents' practices on healthcare for their children rather than just the incident that caused the child's death or disability. The parents may have withheld all preventive and diagnostic measures from their children. They may not have health insurance for their children even though they are able to afford it. Jurors are usually unsympathetic to parents who systematically ignore the medical needs of children while they themselves have often gone to great lengths to get treatment for their own children.

3. In jurisdictions that have some exemption laws, charge using statutes that do not have exemptions. If child abuse laws have exemptions, then charge under manslaughter or criminally negligent homicide. While some convictions have been overturned because of fair notice problems created by religious exemptions, many have been upheld on appeal despite religious defenses in one section of the criminal code (*People* v. *Rippberger* (1991) 231 Cal. App. 3d 1667; *Hall* v. *State* (Ind. 1986) 493 NE 2d 433).

4. Provide copies of literature from medical journals and be prepared to explain why these are to be relied upon and why church testimonials are not. Defenses in these cases often attempt to claim that the parents or others relied on the healing record of prayer in previous cases. Proponents of faith healing will often claim a record of efficacy equivalent or superior to that of modern medicine. They may attempt to deflect blame from themselves by statements such as: "Doctors aren't perfect, either. After all, children die in hospitals, too."

Any physician or medical examiner should be qualified to explain to a jury why anecdotes and testimonials of healing, in most cases in individuals with self-limited disorders or who have not been medically diagnosed, are not evidence of efficacy. The children who have died have not had esoteric or intractable problems, but rather common disorders that would be easily treatable in any community medical facility. This should be explained clearly as well.

5. Be prepared to explain why Christian Science prayer is not "treatment" and why their "nurses" are not what the public would generally recognize as nurses. Most jurors would be appalled at the suggestion that someone without the training to take a temperature or a blood-pressure reading would be sufficiently qualified to care for a seriously ill child.

6. Look for evidence that some forms of medical care had been used by the family or group on other occasions. Jurors will be perplexed by a defense that asserts that obstetric care (allowed by Christian Scientists) is good enough for a parent but somehow other medical care is not appropriate for a child. The father of one infant who died from pneumonia had previously had a vasectomy. After joining a church that encouraged him to procreate for the perpetuation of the group, he had his vasectomy surgically reversed. The irony of such an incident would not be lost on a court.

7. In the case of a stillborn infant in which an unlicenced church midwife attended the delivery, although a coroner or medical examiner may not be able to declare the case a homicide, an investigation should still be completed and the case referred to the local prosecutor for consideration of charges. While the law does not require assistance at delivery, when it is provided it must be competent, otherwise negligence will attach.

8. Strongly consider charges against all whose actions added to delays or prevented access to care in cases of treatable illness. While clergy may have some constitutional protections for their religious speech, their behavior is still subject to the law. Many sects do not have formal hierarchies, but investigations often uncover leadership roles and specific actions by group members that contributed to deaths. In one case an emergency crew was turned away by a church member who stated that a miracle had occurred despite an infant's ongoing distress. Others may have been criminally negligent because of failure to act in an apparent emergency.

9. Two organizations that may be helpful in obtaining relevant literature and case materials are Children's

Healthcare Is a Legal Duty (CHILD) Inc. (www.childrenshealthcare.org), of Sioux City, Iowa and The American Prosecutors' Research Institute of Alexandria (www.ndaa-apri.org), Virginia. Both have records from previous prosecutions and contacts with experts that may be of assistance.

Conclusion

It would be a mistake to consider the investigation and prosecution of child deaths from religion-motivated medical neglect as serving an antireligion purpose. There is no other form of child maltreatment that has religious exceptions in the law. One cannot molest, beat, or starve a child and claim a religious imperative, despite some attempts to do so.

In fact, virtually all theologians and clergy would consider the denial of medical care to a sick child to be incongruous with respect for the divine. The Talmudic scholar and physician Maimonides wrote:

If someone suffers from hunger and turns to bread and, by consuming it, heals himself from his great suffering, shall we say that he has abandoned trust in God? Just as I thank God when I eat for His having provided something to satisfy my hunger ... thus I should thank Him for having provided that which heals my sickness when I use it.

Likewise, the exercise of religious freedom is not to be confused with license to disregard the welfare of others. The US Supreme Court has best expressed the responsibility of a parent for the welfare of a child and the interest of the state to intervene when that responsibility is unmet. In *Prince* v. *Massachusetts* ((1944) 321 US 158) the court ruled: "The right to practice religion freely does not include the liberty to expose the ... child to ... ill health or death. Parents may be free to become martyrs themselves. But it does not follow they are free, in identical circumstances, to make martyrs of their children."

See Also

Autopsy: Pediatric; **Children:** Legal Protection and Rights of Children; **Crime-scene Investigation and Examination:** Death-scene Investigation, United States of America; Suspicious Deaths; **Neonaticide**

Further Reading

American Academy of Pediatrics Committee on Bioethics (1997) Religious objections to medical care. *Pediatrics* 99: 279–281.
Asser SM, Swan R (1998) Child fatalities from religion motivated medical neglect. *Pediatrics* 101: 625–629.
Dwyer JD (1996) The children we abandon: religious exemptions to child welfare and education laws as denials of equal protection to children of religious objectors. *North Carolina Law Review* 74: 1321–1478.
Dwyer JD (2000) Spiritual treatment exemptions to child medical neglect laws: what we outsiders should think. *Notre Dame Law Review* 76: 147–177.
Fraser C (1999) *God's Perfect Child: Living and Dying in the Christian Science Church*. New York: Holt.
Merrick JC (2003) Spiritual healing, sick kids and the law: inequities in the American health care system. *American Journal of Law and Medicine* 29: 269–299.
Rosato JL (1994) Putting square pegs in a round hole: procedural due process and the effect of faith healing exemptions on the prosecution of faith healing parents. *University of San Francisco Law Review* 29: 43–119.
Simpson WF (1991) Comparative mortality of two college groups. *MMWR. Morbidity and Mortality Weekly Report* 40: 579–580.
Skolnick A (1990) Christian Scientists claim healing efficacy equal if not superior to that of medicine. *Journal of the American Medical Association* 264: 1379–1381.
Sloan RP, Bagiella E, Powell T (1999) Religion, spirituality, and medicine. *Lancet* 353: 664–667.
Spence C, Danielson TS (1987) The Faith Assembly: a follow-up study of faith healing and mortality. *Indiana Medicine* 80: 238–240.
Swan R (1997) Children, medicine, religion, and the law. *Advances in Pediatrics* 44: 491–543.

RESTRAINT TECHNIQUES, INJURIES AND DEATH

J D Howard, Tacoma, WA, USA

Introduction

A variety of methods are commonly used to physically restrain individuals taken into police custody, to control severely agitated persons, and to help manage the care of mentally or physically debilitated patients. The restraint process often results in injury to the person being restrained. Death, by a variety of causes, may occur while someone is restrained, prompting major forensic concern. With significant frequency the restraint is the cause of, or directly contributes to, the death of the individual being restrained.

Restraint-associated injury and deaths require in-depth investigation and careful interpretation.

Handcuffs

Handcuffs are the most commonly used restraint device employed by law enforcement agencies worldwide. It is standard policy for most law enforcement agencies to place a person being taken into custody into handcuffs, no matter how cooperative the person may be initially. The handcuffs are mostly metal devices, consisting of two hinged, mirror-image, circular-ratcheting, and self-locking pieces, one for each wrist. The two pieces may be joined by rigid metal pieces, hinged metal pieces, or metal chain. Standardized keys are needed to unlock each wrist piece individually. Use of flexible nylon or plastic wrist restraints is increasingly common. The most common of these devices consists of a single long, thin piece of synthetic material with one molded locking-device end and a tapered opposite end. The device is looped once around crossed wrists, the tapered end is inserted in the opening of the locking piece, and the free protruding end is pulled tight, closing the loop about the wrists. The flexible material is lightweight, strong, and inexpensive. Double-loop versions are also commercially produced. Most of these devices are intended for one-time use only, and must be cut to release.

Handcuffs may be applied with the arms of the restrained person in front or to the back; the latter technique is most commonly used as it limits the range of motion of the person's arms and hands, increasing security. Handcuffs are often joined to a chain that encircles the waist of the restrained person, also to limit arm mobility. A common chain may be attached to the waist chains in order to restrain several prisoners at the same time. This is also commonly accomplished by use of a series of handcuffs, one set of cuffs holding a prisoner's wrist to that of the next prisoner in line. Ankle restraints, similar in design to handcuffs and commonly called leg irons, with attached chains are often applied in addition to handcuffs during the transportation of prisoners. When in place, the restrained person can shuffle the feet, but does not have enough freedom of movement to walk or run in a normal fashion. A common chain between prisoners forming a work crew, the source of the expression "chain gang," may link leg irons.

Handcuffs may cause patterned abrasions around wrists (**Figure 1**), with parallel margins approximating the width of the cuffs, and are associated with wrist contusions of less specific shape. Leg irons produce similar injury patterns in the ankle areas.

Localized soft-tissue swelling at the site of handcuff application is common. Abrasions are often

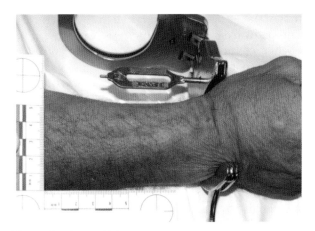

Figure 1 Handcuff injury.

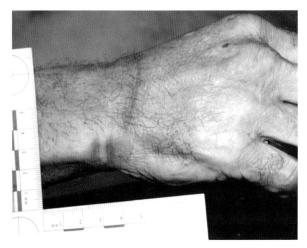

Figure 2 Handcuff abrasions.

prominent at the radial and/or ulnar aspects of the wrists (**Figure 2**).

Compression neuropathies at the wrist may result from the application of handcuffs. Long duration of application of the handcuffs is the principal risk factor for the development of handcuff neuropathy. Intoxication by alcohol or drugs is also a predisposing factor. It has been estimated that 6% or more of prisoners who have been handcuffed experience some degree of compression neuropathy. The superficial radial nerve is most frequently involved. The radial nerve, the median nerve, or the ulnar nerve individually, or any combination of the three, may be injured by handcuff compression. Sensory impairment is common; numbness, paresthesias, and pain are typical symptoms. Motor deficits, with impaired grip, are less common than sensory impairment, but occur with significant frequency. When handcuff neuropathy occurs, involvement of both wrists is common. Neurologic deficits can persist for considerable periods of time, sometimes for years. Nerve conduction studies may differentiate true handcuff compression neuropathy from other conditions or malingering.

While contusions, abrasions, and pain are often reported in association with the use of leg irons, significant neurologic impairment is uncommon. Falls while walking in leg irons may occur and result in an assortment of nonspecific contusions, abrasions, and lacerations, often involving areas of the body other than the ankles.

Carotid Sleeper Hold

Neck holds have been employed in modern times by police and prison personnel, but date back to martial arts teachings in past centuries. Use of neck holds is intended to subdue a physically violent person quickly. One technique involves the approach to the violent person from behind by the person attempting to place a subduing hold. The subduing person places his/her arm around the neck of the person to be subdued. The forearm is positioned in contact with one side and the front of the person's neck, and the biceps surface of the arm is positioned in contact with the opposite side and front of the neck. The subduing person pulls his/her arm and forearm together and backwards, squeezing the neck. The skin and soft connective tissues of the neck are compressed inward, causing the jugular veins and the carotid arteries also to be compressed. Blood flow through the carotid arteries is diminished or stopped entirely. While some blood flow to the head continues through the vertebral arteries, there is not enough blood flow to the brain to provide an adequate oxygen supply for full consciousness, and if the carotid sleeper hold is maintained, the person to which it is being applied loses consciousness and is rendered incapacitated, at least briefly. Once the carotid arteries are compressed to the point of occlusion, the person is expected to lose consciousness in 3–15 s. When properly applied, the carotid sleeper hold places little pressure at the anterior midline of the neck, and does not impair the airway.

The mechanism of action of the carotid sleeper hold is an ischemic/hypoxic insult to the brain, leading to loss of neural function. The mechanism is identical to manual or ligature strangulation, being an impairment of blood circulation to and from the head (and therefore the brain). The degree of dysfunction of the brain and any lasting brain damage or death depends directly on the duration of the carotid sleeper hold. As with any form of compression of the neck, pressure on the carotid bodies has the potential of inducing, through nervous system feedback to the heart, an arrhythmia-inducing sudden cardiac arrest and death. Precipitation of an ischemic stroke and

promotion of a seizure are also potential risks of this type of neck hold.

Chokehold

Another type of hold applied to the neck is the chokehold. This maneuver involves placing the forearm transversely across the front of the neck and pulling backward; pressure is applied to the midline of the neck, resulting in compression of the airway. This restraint method is also referred to as the bar arm control. Airway compression causes pain and impairs the ability to breathe. Blood flow to and from the brain is generally not a significant factor. The pain and struggle to breathe may cause the person to fight the subduing person even more violently. Incapacitation occurs after the collapse of the airway has lasted long enough to cause hypoxia, and is not a rapid event.

When a chokehold results in crush injury to the airway, impairment of breathing may persist after the forearm pressure is released. The duration of hypoxia is the principal determination of degree of central nervous system injury that may follow the use of a chokehold. Acute airway obstruction may result in fulminant pulmonary edema. Hypoxia may exacerbate preexisting ischemic heart disease, resulting in myocardial infarction or cardiac dysrhythmias. Fatal hypoxic brain injury may result from application of a chokehold in the same way that death occurs from any other type of airway obstruction or suffocation. In cases of death following a chokehold, autopsy may reveal fractures to the thyroid cartilage. Injury to the cricoid cartilage and the rings of the trachea may also be identified. Irregular abrasions and contusions may be seen in the skin of the neck after forearm/arm holds have been applied.

Manual Body Restraint Holds

A variety of other manual methods may be used to subdue and maintain physical control over a violent, agitated person in the setting of a mental health facility, emergency room, jail, or street situation. One or more subduing persons may grasp the person to be subdued from behind, placing an arm over one shoulder and the chest. A "takedown" is done in the form of a partially controlled tripping of the individual's legs by the person grasping from behind or with the aid of another person. The individual is placed and held in a prone position, with the weight of the subduing person resting, in part, on the back of the person on the ground. Some degree of compression of one side of the neck is likely with this maneuver. A variation of this involves the person on the ground being held by the wrists with his/her arms crossed over the chest. The person holding the wrists is positioned behind the person on the ground, applying some or most of his/her weight to the back. Pulling on the wrists controls the person's arms. This is sometimes referred to as a "therapeutic basket hold." While far less common than in the past, a straitjacket may still occasionally be used to control a mental patient, putting the patient's arms in a cross-chest position, similar to the basket hold.

When multiple individuals are participating in the takedown and control of one agitated person, it is common for each of the person's limbs to be grasped and controlled by one or more subduing individuals. It is not uncommon when dealing with a particularly violent person that a "piling on" occurs, with multiple individuals holding the limbs and others grasping the person from behind. The person ends up prone on the ground at the bottom of the pile, with the weight of multiple people on his/her back. Neck holds may be used as a part of the takedown process.

A variety of nonspecific contusions and abrasions can occur during a takedown and the application of manual holds to maintain control of an individual. Blunt injuries to the face and anterior chest are common, due to the person ending up in a prone position in contact with the ground. Neck compression and partial or complete impairment of the airway or blood circulation to the head may occur. If the restrained person is held prone on a relatively soft surface (e.g., thick carpet, dirt, bedding, or couch cushion) obstruction of the nose and mouth may occur, resulting in some degree of suffocation. Maintaining weight on the subdued person's back can result in mechanical asphyxia. Combinations of these mechanisms are at play in many cases. Death from this mode of restraint, with weight on the back producing mechanical asphyxia, has occurred following the holding of a person for as little as 4 min. Mechanical asphyxia may also result from very tight application of a straitjacket.

Restraint Chair

An unruly or violent person may be confined to a sitting position in a chair equipped with restraint straps. The arms, legs, and trunk of the individual are each secured to the chair. The head may also be secured in some fashion. When fully secured in a restraint chair, the person is effectively immobilized and has little chance of hurting him/herself, or anyone else. Contusions and abrasions may result from the person struggling with arms or legs against the straps.

If immobilization by any form of restraint is maintained for a significant period of time, there is a risk of development of deep-vein thrombosis, particularly in the legs, and subsequent pulmonary thromboemboli.

Restraint Belts and Vests and Bedrails

It is common practice to restrain hospital and nursing facility patients with an abdominal restraint belt or a restraint vest (also called a "posey"). The belt or vest is secured to the wheelchair, the fixed chair, or the patient's bed. The restraints stop patients from ambulating. The intention is to prevent injury from a fall or to keep the person from wandering away and getting lost. Metal bedrails (side rails) are often used in hospital-type beds to prevent a patient from falling out of bed to the floor.

Restraint vests may result in shoulder compression sufficient to cause brachial plexus injury with varying degrees of persistent nerve function impairment. Belt and vest restraints do not prevent all movement of the patient, and the patient may slide or partially fall from a chair or bed in such a way that much of the body weight is suspended by the belt or vest. The belts can migrate upward and compress the chest; fatal mechanical asphyxia may result. The upper edge of the vest can compress the neck, causing fatal strangulation. Entrapment of patients in bedrails or between the bedrails and the mattress has led to fatal mechanical asphyxia and strangulation.

Excited Delirium

Various forms of mania characterized by marked physical agitation often lead to an individual being physically restrained by others. Physical violence against others and bizarre behaviors, such as running naked through traffic, are often seen in such cases. "Excited delirium" or "agitated delirium" are apt descriptors of the condition. Schizophrenia, other mental disorders, and drug or alcohol intoxication are associated with excited delirium. Cocaine, methamphetamine, and phencyclidine (PCP) have frequently been identified in drug-associated cases. Hallucinogenic drug use (e.g., lysergic acid diethylamide (LSD) and mescaline) may also be associated with excited delirium, although laboratory detection is more difficult than with the more commonly encountered drugs; routine toxicology screening may yield false-negative results.

Excited delirium is observed to be associated with an apparent increased pain threshold; individuals seemingly are unaware of injuries in many cases, and may not react to a delivered blow (such as being struck with a police baton or "night stick") as a normal person would. The degree of agitation is often such that an individual ignores commands and is able to resist the efforts of multiple people to subdue him/her, literally throwing people off his/her back in some instances.

The agitation and violent actions of individuals in a state of excited delirium frequently result in the person sustaining a multitude of contusions, abrasions, lacerations, and cuts. The injuries often occur both well before and during efforts to restrain them. The extremities, the face, and the scalp are usually involved, with no particular pattern recognized. The marked degree and duration of excited delirium may result in considerable physical exertion, with associated changes in heart rate and blood pressure, oxygen debt, metabolic acidosis, and catecholamine release.

Hobble Restraint

Because of the extreme agitation that is often associated with excited delirium, a person may have restraint devices applied to both the arms and the legs in order to be adequately controlled. Hobble restraint is used in reference to a variety of restraint techniques intended to limit a person's leg movements. Commonly this refers specifically to the simultaneous use of handcuffs and leg restraints, a technique that is also called "hog-tying." Hog-tying involves handcuffing a person's wrists behind the back and binding the ankles together. The wrists and ankles are then pulled together and tied to one another. The person most often ends up in a prone position (**Figure 3**). The person putting the handcuffs and ankle bindings on the person being restrained often places a knee, and weight, on the back of the individual during the process, resulting in chest compression.

The hobble restraint results in constant pressure on both the wrists and the ankles. Pain, contusions, and abrasions at the wrists and ankles are common. There are numerous cases of people dying while being subjected to hobble restraint. Research into the possible mechanisms contributing to such deaths has been conducted. Statistically significant decreases in mean

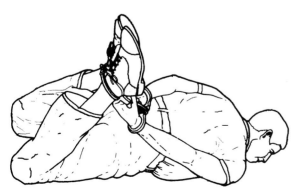

Figure 3   Hobble restraint position.

forced vital capacity and mean forced expiratory volume (restrictive pattern of impaired pulmonary function) has been found in healthy volunteers subjected to hobble restraint in the prone position. Changes in heart rate and blood pressure have also been observed. Two independently conducted studies have shown that recovery of heart rate (pulse rate) following exercise can be prolonged (statistically significant differences) when a person is restrained in a face-down (prone) position, compared to other positions. The characterizations of research findings vary from "not associated with any clinically relevant changes" to "dramatic impairment of hemodynamics and respiration." Further research is urgently needed in this area.

Investigating Restraint-Associated Deaths

When a person who has been restrained is pronounced dead, the death scene should be immediately secured and the body and all items on the body should be left as they are. A trained death investigator should examine the body and all items on the body at the scene. The body and all restraint devices (and all other items) on the body should be photographed and packaged together as evidence. When police were directly involved in the restraint of a person who dies, a scene response by the medical examiner, the coroner, or one of his/her representatives (medical investigator or deputy coroner) is warranted and should be made as quickly as possible. If restraint devices have been removed for any reason prior to the arrival of the death investigator, the items need to be found, taken into evidence, photographed, and examined in detail.

An experienced forensic pathologist should perform a thorough autopsy. Anterior and posterior neck dissections and dissection of the back are recommended to search for injuries that may not be seen at the skin surface. Toxicology is essential, even if drug use history is unknown. Photographs should be taken, recording all areas of the body, even when no injuries are visible. Radiographs (X-rays) should be considered. The deceased's medical history should be ascertained.

An effort to develop a timeline of the activities and actions of the deceased and all individuals involved in the restraint should be made. Surveillance photographs or video images may be available and should be reviewed. Videos should be timed.

Deductive reasoning and a detailed knowledge of the facts of a particular case are needed in order to draw appropriate conclusions as to the cause and manner of an individual's death. Inductive reasoning is to be avoided; the isolated extrapolation of any one animal or human study or case report to the investigation of a particular restraint-associated death is unwise. Statements made by those involved in the restraint must be evaluated carefully; there is a tendency to underestimate both the amount of force used and the duration of the restraint.

Neural inducement of cardiac arrhythmias, catecholamine release and toxicity, rhabdomyolysis, impaired breathing, impaired blood circulation, metabolic acidosis, coexisting natural disease, blunt and sharp injuries, and drug toxicity should all be given consideration in identifying mechanisms of death in cases involving restraint. If one or more physiologic effects stemming from restraint are considered to contribute to death, then the physical restraint should be identified as the cause or one of the causes of the death. If restraint is identified as one of the causes of death, the manner of death should be classified in an unnatural category, even if natural disease is present. Suicide is not applicable when restraint is applied by someone other than the deceased, leaving accident, homicide, or undetermined (or unclassified) to be used to define the action leading to death, according to the circumstances of the individual case.

The fact that a person was in a hobble restraint (hog-tied) is not sufficient evidence by itself to conclude that fatal asphyxia occurred. However, the multitude of physiologic effects of restraint should not be underestimated or quickly dismissed as making a contribution to death, just as modest changes in heart rate and blood pressure recorded in test subjects in controlled low-dose cocaine studies should not lead one to conclude that cocaine is never toxic and not a causative factor in some deaths. Knowing the morbid anatomy in a particular case alone will not allow for proper understanding of the death; physiologic alterations must be taken into account. Restraint need not produce systemic hypoxia to contribute to death. Restraint stress, not just the possibility of asphyxia, must be given due consideration. Following careful investigation, most restraint-associated deaths are determined to be multifactorial.

Police and others using restraint techniques must be aware of and trained in the possible risks of all types of physical restraint, and to monitor closely individuals who are being restrained by any method. If there is any doubt about the restrained person's condition, emergency medical services should be summoned immediately to evaluate and treat as needed.

See Also

Custody: Death in, United Kingdom and Continental Europe; Death in, United States of America; **Detainees:** Care in Police Custody, United Kingdom; Care in Prison Custody, United Kingdom; **Excited Delirium**; **Injuries and Deaths During Police Operations:** Special Weapons and Training Teams

Further Reading

Cannon A (2000) The mystery of a midair homicide. A raging teen dies after air passengers react. *US News and World Report* October 2, 129: 42.

Chan TC, Vilke GM, Neuman T, Clausen JL (1997) Restraint position and positional asphyxia. *Annals of Emergency Medicine* 30: 578–586.

Corey TS, Weakley-Jones B, Nichols GR, Theuer HH (1992) Unnatural deaths in nursing home patients. *Journal of Forensic Science* 37: 222–227.

Emson HE (1994) Death in a restraint jacket from mechanical asphyxia. *Canadian Medical Association Journal* 151: 985–987.

Hick JL, Smith SW, Lynch MT (1999) Metabolic acidosis in restraint-associated cardiac arrest: a case series. *Academic and Emergency Medicine* 6: 239–243.

Hiss J, Kahana T (1996) Medicolegal investigation of death in custody: a postmortem procedure for detection of blunt injuries. *American Journal of Forensic Medicine and Pathology* 17: 312–314.

Luke JL, Reay DT (1992) The perils of investigating and certifying deaths in police custody. *American Journal of Forensic Medicine and Pathology* 13: 98–100.

Parkes J (2000) Sudden death during restraint: a study to measure the effect of restraint positions on the rate of recovery from exercise. *Medicine, Science and the Law* 40: 39–44.

Pollanen MS, Chiasson DA, Cairns JT, Young JG (1998) Unexpected death related to restraint for excited delirium: a retrospective study of death in police custody and in the community. *Canadian Medical Association Journal* 158: 1603–1607.

Pudiak CM, Bozarth MA (1994) Cocaine fatalities increased by restraint stress. *Life Science* 55: 379–382.

Reay DT, Eisele JW (1982) Death from law enforcement neck holds. *American Journal of Forensic Medicine and Pathology* 3: 253–258.

Reay DT, Howard JD, Fligner CL, Ward RJ (1988) Effects of positional restraint on oxygen saturation and heart rate following exercise. *American Journal of Forensic Medicine and Pathology* 9: 16–18.

Roeggla M, Wagner A, Muellner M, *et al.* (1997) Cardiorespiratory consequences to hobble restraint. *Wiener Klinische Wochenschrift, The Middle European Journal of Medicine* 109(10): 359–361.

Roggla G, Roggla M (1999) Death in a hobble restraint. *Canadian Medical Association Journal* 161: 21.

Ross DL (1998) Factors associated with excited delirium deaths in police custody. *Modern Pathology* 11: 1127–1137.

Ross EC (1999) Death by restraint: horror stories continue, but best practices are also being identified. *Behavior and Health Tomorrow* 8: 21–23.

Siebert CF, Thogmartin JR (2000) Restraint-related fatalities in mental health facilities. *American Journal of Forensic Medicine and Pathology* 21: 210–212.

Vanezis P (2000) Deaths in custody. In: Mason JK, Purdue BN (eds.) *The Pathology of Trauma*, 3rd edn., pp. 103–122. London and New York: Oxford University Press Inc.

Restraint, Excited Delirium *See* **Excited Delirium; Substance Misuse:** Cocaine and Other Stimulants

---

RITUALISTIC CRIME

D Perlmutter, Institute for the Research of Organized and Ritual Violence LLC, Yardley, PA, USA

Defining Ritualistic Crime

Ritual crime entails a wide variety of both sacred and secular acts committed by groups and individuals and is most often attributed to practitioners of occult ideologies such as Satanism, Palo Mayombe, Santería, and other magical traditions or to serial killers and sexual sadists who ritually murder their victims. Due to many legal, practical, and ethical controversies the investigation, research, and study of contemporary religious violence are in their infancy. There have been no serious empirical studies of ritualistic crimes or classifications that adequately distinguish ritual homicides committed for sacred versus secular motivations. Problems arising from investigating ritualistic crimes are generally beyond most investigators' typical experience. Due to the lack of standardized categories, law enforcement professionals cannot agree on the extent of ritualistic crime, the types of crimes committed by individuals and religious groups, or the motives of the perpetrators. Hence, ritual violence is not often recognized, reported, or investigated accurately. Additionally certain other crimes or events may be overinterpreted or misinterpreted as ritualistic crime when they are not.

In the law enforcement community illegal ritual activities are typically referred to as occult crimes. However, occult crime is an inaccurate and pejorative designation because occult is applicable to many religions and practices that are fundamentally nonviolent. Furthermore, not all violent ritual acts are committed in the worship of a religion. A more objective and accurate expression is ritualistic crime because it encompasses crimes that may entail ritualistic behavior and that are completely unrelated to the occult or any religious tradition. There is no agreed-upon definition of ritualistic crimes. Building upon a 1989 California law enforcement study of occult crime, ritualistic crime is most precisely defined as any act of violence characterized by a series of repeated physical, sexual, and/or psychological actions/assaults combined with a systematic use of symbols, ceremonies, and/or machinations. The need to repeat such acts can be cultural, sexual, economic, psychological, and/or spiritual (**Table 1**).

Forensic Evidence Specific to Ritualistic Crime

Analyzing ritual crimes not only entails all the forensic, investigation, and legal issues associated with violent crime but also posits its own unique problems. In ritualistic crime, locations are always designated as either sacred (holy) space or profane (ordinary) space. Violence in the form of occult religious ritual always has to occur in sacred space; even mass murder/suicides have to occur in sacred space. Outdoor secluded locations are typical of ritualistic crime scenes due to the nature-based ideologies of most occult religions. They also provide enough privacy to prolong torture and conduct rituals. Indicators of occult outdoor crime scenes include trail markers, unusual tree marking, and anything that is out of place, for example, a circular clearing, an arrangement of tree stumps, or unusual holes in the ground. Natural objects are frequently part of the crime scene and should be checked for blood stains and other forensic evidence. The presence of unusual artifacts,

Table 1 Ritualistic crimes

Trespassing

Trespassing related to ritual violence or, more specifically, occult activity usually involves persons entering private areas such as wooded and forested lands, barns, and other old or abandoned buildings. The purpose of such trespassing is to worship either in the area as it is naturally arranged, or to arrange it so that it becomes a place of worship with the appropriate altars and symbols. Occult-related trespassing of this nature is committed by persons who seek a private and isolated place to worship

Vandalism

Vandalism most often associated with ritualistic crime includes cemetery and church desecration. The most common types of cemetery desecration attributed to occult groups are overturning, breaking and/or stealing headstones; digging up graves; grave-robbing; and tampering with human corpses or skeletons. This is frequently motivated by religious beliefs that require cemetery desecration and human bones to fulfill certain rituals

Church desecration

Church desecration frequently includes the following actions: destroying bibles; urinating and defecating on holy objects and furniture; tearing crucifixes off walls; and destroying rosaries and crucifixes. It is important to note that the motivations behind such vandalism can also be attributed to hate crimes

Theft

Thefts from Christian churches, Jewish synagogues, hospitals, morgues, medical schools, and funeral homes are often linked to ritual violence. Items that are most often taken include cadavers, skeletal remains, blood and religious artifacts that are considered sacred; crucifixes, communion wafers, wine, and chalices. Frequent motivations for these thefts are that particular groups require actual holy artifacts or human organs and bones for their rituals

Graffiti

Graffiti is one of the most common offenses related to ritualistic crime. While a small amount of graffiti is related to other occult groups, the vast majority is directly related to involvement in satanic groups. Nearly all instances of Satanic-related graffiti, which frequently depict Satanic symbolism, are committed by juveniles and young adults, most of whom are dabbling in the occult

Arson

Occult-related arson is almost always attributed to satanists, especially juveniles and young adults. Among the most common places for juveniles to commit arson are churches and synagogues in which particularly holy sections or artifacts are burned, and houses or buildings where damaging evidence could be uncovered by investigators. Additionally, some law enforcement officers have found satanic graffiti at some arson scenes. It is important to note that the motivations behind the arson of churches and synagogues can also be attributed to hate crimes

Animal sacrifice

Animal sacrifice is primarily practiced by believers in Afro-Caribbean religions, principally practitioners of Santeria, who sacrifice animals as part of rituals designed as offerings to their gods to intervene in the universe through magic. However, animal sacrifice can also be attributed to practitioners of Satanism. The symbolic objects at the crime scene, type of mutilation, and other forensic evidence generally indicate which belief system is practiced

Extortion

Although group practice of extortion is not a known activity of any occult group, individual practitioners of some occult belief systems have used their religious involvement as a method of extoring money and information. Investigators have noted that such crimes are especially difficult to prosecute because the victims will not come forward. More often than not, the victims do not perceive themselves as victims because they trust the santero and believe that their economic sacrifices are being used to protect them

Suicide

Occult-related suicide appears to be the primary domain of juveniles and young adults involved in Satanism who are often true believers, but sometimes dabblers. Satanic-related teenage suicide is a major concern among many criminal justice practitioners

Kidnapping

Although extremely difficult to prove, kidnapping people of all ages, but especially children, is thought to be a prevalent crime among some occult practitioners. Especially accused are traditional/cult satanists who are said to kidnap victims needed for ritual sacrifice, self-styled juvenile Satanists whose dabbling has taken them ''to the point of no return,'' and mayomberos, whose rituals require a human skull to add to their nganga

Ritual homicide

Probably the most controversial crime allegedly committed for occult purposes is murder perpetrated for spiritual reasons and sometimes as a human sacrifice. Sacrificing a human being has occurred in almost every culture throughout history and contemporary incidents have been documented. Currently, both Palo Mayombe practitioners and Satanists are often linked to human sacrifice. There is evidence that juvenile and young adult Satanists who have become true believers commit murder for sacrificial reasons required of their spiritual beliefs

Ritual abuse

This is a particularly heinous and controversial crime, which is known as ritual abuse, ritual child abuse, or, more specifically, satanic ritual abuse. The alleged perpetrators of such abuse are most often Satanists. In the broadest sense, ritual abuse of children, adolescents, and adults involves repeated physical, sexual, psychological, and/or spiritual abuse, which utilizes rituals. Currently, there is probably no more divisive issue within the criminal justice community than that of Satanic ritual abuse. While no one disputes the existence or increase of ritualistic abuse, few agree about several other aspects: the extent of ritualistic crimes committed specifically by satanists; the motivations of perpetrators; and the veracity of the victims who claim to have survived ritual abuse at the hands of satanists drawings, graffiti, or other items is especially prevalent in ritualistic crimes. Symbols and artifacts found at the crime scene can help the investigator determine if the crime was conducted by an individual or members of a group, and identify the type of religious ritual and whether that belief requires additional similar rituals which may signify future crimes.

Ritualistic crimes can be committed by one or more offenders who may be members of a religious group or by a lone offender who is following the ideology of a group. However, some lone offenders enact rituals that do not conform to any organized group. Disorganized crime scenes will generally be indicative of dabblers and teenage offenders; they frequently leave trash, food, and bottles in the area near the ritual site. Members of an established group will be highly organized and the crime scene will be particularly clean; because it is sacred space it would be treated with the same respect as the space around the altar of a church. The weapon of choice for ritualistic crime is a knife; it would be magically ineffective to shoot someone in a ritual. A ritual knife (athame) is one of the most sacred items of the offender and would rarely be left at a crime scene unless the perpetrator was interrupted in the act and had recently fled the scene; usually a ritual knife or sword is found during searches of personal areas or on the suspect.

The use of blood in ritualistic crimes is more revealing than any other form of evidence, not to be confused with blood stain pattern analysis. In ritualistic crime the physical pattern is not as important as the symbolic meaning of blood. In addition to many other ritual uses, blood is anointed, exchanged, and imbibed in magical rites of initiation, transformation, and sacrifice. Victims are frequently the result of a ritual sacrifice and should be examined for unusual loss of blood. The level of experience of the perpetrator is immediately evident in the cleanliness of the crime scene or victim; for example, it takes a high level of skill to remove blood from a person or animal without soiling the scene. A juvenile dabbler will not be able to remove blood in the same manner as an experienced high priest who could have the skills of a surgeon. Additionally dabblers do not always treat the scene with the proper regard for sacred space as true believers. Both historically and today the role of the sacrificer is an honored and privileged position and will most likely be the leader of the group.

Body disposition is one crime-scene indicator whose psychological and symbolic interpretations can substantially differ from each other. In ritualistic crimes the body may be positioned in a manner that holds specific magical meaning for the group, as a

necessary function of the ritual, and has nothing to do with avoiding discovery or leaving a message. Also in ritualistic crimes bodies or body parts may be buried for magical purposes that have nothing to do with eluding the police. There is rarely evidence of staging in ritualistic crimes. Perpetrators of ritualistic crimes will not interfere with their crime scenes because in many occult traditions any alteration of the ritual is a form of sacrilege and renders the magic ineffective. If a ritual crime entailed staging it would be indicative of a criminal who is not a true believer and whose primary motive has nothing to do with a group belief system.

Forensic findings are especially relevant to ritualistic crimes due to the amount of trauma, the symbolic nature of physical mutilations, and the prominence of pre- and postmortem sexual assault. The cause of death in murders that are the result of sacrificial ideologies will frequently be from torture, blood loss, or dismemberment caused by knife wounds committed during the ritual. Murders committed for the purpose of millennial group beliefs can entail everything from poison and immolation to gunshot wounds. Ritual homicides committed by serial killers will not correspond to any specific occult tradition and there is no particular cause of death. In ritualistic crimes committed by true believers the motivations for sexual assault differ substantially from other crime classifications. In some occult traditions sexual assault is perceived as a form of sexual magic and has less to do with the gratification of the offender than with achieving magical power and/or as an indoctrination technique. This is based on the magical concept that any form of severe extreme emotion caused by either torture or sexual pleasure will increase the magical power of the offender. Mutilation is extremely common for ritualistic crimes, including symbols cut into the body, bite marks, particular forms of dismemberment, and bloodletting (Table 2).

Contemporary Blood Rituals

Across cultures and throughout history the one practice common to all religions is sacrifice and the most potent form of sacrifice is achieved through blood rituals. Whether animal or human, blood historically is the mandatory substance for religious ritual and sacrifice is the ultimate religious experience. Historically people attributed sacred and magical qualities to blood, and blood rituals entailed everything from drinking, pouring on the body, and a variety of uses in ceremonies. In some cultures it was believed that

Table 2 Forensic ritualistic evidence in general

- Mockery of Christian symbols (inverted cross, vandalized Christian artifacts)
- Use of stolen or vandalized Christian artifacts
- Discovery of candles or candle drippings
- Unusual drawings, symbols on walls/floors (such as a pentagram)
- Nondiscernible alphabet
- Drawings of occult symbols
- Animal mutilations, including removal of specific body parts (anus, heart, tongue, ears)
- Use of animal parts (feathers, hair, bones) to form symbols on ground
- Absence of blood on ground or in animal
- Altar containing artifacts (candles, chalice, knife)
- Effigies like voodoo dolls stuck with pins or otherwise mutilated
- Bowls of powder or colored salt
- Skulls with or without candles
- Robes, especially black, white, or scarlet
- Rooms draped in black or red
- Occult books on Satanism and magic rituals
- Calendars with peculiar days marked
- Computer used to visit occult sites
- Handwritten occult essays or diaries
- Animal or human body parts found in refrigerator

drinking the blood of a victim would endow you with his/her strength; similarly, in drinking the blood of an animal you would acquire its qualities. Today there is a revival of magical ideologies that entail a variety of individual and group blood rituals. The most familiar examples are evident in the current popularity of tattooing, piercing, branding, and body modifications. These and other forms of self-mutilation comprise the basic prerequisites for entry into the contemporary subcultures of modern primitives, the body modification movement, vampire culture, and the fetish scene. The modern primitive movement is a term that is used in the avant-garde art world to refer to visual artists who distort, manipulate, mutilate, and mark their bodies as a form of ritual performance. The modern primitive movement blends tribal traditions with technology to combine magic and science. The body modification movement includes people who are involved in piercing, tattooing, branding, implants, and extreme body modification but do not have a unifying ideology. They differ from modern primitives who claim their performances are a spiritual experience of transformation. Vampire culture is the fastest-growing manifestation of the occult and entails the practice of what is referred to as "blood sports" – the exchange of blood for both ritual and sexual purposes. Finally the fetish scene entails nightclubs where members of all of the previously described movements come together to engage in all manner of sadomasochism, sexual bondage, and blood rituals. Acts of self-mutilation include

everything from cutting the body with razors, burning the flesh, having nails hammered through limbs, being suspended from the ceiling with hooks attached through the skin, being pierced with heavy weights, having objects implanted under the skin, and self-amputation. Every kind of body modification imaginable is being performed, sometimes resulting in death.

When analyzing ritualistic forensic evidence it is important to distinguish mutilations that are the result of willing participation in the many new subculture trends of self-mutilating the body or unwilling victims of group religious rituals and individual occult crimes. This can be accomplished by distinguishing between the types of crime scenes, victimology, and trauma associated with particular occult traditions. There are distinct and discernible forensic differences in the blood rituals, animal and human sacrifices perpetrated by practitioners of Vampirism, Santería, Voodoo, Palo Mayombe, Satanism, serial killers, and natural animal predators.

Vampire Culture and "Blood Sports"

Vampire culture, more commonly called the "vampire scene," refers to individuals, group organizations, events, and businesses which all share an interest in the vampire lifestyle. Currently, there is a prevailing phenomenon of modern vampires whose serious commitment to their beliefs, community, and culture meet the criteria to be designated a contemporary new religious movement. Since there is no agreed-upon definition of what constitutes a vampire, the modern vampire is an amalgamation of characteristics derived from a variety of historical and cross-cultural archetypes. The subculture, like the vampire, evolved from a combination of folktales, cultural myths, legends, and eventually the romanticized images found in Hollywood films and popular novels. There are many facets to vampire culture and members range from dabblers such as participants in role-playing games to the extremely devoted, who are referred to as "real vampires" within the vampire community. Vampire belief systems are dependent upon the personal or group interpretation of a vampire and may manifest simply as an esthetic choice or an entire lifestyle based on a sophisticated vampire philosophy. Vampire culture is a serious and growing phenomenon that has gatherings where thousands of vampires attend. Vampirism, like other religions, consists of people who have committed themselves to an ideology, who maintain ethical tenets within a hierarchical system, and who participate in rituals specific to their clans. Practitioners of Vampirism are referred to as vampires and are part of an extensive subculture.

The practices that are most relevant to forensics in the vampire scene are blood-drinking and bloodletting. For modern vampires, the use of blood is what separates the dabblers from the real vampires. In vampire culture the use of blood is commonly referred to as blood sports, blood play, blood lust, and blood fetishism and is an expression of sexual, spiritual, recreational, or artistic activities that involve cutting and drinking blood. Blood rituals in the form of sacred acts of worship are fundamental to real vampire religious beliefs. Blood sports in the form of recreational and/or sexual activities are one of the most dangerous aspects of vampire culture and are noticeably increasing in popularity. Blood play involves cutting the body, then having another person licking or sucking the blood from the cut. Cutting is most often done with a surgical scalpel or fine razor blade, making shallow cuts in the top layer of the skin. At many of the vampire nightclubs it is not unusual to see a group of people cutting and sucking each other's blood in what is referred to as a feeding circle. Blood play is frequently intertwined with sexual activities and becomes an integral part of the intimacy shared. Occasionally blood sports entail using a syringe to draw blood and then imbibing it or sharing the blood with your partner. Essentially blood sports involve any sadomasochistic practice that involves blood and encompasses all forms of body mutilation such as self-scarring and play-piercing in addition to cutting.

The immediate and obvious dangers in blood sports are bloodborne diseases and accidental deaths caused by sadomasochism gone wrong. A general principle for determining how deeply individuals are involved in vampire culture or any form of occult religion is their use of blood. Once blood is being exchanged, imbibed, extracted, or used in any manner whatsoever in ritualized activity, the person has now committed to that religion or group. Additionally blood rituals are addicting, both psychologically and physiologically. Physically, when someone is experiencing pain, endorphins (natural painkillers) are released; however, eventually more pain is needed to achieve the same endorphin high. Psychologically, individuals feel that without blood their vitality will diminish, magical powers will subside, or they simply are not themselves. It is not unusual for participants of vampire culture who are in this situation to carry around vials of blood. The more insidious danger of blood play is that occasionally self-mutilation is not a sufficient religious experience and can escalate into blood rituals that entail harming others.

Vampirism, the most recent manifestation of the occult, has led to many crimes ranging from vandalism to murder. Many juveniles and young adults dabbling in the occult are seduced into the more

Table 3 Forensic evidence unique to the vampire scene

- Human blood (in vials)
- Hypodermic needles used to remove blood
- Razor blades
- Fangs (false teeth)
- Knives, swords
- Dramatic clothing, robes
- Metal claws that attach to fingers
- Whips, leather restraints, chains, sexual bondage items
- Unusual contact lenses
- Skulls, coffins, and other gothic items
- Symbolic silver jewelry with precious stones

serious level of the subculture, the vampire and fetish scenes, where blood rituals, sexual sadomasochism, and bondage discipline are regular occurrences. The dangers implicit in drinking and exchanging blood and violent sexual activities are more insidious when they are viewed as sacred rituals that are required for initiation, membership, and status in the group (**Table 3**).

Santería and Voodoo "Blood Offerings"

Afro-Caribbean faiths originated in the eighteenth and nineteenth centuries during African slave trading when owners imposed Catholicism on to their slaves and forbade traditional religious practices. In an attempt to maintain their cultural and religious beliefs, Africans disguised their religion by assigning each of their gods the image of a Catholic saint. Over the years the religions and cultures synchronized into new religions. Syncretic belief systems refer to religions that have combined two or more different cultural and spiritual beliefs into a new faith. Santería, Voodoo, Palo Mayombe, Candomble, and Shango are some of the syncretic Afro-Caribbean religions. Magic and the belief in supernatural intervention occupy a significant place in the worship of all occult syncretic religions.

Santería combines the cultural and spiritual beliefs of the southwestern Nigerian Yoruba tribe with the religious practices of the Catholic faith and consists of using magical rituals to worship or satisfy a pantheon of gods and goddesses, known as orishas. Santería is an earth religion, a magical religious system that has its roots in nature and natural forces. Santería retains the fundamental precepts of the ancient Yoruba tradition, including the concepts of ashe and ebbo. The gods of Santería are the repositories of ashe, the divine power/energy, and santería spells, rituals, and invocations are all conducted in order to acquire ashe (energy) from the gods. This energy is the power to change things, to solve all problems, subdue enemies, and acquire love and money. Ebbo is the concept of sacrifice and is the way that the orishas are worshiped so that they will give their ashe. Every rite and spell of Santería is part of the ebbo concept. Fortunately sacrifice does not always require a sacrificial victim. Ebbo can be an offering of fruits, flowers, candles, any of the favorite foods of the orishas, or a blood offering.

Voodoo is also known as vodun, voudou, vodoun, and hoodoo and is derived from the African language of the Fon word vodu, which means spirit or deity. The term voodoo and its derivative hoodoo originated as derogatory expressions to refer to systems of sorcery and magic, or to specific spells or charms stemming from these systems. Similar to Santería, Voodoo is a syncretic religion that developed as a response to the African slave trade; however, Voodoo evolved among the slaves who were taken to Haiti. Although some of the rituals and ceremonies of voodoo are comparable to Santería, there are marked differences. The African tribes from where the religious movements originated were different and the rites varied with each tribe. The Haitian form of Voodoo has many deities, known collectively as loa, who participate in ritualistic ceremonies in several different ways. Rituals are most commonly held to invoke a particular god who best fits the need of the moment and gods are known either as rada or petro. There are many different types of Voodoo rituals, including individual acts of piety such as lighting candles for particular spirits and large feasts, sometimes lasting several days. Similar to Santería, initiation, divination, sacrifice, and spirit possession are fundamental Voodoo rituals (**Figures 1–6**).

Currently there are several million people living in the USA who practice some sort of Afro-Caribbean faith, most of whom are not involved in criminal activity. Controversies associated with the practice of Santería and Voodoo most often entail the misunderstanding of the use of magical spells, amulets, food offerings, and debates surrounding the practice of animal sacrifice. Due to the growing population of Santería and Voodoo practitioners, many officers routinely discover the remains of sacrificed goats, chickens, roosters, and other animals covered in sacrificial matter, in areas such as cemeteries, beaches, near railroad tracks, and other places that have magical significance to believers. Although it is illegal to discard animal corpses in public places, most of these cases are not indicative of violent criminal behavior but are remnants of ritual ceremonies. A general rule of thumb for investigators is that Santería and Voodoo devotees will not torture their sacrificial animals and most often either quickly slit the throat or break the neck of an animal. If an animal is discovered that has obviously been mutilated or tortured then it is a practitioner of one of the black magic traditions, another occult religion, or a nonreligious act of sadism. A basic knowledge of Santería and Voodoo beliefs can assist in distinguishing between violent crimes and typical Santería and Voodoo worship. Knowledge of these practices can also help investigators avoid inadvertently offending practitioners or violating their rights during searches, such as disturbing items without realizing that they may constitute a religious altar, amulet, or other religious artifact (**Table 4**).

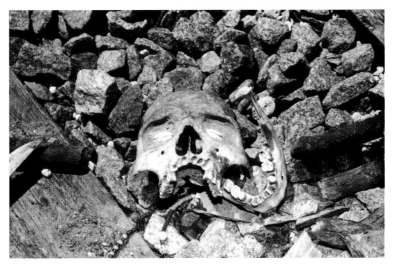

Figure 1   A human skull, cauldron, animal skulls, blood-soaked bag, beads and other religious artifacts were ritually discarded on railroad tracks and are indicative of the Palo Mayombe religion. Courtesy of Detective Christine Kruse-Feldstein, Miami Dade Police Department, Crime Scene Unit, Miami, Florida.

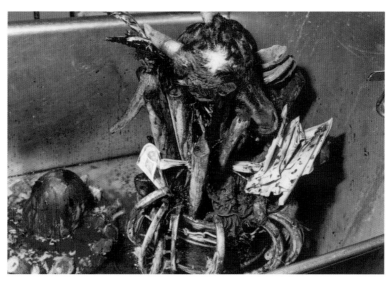

Figure 2 Palo Mayombe nganga (sacred cauldron) containing 21 sticks, horseshoes, handcuffs, gun, money, letters, goat's head, blood and other ritual items. Courtesy of Detective William Pozalante, Ocean County Sheriff's Department, Criminalistics Investigative Unit, Toms River, NJ.

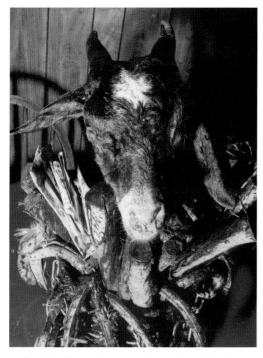

Figure 3 Palo Mayombe nganga (sacred cauldron) containing 21 sticks, horseshoes, handcuffs, gun, money, letters, goat's head, blood and other ritual items. Courtesy of Detective William Pozalante, Ocean County Sheriff's Department, Criminalistics Investigative Unit, Toms River, NJ.

Palo Mayombe "Blood and Human Remains"

Palo Mayombe is a syncretic Afro-Caribbean belief system that combines the cultural and spiritual belief systems of the ancient African Congo tribes with the religious practices of Yoruba slaves and Catholicism. It uses magical rituals that manipulate, captivate, and/or control another person, most often for the practitioner's malevolent purposes. Like the people from Nigeria, the Congo slaves were forcibly brought to the Caribbean and subsequently forced to adapt their cultural and religious beliefs to the culture and Catholic religious tradition of the new land. Through their assimilation process, the Congo slaves also incorporated some of the beliefs, symbols, and rituals of Santería. The result of this particular syncretism was Palo Mayombe, derived from the Spanish palo, meaning "wooden stick" or "branch," and referring to the pieces of wood practitioners use for their magic spells.

Priests of Palo Mayombe are known as paleros or mayomberos. Although the origins of the Mayombero and Santero share similar roots, there are two features that distinguish the rituals and beliefs of these different and individualistic belief systems. First, although many Mayomberos are originally initiated into Santería, very few Santeríans also practice Palo Mayombe. In fact, most Santería practitioners fear the Mayombero, claiming he practices a sinister form of Santería, which they call brujería, black magic, or witchcraft. Second, the rituals of Santería most often focus magic on positive actions designed to improve one's personal position or please an orisha. Palo Mayombe, on the other hand, centers its rituals around the spirit of the dead, often using magic to inflict misfortune or death upon an enemy. In fact, the Mayombero does not use the orishas but rather invokes the spirit of one

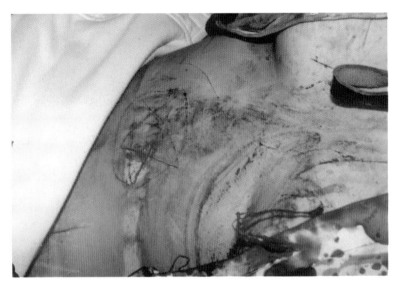

Figure 4 Satanic pentagrams cut into stomach and arms, deep lacerations on body and chain tied around neck when victim was found in a car in an isolated wooden area of Waco, Texas. Upon medical examination it became apparent that this was an incident of self mutilation. Courtesy of Detective James Blair, Waco Police Department, Waco, Texas.

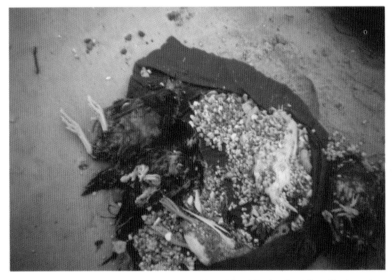

Figure 5 Headless chickens, food and other ritual items wrapped in a blue blanket found on the beach are remnants of a Santeria ritual sacrifice. Courtesy of Bradford K. Varney, Pennsylvania State Constable, Bucks County, PA.

specific patron who resides in his nganga, the cauldron used during most rituals. Some practitioners of Palo Mayombe claim that, although they are evoking the spirits of the dead, their intentions are not to harm but rather to use Palo in particularly difficult cases because it works much faster and is more effective than Santería rituals. Regardless, Palo Mayombe essentially is the practice of magic in the context of myths and rituals of Congo origins and its magic is accomplished with the use of human bones.

The forensic aspects of Palo Mayombe stem from the ritual requirement of human bones in the making of the sacred cauldron. The following is a detailed description of the Palo Mayombe rituals involved in making the sacred cauldron. The mayombero waits until the moon is propitious, and then he goes to a cemetery to a prechosen grave. The grave is opened, and the head, toes, finger, ribs, and tibias of the corpse are removed. After the human remains are removed from their graves a ceremony is conducted

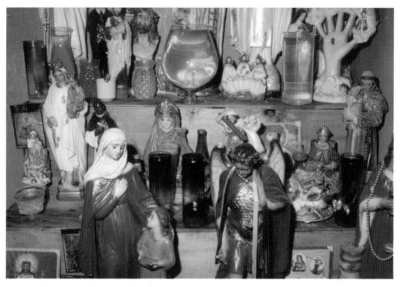

Figure 6 Santeria alter containing statues of Catholic saints, glasses of water, candles, food, cigars and other ritual items.

Table 4 Forensic evidence unique to Santeria

- Coins in multiples of seven
- Seashells
- Corn kernels
- Pieces of fruit (coconut, oranges, apples)
- Mutilated and beheaded chickens, hens, cows, goats, roosters (heads torn off)
- Scarves or pieces of clothing in specific colors (determines saints being worshipped)
- Necklaces in specific colors (also determines saints)
- Dolls with pins or strange symbols or writing
- Head of homicide victim missing from the scene
- Herbs, roots, flowers
- Parts of celba tree, or palm and cedar
- Animal blood and feathers
- Body oils
- Iron tools and objects
- Catholic saint statues
- Goblets of water

at the mayombero's house to determine if the spirit is willing to work for the mayombero. Once the spirit accepts the pact, the mayombero writes the name of the dead person on a piece of paper and places it at the bottom of a big iron cauldron, together with a few coins, which are the price of the spirit's help. The body's remains are added to the cauldron, together with some earth from the grave. The mayombero then makes an incision on his arm with a knife and lets a few drops of blood fall into the cauldron, so the spirit may drink and be refreshed. After the human or animal blood has been sprinkled on the remains, the mayombero adds to the cauldron the wax from a burnt candle, ashes, a cigar butt, and some lime. Also added to the mixture is a piece of bamboo,

sealed at both ends with wax, and filled with sand, sea water, and quicksilver. Frequently the body of a small black dog is also added to the cauldron to help the spirit track down it victims. Next to the dog, a variety of herbs and tree barks are placed inside the cauldron. The last ingredients to be added are a variety of herbs, spices, and insects. The initiate in palo is known as mpangui, nganga nkisi, or tata nkisi. The nganga (sacred cauldron) does what its owners order it to do and working with it is referred to as "playing" with it. When the spirit of the nganga carries out its owner's wishes, the owner gives it blood as an expression of gratitude, hence animals are frequently sacrificed and placed in the cauldron.

Similar to Voodoo and Santería practitioners, paleros claim that they are being persecuted for their religious beliefs and stigmatized for their ritual practices. There is a significant difference, regardless of whether the palero's intent is to heal or harm. Palo Mayombe ritually requires the use of human bones, hence this practice always entails the theft of human remains. Additionally the types of animals sacrificed for palo include domesticated pets such as dogs. The sacred cauldron is routinely fed with blood so sacrifice occurs much more frequently than in Santería rituals. Finally the religion of Palo Mayombe appeals to drug traffickers who believe that it has the power to protect them and paleros are hired to conduct special protection rituals. Palo Mayombe is frequently brought to the attention of medical examiners to identify human remains. Crimes frequently associated with the religion include grave robbing, extortion, and animal sacrifice (**Table 5, Figures 1–3**).

Table 5 Forensic evidence unique to Palo Mayombe

Sacred cauldron (nganga) contains:
- human bones (invariably a human skull)
- wooden sticks (21)
- various herbs, feathers
- animal bones (skulls or other bones of various birds)
- small iron agricultural tools (rakes, picks, hoes)
- sacred stones
- often a chain with a padlock will be wrapped around it
- other items that may be of special significance to the palero

Satanism: "Mutilation, Cannibalism, Ritual Abuse, and Dismemberment"

Satanism is a religion acknowledged by the US federal government and it maintains a doctrine of ethical tenets, specific rituals, and true believers. This religion is widely practiced in western society both individually and communally through satanic churches, covens, and grottos. Similar to other organized religions, beliefs vary among different sects and, according to church leaders, range from a form of ethical egoism through worshipping a particular deity. In most sects Satanism is a reversal of Christianity and similarities are found in the symbolism and ritual practices of each group.

Contemporary Satanism entails either worshipping Satan as a personified evil being (theistic Satanism) or glorifying what he represents, which includes, among other things, indulgence, vengeance, and engaging in all sins as long as they lead to self-gratification or self-deification (atheistic Satanism). Other characteristics of Satanism include beliefs based on a form of hedonism (pleasure-seeking) or egoism (putting oneself above all others). There are four general categories of Satanism: (1) religious/organized satanists; (2) traditional/intergenerational satanists; (3) self-styled satanists; and (4) youth subculture satanists. These classifications are generalized and not mutually exclusive. Although specific ideologies and rituals vary among different groups, all satanists practice magic. In fact, variations in magical rites are the core of satanic religions and what differentiates them from each other and other occult traditions.

Traditional satanists are proposed to be a highly organized, international, secret cult network that is actively engaged in a variety of criminal activities, including arson, ritual abuse, sexual abuse, incest, kidnapping, child pornography, and ritual murder, involving mutilation, dismemberment, and sometimes cannibalism. Also referred to as generational or intergenerational satanists, many members contend that they were raised in this belief system going back several generations. Self-styled satanists are either individually involved with Satanism or belong to small loosely organized groups and are either intermittently and experientially involved in occult activities and/or use the occult as an excuse to justify or rationalize their criminal behavior. Their rituals and belief systems are completely self-invented, a combination of a variety of traditions, or are emulated from media/cultural images of satanic practices. Self-styled satanists' primary interests usually entail the acquisition of personal power, material gains, or gratification through criminal interests and not spiritual satanic worship. Some self-styled satanists engage in criminal activities ranging from child molestation and animal mutilation to homicide, and their crimes conform to their self-invented ideologies.

Youth subculture satanists are similar to self-styled satanists; however their interest in Satanism is usually transitory and may not evolve into criminal activities. Youth subculture satanists are teenagers and young adults who are usually introduced to Satanism via music, film, the internet, and other media influences. Most often these young adults turn to the occult because of a deep sense of alienation from mainstream culture and spiritual traditions. They either eventually return to more traditional beliefs or they can easily be recruited into one of the many satanic religious organizations. Their rituals usually escalate depending upon the length of time they are involved in Satanism, beginning with simple magical incantations and evolving to animal and human sacrifice. Common crimes of youth subculture satanists include vandalism, arson, grave desecration, animal mutilation, school violence, and sometimes murder (**Table 6, Figure 4**).

Animal Sacrifice

Animal sacrifice is practiced by believers in Satanism, Santería, Voodoo, Palo Mayombe, Vampirism, and by young serial killers. The symbolic objects at the crime scene, types of mutilation, and other forensic evidence generally indicate which belief system is practiced.

In Santería, Voodoo, and Palo Mayombe, animal sacrifice is a fundamental aspect of the belief system and ritually required offerings for gods, ancestors, and spirits. For most satanic and vampire religions animal sacrifice is viewed more as an assimilation of power through the torture, pain, and blood of the victim and frequently escalates to larger animals and occasionally humans. In Satanism the torturing and killing of animals are also common indoctrination methods. For serial murderers the killing of animals is not

Table 6 Forensic evidence unique to Satanism, however these examples may not in isolation be indicative of Satanism

- Animal and fowl mutilations, including the removal of specific organs (genitals, anus, heart, tongue, ears)
- Altar upon which stones or other implements are placed
- Occult writing, biblical passages (sometimes written in blood)
- Circle on the ground (approximately 2.4–2.7 m (8–9 ft) in diameter, may contain a pentagram)
- Symbols: inverted cross, pentagram (a single point down signifies Satan), 666 (sign of the anti-Christ), NATAS (teen symbol of Satan (satan spelt backwards)), nondiscernible alphabet
- Goat's head (real or mock), symbolizing the devil
- Black candles and incense
- Robes, detached hoods
- Inverted cross, serpent, serpent with horns
- Skull with eyes hollowed out and red stones, rubies, or candles placed in the sockets
- Tattoos (pentagram or goat's head)
- Human cadavers and/or body parts
- Human or animal blood
- Wax drippings on the cadaver and/or in body orifices
- Positioning of bodies (north indicates Satan's supremacy)
- Slashes or cuts in patterns on the cadaver

connected to any theology. Although the crime scene may initially appear similar, serial killers' motivation for torture and slaughter is primarily a secular experience and the honing of one's skills that also frequently escalates to humans.

Animal sacrifices for Santería and Voodoo rituals are the relatively least disturbing and least heinous. There are three basic types of sacrifice in Santería: (1) ritual cleansings; (2) offerings to the egun or the orishas; and (3) initiation offerings. Ritual cleansings, known as "despojos," are when the animals are believed to take on the negative vibrations surrounding an individual and therefore cannot be eaten. During a ritual cleansing the blood of the animal is offered to the saints and the remains of the animal are disposed of in accordance with the wishes of the saint. Cleansing rituals are best explained as cathartic techniques in which the bad feelings caused by the evil in the person are passed into a bird, and the herbs' curative properties pass into the consultant. Many of the sacrificed animals that are routinely found along the beach, rivers, or railroad tracks are often the result of ritual cleansings. The other two types of offerings are made to eggun and the orishas and are known as ebbos and initiation offerings. During initiation offerings the blood is always given to the saints and the meat is always eaten because it is believed to be full of the energy of the gods, as opposed to ebbo offerings, where the meat is not always eaten. Many of the animals used in ritual sacrifice are fowl and include male and female chickens, roosters, ducks, guinea

hens, and pigeons. They are known collectively as "plumas," feathers. Other animals sacrificed in Santería include goats, sheep, pigs, and occasionally cows. Sacrifice to particular orishas is also used in a variety of magical spells for very specific results. In communities with large populations of Santería and Voodoo practitioners it is not unusual to find headless chickens on the doorways and steps of courthouses and government buildings where practitioners discard the sacrificed bird as part of a spell that will protect them from being prosecuted.

Animal sacrifice in the worship of Palo Mayombe is much more disturbing because it entails the use of domesticated pets such as dogs. Since Palo Mayombe focuses its rituals around the spirits of the dead instead of the palo gods, rituals require human remains, specifically the human skull and other body parts. The central theology of palo is that the spirit of the person whose bones are placed in the nganga, the sacred cauldron, carries out the owner's wishes. Animal sacrifice occurs because the nganga must be initiated and continually "fed" blood. Although penalties for animal abuse and grave desecration vary from state to state, the more serious ritualistic crime is generally the theft of human remains.

Although animal sacrifice for Santería and Voodoo is disturbing to persons unfamiliar with these practices, it pales in comparison to animal sacrifice that occurs for particular satanic and vampire religions. In syncretic religions animals are sacrificed by either quickly slitting their throats or by snapping their necks; at worst the heads of pigeons or other birds may be bitten off by the priest. However, in Satanism animals are slowly tortured and heinously mutilated. In most occult traditions blood consists of life-force energy. For satanic and vampire religions bloodletting or imbibing blood from a victim represents the assimilation of raw power. Ritual torture is viewed as a powerful form of magic that releases energy that can be directed by the perpetrator and used for specific goals. A basic magical principle is that intense emotion releases energy: in nonviolent groups such as neopaganism this emotional energy is achieved through sexual magic and in traditional Satanism it is achieved through pain. In many cases traditional satanic and vampire practitioners will commit sexually sadistic acts to increase their power by harnessing the energy of both.

Cats are frequently the victims of satanic crimes and it is common to find dismembered and skinned animals that were used in satanic rituals. It is important to determine if mutilations are attributed to human or animal predators. This can be difficult because certain mutilations resulting from animals resemble surgical cuts. Evidence of animal predators include hair fibers from foxes or coyotes found in the claws of the mutilated animals or the head or body will be found randomly discarded near the scene, as opposed to animal remains being symbolically placed by human perpetrators of ritualistic crimes. Investigators can also look for hairs of mutilated cats in animal dens that may be near the crime scene and consider weather conditions such as a drought, which may change migration patterns and cause animals to migrate to residential areas. There have also been numerous incidents of cows and horses that have been ritually mutilated and it is much more difficult to attribute their deaths to animal predators. Forensic findings are extremely important in determining the cause of large-animal deaths and common indicators of ritualistic crimes are the removal of organs, the level of skill used in dismemberment, unusual mutilations, and inexplicable loss of blood (**Figures 7–10**).

Another indicator of animal sacrifice resulting from ritualistic crimes is the dates on which the incidents occurred. Since Satanism, Santería, Voodoo, Palo Mayombe, and Vampirism constitute organized religions they practice specific rites on particular holidays. Originating from ancient agricultural timetables occult religions celebrate the phases of the sun, the moon, the earth, and the changing of the seasons. There are eight major holidays (sabbats) common to the hundreds of satanic, vampire, and neopagan

religions, and many lesser holidays are celebrated, including what is known as esbats (full moons). Syncretic traditions such as Santería, Voodoo, and Palo Mayombe holidays concentrate on the worship of individual gods and often require animal sacrifice on those days. Occult holidays such as Samhain, an ancient Celtic harvest festival honoring the Lord of the Dead which evolved into Halloween (October 31) are worshipped by many occult religions; however, the rituals are unique to each group and are useful methods of identification. For example, traditional satanic groups celebrate samhain with an animal or human sacrifice, while vampire groups hold huge gatherings at formal vampire balls in cities across the country and have ceremonies entailing bloodletting and drinking. Dabblers in many of the occult groups choose samhain to hold their first blood sacrifice and many humane societies will not allow people to adopt cats in October due to the large number of animals killed on October 31. In addition to general occult holidays each group also has its own unique rites requiring specific types of violence, ranging from animal sacrifice to ritual murder (**Table 7**).

Ritual Murder

Human sacrifice entails the killing of humans or the use of the flesh, blood, or bones of the human body for ritual purposes. This has been a widespread and

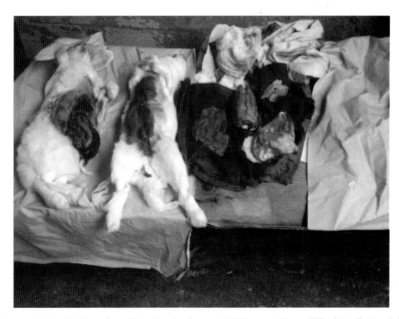

Figure 7 Animals that were tortured, skinned, mutilated and eviscerated. It is sometimes difficult to distinguish whether animals were mutilated due to sadism or Satanism. Significantly, in Santeria and other syncretic religions animal sacrifice never entails torture. Courtesy of the Animal Cruelty Section, Palm Beach County Animal Care and Control Division, West Palm Beach, Florida.

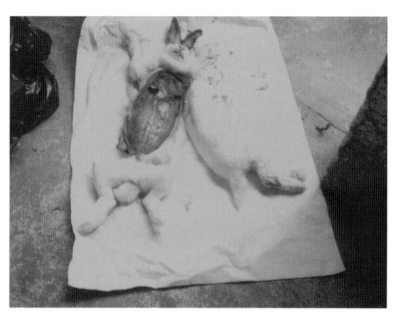

Figure 8 Animals that were tortured, skinned, mutilated and eviscerated. It is sometimes difficult to distinguish whether animals were mutilated due to sadism or Satanism. Significantly, in Santeria and other syncretic religions animal sacrifice never entails torture. Courtesy of the Animal Cruelty Section, Palm Beach County Animal Care and Control Division, West Palm Beach, Florida.

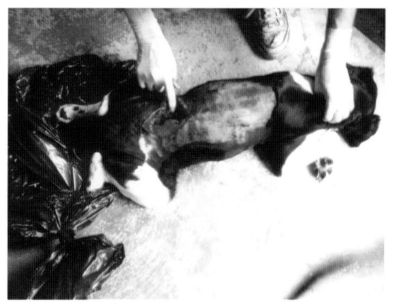

Figure 9 Animals that were tortured, skinned, mutilated and eviscerated. It is sometimes difficult to distinguish whether animals were mutilated due to sadism or Satanism. Significantly, in Santeria and other syncretic religions animal sacrifice never entails torture. Courtesy of the Animal Cruelty Section, Palm Beach County Animal Care and Control Division, West Palm Beach, Florida.

complex phenomenon throughout history. The significant ideology behind sacrificial ritual is that blood consists of life-force energy constituting the highest offering to the gods or ancestors. In specific occult worship, bloodletting or imbibing blood from a victim represents the assimilation of raw power. Additionally, the longer a victim is tortured and the pain is prolonged, the more life energy/power is emitted. In this manner ritual torture, cannibalism, and eventually ritual homicide are contemporary acts of human sacrifice and for the perpetrator it is a sacred communion meal in which the power of life is assimilated and regenerated. Ritual murder becomes a method of achieving immortality and/or becoming a god by

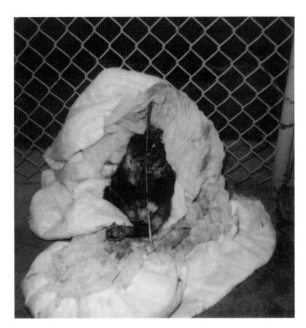

Figure 10 Animals that were tortured, skinned, mutilated and eviscerated. It is sometimes difficult to distinguish whether animals were mutilated due to sadism or Satanism. Significantly, in Santeria and other syncretic religions animal sacrifice never entails torture. Courtesy of the Animal Cruelty Section, Palm Beach County Animal Care and Control Division, West Palm Beach, Florida.

unifying the divine and the mortal. The theology of many contemporary occult groups describes their most sacred rituals in sacrificial terms and they have specific rituals and degrees of initiation that culminate in achieving some level above human, such as godlike or superior beings.

Currently, Palo Mayombe practitioners, satanists, vampires, disturbed individuals, and serial killers have been linked to ritual murders. Although sacrificial magical ideologies of various occult traditions have fundamental principles in common, the rites and theologies differ between religions and individual religious sects. Common goals include the acquisition of power to manipulate events that result in harm, healing, protection, or as a form of initiation, transformation, achieving knowledge, or the ultimate goal of self-deification. The least common motivation for human sacrifice and the one most people associate with Satanism is to draw down dark forces or entities.

Numerous ritual murders have been committed by juvenile and young adult satanists who are dabbling in magical ideologies. In many of the cases the perpetrators previously engaged in some form of blood-ritual by cutting/mutilating themselves, drinking and/or exchanging blood during initiation ceremonies, sacrificing animals, or all of the above. There have also been a number of ritual homicides committed in the vampire religious tradition. Typically the magical goal is connected to achieving power and immortality. Drinking blood and cannibalism frequently occur in vampire murders for the reason

Table 7 Occult calendar

The Greater Sabbats
Samhain (aka Halloween): October 31
Imbolc (aka Candlemas): February 2
Beltane (aka May Day): May 1
Lammas (aka Lughnasadh): August 1

The Lesser Sabbats (date varies each year)
Yule (aka winter solstice): December 21–23
Ostara (aka spring equinox): March 21–23
Litha (aka summer solstice): June 21–23
Mabon (aka autumn equinox): September 21–23

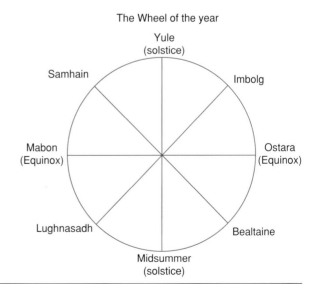

that blood is a fundamental aspect of the religious tradition. The symbolic evidence found at the scene helps differentiate between these two religions.

In most juvenile cases the perpetrator's method of operation is indicative of "dabbling." Dabbling involves people who are intermittently and experientially involved in occult activities. These perpetrators most often act alone or in small, loosely organized groups.

Another important distinction when investigating ritualistic crimes is the difference between motives of true believers and true criminals. True believers are religious practitioners who commit crimes because such acts fit into and/or are required by their particular belief system. These persons are involved in crime primarily because the ideology, rituals, and tenets of their beliefs require them to do so. Dabblers most often are true believers who are emulating a particular tradition or theology but are not yet experienced enough to conduct the ritual accurately and the crime scene reflects a lack of knowledge or skill involved in sacred rites.

True criminals are persons who use the occult as an excuse to justify or rationalize their criminal behavior. They are committed not to the belief system but to the criminal action. True criminals are not as concerned about the accurate symbolism, place, date, or victim of the rituals and are not connected to any organized group or specific tradition; consequently the symbolic evidence will be unique to that person.

Ritual murders committed by true criminals are individual secular (nonreligious) ritual acts and are often mistaken for sacrifice. Secular ritual murder is often the work of a lone offender and typically attributed to a serial murderer. Ritual murder occurs when criminal conduct goes beyond the actions necessary to perpetrate the crime and some type of nonreligious ritual behavior is expressed in the form of a "signature" or "calling card." The victim will be chosen according to the ritual need of the offender. Sexual assault, use of restraints, and depersonalization are often present. Forensics often include mutilation to the face and specific body parts, objects inserted into the victim's body orifices, and sexual acts after the victim's death. Body parts or other souvenirs such as personal items may be missing from the scene. The purpose of the ritual often fulfills a personal spiritual and/or sexual need of the offender. Offenders often make up their own belief system and perpetrate criminal activity that conforms to that ideology (**Figures 11–15**).

Ritual homicides committed by true believers reflect a serious knowledge of the particular theology, high level of skill, and meticulous attention to detail. Essentially ritual murders committed by true believers are contemporary acts of human sacrifice. The perpetrator considers the murder to be a sacred holy act and the crime scene will reflect this. The victim is selected according to the purpose of the ritual and

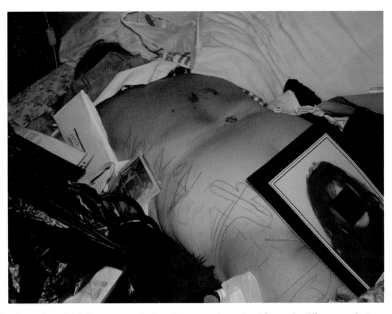

Figure 11 Although ritual murders initially appear similar, there are important forensic differences between murders committed for sacred versus secular motivations. In sacred ritual murder (sacrifice) mutilation always occurs while the victim is alive and the cause of death is typically from injuries acquired during torture. In this example of secular ritual murder the mutilation was postmortem and the cause of death was strangulation. Courtesy of Dr. Bernard Marc, medical examiner, Paris, France.

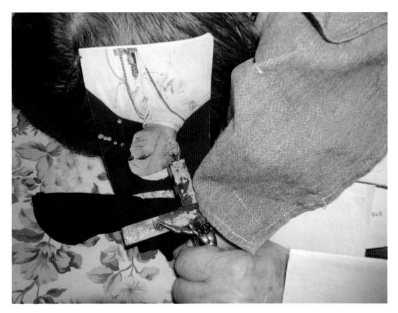

Figure 12 Although ritual murders initially appear similar, there are important forensic differences between murders committed for sacred versus secular motivations. In sacred ritual murder (sacrifice) mutilation always occurs while the victim is alive and the cause of death is typically from injuries acquired during torture. In this example of secular ritual murder the mutilation was postmortem and the cause of death was strangulation. Courtesy of Dr. Bernard Marc, medical examiner, Paris, France.

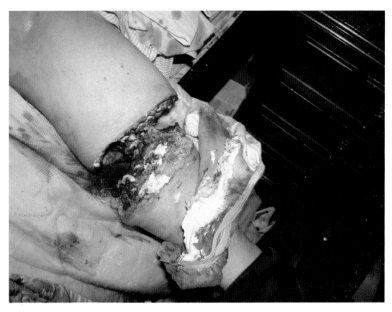

Figure 13 Although ritual murders initially appear similar, there are important forensic differences between murders committed for sacred versus secular motivations. In sacred ritual murder (sacrifice) mutilation always occurs while the victim is alive and the cause of death is typically from injuries acquired during torture. In this example of secular ritual murder the mutilation was postmortem and the cause of death was strangulation. Courtesy of Dr. Bernard Marc, medical examiner, Paris, France.

can be a stranger or a member of the group. The death will occur in a designated sacred space, determined by the group's doctrine, often an isolated outdoor area. The date is often significant and may correspond to an occult holiday or a group holiday. Since human

sacrifice is a blood ritual, the most common weapon is a ritual knife. Depending on the group's doctrine, death may be slow and torturous or a quick slitting of the throat. A common forensic indicator of ritual sacrifice is for blood to be drained from the victim.

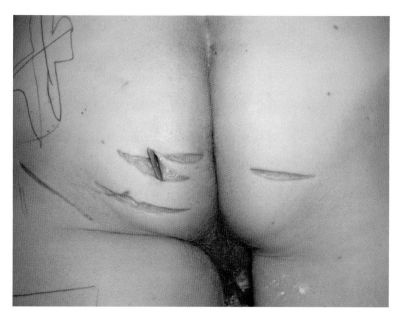

Figure 14 Although ritual murders initially appear similar, there are important forensic differences between murders committed for sacred versus secular motivations. In sacred ritual murder (sacrifice) mutilation always occurs while the victim is alive and the cause of death is typically from injuries acquired during torture. In this example of secular ritual murder the mutilation was postmortem and the cause of death was strangulation. Courtesy of Dr. Bernard Marc, medical examiner, Paris, France.

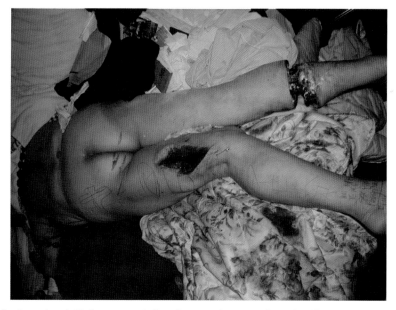

Figure 15 Although ritual murders initially appear similar, there are important forensic differences between murders committed for sacred versus secular motivations. In sacred ritual murder (sacrifice) mutilation always occurs while the victim is alive and the cause of death is typically from injuries acquired during torture. In this example of secular ritual murder the mutilation was postmortem and the cause of death was strangulation. Courtesy of Dr. Bernard Marc, medical examiner, Paris, France.

Other indicators are mutilation, carving symbols into flesh, cannibalism, sexual abuse, and dismemberment. The purpose of sacrifice is to increase personal power and/or fulfill the requirements of the belief system. True believers are the most dangerous perpetrators of any kind of religious violence because of the degree of their commitment to their beliefs, their disregard for civil authority, and their nontraditional world view that permits them to murder without remorse (**Table 8**).

Table 8 Forensic evidence unique to ritual murder, however these examples may not in isolation be indications of ritual murder

- Location and position of the body
- Missing body parts
- Cannibalism or absence of blood in victim or at scene
- Decapitation/mutilation or removal of specific organs (head, heart, tongue, tibia, eyes, fingers)
- Location of stab wounds or cuts
- Branding-iron or burn marks
- Wax, powders, oils on or around body or crime-scene area
- Human or animal feces consumed or found on victim
- Indications of bloodletting
- Stomach contents analyzed for urine, drugs, wine, potions
- Any sign of semen on or in the cadaver
- Evidence that the hands or feet have been tied or shackled
- Any jewelry, charms, amulets, stones, on, near, or inserted in the cadaver

See Also

Deliberate Self-Harm, Patterns; **Forensic Psychiatry and Forensic Psychology:** Sex Offenders; **Serial Murder**; **Torture:** Physical Findings

Further Reading

Canizares BR (2002) *The Book on Palo, Deities, Initiatory Rituals and Ceremonies.* Old Bethpage, NY: Original Publications.

Galanter MMD (ed.) (1989) *Cults and New Religious Movements, A Report of the American Psychiatric Association, from the Committee on Psychiatry and Religion.* Washington, DC: American Psychiatric Association.

Gonzalez-Wippler M (1996) *Santería: The Religion.* St. Paul, MN: Llewellyn Publications.

Hewitt K (1997) *Mutilating the Body: Identity in Blood and Ink.* Bowling Green, OH: Bowling Green State University Popular Press.

Lifton RJ (1999) *Destroying the World to Save It, Aum Shinrikyo, Apocalyptic Violence, and the New Global Terrorism.* New York: Metropolitan Books/Henry Holt.

Montenegro CG (1994) *Palo Mayombe, Spirits, Rituals, Spells, The Dark Side of Santería.* Plainview. New York: Original Publications.

Moynihan M, Soderland D (2003) *Lords of Chaos, The Bloody Rise of the Satanic Metal Underground*, 2nd edn. Los Angeles, CA: Feral House.

Perlmutter D (2000) *The Sacrificial Aesthetic: Blood Rituals from Art to Murder.* Electronic journal article http://www.anthropoetics.ucla.edu/ap0502/blood.htm, Anthropoetics. *Journal of Generative Anthropology*, Gans E (ed.), Fall/Winter Issue 5 No. 2, UCLA: Los Angeles, CA.

Perlmutter D (2002) *Skandalon 2001: The Religious Practices of Modern Satanists and Terrorists.* Electronic journal article http://www.anthropoetics.ucla.edu/ap0702/skandalon.htm. *Anthropoetics, Journal of Generative Anthropology*, Gans E (ed.), Fall/Winter Issue 7 No. 2. UCLA: Los Angeles, CA.

Perlmutter D (2004) *Investigating Religious Terrorism and Ritualistic Crimes.* Boca Raton, FL: CRC Press.

Ramsland K (1998) *Piercing the Darkness, Undercover with Vampires in America Today.* New York: Harper Prism.

Sakheim DK, Devine SE (eds.) (1992) *Out of Darkness: Exploring Satanism and Ritual Abuse.* New York: Lexington Books.

Vale V, Juno A (eds.) (1989) *Modern Primitives, An Investigation of Contemporary Adornment and Ritual Research*, vol. 12. San Francisco, CA: Re/Search Publications.

Wood D (ed.) (1999) *Body Probe: Torture Garden 2. Mutilating Physical Boundaries.* London: Creation Books/Velvet Publications.

Zusne L, Jones WH (1989) *Anomalistic Psychology, A Study of Magical Thinking*, 2nd edn. Hillsdale, NJ: Lawrence Erlbaum.

ISBN 0-12-547970-0

9 780125 479707